DATE DUE

DEC 1 3 1994	APR 0 3 1998
	APR 2 0 1998
FEB 2 0 1995	SEP 2 4 1998
	OCT - 8 1998
MAR 0 6 1995	JAN 1 5 1999
MAR 2 0 1995	
	DEC - 2 1999
APR - 8 1995	APR 0 1 2008
AUG - 8 1995	APR 1 7 2008
	OCT 1 4 2
APR 1 1 1996	
JAN 2 1 1997	
Feb 2	
MAR 2 7 1997	
Apr 10	
JAN 2 6 1998	
FEB 18 1998	
MAR 0 5 1998	
MAR 1 9 1998	

Learning Disabilities and Brain Function

A Neuropsychological Approach

Third Edition

To the children and adults seen clinically at the Neuropsychology Laboratory of the University of Victoria for the past thirty years, and the many children assessed and treated at the Queen Alexandra Centre for Children's Health over the past decade, with sincere gratitude. They have been our most valuable teachers.

William H. Gaddes   Dorothy Edgell

Learning Disabilities and Brain Function

A Neuropsychological Approach

Third Edition

With a Foreword by George W. Hynd

With 53 Figures

Springer-Verlag

New York Berlin Heidelberg London Paris
Tokyo Hong Kong Barcelona Budapest

William H. Gaddes
Professor Emeritus
Department of Psychology
University of Victoria
Victoria, British Columbia
Canada V8W 2Y2

Dorothy Edgell
Clinical Child Neuropsychologist
Queen Alexandra Centre for Children's Health
Adjunct Assistant Professor
Department of Psychology
University of Victoria
Victoria, British Columbia
Canada V8W 2Y2

Graphic design on cover by William D. West

Library of Congress Cataloging-in-Publication Data
Gaddes, William H.
    Learning disabilities and brain function : a neuropsychological
approach / William H. Gaddes, Dorothy Edgell. — 3rd ed.
      p.   cm.
    Includes bibliographical references and index.
    ISBN 0-387-94041-3. — ISBN 3-540-94041-3
      1. Learning disabilities.   2. Learning—Physiological aspects.
    3. Neuropsychology.   I. Edgell, Dorothy.   II. Title.
      [DNLM: 1. Learning Disorders—physiopathology.
    2. Neuropsychology.   WS 110 G123L 1993]
    RJ496.L4G33   1993
    618. '85889—dc20
    DNLM/DLC   93-28185

Printed on acid-free paper.

Production coordinated by Chernow Editorial Services, Inc., and managed by
    Christin R. Ciresi; manufacturing supervised by Jacqui Ashri.
Typeset by Best-set Typesetter Ltd., Hong Kong.
Printed and bound by R.R. Donnelley & Sons, Inc., Harrisonburg, VA.
Printed in the United States of America.

9 8 7 6 5 4 3 2 1

ISBN 0-387-94041-3 Springer-Verlag New York Berlin Heidelberg
ISBN 3-540-94041-3 Springer-Verlag Berlin Heidelberg New York

Prelude

And now, I said, let me show in a figure how far our nature is enlightened or unenlightened: Behold! Human beings living in an underground den, which has a mouth open towards the light and reaching all along the den; here they have been from their childhood, and have their legs and necks chained so that they cannot move, and can only see before them; being prevented by the chains from turning round their heads. Above and behind them a fire is blazing at a distance, and between the fire and the prisoners there is a raised way; and you will see, if you look, a low wall built along the way, like the screen which marionette players have in front of them, over which they show the puppets. . . .

Like ourselves, I replied; and they see only their own shadows, or the shadows of one another, which the fire throws on the opposite wall of the cave.

Plato, *The Republic*, Book VII

Modern psychology takes completely for granted that behavior and neural function are perfectly correlated, that one is completely caused by the other. . . . One cannot logically be a determinist in physics and chemistry and biology, and a mystic in psychology.

D.O. Hebb (1949)

Foreword to the Third Edition

Now in its third edition, this time coauthored with Dr. Dorothy Edgell, *Learning Disabilities and Brain Function* has clearly become a classic text. Rarely do I visit colleagues who do not have a copy in their professional libraries. There are a variety of reasons why this particular volume has been so widely and enthusiastically received. I suspect, however, that the primary reason is that Dr. Gaddes, in the previous editions, achieved exactly what he intended to accomplish despite well-intended advice to pursue other, more modest goals in preparing a text on the presumed relationship between learning disabilities and neurological function.

In the preface to the first edition, Dr. Gaddes stated his goal to prepare a book that would be of interest to both neuropsychologists and educators. He was warned that it would be impossible to write such a book, because of the potential risk associated with over-simplification for those with little background in brain-behavior relations. At the same time, confusion might result from trying to adequately integrate the vast and often conflicting literature on the neuropsychological basis of learning disabilities. Drs. Gaddes and Edgell, however, have accomplished what many would have hesitated to attempt. They have produced a comprehensive volume that precisely addresses the relationship between brain function and the behavioral manifestations associated with learning disabilities.

Despite those who would attempt to enforce their belief that the study of behavior can be divorced from the study of its neurological origins, the study of behavior necessarily is the study of the brain. The behavior we observe is obviously the end product of the integrated functioning of the central nervous system. With regard to learning disabilities, a careful reading of the seminal reports of Dejerine, Hinshelwood, Bastian, and other investigators at the turn of this century reveals evidence in support of the genetic and neurological bases of the behaviors we clinically characterize as manifestations of learning disabilities. The clinical reports included in this volume provide a meaningful understanding that best exemplifies the research reported in this book. And it is in this manner that psychologists, educators, and other clinicians will find the contents their of this volume not only readable, but articulate in presentation.

Although the study of individuals with learning disabilities has continued for well over a century, only within the past several decades have learning disabilities been formally acknowledged through laws and regulations that require the provision of services to those who experience severe difficulties in learning. In addition to national definitions and state or provincial regulations regarding the diagnosis and treatment of learning disabilities, various nosologies now include definitions and diagnostic criteria. Further, the presumed neurological basis of learning disabilities has received considerable attention from clinicians and researchers. In large part, this increased interest has been sustained and fostered by research methodologies not previously available. Only in the past two decades have postmortem, neuroimaging, and sophisticated neuropsychological procedures been available to study brain-behavior relationships in individuals with learning disabilities. These research endeavors have been wonderfully productive in providing evidence that the brains of learning disabled persons may be morphologically and functionally different than those of normal controls. Importantly, evidence now suggests that people with acquired and developmental learning disabilities may indeed share a disruption of the same neurological systems. In other words, whether of developmental or acquired origin, learning disabilities result from a disruption of known systems in the brain. Although the etiology may be different in each case, the behavioral symptomatology observed is consistent with our rapidly evolving understanding of brain-behavior relations. This is why this volume is so important. Drs. Gaddes and Edgell approach this literature not only from the point of our theoretical understanding of brain-behavior relations, but they provide a meaningful integration of this literature with our clinical and educational experience. Simply put, they have successfully taken on the normously difficult task of showing how our understanding of the central nervous system supports and extends our ability to effectively identify and work with persons who have learning disabilities.

To accomplish this task, they have had to carefully present research from neurology, psychiatry, psychology, and education in a way that provides a unified conceptualization of learning disabilities. Of course this is appropriate as the most recent definition of neuropsychology acknowledges the multidisciplinary nature of the field. That is why this volume has been so widely received and cited—it is a theoretically consistent and multidisciplinary presentation of a complex literature in a concise and clinically relevant format.

Further, this volume provides new and updated information on comorbid disorders that may be observed in individuals with learning disabilities. As an example, this volume now includes a fine chapter on "Attention Deficit Disorder," prepared by Dr. Edgell. Research conducted over the past several decades has produced a rapidly evolving literature not only on the deficits in attention that many persons with learning disabilities experience, but on the presence of comorbid disorders that may accompany learning disabilities. Understanding the complexities in arriving at a diagnosis of attention deficit disorder and its possible relationship to learning disabilities is important in providing appropriate psychological, educational, and medical treatment. In this regard, this edition is indeed new and improved.

Significant challenges exist on our horizon. Educators must be vigilant that the recent move toward inclusion of special education students within regular classroom settings does not adversely impact on the provision of relevant and quality services to these pupils. Psychologists must address the need for more accurate and relevant diagnostic procedures aimed at providing information that can be translated into documented treatment procedures that are effective and targeted at all of the educational and emotional needs of these individuals. Neurologists must continue their efforts to interface with the educational process by becoming more involved in monitoring medical treatment required by some learning disabled students. Finally, researchers must effectively present their findings to the broad range of professionals who may most profit from them. The information provided in this volume by Drs. Gaddes and Edgell make a great stride forward in this larger context.

It has been an honor to provide this Foreword. Little did I suspect that when Dr. Gaddes and I first corresponded two decades ago that I would be asked to prepare these comments. His early writings had a very significant impact on my own understanding of learning disabilities. I am sure that this volume will likewise influence those who seek to understand brain-behavior relations in persons with learning disabilities. This volume is a landmark in the literature on learning disabilities and consequently commands our incorporating the knowledge shared herein in our daily experience.

George W. Hynd, Ph.D.
University of Georgia

Foreword to the Second Edition

Reading this volume, chapter by chapter, I had a feeling of exuberance and exhiliration. It is both a privilege and a challenge to write a foreword for this second edition of *Learning Disabilities and Brain Function*. The scope and quality of the scientific and clinical insights expressed are unusual. It is difficult to do justice to the book within the constraints of a foreword. I can only reflect its significance to instructors, scientists, and clinicians in education, psychology, psychiatry, pediatrics, speech pathology and neurology.

In the early chapters there are discussions of brain function as it relates to learning and learning disabilities, with many implications for better understanding of the neurology of behavior. These chapters are followed by an articulate consideration of neuropsychological disorders, definition, identification and diagnosis of the cognitive dysfunctions that underlie learning disabilities. There is an analysis of the role of perception, as well as of the significance of impared sensory and motor-cognitive processes. The concluding chapters comprise a clear, erudite, yet practical discourse on the spectrum of language disorders, including the spoken, read, and written forms. Dr. Gaddes provides a constructive review of what it means when children have aphasia, of how this language disorder has implications for other types of learning. He elucidates and evaluates the status of our knowledge relative to childhood dyslexia and dysgraphia. This analysis holds promise for clarification of the issues that have been disconcerting, especially to educators and psychologists.

Dr. Gaddes adheres to the scientific evidence but in so doing he reveals the various ways in which carefully programmed remediation can benefit many children throughout the school years. I found this emphasis especially noteworthy for special educators and for regular teachers as well. Because of his wide experience as an educator and neuropsychologist, Dr. Gaddes does not simply present scientific evidence and overlook the pressing problems confronting those who are responsible for evaluating and teaching children who have learning disabilities. He presents evidence with a frame of reference, a point of view, that recognizes the urgency of being able to remediate and alleviate the total complex of circumstances that surround children, educationally and socially. He urges that all who are involved share knowledge so that these children can be better understood, their well-being fostered more effectively, and the confusions that commonly are associated with them be relieved. And if we professionals do not interact and share knowledge, the result will be less, not better services for the children we serve.

In studying this volume one cannot but be mindful of the ways that the learning-disability concept has prevailed upon other fields which focus on children. As manifested by this volume, this concept has significantly influenced education. It has enhanced and fostered special education, as can be observed in any school. Less obvious is the fact and the manner in which it has penetrated general education. There is a movement toward greater awareness of individual differences and needs, of how patterns of learning differ, verbally and nonverbally. Moreover, learning itself as a manifestation of cognitive behavior, and its role in the acquisition of meaning has taken on new significance. This volume, through its interdisciplinary contributions, broadens this salient new emphasis in our schools and in society.

Perhaps we can see an even greater impact of the learning-disability concept in the fields of psychology, psychiatry and neurology. Neuropsychology now is one of the prominent branches of psychology. But the construct that cognitive dysfunctions result in disturbed learning processes has been recognized by other specialties in psychology. The division of clinical child psychology has presented monographs that are important contributions. Pediatric and school psychology are both heavily involved in meeting the needs of children with psychoneurological cognitive disturbances. Psychologists working in these specialty areas will find that this volume has many observations and suggestions that bear directly on the ways children with learning disabilities can be evaluated and helped through programs designed specifically for the dysfunctions defined through careful, systematic, objective analysis of the impositions on learning.

This volume, the theme of which is cognitive functions as they relate to the neurology of learning, is relevant and purposeful also in other respects. As the science of learning disabilities develops, it might be that its most consequential influence will be in cognitive psychology. The concept of learning disabilities itself is based primarily on constructs evolved by cognitive psychologists during the past several decades. Many scientists agree that the most fundamental behavioral manifestation of a learning disability is the dysfunction of otherwise normal cognitive processes. Throughout this volume an underlying theme is that this construct must not be overlooked. Rather, the emphasis is that this basic character of learning disabilities be recognized as the true meaning of the problems confronted by many children; a neurocognitive deficit is a severe imposition on both academic learning and social adjustment.

The learning-disability concept also has been relevant to developments in the fields of pediatric neurology and child psychiatry. Not many years ago there was little awareness of the childhood aphasias, the childhood dyslexias and dysgraphias; these and other neurogenic involvements now are appraised and treated routinely. Although these language disorders often are subtle symptomatically, pediatric neurologists and child psychiatrists are aware that these neuropsychological conditions must be identified before children who have these learning disabilities can profit from available programs. These specialists play a vital role in diagnosis and program planning, medically and educationally. It is gratifying that scientists in neurology, psychiatry and psychology are evolving what is essentially a new field of endeavor, referred to as behavioral neurology. The learning-disability concept has been an important frame of reference for these developments. Year by year the ways in which even minor brain dysfunctions result in constraints on learning and behavior are demonstrated. This volume makes a significant contribution in this regard as we pursue greater and greater recognition of the meaning of behavior, both normal and abnormal. Finally, it seems purposeful to reflect briefly on how the science of learning disabilities relates to the concept of *mind*. That a learning disability impedes development and use of the mind must be stated and emphasized. Although rarely mentioned, this is the most imperative of all of the implications of this disorder. Investigation of the nature of learning disabilities has made a meaningful contribution to further definition, to further elucidation, of the concept of mind. Deficiencies in perception, in memory, in verbal and nonverbal symbolic representational learning, that is, in cognition, provide rich opportunities for us to gain insights into the brain-behavior relationships that comprise the construct we refer to as mind. These implications are a predominant concern of this book. As such, this volume can be used effectively by students in neuropsychology, and by those specializing in other branches of child psychology, in pediatric neurology, in child psychiatry and in special education. Practitioners in these and other fields will find it to be a practical guide in their day-to-day responsibilities. In fact, all of us who are concerned about learning, with the urgent consequences of what it means to have impositions on the development of the minds of a large number of children, should study it carefully.

Helmer R. Myklebust
Northwestern University

Foreword to the First Edition

Some may say that this book is long overdue; others, including myself, will state that the book appears at just the right time. The latter is likely more true, for it is doubtful that many in the professions would, until now, link issues of learning disabilities with those of neurophysiological dysfunction in the manner in which ultimately must be the case. As a matter of fact, there are those who deny the relationship completely. Lee Wiederholt (1974)[1] in his short, but excellent, review of the historical perspectives of learning disabilities, traces the early interest in this problem to the work of Gall (1802), and to his successors Broca (1861), Jackson (1864), Bastian (1869), and a few others. Each of these men would, at the time of this writing, be considered to have interests in the field of neurology, although at the time of their investigations, neurology per se was but a gleam in the eye of the anatomical beholder.

A relative detour then took place. Cerebral palsy, in the decades of the 1940s and 1950s, caught the attention of researchers through the work of Winthrop Morgan Phelps (orthopedist) and George Deaver (physiatrist) and one or two other medically oriented individuals. This was related to the writing of W.J. Little (1810–1894). It was, however, Kurt Goldstein, Heinz Werner, both eminent German scientists, and Alfred A. Strauss, a distinguished German neuropsychiatrist, who, as refugees of Hitler's Germany, emigrated to the United States and stimulated several psychologists to further investigate the issues of psychological dysfunction in children with identifiable neurological dysfunction. At this point, interest in the problem of psychological dysfunction essentially moved from the field of neurology to that of clinical psychology, and for nearly two decades, all but a few of the investigators who were working in this area ignored the neurological foundations of the problem. Exceptions to this statement were Newell Kephart and myself, both psychologists working closely with Werner and Strauss.

---

[1] With the exception of Wiederholt (1974), and Cruickshank et al., (1957/1965), no other dates included in parentheses here are listed as references. They are included in the Foreword solely as benchmarks in the brief historical sketch included herein.

Ruth Melchior Patterson, Bluma Weiner, Charlotte Philleo, and, to a lesser extent, the late Thorlief Hegge, all members of the psychological research group of the Wayne County (Michigan) Training School, kept alive the basic research direction of Werner and Strauss (1935–1955). Arthur Benton (Iowa) approached the problem from the point of view of the motor components of neurophysiological dysfunction. The unusual perceptual psychopathology observed by these researchers in the performance of exogeneous types of mentally retarded children were later determined to be identical to those of the athetoid and spastic types of children and youth with cerebral palsy (Cruickshank, Bice, Wallen, & Lynch, 1957/1965), by Shaw (1955) with some epileptic children, and with other clinical groups of children with neurological problems studied by the group of students working under me at Syracuse University between 1950 and 1965. Kirk's famous efforts with the Illinois Test of Psycholinguistic Abilities (1960) again focused the perceptual problems of some children on the malfunction of the neurological system, and his work, along with that of myself, Joseph Wepman (1960), and Mildred McGinnis (1963), again brought the issue full circle to the early efforts and interests of the 1800s of Gall, Broca, Bouillaud (1825), Wernicke (1881), Marie (1902), and Head (1926).

In 1980, if the education of these children is to be carried out within an appropriate milieu, it will be done so by teachers, psychologists, pediatricians, and parents who are thoroughly familiar with the interrelationships between neurological dysfunction and perceptual processing deficits. This is the theme of this book. Neurological dysfunction leads to perceptual processing deficits which, in turn, result in a variety and complexity of learning disabilities.

In more than 175 years, between the first published work of Gall in the area of phrenology and the publication of the current book by William Gaddes, there has been a waxing and waning of interest in this significant problem of childhood growth and development. The problem has been characterized by ignorance and ignoring, by attitudes of *laissez faire*, and by a manifestation of permissiveness in child rearing. Only lately, through the research that began appearing about 1950, has this problem been closely related by some to the work of the early "neurologists," and to a problem embedded in unique characteristics of perceptual processing deficits and pathology.

William Gaddes has written an important and very timely book. It puts forth a number of changes in educational and child management that will be required of all in teacher education and subsequently by those educators who are at the firing line with children and youth. *Learning and perception are neurological.* Herein is the basis for the preparation of a new type of educator—the neuro-educator. The neurophysiological structure and intactness of the human organism are fundamental to learning and adjustment. The late Alexander Luria pointed this out, but too few people recognized the truth of what he said so well. Instead, a great gulf existed. Educators did not really see or understand the importance of neurons to spelling, for example. Motor activities involved in handwriting were not viewed by the average educator as being intimately related to neurophysiological growth and development, except in the most gross manner. Clumsiness in the gymnasium, poor coordination in running, or inability to target in baseball were seldom seen to have any relationship to reading, number concepts, or writing.

For years, some of us have been stressing the interrelationship of figure-ground pathology, dissociation, failure to sequence, inability to obtain closure, disabilities of intersensory organization, forced responsiveness to stimuli extraneous to the task, and a myriad of other manifestations of perceptual processing deficit as fundamental aspects of perceptual pathology—each alone and more often in multiples as related to learning and to learning disabilities. Dr. Gaddes understands these interrelationships, too, and he has prepared here a book so fundamental as to insure that it will have an impact on the future of education, not only for those with learning disabilities, but for all children and youth.

There are those who will not accept this book. Among them are those who advocate the education of the "whole child" without recognizing that the whole child is a complex neurological structure. There will be those with pet recipes for teaching reading or arithmetic, yet who fail to understand that the concepts of sets, borrowing, and subtracting, memory involved in multiplication and division, and the capacity to make fine discriminations in the orthographic forms required in reading, each and all have a neurological base. There are those who reject the school entirely as a source of education and learning. Another group of educators who will reject this book are those who advocate, along with Patrick Dennis, permissiveness. They are those who fail to see structure as an effective tool of learning—structure encompassed in the neurophysiological system of the organism. This book is going to require an effort on the part of these groups of people to reorient themselves to education per se and to become familiar with the basic elements out of which learning is made possible.

This book contains within its covers elements that are basic to the learning of all children. Until educators incorporate them thoroughly into their understanding of the total educational process, the needs of children will not be adequately served. The emphasis in this book is not on how to teach arithmetic, reading, or spelling, but on the basic neurological ingredients that make such learning possible. It is the considered opinion of the under-signed that this is one of the most fundamental books to have appeared in the lengthening list of those concerned with the field of both general and special education. It is a keystone in the profes-sional library and in the growing literature on learning disabilities.

William M. Cruickshank, Ph.D.
University of Michigan

Preface

The present edition of this book is a revision and expansion of the first two editions which appeared in 1980 and 1985, and in German translation in 1991. More than half of the present volume includes new material, and what has been retained from the former editions has been largely rewritten and updated with new research findings. A completely new chapter has been added on "Attention Deficit Disorder."

The author of the earlier editions (W.H.G.) has been joined by a coauthor (D.E.), and their combined elementary, high school, and university teaching and clinical experience totals approximately seventy-five years. Both of us have directed our professional energies to understanding the puzzle of human learning, especially academic learning, of those students who, despite apparently normal intelligence and opportunity, have varying degrees of difficulty in acquiring ideas and skills that are easily mastered by others.

Until about fifty years ago there was a common tendency to equate academic success with intelligence, and those students who could not meet the demands of the prescribed program were usually required to repeat the same grade with a repetition of the same discouraging treatment that had been unsuccessful the first time. Attempts to analyze or understand the individual child's aptitudes, learning skills, or strategies were rare; each child was expected to fit the Procrustean system. A few enlightened educators looked to clinical psychology for answers to the problems of learning disorders because it was less authoritarian and more experimental. But while it appeared to offer more promise in understanding the individual child, it still was unable to deal with many learning problems because it recognized only psychological variables and ignored the biological bases of cognition and behavior.

In the late 1950s neuropsychology was just emerging as a research and clinical discipline, and it gave promise of a more complete account of behavior and learning. In the next thirty years this new professional approach gained international recognition and acceptance by many researchers interested in relating neurological function and academic learning. The first edition of this book was designed for educators and others with this interest, and with little or no knowledge of neuropsychology. In the preface of the first edition there was a need to argue the legitimacy of a neuropsychological approach in the field of education because of its novelty at that time. But very soon, large numbers of educators became aware of the value of recognizing a more complete account of the learning student. Neuropsychology has become a respected and established discipline not only in universities, in medical research laboratories, and in hospitals across the continent, but also in many educational diagnostic centers.

Developmental neuropsychology is of more recent origin and has grown out of an alliance of several disciplines, such as neonatology, teratology, neurobiology, and biochemistry, with a core of theory and information that emphasizes a psychobiological model on a continuum of time and development. Clinical child neuropsychology, a more recent and growing field, has evolved from an understanding of developmental neuropsychology and stresses the important differences in brain-behavior relationships between children and adults.

In 1872 Hughlings Jackson, the eminent British neurologist, in presenting the Hunterian Oration at Oxford University, had urged his listeners to bring mind and body closer together in their inquiries into education and physiology. In the preface of the first edition, it was stated that the book was an attempt to accept his challenge. Judging from the increase since 1980 in research studies, new periodicals, educational conferences, and new books that attempt to integrate neuropsychology and education in their theories and applied procedures, it is encouraging to find that this challenge is being accepted more widely.

William H. Gaddes
Dorothy Edgell
Victoria, British Columbia

Acknowledgments

William M. Cruickshank (1915–1992) has encouraged the development of a program in educational neuropsychology at the University of Victoria since 1963. He was a gifted researcher, scientist, administrator, humanist, and loyal friend. His theories and practices in learning disabilities have been and will continue to be a major influence in the field. We are also singularly indebted to Helmer H. Myklebust for his interest and support for the past thirty years. The major impact of both these men is evident in all editions of this book.

Che Kan Leong of the University of Saskatchewan has been particularly helpful in reading the new sections on the psychology of reading, linguistics, and psychometrics, and providing scholarly advice. Ralph M. Reitan, as always, has been supportive and encouraging in providing us with detailed accounts of his current research.

We are grateful to George W. Hynd and Noel Gregg, both of the University of Georgia, for their detailed suggestions about new topics to be included in the planning of the present volume. We are also indebted to George W. Hynd for agreeing to write the foreword for this edition of the book. Other scholars who have helped us are George O.B. Thomson of the University of Edinburgh; David H. Ingvar of the University Hospital in Lund, Sweden; Janette Atkinson of the University of Cambridge; Patricia K. Kuhl of the University of Washington; Doris Johnson of Northwestern University; Henrietta C. Leiner of Channing House, Palo Alto, California; George Middleton of Lake Charles, Louisiana; and Michael A. Cornell of the Spotsylvania Vocational Center in Virginia.

Dr. D'Arcy D. Lawrence, Chief of Imaging Services at the Royal Jubilee Hospital, Victoria, advised us on the CT amd MRI, and read critically those sections in the book. Campbell Clark of the University of British Columbia Triumph PET Core Group and the Department of Psychiatry read the section on the PET scan and provided useful comments. Robert M. Peet, neurologist, supplied information on some points of clinical neurology. Sheri McIntyre, Director of Communication Disorders at Queen Alexandra Centre for Children's Health, provided information on the role of the speech and language specialist; she read that section and made useful suggestions.

Colleagues at the University of Victoria to whom we are indebted include Otfried Spreen, Frank Spellacy, Esther Strauss, Bram Goldwater, Lorne Rosenblood, and Harry Scargill. Lisa Carswell, graduate student in neuropsychology, assisted ably in checking the reference list against the complete text.

The staffs of Springer-Verlag New York have been helpful throughout.

Contents

Contents

1 Neurology and Behavior: Background and Assessment

Models [of human behavior] which leave out man's physical organism are bound to be inadequate for the task of making behavior intelligible.
Edwin R. Guthrie (1950)

. . . I prefer to think of man's humanity as vested in his bodily structure and function, not least, in the activities of his brain.
Oliver L. Zangwill (1976)

This book is expressly written for educational diagnosticians, clinical psychologists, school psychologists, and remedial teachers who are committed to developing for their learning impaired students prescriptions based on a broad spectrum of relevant diagnostic knowledge. This knowledge should include, in addition to the social history of the student, a record of academic achievement, a psychological assessment of perceptual, motor, and cognitive strengths, and, in those cases of known brain damage or suspected central nervous system dysfunction, a neurological examination. The in-depth study of the neurologically impaired learning disabled student should include a synthesis of educational, psychological, social, and neurological data. Such an approach is ambitious and requires educational diagnosticians to learn some basic neurology and neuroanatomy and a useful body of neuropsychology, in addition to their expertise in professional education and psychology. Their knowledge of neuropsychology need only be at an introductory level, which will not qualify them to make diagnostic statements about the neurological functioning of their learning disabled (LD) students, but it will provide them with a broader and more productive hypothetical concept of their learning processes. Greater knowledge is more likely to lead them to produce better remedial treatment.

School psychologists who have found an applied behavioristic model (such as behavior modification) with which they can quickly and practically produce remedial prescriptions, may wonder why anyone would think it necessary to learn a whole new body of knowledge such as neuropsychology. Not only do many professionals question this proposal but some oppose it and deny its value. The whole question relates to one's theoretical concept of child behavior and whether a within-child model or a behavioral model is preferred. It seems evident that these two models reflect the historical conflict between phenomenology and behaviorism (Wann, 1964); that is, between a within-subject view that of necessity was subjective, mentalistic, and speculative, and behaviorism, which because it dealt with observable behavior, was objective and scientific. The rising interest in the rapidly increasing study of neuropsychology during the 1960s added a dimension to the concept of the within-child model by increasing its objectivity and reducing some of its speculative aspects. Along with perceptual and dynamic forces operating within the child, neurology and neuropsychology were able to provide new knowledge about neurophysiological correlates of behavior, many of which could be identified physically. Where the hypothetical constructs of dynamic personality theory were completely speculative, the findings of neurophysiology were largely observable, and the discoveries emerging from neuropsychology were in many cases demonstrable. This meant that the speculative component that dominated dynamic psychology was much reduced and hence implied scientific progress in the study of human behavior.

Many psychologists welcomed the objectivity of neurophysiological measures and were impressed with the new opportunity to validate neuropsychological methods for measuring behavior (Reitan, 1955b). Several new journals appeared in neuropsychology in the early 1960s, Kirk coined the term "learning disabilities" in 1963, and planners of conferences in special education began to invite neurologists and neuropsychologists to tell them about their research activities. Teachers began to see a new avenue of help, and some may have embraced the new neurological model prematurely, with more enthusiasm than knowledge. No doubt some harm was done by those who labeled children "brain injured" or "minimally brain damaged," just two of the 2000 terms that appeared about this time (Spreen, 1976, p. 450). Whereas some professionals may have used this knowledge unwisely, it did provide a more complete account of the child. The within-child variables were now both psychological (inferred) and neurological (in some cases directly observed and sometimes inferred). The environmental forces were still identifiable, which meant that the child now could be observed more accurately physically, psychologically, and socially. It soon became evident that the neuropsychological data that could be obtained were invaluable in providing fuller understanding of the child with a chronic perceptual deficit, a perceptual–motor dysfunction, or some type of chronic and severe learning problem (Gaddes, 1968).

Assessing the Use of the Neuropsychological Model in Education

Many educators with no knowledge of neuropsychology frequently warn against its use and label it "a medical model." This practice, they will tell you, has frightening dangers for school children and serious professional problems for school personnel. But any theoretical model of behavior must be assessed critically in terms of its objective values and weaknesses; otherwise it may be accepted or maligned by an observer more for its emotional compatibility or dissonance with his or her perceptual and cognitive satisfactions.

Let us look at some of the frequent objections to and the *alleged* weaknesses of the neuropsychological model of learning disabilities. Most of these do not stand up to close, logical scrutiny.

1. The model stresses disease and pathology, its opponents will tell you, and it ignores the potential for change that is inherent in dynamic theories of personality and current learning theories. It is true that in the past some medical doctors, with little or no training in psychology and education, and reinforced with the concept of the correlation between pathological, physical conditions and deficit behavioral syndromes, have advised parents of mentally impaired children of the hopelessness of their child's condition. This point is related to the next two.

2. It stresses chronicity, persistence, and permanence.

3. Hence, it is unduly pessimistic. The reader will recognize that all three of these "objections" are not inherent in the theoretical model, but are misinterpretations of it by inept professional workers. Many able pediatricians are aware of these practical weaknesses and stress the importance of psychosocial factors. One pediatrician has warned that looking for "soft neurological signs" may even "distract [the physician] from looking at environmental factors" (Schmitt, 1975).

4. It encourages drug therapy, its opponents will tell you, and minimizes the value of psychoeducational intervention. It is true that some extreme proponents of drug treatment tell us that "these drugs can produce immediate psychological growth" and such a child showing these dramatic changes "thus refutes Skinner and Pavlov" (Wender, 1976). Pihl (1975) has told us that "the physical model begets physical intervention" and Schmitt (1975) has echoed this view. Again the reader will recognize this as a poor use of a

model rather than an inherent weakness in its theory. The neuropsychological view of human behavior does not encourage indiscriminate drug therapy; use or abuse depends on the knowledge and skill of the attending consultant. The authors have knowledge of a residential treatment center using a neuropsychological diagnostic approach to learning disabled children where all children on admission are removed from medication unless a carefully researched medical reason can be provided for its prescription.

5. Neurological knowledge is incomplete. This statement is true, but that is no reason to refuse to apply what we do know about brain–behavior relationships. "We can take for granted that any theory of behavior at present must be inadequate and incomplete. But it is never enough to say, because we have not yet found out how to reduce behavior to the control of the brain, that no one in the future will be able to do so" (Hebb, 1949, p. xiii). This same idea has been stated by Cruickshank in an educational context: "One excuse for lack of activity in the area of education of brain-injured children is that too little is known to do an adequate job with the children. This is not true. Much is known and much can be accomplished immediately. Educators cannot await the arrival of every piece in the mosaic before beginning to assemble the puzzle. Education must . . . begin to work now, where it is, and with what it has" (Cruickshank, 1966, p. 311).

6. Some known brain-damaged children are free of learning disabilities, and most learning disabled children have no conclusive evidence of brain damage or dysfunction. These statements are true, and their seeming contradictions may be explained as we get into the discussions of neurology and neuropsychology later in the book.

7. Labeling a child "brain-damaged" or "MBD" (minimal brain dysfunction) is damaging to the child, frightening to the parents, and confusing to the school. True, but this is unnecessary and ill advised. Again, it is not recommended by the neuropsychological approach, but such labeling may be done unwittingly by inexperienced or poorly trained professional personnel.

8. Some critics of the use of neuropsychological knowledge in education believe that giving a child an organic label permits the school to shift the responsibility for evaluation to the physician (Schmitt, 1975) and to neglect the child, at least partially. This tactic has not been our experience because in working with children we do not give them medical labels. We report the nature of the child's learning problems to the parents and to the school, and recommend what might be done to alleviate them. It has also been our experience that the medical specialists, after making their medical reports on the child, are happy to have the clinical psy-

chologist and the educators take over the behavioral and educational management of the case.

9. A search for organic factors may blind the diagnostician to the presence and importance of psychosocial etiological forces. If this happens it is more likely to result from the limited skill of the clinician than from a weakness in the theoretical model. A team approach to the study of the child, which includes at least the teacher, the parent, and the neuropsychologist, should guard against ignoring the important causal psychosocial forces.

10. Much research comparing behavioral and neurological variables is oversimplified. True, "studies in which groups of children labeled as children with learning disorders, hyperactives, MBD cases, etc. are compared with controls . . . suggest behavioral and neurological 'homogeneity' within such groups and simple one-to-one relationships between neurological factors on the one hand and behavioral and learning problems on the other" (Kalverboer, 1976). Again, however, the presence of poorly designed research in any area is a weakness not of that area of knowledge but of the methods used by the people investigating it.

Let us now look at the promising advantages of and the basic reasons for a neuropsychological diagnostic approach to human behavior and learning disabilities in particular.

1. Neuropsychology is an established science in its own right; it began with the research of the neurophysiologists during the nineteenth century and grew with the added impetus of the two world wars in the twentieth century. This large body of knowledge, which is increasing rapidly, is relevant to all human behavior, and educators should be aware of it if they are to have maximal understanding of any learning disabled child.

2. All behavior is mediated by the brain and central nervous system, and an investigator is better prepared to understand a child's disturbed behavior if supplied with neuropsychological information about that child. The reader will recognize that in the past this statement has not enjoyed complete agreement from everyone. Behavioristic psychologists in particular have recommended an "empty organism" approach, in which an accurate measure of stimulus and response is all that is needed. In 1938, Skinner proposed a completely dualistic position.

There are two independent subject matters (behavior and the nervous system) which must have their own techniques and methods and yield their own respective date. . . . I am asserting, then, not only that a science of behavior is independent of neurology but that it must be established as a separate discipline whether or not a rapprochement with neurology is ever attempted. (B.F. Skinner, 1938)

Although this statement was very clear and proved strongly influential with thousands of psychologists all over the world, Skinner did recognize the value of knowing about a brain lesion in a case of aphasia (B.F. Skinner, 1938, p. 424). If we were to paraphrase Skinner in this regard, we might conclude that neuropsychological knowledge is redundant or irrelevant in the understanding and treatment of normal behavior, where the physiological systems of the person are normal and healthy both structurally and functionally, *but is required for understanding and treating impaired behavior* resulting from a lesion or lesions in the brain and central nervous system. And we concur basically with this view. However, neuropsychological studies of *normal* brain function are already adding significantly to the understanding of learning strategies of *all* academic learners with or without evidence of neurological dysfunction (such as the cognitive processes in reading).

Skinner's support for an exclusively behavioristic view of normal behavior in the 1930s and 1940s was a powerful voice. An equally powerful voice, objecting to this restrictive view, proposed a neuropsychological theory of behavior for understanding not only deficit behavior but also normal behavior. Hebb (1949), in his classic book, recognized Skinner's influential support of a positivistic view of behavior, but he wrote, "The present book is written in profound disagreement with such a program for psychology" (Hebb, 1949, p. xiv). Although he supported a neuropsychological view of behavior, he made it clear that psychology is not physiology: "The problem of understanding behavior is the problem of understanding the total action of the nervous system, and *vice versa*" (p. xiv), and "this does not make the psychologist a physiologist, for precisely the same reason that the physiologist need not become a cytologist or biochemist, though he is intimately concerned with the information that cytology and biochemistry provide" (p. xv).

It is not just the recognition of neurological data that is useful but also its application in deciding on an appropriate treatment program. Diagnostic understanding of the status of the child's brain and nervous system, coupled with skilled remedial teaching, has facilitated, in numerous cases, marked cognitive improvement. Maria Montessori, a medical doctor, was one of the first to use this medical–pedagogical approach and, as a result, electrified the worlds of both education and medicine at the turn of the century with her success in teaching mentally retarded children (Montessori, 1964). With our recent improved knowledge of neuropsychology and its relation to remediation, many severely impaired children who might have been abandoned 30 years ago to the back ward of a mental hospital are now being successfully trained, many to be relatively self-sufficient in a sheltered workshop or other special environment. Others, less severely impaired, are being educated and trained, sometimes in highly skilled trades or crafts.

3. Neuropsychological data are essential to a diagnostic understanding of a child with a perceptual, cognitive, or motor deficit. Those educators who consider neuropsychology irrelevant to teaching are likely to be stressing symptoms and neglecting causes. Although they might freely advise *against* neurology and *for* behavior modification, it is highly likely they would avoid choosing a family doctor interested only in symptoms. The medical student is typically taught to recognize a pattern of symptoms as reliable signs of a particular disease condition. Once having recognized the disease from its symptoms, a doctor knows the probable cause or causes gained from medical research and the large body of empirically supported related knowledge and *treats* the *cause*. In other words, the doctor possesses knowledge, beyond the actual symptoms, which is theoretically related to the basic cause, and this knowledge enables provision of a better and quicker treatment.

Teachers are practitioners who are looking for successful methods to teach their students. Similarly, most people who drive cars do so with reasonable success without knowing the principles of the gasoline combustion engine. So long as the car is operating normally, this type of driver has no problem, but as soon as it stops because of mechanical failure then a mechanic must be called in to make it run again. The mechanic has detailed knowledge about the structure and functions of the automobile, is able to make a diagnosis on the basis of this knowledge, and with this same knowledge is able to repair the car. A professional racing driver is also required to have thorough mechanical knowledge about the car as well as expertise in driving it; being able to drive is not enough. The teacher, like the average car driver, may not have the knowledge to diagnose a complex learning problem and will need to call on the school psychologist to diagnose the problem and prescribe possible remedial measures. It is our thesis in this book that the psychologist who is a neuropsychologist will be better equipped to diagnose.

Also, the teacher with an introductory knowledge of neuropsychology will be better able to read medical and psychological reports, and may have more hypotheses to choose from in deciding on a possible treatment program.

The astute reader may have detected a procedural difference between the problems facing the educational diagnostician and those confronting the physician. A physician is dealing with a changing physical condition the etiology of which may be understood. Most disease conditions, such as infections, react in a homeostatic pattern; that is, the infection gradually decreases with treatment, and the body regains its normal levels of equilibrium. However, some physical problems faced by the physician are static. Orthopedic problems, such as broken legs that result in different leg lengths, may require physiotherapy and remedial shoes to correct them. Such remedies are not cures but attempts to deal with a chronic state of physical abnormality. In these cases there is no disease condition, but a deficit in organic structure and function.

Children with traumatic brain damage or underdeveloped brain structure (agenesis), like those with orthopedic problems, possess a continuing and permanent structural deficit in their brains that may alter their normal sensory, cognitive, or motor responses. A knowledge of brain–behavior relationships will help the school or clinical psychologist to alert the teacher to the nature of these changes.

4. Because a neuropsychological examination of the child provides a systematic description of his or her behavioral and cognitive strengths and weaknesses and so provides information on the *nature* of the learning disability, it helps to realize that all learning disabled children are different; they are not a homogeneous population and should not be treated alike (Myklebust, 1967a). A battery of neuropsychological tests can provide detailed information about the various characteristics of a child's learning disorder whether or not there is evidence of brain damage or dysfunction.

5. The neuropsychological approach to learning disabilities should not supplant other successful theories or methods but should be used along with them. In fact, thorough understanding of organically impaired learning disordered children and adults needs the best aspects of a behavioral, a psychosocial, a cognitive, and a neuropsychological approach. Neuropsychology should never be used exclusively in educational diagnosis, but should be applied along with other models of behavior to enrich them. Exact knowledge of human behavior is still so minimal that no one who wishes to learn about it can afford to exclude any segment of reliable knowledge related to it. If clinical psychologists or educational diagnosticians choose to blind themselves arbitrarily to major segments of knowledge about human behavior, their understanding and hence their diagnoses and prescribed treatments will be sadly limited and in some cases may be ineffective and even damaging to a child's well-being.

6. Competent in-depth neuropsychological study of the child can relieve parental anxieties and doubts and provide additional help to the school.

7. A neuropsychological anproach to understanding perception, cognition, and motor behavior has been actively supported by a large number of eminent researchers and scholars. Hebb has told us that "modern psychology takes completely for granted that behavior and neural function are perfectly correlated, that one is completely caused by the other" (Hebb, 1949). A.R. Luria, the distinguished Russian neuropsychologist, has not only examined sensorimotor and cognitive functions in detail in brain-damaged patients but has produced brilliant insights in the teaching of spoken language, reading, writing, spelling, and arithmetic (Luria, 1966, 1970, 1973). Myklebust, one of the most prolific writers on learning disabilities, has clearly stated his approach: "It is our presumption that learning disabilities as defined here are the result of minor disturbances of brain function" (Myklebust, 1967a). Cruickshank (1979), an equally prolific and influential writer in special education, conceives of learning disabilities as "the result of perceptual processing deficits which, in turn, are or may be the result of a (diagnosed or inferred) neurophysiological dysfunction."

By the late 1960s and during the 1970s, several young and very able researchers were following the early examples of Benton, Cruickshank, Myklebust, Reitan, and others and began to use a neuropsychological model for analyzing the nature of learning disabilities in children and adults (see Knights and Bakker, 1976).

During the 1980s an increasing number of research and applied psychologists, impressed with the rapidly increasing research interest in educational neuropsychology, began to adopt and recommend its use in educational practice (e.g., a whole issue on Neuropsychology in the Schools, *School Psychology Review*, 1981, X[3]).

Although appeal to authorities and popularity does not validate a theory, it is encouraging to know that a number of highly competent scholars have tested the neurological approach for more than 50 years, and more recently a large number of research and applied professionals have found it highly useful in practice. Until knowledge is near completion in any area, no more can be expected of a theory.

Degrees of Brain Dysfunction

In the previous discussion, we have referred to children with brain dysfunctions and, although we stated that this was not a homogeneous population, few attempts had been made to examine the various categories of brain damage and cerebral dysfunction. That attempt will now be made.

The essential concept professed here is that all human subjects represent varying degrees of cerebral function from exceptional through normal to severely impaired. Some people presumably possess brains and nervous systems that are perfect in structure and healthy and optimal in function. Others unfortunately inherit imperfect brains with genetic defects, or they may suffer traumatic injury, pre- or postnatally, to their previously normal brains. Still others may be free of pathology but may have inherited a brain structure and function with a weak aptitude for processing written language or spatial or numerical stimuli. Because of the massive complexity of cerebral neural structure, the infinite possibilities of loci of damage, and the almost limitless continuum of intensity and extent of dysfunction, the nature of cognitive impairment resulting from central nervous system (CNS) dysfunction or genetic uniqueness is incalculable. This statement means that no two brain-injured children or adults are similar, and any group research with these subjects includes a heterogeneous population. For this reason many comparisons of "brain-injured" and "normal" children have been unreliable, frequently insignificant, and essentially meaningless. To avoid this weakness it is necessary to identify different groups of children with basic similarities, such as the same range of intensity of dysfunction or the same lesion locus.

In our own laboratory the following clinical classification was established some years ago to assist in selecting individual cases for intensive study. The classification grew from what we found in the referral stream and is based on the empirical distribution of subjects with the presence or absence of varying types and degrees of CNS damage and/or dysfunction. This classification can be useful in neuropsychological research. In educational research a classification based on the degree or nature of cognitive deficit would be more likely to be chosen, although knowledge of the neuropsychological status of the LD child or adult is still essential in a comprehensive understanding of a case.

Clinical Classification (Table 1.1)

1. Brain-damaged, learning disabled with "hard signs."
2. Borderline dysfunction (MBD), learning disabled with "soft signs."
3. Learning disabled with no positive neurological signs.
4. Normal.
5. Psychiatric.

Constitutionally based learning problems will appear in 1, 2, or 3. Learning problems, when they appear in 4 or 5, are usually en-

Table 1.1. Neuropsychological Clinical Classifications

Brain-Damaged	MBD	Specific Learning Disability	Normal	Psychiatric
Learning disabled with Hard Signs	LD with Soft Signs	Learning Disability with No Positive Neurological Signs	No Learning Problems	Emotional Disturbance
Conclusive signs of brain tissue damage or dysfunction Examples: brain tumor, bleeding, penetrating injury, EEG, grade iii[a]	Developmental delay, language retardation, motor clumsiness, perceptual deficits, right–left problems, hyperactivity, poor body image, poor hand–eye coordination	Cause may be: a. Genetic deficit, b. Subtle brain dysfunction not detectable on standardized neurological examination c. anatomical variations in brain development Resulting in: reading or arithmetic deficit	No conclusive neurological or behavioral signs	Learning disability is secondary to inattention, anxiety, or other correlate of emotional disturbance; it may have an organic cause or may result from a biochemical dysfunction, or it may be psychogenic
Hemiplegia (half–paralysis) Hemiparesis (half–partial paralysis)	EEG, Grade i or ii[a] (see Spreen, 1988, pp. 149–150)			

[a] EEG, electroencephalogram: grades i, ii, and iii indicate minimal, moderate, and severe pathology, respectively (see Chapter 2).

vironmentally produced or secondary to emotional disturbance. Learning problems thus can occur in all five of these clinical categories.

The reader should understand that the categories of learning disabled patients listed above represent a clinical distribution based on the presence, absence, or degree of cerebral dysfunction. This type of grouping is useful in medical and neuropsychological research where a knowledge of the neurological damage and/or dysfunction is needed. It is not a classification of subtypes of LD subjects based on a cluster analysis of their competence or failure on a large battery of neuropsychological tests. The latter type of grouping has been well developed by Rourke and his associates (1985) and is useful in understanding the nature of an individual's learning problems and how they might be treated.

This section includes a symptomatic description of MBD children that is designed to help the teacher. In the Clinical Addendum at the end of Chapter 2 appears a discussion of the problems of definition faced by the clinical research psychologist.

It may help the teacher to remember that:

1. His or her[1] responsibility is to be aware of the child's cognitive and behavioral strengths and weaknesses and to design an appropriate remediation program regardless of the clinical category in which the child may be placed by the psychologist.

2. The type of child clinically categorized as MBD reflects a pattern of behavior on a continuum ranging from (a) brain-damaged (documented medically) to (b) MBD (many "soft neurological signs" and no "hard" or strongly conclusive ones) to (c) learning disabled, with no neurological signs, either "hard" or "soft," to (d) normal (no learning problems, except those which can be resolved by completely motivational management). See Table 1.1.

1. Brain-Damaged Subjects

For a subject to be included in this class there must be conclusive medical or clinical evidence of tissue damage and resulting behavioral deviation. Brain surgery, postmortem study, and a variety of medical tests enable the surgeon to report the nature, extent,

---

[1] Throughout this book, specific social roles that may be assumed by either sex (e.g., teacher, doctor, parent) will be referred to by the pronouns "he or she." However, particular syndromes or specific forms of behavior (e.g., the epileptic patient, the elementary school student, the learning disabled child) will be described as a hypothetical person, and frequently may be referred to by the pronoun "he" in its generic sense, to indicate a person of either sex. This practice avoids a tedious repetition of "he or she" and promotes greater clarity of meaning and economy of sentence structure.

and intensity of the tissue damage. Other sources of unequivocal signs of central nervous system damage include "stroke" (cerebral bleeding); hemiplegia (paralysis on one side of the body, such as left arm and left leg); brain tumor (detected by imaging techniques); or penetrating head injury. Severe and localized dysrhythmias revealed on the electroencephalogram (EEG) may indicate the presence of actual damaged or scar tissue, or an area of the brain where electrochemical functions are abnormal. The last named may result in intermittent epileptic seizures.

In severe bilateral brain damage the person may be unable to walk, handle things, move about, or talk normally. In cases of brain damage that is highly localized and outside the cerebral speech and sensorimotor areas, mental impairment may be minimal or nonexistent. *Some brain-damaged people are intellectually superior.*

2. Borderline Dysfunction or MBD

During the past quarter century, the diagnostic term "minimal brain dysfunction," or MBD, has become common in medical and clinical psychological practice. This description has referred to the child with no conclusive "hard" neurological signs on medical examination, or very minimal indications, and the presence of "soft signs." It has been a confusing label for most teachers because it appeared in the late 1940s from medical studies as "minimal brain damage" in children with learning and behavior problems and the concept has been changing, both medically and psychologically, as more precise neuropsychological knowledge has emerged.

This condition has been frustrating for educators and has led many of them to discard a neurological approach as unworkable and confusing. Teachers and school psychologists need some clarification for this category of students, who along with the next group who have no positive neurological signs make up the largest group of learning disabled students.

A list of the most common soft signs includes:

1. Signs that reflect a developmental delay: speech and language retardation, motor clumsiness, perceptual deficits (e.g., visual rotations, reversals, or inversions; auditory phonetic imperception; poor finger localization), poor right–left orientation, meaningless and hyperactive motor activity, and being aware of only one hand being touched when, in fact, both have been simultaneously stimulated. The teacher will recognize that some of these behaviors are common among children up to about age 8, but if they persist in large numbers beyond that age, it may be useful to refer the child for neurological and neuropsychological examination.

2. Inability to copy simple geometric forms, "sloppy" writing and copying, faulty hand–eye coordination. The teacher will recognize that boys, until about age 9 or 10, are usually inferior to girls of the same age in writing and drawing, and these differences are generally believed to result from a different pattern of neural maturation in boys.

3. For a neurologist's list of soft signs see Spreen, 1988, pp. 149–150.

Frequently, but not always, the presence of a number of soft signs coexists with hyperactivity and a severe learning disability, but we cannot conclude that soft signs necessarily cause either hyperactivity or a learning disability. Any experienced teacher can think of some learning disabled children who are quiet and amenable to direction and some physically clumsy children who are competent students.

Although the physician or psychological researcher may continue to use the MBD label because it is useful for categorizing a clinical group of children, the teacher is better advised to avoid the label and to deal only with the child's learning problems. The school psychologist's interpretation of the possible limiting effects of the soft signs should be useful for the teacher in providing more detailed understanding of the child's skills and potential.

Soft signs appear to be permanent and may increase as the child grows. Spreen (1988, 1989b) in a 15-year follow-up study of 226 boys and girls between ages 10 and 25 found that neurological soft signs identified at age 10 actually increased in most cases by age 25. A large number of soft signs were observed, including slight ataxia, slight anosmia, unsustained bilateral nystagmus, slight choreiform movements, mild spasticity, slight bilateral weakness, mild uni- or bilateral exaggeration of tendon reflexes, slight heel/knee testing, moderate or slight anesthesia, bilateral simultagnosia, and slight position sense.

3. *Learning Disabled with No Positive Neurological Signs*

This group of children is particularly interesting because its members are usually of average to above-average global intelligence and may or may not be free of perceptual and/or motor deficits. But for no clear reasons they have great difficulty in processing and learning academic material. This is the child with a "developmental or specific learning disability," sometimes labeled a "congenital learning problem."

Because of the persistence of the problem and its lack of response to normal educational measures to which the majority of children respond positively, a constitutional cause is suggested as a fixed etiological force underlying the psychological influences of the child's social environment. Such chronic causes are not fully understood at present but they may result from (1) an abnormal brain structure (Galaburda & Kemper, 1979; Galaburda et al., 1985); or (2) genetic deficits (DeFries & Gillis, 1991; Regehr, 1987); or (3) some form of neurotoxicity (Fulton et al., 1987; U.S. Government Printing Office, 1990) or body–chemistry imbalance; (4) minimal brain dysfunction so obscure as to be undetected on a standard neurological examination; or (5) some other neuro-physiological cause unknown at present.

The supposed cause in (4) is inferred from the scientific assumption about the unity of nature and the stable comparative pattern of cognitive measures of different clinical groups. Data from many clinical studies of groups of brain damaged, of subjects with soft signs (a MBD group), and of LD subjects without neurological signs, have shown that the BD group, on average, was most impaired cognitively, and that the MBD and the LD groups were less affected, but still worse than normal control subjects (Reitan & Boll, 1973; Spreen, 1988, 1989b). Also, because the "nonneuro-logical" LD students frequently show the same types of learning problems as the BD and MBD groups, although often to a lesser degree, inferring an obscure, fixed, and unidentifiable neurological dysfunction affecting their LD problems has seemed logical.

It is this group that opponents of educational neuropsychology like to use to support their arguments. One such discussion (Reschly & Gresham, 1989) deliberately avoided the diagnosed BD and MBD groups, the cases in which brain–behavior relationships in LD can be demonstrated. Selecting data to support one's argument might win in some applied fields, but it is not an acceptable pro-cedure in science. A more persuasive approach is that of Spreen (1989b), who after exhaustively studying a large sample and exam-ining *all* clinical groups of LD subjects has urged a cautious and careful approach to educational neuropsychology.

4. Normal

Normal children are free of neurological deficits for the most part and show normal learning skills.

5. Psychiatric

Children whose learning disabilities are psychiatric in origin may show no perceptual, cognitive, or motor deficits nor any conclusive neurological signs. Their learning problems are believed to result from inattention, emotional disturbance, cultural deprivation, parental rejection, or environmental deficiency.

Three Levels of Neuropsychological Investigation

1. The first and most scientifically valid level of neuropsychological investigation includes direct observation of the learner's brain by the neurosurgeon during brain surgery, by the pathologist at autopsy, or by the medical researcher using technically complex medical tests (e.g., angiography, a brain scan, a Wada amytal test, etc.). These data are correlated with the assessment scores of the psychologist, the educational records of the teacher, and the social history of the parents or the family. This level of investigation permits the most accurate method for observing the brain–behavior relationships of a student because it correlates two independent sets of data (neurological and behavioral), and these data can be correlated objectively. For example, a massive left-hemisphere stroke will result in serious language impairment (aphasia) in most adults and some language problems in school-age children.

2. Although level 1 is scientifically the most desirable observational approach, the majority of students are never subjected to brain surgery or advanced neurological investigating techniques, and for these reasons nothing is known directly about the details of the structure or function of their brains. Whereas in level 1 there were two sources of objective observations, in level 2 there is only one. All that the educational diagnostician knows for sure is the behavioral data reported by the teacher, parent, and/or school psychologist. Any ideas about brain function in these cases are speculations usually made by the medical specialist or the experienced neuropsychologist. Although the diagnostician in this approach must speculate about possible cerebral function or dysfunction from observable behavioral signs, this is an acceptable method of diagnosis by neurologists and neurosurgeons, who call it "presumptive diagnosis" (Penfield, 1977, p. 46). But to attempt this type of neurological prediction requires advanced training and experience in clinical neurology or neuropsychology. It is usual that only a medical practitioner can make definitive statements publicly about brain function. Thus the clinical neuropsychologist, who may have opinions about the cerebral dysfunction of a patient, will communicate these predictions privately to the medical doctor

or to the court that has requested this opinion. In the latter case, the neuropsychologist may have to make a statement such as, "This patient has shown a number of behavioral signs similar to medically documented cases with known right-hemisphere lesions." In clinical reports to school personnel or parents about a learning disabled child, the school psychologist should never make statements about the child's brain function or dysfunction, but only about observed cognitive, perceptual–motor, or behavioral deficits. Level 2 allows reliable statements only about behavior and speculation about brain function. In this connection, Benton (1982) wisely cautions us, "Much of the research and clinical and educational service that we categorize as neuropsychological is in fact, *purely behavioral in nature* [our italics].

3. Level 3 includes what is frequently called erroneously "neuropsychological screening" by some school psychologists. As we shall see, it is actually "psychoeducational assessment" or screening. Because of the recent invasion of school psychology by neuropsychology, very few university special educators are qualified to teach developmental neuropsychology (Moss, 1979), hence most teacher trainees still receive little or no exposure to it. Their information must be gleaned from popular writers, from one- or two-day workshops, or from professional educational journals that sometimes present material that is confusing, or sometimes actually misleading. As a result of their sketchy knowledge, some educational diagnosticians feel free to make statements about brain function using a few tests (e.g., a Wechsler, a Bender–Gestalt, a Frostig, and maybe two or three subtests from the Halstead–Reitan Battery), and this type of practice has led to legitimate criticism (Coles, 1978). "If some school psychologists or teachers with little or no training in clinical neuropsychology are willing to make diagnostic statements about a child's brain, using an incomplete battery of tests, most of which were never intended as discriminators of abnormal brain function, then they are inviting a vigorous and justified attack such as Coles's" (Gaddes, 1981a). Not only are test batteries frequently too brief and inappropriate, but the investigator may confuse "neuropsychological assessment" with "psychoeducational asessment." As we have seen in level 1, "the behavioral relationship is empirically validated (i.e., based on 'hard data') and in the direction of *brain-to-behavior*" (Gaddes, 1981b), while in level 2, which includes closed head injuries (e.g., hemorrhages, infections, tumors, concussion), or a number of "soft" neurological signs, or a developmental learning problem (e.g., dyslexia) with no neurological signs on a standard neurological examination, the direction of presumptive diagnosis is from

behavior-to-brain. In level 3, the diagnostician with little training in neuropsychology is advised to accept the test and interview findings as a *psychoeducational* problem because that is what it is. Using a few neuropsychological tests can enrich the behavioral data, but their use does not necessarily make the report a "neuropsychological assessment." Legitimate statements can be made regarding cognitive and behavioral strengths and weaknesses and learning strategies, but no public statements should be made about neurological functions because of the lack of a comprehensive test battery and the meager training and experience of the diagnostician.

This is not to imply that the diagnostician should not indulge in private speculations about the *possible* brain functions or dysfunctions of the child or adult being examined. Such speculations are to be encouraged because this is how one learns the complex processes involved in neuropsychological diagnosis. School psychologists who wish to add neuropsychological knowledge and clinical procedures to their present repertoire of professional skills will need to find some experienced person to monitor and direct their attempts in neuropsychological diagnosis. They may do so formally during a sabbatical study year or informally in a continuing professional relationship in their place of employment. Once the school psychologist has reached a level of competence, then he or she can move from level 3 to 1 and 2, but as long as the chief responsibility is to provide definitive information for diagnosis and remediation in a school setting, it is best to keep it as a psychoeducational exercise (i.e., level 3).

Some Professional Problems

To be able to identify a syndrome we need an explicit definition, and to arrive at a complete and accurate definition we must understand the causes or etiology of the condition being defined.

At the outset, the reader should be clear about the difference between epidemiology and etiology. The first refers to studies of a community that tell us how many children are affected by an infectious disease or abnormal physical condition. The parallel in the present problem is to try to make a count of how many children are learning disabled in a community or population and of the various types of learning problems and their locations in the community. By contrast, etiology refers to the causes of the deficit condition, which for learning disorders may be physical, psychological, social, or a combination of some or all of these.

Prevalence Estimates of Learning Disabilities

Because of the methodological difficulties in producing a comprehensive prevalence study of LD subjects, there are very few. In
fact, Cruickshank (1983) has claimed that "there is not a single
adequate epidemiological study of learning disabilities in the world
literature," and this is true if one is looking for a study with
international application. However, it is unlikely that such a study
will ever appear because of the varieties of definitions of learning
disabilities and the differing cultural demands in different countries.

Nevertheless, a survey of estimates from different countries
shows some reliability, for example: United States, 10%–15%;
Canada, 10%–16%; Great Britain, 14%; and France, 12%–14%
(Gaddes, 1976). Unfortunately, just a small fraction of these children are in special classes. In 1970 in the United States from 1.4%
to 2.6% of school-age children were in special classes (Silverman &
Metz, 1973), but such classes were needed for 15% (Myklebust &
Boshes, 1969). In Canada the picture was equally dismal. In 1966,
fewer than 2% of children were receiving specialized help, and
presumably the current obsession with 'normalization" has resulted
in some new and different problems.

Incidence figures in Canada reported in a government survey covering 1982 and 1983 showed that 15.5% of public-school
children were receiving some form of special education, and of
these the LD segment comprised 4.4% of the total school population (Kendall & Wong, 1987). However, because some of the
other categories (LD was only one of eight groups of excep-
tionality) also included some students who were mildly learning
disabled, Kendall and Wong speculated that the actual LD population might be as high as 8% to 10%. The reduction in estimates
of LD students in the 1980s, compared to those in the 1960s, seems
to be the result of more refined diagnostic procedures and better-
informed definitional concepts.

In spite of the difficulties in estimating the number of LD children there is rough agreement among estimates from different
countries suggesting the possibility of an organically based etiology.
Rutter, Tizard, and Whitmore (1970) concluded from a study of
2300 children aged 9 to 12 years, on the Isle of Wight, that 7.9%
were both mentally impaired and educationally retarded. Because
theirs was a medical study, they included all Ss who were mentally
retarded (i.e., 2.5%), and so this figure suggests that about 5.4%
of children with IQs above 70 were educationally retarded. A
much-quoted American study by Myklebust and Boshes (1969)
showed that 7.5% of more than 2700 third- and fourth-graders

with IQs higher than 90 were underachieving. These children had evidence of some type of neurological dysfunction. A more recent study (Stevenson & Richman, 1976) estimates that in the population of 3-year-old American children, more than 3% have some form of language disorder and 2.3% are severely impaired in their language expression. Follow-up studies of these children showed that most of them were still having oral language and naming problems at age 9 (Stominger & Bashir, 1977). Kaufman and Kaufman (1983, p. 70, Table 3.9), studying a standardization sample of 2000 American children aged 6 to 16 years, found that 2% were speech impaired and 2.3% were learning disabled.

These data suggest that the average elementary school population may include about 15% of children who are underachieving academically. Of these, about half have some degree of central nervous system (CNS) dysfunction (i.e., approximately 7%). This means that in Table 1.1 (p. 11), category 1 (hard signs) may have about 2.5% of the average elementary school population, and category 2 (soft signs) may have about 5%. These estimates appear to be both conservative and stable, and they can be useful if used cautiously and until estimates based on better data become available.

Etiology

The major causes of learning problems are (1) physiological, (2) psychological and psychiatric, and (3) sociological or environmental. The physiological causes easiest to identify are neurological dysfunctions, which are the main subject of this book, and genetic determinants and malnutrition. Of the approximately 15% of underachievers in our public schools, about half appear to have some type of neurological or genetic deficit and half have purely motivational problems (Myklebust & Boshes, 1969). A huge body of literature has appeared on the MBD child (Birch, 1964; Clements, 1966; Hern, 1984; Paine, 1962, 1965; Rutter, Graham, & Yule, 1970; Tupper, 1987; Wender, 1971, 1973); and although some of these sources use the terms "minimal brain damage or dysfunction" and "learning disorder" synonymously, that is not the view taken by the present authors. As already described, there is a recognition of a learning disability category *without neurological signs*, and also a number of children with several soft signs may have no learning difficulties. Although children in both categories will have their learning disabilities analyzed and treated remedially, the medical data or soft signs in the MBD case may provide a more complete understanding and a *better basis for prediction* in pre-scribing treatment. The learning disabled child with no positive evidence of neurological dysfunction, once it is evident that the problem is not psychological or motivational, may be hypothesized to have some genetic disorder, or developmental problem or possibly a very minimal neurological dysfunction, so subtle as to be missed on a standard neurological examination.

Or in some other cases, neurological function is normal and academic learning deficits may be associated with anatomical variations in brain development in different children. Geschwind (1979b) has proposed the hypothesis that in some children the normal asymmetrical structure of the temporal lobes develops dif-ferently both structurally and sequentially during fetal life. When this cerebral structure is such as to facilitate verbal processing, the child may learn to read and write with ease; when it does not, the child may have verbal learning difficulties. This is an interesting theory because it does not imply neural damage, but a particular structural development not conducive to a particular aptitude. As Geschwind wisely points out, we can accept a lack of aptitude for music, drawing, or athletics without associating neurological dysfunction; it is reasonable to include reading in the same be-havioral model.

Malnutrition has been known for a long time to impair mental development, but little controlled research has been done, nor has the knowledge been relayed to the professionals who might make good use of it. Physicians, psychologists, teachers, and parents rarely have had instruction in the relation between nutrition and mental development. In the past a number of studies have shown that malnutrition in animals (Cravioto, De Licardie, & Birch, 1966; Stewart & Platt, 1968) and at critical periods of early growth in children (Stoch & Smythe, 1968) may result in reduced brain size and impaired intellectual development. Central nervous system damage from malnutrition during the last trimester of intrauterine life or during the first year of postnatal life is usually permanent (Birch, 1970).

During fetal development, tissues that undergo the most rap-id development are most vulnerable. This fact corresponds to Dobbing's hypothesis of critical periods of growth (Dobbing, 1968). These rapidly developing tissues are particularly susceptible to the effects of maternal malnutrition.

The brains of fetuses obtained from therapeutic abortions per-formed on malnourished women were examined by one group of researchers (Winik et al., 1972). They also examined the brains of infants who died of severe malnutrition or who died accidentally during the first year of life. They found that the number of cells in the human brain increases linearly until birth, then more slowly until six months of age. After the first year, there is no increase in the number of cells, only increase in brain weight. They found that the brains of the malnourished infants contained only 60% as many cells as those of normal infants. In addition to the reduction in gross brain weight that accompanies severe maternal malnutrition, there is a reduction in brain cell number (Zamenhof & van Marthens, 1978).

Other physiological causes of learning disabilities include endocrine gland imbalances in which one or more of the glands in this interrelated system produce too little or too much of some of their chemical secretions. The "master gland," or pituitary gland, located near the thalamus, secretes several hormones directly into the bloodstream, and at least two of these control physical growth and sexual behavior. The thyroid gland, located in the neck, secretes thyroxin, a strong chemical agent that controls the basal metabolism rate of the body, or the rate of oxygen consumption and energy output. The effect of abnormal thyroid function on physical growth has been known since the turn of the present century, and Mateer in the 1920s related underproduction of thyroxin (hypothyroidism) with poor memory, low IQ, overweight, and lack of energy (Mateer, 1935). Overproduction of thyroxin (hyperthyroidism) can produce hyperactivity, irritability, loss of weight, and difficulty in concentrating. A marked rise in IQ and improvement in social behavior can result from competent medical treatment of the hypothyroid child.

The other endocrine glands are not usually as controllable in their relation to cognitive function, although pancreatic dysfunction, resulting in abnormal blood sugar levels, can be disruptive to academic learning, and pancreatic function may be modified by diet to some extent. Parents should be advised if their child suffers from diabetes mellitus (hyperglycemia) and the teacher should be advised of its possible behavioral effects. Too little sugar in the blood (minimal hypoglycemia) can result in word-finding difficulties, increased spelling errors, and other problems of language competence.

The other ductless glands, including the adrenals, parathyroids, pineal, and gonads, are equally important to normal physical and mental functioning, and any unusual and otherwise undiagnosed behavior that persists in a child should lead to an examination by a competent internal medical specialist. Should an endocrine imbalance be discovered, the parents, the school psychologist, and the child's teachers should be informed of its possible effects so that adequate adjustive or remedial action can be taken.

Exposure of the mother or fetus during pregnancy to various toxins (teratogens—i.e., substances that produce defects in the developing embryo) may result in short- and long-term impairment during childhood.

For example, using drugs during pregnancy may harm the fetus. These include a range of potentially harmful agents, from the hard drugs such as heroin, to prescription and nonprescription drugs, to nicotine and alcohol. Women addicted to narcotic drugs such as morphine or heroin are likely to give birth to premature infants who themselves have become addicted to the drugs during fetal development. Many suffer a number of difficulties, including seizures and CNS damage (Rosenblith & Sims-Knight, 1985). In one study a group of such children at ages 3 to 6 were found to be of shorter stature and lower weight, and they performed poorly on tests of perception and learning (Houselander et al., 1982). Similarly, infants of mothers who use cocaine during pregnancy begin life with many problems. Many of these infants are premature, abnormally underweight and undersize, and they may have a variety of neurological problems (Bingol et al., 1987).

A cluster of symptoms known as Fetal Alcohol Syndrome (FAS) may afflict infants born to mothers who drink excessively during pregnancy. The condition varies in intensity, outward expression, and degree of cognitive impairment, but it affects the whole-body systems leading to malformations and anomalies of the nervous system, musculoskeletal structure, and internal organs, including the heart and urinogenital tract. Alcohol appears to hamper fetal growth and produces small infants with small brains. Damage to the fetal brain is caused when the ethanol in the alcohol takes fluid from the developing brain, causing the death of brain cells (Winzer, 1990). Although ingestion of alcohol seems to interfere with normal fetal brain growth, the occurrence of defects depends upon the basic metabolism of the mother and infant.

The syndrome can be seen along a continuum of deficits from full-blown FAS to selective deficits, or Fetal Alcohol Effect (FAE). FAS to minor developmental effects (Fetal Alcohol Effect, or FAE). About 1 in every 750 newborns in the United States suffers from full-blown FAS. Symptoms in childhood occur along a continuum of mental impairment and physical anomalies to milder effects, including short attention span, restlessness, irritability, hyperactivity, learning disabilities, and motor incoordination (March of Dimes Birth Defects Foundation, 1983a; Rosett & Sander, 1979; Barkley, 1990). The teratogenic effects of anticonvulsants taken by pregnant mothers with seizure disorders was first presented by Meadows in 1968. Further studies (Speidel & Meadow, 1972; Hanson & Smith, 1975; Janz et al., 1982), reveal a pattern of physical malformations and cognitive deficits referred to as Fetal Dilantin Syndrome. Varying combinations of abnormalities can be found along a continuum from the more severe to the milder cases. Characteristic features include varying degrees of shortened stature, craniofacial anomalies, anomalies of the hands and feet, mental deficiency, attention deficit, and hyperactivity. About 10% of exposed infants may be sufficiently affected that the condition is recognizable in infancy, and an additional 30% may show lesser degrees of alteration.

Mothers who smoke during pregnancy may contribute to a range of problems in their infants, including growth retardation, prematurity, and behavioral problems (Dunn et al., 1977). Nicotine causes a rise in heart rate, blood pressure, and respiration and constricts blood flow, thus reducing the amount of oxygen available to the fetus. The effects of nicotine are dose related. The clearest finding is the tendency of pregnant smokers to produce smaller babies. Some researchers have identified a "fetal tobacco syndrome" characterized by slow fetal growth (Nieburg et al., 1985). There is evidence to indicate that smoking during pregnancy can affect a child's later cognitive and psychological development. At 4 years and 11 years, children whose mothers smoked during pregnancy showed poor attention span, hyperactivity, and problems with reading, spelling, mathematics, and perceptual and motor skills. They scored lower on tests of intelligence than matched groups of subjects (Ss) from nonsmoking mothers and they were more likely to be classified MBD by neurologists (Naeye & Peters, 1984). All parents should consider marijuana use during pregnancy hazardous because the drug may compromise central nervous system integrity (Osofsky, 1978).

Acquired Immune Deficiency (AIDS) may be contracted by a fetus if the mother is infected. Infants born with AIDS may exhibit growth failure, hand and face abnormalities, and incomplete brain development (Iosub et al., 1987).

Lead poisoning is not a common cause of learning disabilities in children except in some deteriorating housing areas. Modern house paints do not have a lead base, but many ghetto areas with older houses where children can peel off chips of older, lead-based paint and eat them, present a threat. Ross and Ross (1982, pp. 83–90) discuss its possible relation to hyperactivity.

Controlled studies of the effects of lead on children's behavior and cognitive achievement have appeared only in the last few years. "In 1979 the first of the general population studies was published" (M. Smith, 1985); this study was done by Needleman and his colleagues at Harvard. Similar studies appeared throughout the 1980s in both North America and Europe (e.g., Brunekreef et al., 1983; Needleman et al., 1979; Yule et al., 1981; M. Smith et al., 1983); and M. Smith (1985) has published a useful comparative examination of nine of these studies carried out between 1979 and 1983.

One of the larger investigations is the Edinburgh lead study, in which a multidisciplinary team examined cognitive function, social behavior, reaction time, and inspection time of 501 boys and girls aged 6 to 9 years. These behavioral measures were related to current blood-lead and tooth-lead levels, and the investigators included careful examination of lead in the drinking water and dust in each child's home. They included eight other possible sources in the child's home environment. To date, four detailed reports from this study have been published (Raab et al., 1985; Fulton et al., 1987; Thomson et al., 1989; Raab et al., 1990). The investigators concluded, "in Edinburgh children with a mean blood-lead value of 10.4 µg/dl (i.e., 10.4 millionths of a gram per deciliter, or tenth of a liter) there is a significant relation between tests of ability and attainment [BASC, a combined score from the British Ability Scales and a number of other cognitive abilities including mathematical and reading scores] and blood-lead when confounding variables are taken into account. The strongest relation is with the reading score" (Fulton et al., 1987).

The effect on children's learning of harmful fluorescent lighting and unshielded television tubes is just beginning to attract research attention. This study has grown out of original and interesting work by John Ott, whose early work in photography led him to experiment with the effects of natural and artificial light on plants, animals, and humans. The possibilities of its importance to physical health, mental health, and classroom learning are just beginning to be realized (Ott, 1976).

All studies have not supported Ott's findings, however. In a carefully controlled study of the effects of cool-white and full-spectrum fluorescent illumination on learning and behavior, Ferguson and Munson (1987) found no significant effects of such lighting on attention and classroom activity level. They found that cool-white and full-spectrum fluorescent lighting had differential effects on neuromuscular performance (e.g., handgrip strength and visual reaction times), reflecting the indirect effects of illumination on physiological functioning.

One of the more controversial questions about possible radiation is the effect of computer video display terminals (VDTs) on fetal development. In the 1980s, groups of mothers who had miscarriages and infants with birth defects were reported in some areas to be using VDTs. However, recent large-scale, well-controlled studies have found no significant association between VDT use and problems in pregnancy (Blackwell & Chang, 1988).

Since the first nuclear bomb was dropped in 1945, the dangers of radiation have become very real to people worldwide. Exposure to radiation has been linked to fetal deaths and structural abnormalities in infants. Studies following the nuclear bombing of

Hiroshima and Nagasaki found that exposure to radiation increased the incidence of spontaneous abortions, miscarriages, and mutations among surviving infants (Annis, 1978).

Pollutants and radiation can adversely affect the unborn child. A tragic example of the effects of environmental pollutants occurred in Japan in the 1950s. A large industrial complex discharged mercury-laden effluent into the Bay of Minamata, contaminating fish that were later eaten by pregnant women. Their infants were born with physical abnormalities and mental retardation as well as other neurological impairments (Miller, 1974; U.S. Government Printing Office, 1990). Polychlorinated biphenyls (PCBs), chemicals widely used in industry before they were banned in 1976, contaminated salmon and trout in Lake Michigan. Pregnant mothers who had eaten the fish two to three times a month gave birth to infants who, when tested at birth, showed poor muscle tone and depressed responsiveness. Later at age seven months, the infants performed poorly on tests of visual recognition and interest in novel stimuli (Jacobson, et al., 1984).

Newborns whose well-being may be in jeopardy are known as high-risk infants. Two conditions that can place the infant at risk are prematurity and low birth weight. Preterm infants are those whose birth weight is appropriate for gestational age, but who are born at or before 37 weeks' gestation. They generally weigh less than 2500 grams (about 5.5 pounds). Small-for-date infants are born below the weight expected for their gestational age. But not every premature infant suffers chronic deficits, and with good care in infancy many of them grow up to be successful children and adults. In general, the lower the birth weight the shorter the gestation period, the more disadvantaged the environment, and the greater the likelihood of developmental problems.

Until about 25 years ago, the morbidity rates for premature infants, especially the smaller ones, were very poor. It is so no longer, and even infants born with very low birth weight (750–1000 grams or 1.7–2.2 pounds) have a 70% chance of survival. Today's dramatic medical advances have made this improvement possible, but the long-term outlook for these children is generally less optimistic. In one study (Sagal et al., 1982), the developmental progress of 294 low birth-weight infants was monitored. Of the 179 survivors, 30 exhibited neurological impairment, including blindness, microcephaly, deafness, and mental retardation. In another major study of infants born between 1975 and 1985, it was found that 26% of survivors weighing less than 800 grams (about 1.8 pounds), 17% of survivors weighing between 800 and 1000 grams (about 1.8–2.2 pounds), and 11% of survivors weighing 1000–1500 grams (about 2.2–3.3 pounds) exhibited major handicaps when assessed at age 1 and 2 years (Ehrenhaft et al., 1989). An Australian longitudinal study of children born between 500 and 900 grams had more optimistic findings (Kitchen et al., 1987). They found that 72% of survivors in their group had no handicaps at all at age 5 years, and only 19% had major disabilities. These findings suggest that age 2 may be too early to evaluate long-term future outlook.

Sensory deficits, such as impaired vision or hearing, may interfere with normal academic learning, but a child with these problems, if he or she possesses at least average intelligence, can usually be taught to read and write with the use of glasses or a hearing aid coupled with special teaching methods. Most sensory deficits are "peripheral"; that is, they result from damage or dysfunction in the sensory nerves outside the brain. However, "central" visual or auditory deficits are more difficult to treat. Should the visual cortices be damaged, the child may have problems interpreting what he sees; similarly, damage to the auditory cortices can result in problems of language interpretation (receptive aphasia). Where brain damage occurs, some form of "central" processing may be disturbed and normal perception, motor response, and learning disrupted. It is these central processing types of learning disabilities that form the chief subject of this book.

The psychological and psychiatric factors influencing learning behavior are frequently difficult to tease out, although it is clinically evident that large numbers of children with emotional problems do badly in school. Glasser (1969) has stressed the need for love, self-worth, and successful achievement for competent learning, and the large-scale Isle of Wight study carried out in England has shown the important relationships between education and good physical and mental health (Rutter, Graham, & Yule, 1970).

Sociological factors are difficult to relate specifically to academic competence, but the studies of ghetto children show them to be at high risk for biological and social–environmental deficits (Hallahan & Cruickshank, 1973; Walzer & Richmond, 1973). Poor living conditions and malnutrition encourage and perpetuate ill health in all its aspects—physical, psychological, and social. It acts as a feedback process so that, "To him that hath shall be given and to him that hath not, even that which he hath shall be taken away" (paraphrase of Matthew 25:29). Eisenberg (1966) has shown larger numbers of poor readers in large urban centers and fewer in suburban residential neighborhoods. It seems highly likely that ghetto living produces a number of children who fit the definition of learning disabled *in some respects*, but here the etiology is difficult to isolate. Many of these children respond to remedial teaching programs that include strong emotional support and academic skill training. Because in many of them their learning problems result not from a chronic neurological structural or functional abnormality but from an emotional lack that gradually is alleviated, these children may be considered "false positive" LD children. Sometimes these cases, where the basic cause can be altered, are referred to as "learning problems" rather than "learning disabilities" (Frostig, personal communication, 1978; Gaddes, 1978).

The reader will recognize that the discussion above gives much greater attention to the physiological causes of learning disabilities than to the psychological and social causes. This is not to imply they are more important, but to stress the aim of this book. All etiological causes are important, but by briefly acknowledging the psychosocial causes, we can get to the real subject of our discussion sooner.

Problems in Defining Learning Disabilities

The concept of learning disabilities has emerged within about the past 30 years, and numerous definitions have been given, depending on the professional training and experience of the person attempting the definition. Some medical doctors have stressed neurological and physical factors and made little or no attempt to relate them to classroom learning. Most psychologists and educators ignore the physical dysfunctions in learning impairment and some even deny that they exist. Some medical doctors complain that "virtually all definitions of learning disabilities exclude children whose learning problems are due to neurological handicaps" (Schain, 1972). Neither of these extreme views is accurate. There is no doubt that neurological dysfunctions are intimately involved in producing some perceptual, cognitive, and motor impairments, as we show in this book, and it is true that since the work of Alfred Strauss in special education (Strauss & Lehtinen, 1947); Ward Halstead (1947) and Wilder Penfield in neurosurgery (Penfield, 1938, 1947); and Donald Hebb in neuropsychology (Hebb, 1939, 1942a, 1949), increasing numbers of psychologists have begun to see the value in using neuropsychological knowledge in problems of special education (Bakker & Satz, 1970; Benton, 1962b; Cruickshank, 1961, 1966, 1983; Gaddes, 1966b, 1968; Kalverboer, 1976; Knights, 1970; Knights & Bakker, 1976; Myklebust, 1963, 1967a, 1971b, 1975b; Reitan, 1966a). Since the late 1970s, interest has grown at an increasing rate (Chall & Mirsky, 1978; Gaddes, 1980, 1981a, 1982, 1983, 1985; Hartlage, 1975, 1979; Hartlage &

Hartlage, 1977; Hynd, 1981; Hynd & Obrzut, 1981; Obrzut & Hynd, 1991; Pirozzolo, 1979, 1981).

Probably the most important influence is the stimulation of interest and research energies of not only psychologists and educators, but medical researchers in neurophysiology, neurosurgery, genetics, and endocrinology. The work of Geschwind (1962, 1965; Geschwind & Levitsky, 1968) was the beginning of a rapidly increasing interest by a wide variety of medical researchers (Bjørgen et al., 1987; Duara et al., 1991; Galaburda, 1983, 1984; Galaburda & Kemper, 1979).

Most definitions include neurological dysfunctions in their descriptions (Bateman, 1964; Clements, 1966; Kirk & Bateman, 1962; Myklebust, 1963, 1973b; National Joint Committee on learning Disabilities, 1987; Strauss & Lehtinen, 1947), although they are usually recognized as peripheral correlates of the child's psychosocial adaptation within a circumscribed educational program. In simple terms, the child's learning disability is a function of his inability to cope with the demands of the school, so that the degree of academic incompetence relative to his potential ability is the chief evidence that the child has a specific learning problem. Knowledge of a brain lesion will not remove the physical deficit, but it can enrich the understanding of the child's problem and thus help him or her to circumvent the difficulties imposed by the lesion.

The Search for a Definition of Learning Disabilities

With the adoption of the term "learning disabilities" in 1963 came the need to define it. Parents' groups conceived it as a learning disorder in the presence of normal or better-than-average intelligence. Professionals saw it as occurring at any level of intelligence (Cruickshank, 1975b). During the 1960s and 1970s, parents led mainly by the Association for Children and Adults with Learning Disabilities (ACLD), both in the United States and Canada, attempted to promote their concept that, if strictly adhered to, would exclude any child with an IQ below about 85 or 90 from the benefits of their recommended treatment programs. Professionals continued to present a research-based view of learning that included the full spectrum of human behavior. Some researchers in the field who expressed opinions in conflict with the parents' view were maligned personally by a few of the parents who perceived those professionals as unfeeling false witnesses attempting to deprive them of the satisfactions of their perception of Samuel Kirk's definition. (In fact, Kirk's original statement (1963) had said that a learning disability did not result "from generalized mental retardation"). But that definition did not mean that a specific dysfunction in one or two cognitive skills, the characteristic identity of LD, could not occur in some children with an IQ of less than 90.

Numerous conflicting definitions began to appear, and one attempt to resolve the problem proposed, "it may be unrealistic to expect a single definition to hold relevance for many different disciplines. That which is relevant for the neurologist and pediatrician . . . may not be relevant for the educator" (Chalfant & Scheffelin, 1969). In the same vein it was suggested that several kinds of definitions might be necessary to satisfy the various groups intending to use them. Such professional tolerance became difficult to continue in the United States, however, with the passing of legislation (P.L. 94–142 the Education for All Handicapped Children Act of 1975). Now it became administratively necessary to identify clearly those students who were LD so that special services that had been decreed by law could be delivered.

To provide professional input to the U.S. Department of Education, a multidisciplinary advisory group, the National Joint Committee on Learning Disabilities (NJCLD) was formed in 1975 (Abrams, 1987). It had representatives from the American Speech-Language-Hearing Association (ASHA); Association for Children and Adults with Learning Disabilities (ACLD); Council for Learning Disabilities (CLD); Division for Children with Communication Disorders of the Council for Exceptional Children (CEC); Division for Learning Disabilities of the Council for Exceptional Children (CEC); International Reading Association (IRA); National Association of School Psychologists (NASP); and The Orton Dyslexia Society (ODS). Approximately 250,000 individuals were members in 1987 of the organizations represented by the NJCLD (Abrams, 1987). This council was faced with the horrendous task of not only attempting to produce a workable definition of LD to satisfy everyone, but of recognizing and supporting the need for competent clinicians and teachers to provide effective services, to decide how services could be delivered, and to see that communications were successfully shared by all. More detailed accounts of the activities of the NJCLD can be found elsewhere (Abrams, 1987; Hammill et al., 1987).

The confusing situation in the United States led William M. Cruickshank of the University of Michigan to question a large number of professionals in the United States, Canada, and Europe about the advisability of forming an international community of researchers to focus their scientific interests on the field of learning disabilities. Their response was positive and led to the formation of the International Academy for Research in Learning Disabilities (IARLD) in 1975, with Cruickshank as its first president and director. He hoped that this worldwide group of researchers would pool their knowledge, leading to a definition of LD that would enjoy widespread agreement and recognition. Cruickshank was successful in attracting many scholars of international stature and they have agreed on a neurological basis of perceptual, motor, and cognitive deficits, but cultural differences make an international definition unlikely. The IARLD at the time of Cruickshank's death in 1992 had about 270 members from 28 countries around the world; communication is maintained by a regular newsletter and a program of published research studies by the members.

Some of the parents in the Canadian ACLD, formed in the mid-1960s, also were deceived by the same misperception of Samuel Kirk's definition. In 1977 they invited Dr. Cruickshank to Ottawa to meet with Canadian special educators and senior government representatives from all ten provinces. As a result of this conference he wrote an articulate position paper on "a definitional statement" (Cruickshank, 1979) that was to provide the basis for the official definition of the CACLD. However, in Canada responsibility for public education is provincial and not federal. Consequently, special education policies and services differ among provinces and there is no pressure to conform to a national policy. Provinces may use the CALCD definition as a guide, or they may produce their own (Kendall & Wong, 1987).

In preparing any definition of learning disabilities, it is useful to remember that at least three types are possible (D. Kendall, quoted in Cruickshank, 1979).

1. A diagnostic and etiological definition describes the symptoms in relation to recognized or inferred causes. The NJCLD definition, quoted below, is an example.
2. Educational, pedagogical, pediatric, or biochemical definition. This type defines LD within the framework of a particular discipline. Myklebust's learning quotient is an example of an educational definition.
3. Legislative or administrative definition.

> Although a purist clinician might express dismay, a judgment as to whether a child should be designated as learning disabled stems from what is essentially an administrative decision as to how many dollars are to be spent, and therefore how many chil-

> dren are to receive additional specialist assistance. Sometimes
> administrative decisions are made directly as to how many chil-
> dren will be recognized as learning disabled. (McLeod, 1978)

Governments may decide that if 12% of the school population is
underachieving they will allot funds for one-sixth of this group, and
so recognize 2% of the population as learning disabled. Such a
definition exemplifies an administrative designation, and, although
it may be administratively expedient, it may be invalid diagnostically and educationally.

Anatomy of the Definition

In an attempt to deal with the confusion of definitions, the NJCLD
in 1981 adopted this wording:

> Learning disabilities is a generic term that refers to a heterogeneous
> group of disorders manifested by significant difficulties in the acqui-
> sition and use of listening, speaking, reading, writing, reasoning, or
> mathematical abilities. These disorders are intrinsic to the individual
> and presumed to be due to central nervous system dysfunction.
> Even though a learning disability may occur concomitantly with
> other handicapping conditions (e.g., sensory impairment, mental
> retardation, social and emotional disturbance) or environmental
> influences (e.g., cultural differences, insufficient/inappropriate in-
> struction, psychogenic factors), it is not the direct result of those
> conditions or influences (Hammill et al., 1987).

Because the descriptive definition above was produced by the
various professional groups primarily involved in delivering remedial services, it differs in emphasis from the government definition
(P.L. 94–142), whose primary aim was to identify and select LD
students. A major difference is the omission of the etiological role
of neurological factors in P.L. 94–142 and its inclusion in the
definition of the NJCLD (Heath & Kush, 1991). The government
definition stresses academic signs rather than neurological symptoms, no doubt from a pragmatic view. The relationships between
academic scores and LD can be obtained with greater reliability
than between neurological dysfunctions and LD. During the 1980s,
educators began to favor use of a discrepancy between expected
and actual achievement as a criterion for identifying a student as
LD (Heath & Kush, 1991).
    In 1985, the special U.S. Federal Government Work Group on
Measurement, delegated to improve the methods for assessing LD,
declared in a public statement (Reynolds, 1984–1985) that their

definition and the determination of LD is based on (1) whether a child is achieving at or below the level normal for his or her age, and (2) whether a child has a severe discrepancy between achievement and intellectual ability in one or more of seven areas relating to communication skills and mathematical abilities. Although this statement was becoming more operational than the earlier descriptive definitions, serious difficulties remained. One of the most obvious was what constituted a "severe discrepancy." Aware of these difficulties, educators were instructed (Federal Register, 1977) that "These concepts are to be interpreted on a case by case basis by the qualified evaluation team members" (Reynolds, 1984–1985). Because of the potential pitfalls in many psychometric models of selection and because of the difficulties in tying specific neurological signs to LD, the government work group has probably made the safest and most effective recommendation at this time. When the present body of correlational knowledge between brain function and cognitive skills is substantially increased, then a revised methodology for identifying LD students may be considered.

Basic Assumptions in LD Definitions

In spite of the profusion and variability among definitions, Morrison and Siegel (1991) propose that most of them include three basic assumptions:

1. Specificity. The learning problem is the result of the inadequate functioning of one or more cognitive skills in the presence of intact intelligence. Johnny can't read because he is not a good listener, or perhaps because his auditory perception is weak. He is said to have a "specific reading disability."
2. IQ–Achievement Discrepancy. The child's academic achievement, measured by achievement tests, is not commensurate with his or her ability, measured by a standardized IQ test, or it is below the level expected for his or her chronological age.
3. Exclusionary Criteria. Even though a LD may occur along with other handicapping conditions or environmental influences, it is not the direct result of those conditions or influences (Hammill et al., 1987).

The Search for the Severe Discrepancy

Traditionally, students have passed or failed an exam by achieving a score above or below an arbitrarily chosen cutoff point. For grade school it may be 50%, but for college entrance it is usually much higher. Initially, LD students were selected on this basis, but because the very nature of LD implied that the condition was determined by factors within the individual (teaching brain-injured children, Cruickshank, 1966; "Psychoneurological learning disorders in children," Myklebust & Boshes, 1960; "a possible cerebral dysfunction," Kirk, 1963) it soon became clear that some type of self-related measure was needed. Four methods of measuring the discrepancy between ability and achievement are prevalent, and some are psychometrically better in detecting the "severe discrepancy."

Deviation from Grade Level. This is the least sophisticated of the four methods. In its simplest form, constant deviation, it classifies as LD any child whose academic achievement is a predetermined number of years (e.g., one or two years) below the normal level indicated by his or her age. Though simple in theory and easy to use, this procedure has serious defects. It includes only academic deviation and ignores differences in intelligence, and by ignoring intellectual factors it identifies low achievers, including those with low IQs, instead of those whose achievement deviates from their intellectual potential (Heath & Kush, 1991). A further weakness is that various achievement tests have different normative data for the same age level, and within any one test the percentile ranks differ with age. For example, if two years were subtracted from the average reading level of 7-year-olds on the Wide Range Achievement Test (WRAT), 2% of the group would be considered reading retarded; at age 10 the impaired group would include 13%; at age 12, 18%; and at age 18, 25% (Gaddes, 1976). Reynolds has shown the variability of percentile ranks among tests when the WRAT, Peabody Individual Achievement Test (PIAT), Woodcock Reading Mastery Test (WRMT), and Stanford Diagnostic Reading Test (SDRT) are compared (Reynolds, 1981a). In spite of the severe invalidities of this method it continues to be used by some researchers and is accepted as standard procedure in a few states (Cone & Wilson, 1981).

A variation of the constant deviation model is "graduated deviation." This method is a little better than constant deviation in that it does control for increasing errors as students progress to the upper grade levels (see example above), but it fails to control for all other sources of error (Cone & Wilson, 1981) and low-IQ children remain more likely to be identified as disabled than those with higher IQs (Heath & Kush, 1991).

Expectancy Formula. The Federal Work Group on Measurement Issues in the Assessment of LD considered five formulas for calculating expected grade equivalence, but all were rejected because of their mathematical inadequacies (Reynolds, 1984–1985).

One of the formulas that has been used for calculating the Expected Grade Equivalent (EGE) is

$$EGE = \frac{IQ \times CA}{100} - 5$$

Because the child's chronological age (CA) is factored into the formula, five years are subtracted from the overall result to include only the years spent in school.

Expectancy data have also been used for calculating specific quotients or measures of achievement relative to a child's learning potential. For example, a formula widely used in the 1960s and 1970s was the Learning Quotient (LQ), or some variation of it, to indicate the level of competence of a child in a specific academic or cognitive skill. An LQ in reading could be determined with this formula:

$$LQ \text{ (reading)} = \frac{Reading\ age}{Expectancy\ age}$$

A child's "expectancy age" was the average of the mental age, chronological age, and grade age. The LQs were calculated for perception, conception, motor function, language, and nonverbal skills, where reliable normative data were available. The expectancy approach was a marked improvement over the deviation-from-grade-level method because IQ was now included in the formula; nevertheless, it contains serious limitations that can lead to invalid conclusions (Heath & Kush, 1991; Reynolds, 1984–1985).

Standard Score Difference Method. This method involves direct comparison of a child's intellectual potential with his or her academic achievement by converting both the IQ measures and the achievement-test scores into some form of standard scores. Because two sets of standard scores are directly comparable since they are expressed in equivalent units, it is a simple procedure to obtain a child's discrepancy or difference score by subtracting the achievement score from the IQ score, provided that the two distributions have the same mean and standard deviation. When the WISC-R is used as the intellectual measure, a mean of 100 and a standard deviation of 15 is chosen for the distribution of the achievement-test scores. Because of their comparability, standard scores "can be subjected to mathematical calculations and comparisons across tests, subject matter (subtests), as well as age or grade equivalents" (Cone & Wilson, 1981). A variety of formulas, using standard scores, have been developed for identifying LD students, but all have an inherent weakness: they are based on the assumption that the correlation between a child's IQ scores and achievement scores is perfect and positive (i.e., $r = 1.00$), but in fact it is between .50 and .65 (Heath & Kush, 1991; Yule & Rutter, 1976). Because of the effect of regression toward the mean, this system will always have a systematic bias. Children with a high score on one measure (e.g., IQ) will be underestimated on the other measure (e.g., achievement). The reverse is true in which prediction from a low score will over-estimate the other score. Therefore, any measure of underachievement that fails to allow for the statistical effects of regression will find too many bright children and too few dull children identified as "underachievers" (Yule & Rutter, 1976). In spite of these difficulties the standard score difference method is the most widely used to calculate a difference score for suspected LD students (Heath & Kush, 1991).

Regression Model. To avoid the effects of bias, as described above, a regression model is required. This design accounts for the imperfect relationship between IQ and achievement. "It is necessary to define 'underachievement' as discrepancy of actual achievement from the *predicted* value, predicted upon the basis of the regression equation between aptitude and achievement. A failure to recognize this regression effect has rendered question-able, if not meaningless, much of the research on 'underachieve-ment'" (Thorndike, 1963, p. 13). But in spite of this authoritative warning 30 years ago, the model is still rarely used (Heath & Kush, 1991).

The regression method uses a prediction equation based on the correlation between IQ and achievement scores, and as a result it adjusts for the tendency of scores to regress toward the mean. This method, though statistically freer of intrinsic mathematical weaknesses that can distort results than the other three methods, still depends on many prerequisites to produce valid discrepancy scores. Reynolds (1985) provides a useful and comprehensive list of standards for producing high quality input data for assessing a discrepancy. Some of these include selecting tests that are psy-chometrically well designed and constructed; adhering strictly to administrative instructions of all tests being used; selecting and using only valid normative data; selecting traits that are subject to at least ordinal scaling; and choosing a test that can provide an adequate operational definition of the trait being considered. Because the matter of diagnosing LD is the most difficult psycho-educational diagnostic task, only the best-trained clinicians should be delegated to assess LD students. Unfortunately, among the school personnel assigned to this difficult task, many "do not possess the requisite knowledge of tests and measurements to allow them to interpret test scores adequately" (Reynolds, 1985).

For the student not familiar with the application of the regression model, Heath and Kush (1991, pp. 295–303) provide a clear, step-by-step introductory explanation of how to use it to predict achievement from intellectual potential.

In conclusion, it is evident that of the four discrepancy formulas described briefly above, the first two are severely flawed mathematically and psychometrically. The last two are statistically better, although "it is at this stage inappropriate to recommend a single, specific theoretical model from which to assess LD. What is imperative however is that *a clear theoretical rationale is necessary for a coherent diagnosis and evaluation of LD children*" (Reynolds, 1985).

Is IQ Irrelevant to the Definition of LD?

From the preceding discussion it is evident that IQ is one of the two basic measures in calculating a discrepancy score for identifying LD students, and for that reason its validity must be established in this context. Siegel (1989) identifies four basic assumptions inherent in the concept of the IQ-achievement discrepancy. They are: (1) IQ tests measure intelligence; (2) intelligence and achievement are independent; (3) IQ scores predict academic performance; and (4) reading disabled (RD) students of different IQ levels have different patterns of cognitive and information processing skills. She believes that all four of these assumptions are invalid and that the practice of using discrepancy scores for selecting LD students is highly questionable. She supports her argument that IQ is irrelevant to the definition of LD with data that show no differences among children with reading disabilities at four IQ levels (<80, 81–90, 91–109, and >110) on measures of reading single words, reading pseudowords, demonstrating phonological skills, and spelling (Siegel, 1989). Although most investigators consider use of the discrepancy formula for identifying LD students problematic, they do not agree with Siegel's extreme position. Lyon (1989) challenges Siegel on the validity of her data and the logic of her concepts, as does Stanovich (1989). Torgesen (1989), though finding value in her comments, disagrees with her basic contention that IQ is irrelevant to the definition of LD. He quotes from a number of manuals accompanying established tests of general knowledge that show correlations with reading as high as .82 and .85. He believes that IQ is relevant to the definition for purposes of scientific research, but it should not be used to select children for special services. Leong (1989b) believes that Siegel's attempt to deal with "the umbrella term LD subsuming those with reading disabilities, spelling and writing disabilities, and mathematical disabilities" is impossible because it "suffers from lack of clarity because the processes of reading, spelling, composing, and mathematics, though similar and related, are dissociable." He discusses this at more length (Leong, 1987, pp. 10–12).

Still, Siegel's proposals have value. In discussing the first of the four concepts, she complains that IQ tests tend to include items and problems "that traditionally dominate school curricula" (Morrison & Siegel, 1991) and for that reason they appear to predict school success reasonably well for normal children, but they fail to measure general intelligence as the formula demands. This criticism is accurate. Tests like the WISC-R, she thinks, are too dependent on verbal memory and automated academic skills and fail to tap open-ended adaptive types of problem solving. It was just this point that led Ward Halstead, a neurologist at the University of Chicago, to propose almost fifty years ago the concept of "biological intelligence" (Halstead, 1947, 1951). He was investigating the mental deficits that resulted from surgically imposed brain damage, and he found, as Hebb had (Hebb, 1939) that the current intelligence tests were not sensitive to cerebral tissue damage. Most patients following brain surgery, showed little or no decrease in their IQ scores because these tests typically have a high loading of habituated verbal memory. In fact, most traumatically brain-damaged patients characteristically do better on the verbal tests than on the performance tests, and the Vocabulary subtest was found to be most resistant to the effects of brain damage (Wechsler, 1939). Halstead observed clinically that, in spite of the lack of evidence from the IQ tests, his patients did show signs of mental deficits, which led him to construct a battery of tests to measure cognitive skills that were not verbally loaded. He produced a set of 13 tests that were designed to tap mental abstraction, categorical thinking, nonverbal problem solving, spatial memory, stereognosis (tactile form recognition), tactile–visual cross-modal integration and memory, and perceptual and motor accuracy and speed. Because this battery was sensitive to the effects of brain damage where the IQ tests had not been, and because he believed it measured a number of cognitive functions strongly dependent on the efficiency of the human brain, Halstead named it "biological intelligence," as opposed to "psychometric intelligence," the type of mental processes that IQ tests measure (Reitan & Wolfson, 1992c, Chapter 1; 1992d).

A factor analysis of the 13 test results produced four factors: (1) a central integrative field factor C, which appeared to represent the ability of the individual to relate novel experiences to the known or familiar; (2) a factor abstraction A, the ability for abstract reasoning and categorical thinking; (3) a power factor P, the speed and accuracy of perceptual processes; and (4) a directional factor D, the ability for motor–expressive behavior. In subjecting the test battery to a statistical validity study by measuring the performance of a sample of brain-damaged adults against a matched sample of normal subjects, Reitan (1955b) eliminated three of the tests that failed to discriminate between the two groups, and the remaining ten tests became the Halstead-Reitan Neuropsychological Test Battery. An Impairment Index can be calculated (for adults only) by counting the number of tests on which the results fall in the range of scores of brain-damaged rather than normal subjects (Reitan & Davison, 1974). Reitan showed this to be a reliable psychometric method for identifying brain-damaged patients.

Because of the psychometric and conceptual problems inherent in the IQ-achievement discrepancy formula for discriminating LD from non-LD students, Siegel proposes abandoning the IQ test in the analysis of the LD child. We would modify Siegel's proposal by advocating that IQ test input be used for analysis but not for categorizing LD students. Most neuropsychologists may use the WISC-R IQ as an indication of the level of a child's cognitive function relative to the normal population, but its greatest value is that it provides a *profile* of test scores (Lezak, 1988) to be used along with a comprehensive battery of neuropsychological test findings to provide a cognitive analysis of the child. This has been the policy in our laboratory since its inception in 1963.

Whether the school psychologist uses a neuropsychological battery or not, he or she will use clinical judgment to decide the category of any child and the type of treatment to be followed. Clinical judgment by the best-trained personnel and using the most comprehensive clinical test findings, is the official policy advised by the U.S. Office of Special Education (Reynolds, 1985).

If the present discrepancy model has any validity, it would be interesting to test the possibility of improving the "mental potential" side of the formula by introducing subtests that have proven themselves reliable in measuring "biological intelligence." Because Halstead's solution to this problem has had success in classifying brain-damaged patients, it seems a promising area of research to pursue the possibility of producing a battery of tests that would measure *intellectual potential* more comprehensively and in a way that is less curriculum bound than many IQ tests currently used. Such a battery would need to tap visual information processing, speech perception and all phonological processes, word retrieval, short-term memory, and auditory verbal comprehension, along with the cognitive processes included in the Performance tests of the WISC-R and the nonverbal reasoning skills of present neuropsychological test batteries. We say more about neuro-psychological testing in Chapter 3.

Some Professional Problems

Introducing new ideas and practices in any applied professional field is likely to produce some professional difficulties. Some of these are discussed in the following sections.

Communication

Neurology and neuropsychology possess their own medical concepts and language; some might say "jargon." For example, a report on a seven-year-old girl by a neuropsychologist in a medical center might tell us that "her sensory-perceptual tests suggest right-sided involvement," which can mean that her tactile recognition of letters and forms with her right hand is inferior to that of her left hand. Or, "there is evidence for involvement of right-sided motor function," which is jargon for "her right hand is slower and weaker in responding." Or, "there remained evidence of motor involvement of the right upper extremity," which translated into plain language tells us that she is relatively slower in tapping with her right hand.

To avoid discouraging educators and others from reading about neuropsychology, we avoid this type of language in this book, and technical terms, when they have to be used, will be explained. A Glossary is supplied at the back of the book.

Even so, neuropsychology is a complex subject, and trying to explain it in simple language risks the possibility of distortion or serious omissions. Every school psychologist who plans to include neuropsychological findings in a report to teachers and parents must learn to deal with this problem. Successful report writing requires sound knowledge of neuropsychology and learning theory, understanding test results from a comprehensive battery, (ideally) some first-hand classroom teaching experience, and a creative imagination to put all this information together into a meaningful description from which a successful remedial program can come.

Translating Theory to Practice

To understand and treat organically impaired learning disabled (LD) children and adults includes at least four steps: (1) a thorough neurological examination and clinical report from the neurologist; (2) a complete neuropsychological examination and report of the subject's (S's) perceptual–motor and cognitive/behavioral strengths and weaknesses; (3) a comprehensive report of S's academic strengths and weaknesses and an analysis of the nature of the learning problem; and (4) a remedial prescription constructed on the basis of all the information in (1), (2), and (3).

Many neuropsychologists produce a fine synthesis of (1), (2), and (3), but they fail to produce (4), probably because of ignorance about the methods of special education. They sometimes rationalize this professional lack by claiming that they are not teachers but clinical psychologists, and therefore they feel no responsibility for developing educational programs. Others may claim that, because a learner possesses a chronic and hence an incurable brain lesion, no remedial program exists that can correct the problem. Others have claimed that there is no demonstrated relevance between biological factors and the choice of teaching strategies. In this book we propose a thesis in direct contradiction to the negativism of the points of view above. Although no comprehensive and systematic theory has yet been constructed relating biology and learning, a large body of useful teaching techniques for LD students has grown out of knowledge about cognitive deficits associated with specific types of cerebral dysfunctions, and the reader will find them described throughout this book. Along with the present writers, several others have produced evidence to support the use of neurological knowledge in preparing programs of educational intervention (Adams, 1978; Gray & Dean, 1989; Hartlage & Reynolds, 1981; Hartlage & Hartlage, 1977; Hynd & Obrzut, 1981; Leong, 1989a; Obrzut & Hynd, 1991).

A knowledge of an LD student's cerebral areas of dysfunction and their related cognitive deficits can suggest remedial methods that might not otherwise have been considered. For example, a child who has difficulty in learning the alphabet because of a left-hemisphere dysfunction may be taught by singing (see the case of Pearson Morsby in Chapter 9). Such an approach makes use of the knowledge of cerebral asymmetry and supports the belief that the researcher provided with detailed and relevant knowledge is more likely to hit on original and useful solutions. Pasteur told us more than a century ago, "In the fields of observation, chance favors the prepared mind" (quoted by Geschwind, 1982).

Is Educational Neuropsychology Too Time Consuming?

Neuropsychological testing of one subject can take between 5 and 6 hours, and adding consultations with medical personnel and others, it will take much more time. How can this schedule be thought practical in a school setting? First, this level of diagnostic study is needed only for a minority of academic underachievers. Most are allocated to a remedial program by an *administrative* decision with little or no formal testing. However, for two classes of students, neuropsychological information is useful: (1) any child who is obviously neurologically impaired (e.g., a hemiplegic or epileptic child) and who is not responding successfully to the school programs available, and (2) a child with no evidence of neurological impairment who, after several administrative referrals to the school's remedial programs, is still not able to learn.

Examples of the second type are numerous. Frequently, bright children who are poor readers, spellers, and/or arithmetic calculators may be referred for visual and auditory tests, physical examinations, and studies of nutrition. Although the test results are usually negative, the child still has difficulty learning to read, to write, and to do arithmetic, but because of his inferior achievement, the school authorities may have placed him in a special remedial program. He may hate this placement because he speaks fluently and understands ideas better than most of his classmates. Even with the extra help he may make little academic progress because his treatment was based on an administrative decision rather than on understanding the causes behind his learning problems. A case of such a boy, Derrick White,[1] who was kept unsuccessfully in learning assistance classes for five years until accurately diagnosed, is described in detail in the addendum to Chapter 8.

Are the Professional Demands of Neuropsychology Too Heavy?

Senf (1979) comments very clearly on the professional problems in recommending additional graduate training to the already heavy curriculum of the trainee in special education. To add training in adult neuropsychology, developmental neuropsychology, behavioral neurology, and psychometric assessment will result in a demanding program for the graduate student and an exacting task for the curriculum planner. Hynd (1981) discusses four possible models for teaching neuropsychology to graduate students in education, and if the two disciplines are to be merged successfully, standards of training and training programs will have to be estab-

---

[1] The names in all case histories are fictitious, and other details have been changed to guard the anonymity of each individual.

lished to ensure that the population of organically impaired LD students will be optimally served.

Conclusions

The advantages and potential weaknesses of the neuropsychological approach to learning disabilities have been described. Unfortunately, more writers have presented the weaknesses of its definition and the risks in its application than have described its value, but most of the objections by professionals who oppose it are criticisms of its clinical abuses and not of the theory itself or of its valid clinical practice. Frequently these are educators with little or no knowledge of neuropsychology and no diagnostic experience in a neuropsychology laboratory. Clinicians and teachers with training in neuropsychology usually become enthusiastic converts when they see the diagnostic possibilities and their applications.

The causes of learning disabilities are complex and varied and may interact in subtle ways to render etiology difficult to determine. Generally they can be grouped in three major categories: organic and biological, genetic, and environmental. Children with organically determined problems may exhibit clear, hard neurological evidence. In some cases the neurological signs are not so evident or reliable, and these children are described as borderline LD with suspected neurological deficits. Also, some LD children who show no positive neurological signs may have minimal neurological dysfunctions that do not show on a standard neurological examination, or their disabilities may be a result of genetic deficits. Finally, some children have learning difficulties because of social–emotional problems.

The term MBD, although still used by researchers in medicine and the behavioral sciences, may be confusing for the educator. Because of the lack of organic evidence, the chaotic variability of the symptoms, and the frequent presence of some or all of these symptoms in all children up to age eight, the term is usually difficult for the researcher to validate and of little or no direct value for the educator. Borderline LD children with suspected neurological dysfunction may be a more useful description.

No one theory is complete or necessarily valid, but the best available knowledge should be used to develop a theory constantly open to review and revision in light of new experimental evidence. Similarly, no one remedial practice is appropriate for treating all behavior or learning problems. For the child with a serious or subtle learning disorder, neuropsychological diagnosis for understanding the nature of the child's problem and behavior-management techniques for treating it are probably the best at this stage in our knowledge.

Suggested Readings

For a more extensive discussion of the need for and the problems inherent in developing a definition of learning disabilities, see:

Cruickshank, W.M. Learning disabilities: A definitional statement. In Cruickshank, W.M. *Concepts in learning disabilities: Selected writings, vol. 2.* Syracuse: Syracuse University Press, 1981, 80–110.

Heath, C.P. & Kush, J.C. Use of discrepancy formulas in assessment of learning disabilities. In Obrzut, J.E. & Hynd, G.W. (Eds.), *Neuropsychological foundations of learning disabilities.* San Diego: Academic Press, 1991, 287–307.

Lyon, G.R. IQ is irrelevant to the definition of learning disabilities: A position in search of logic and data. *Journal of Learning Disabilities,* 1989, *22*(8), 504–507.

Morrison, S.R. & Siegel, L.S. Learning disabilities: A critical review of definitional and assessment issues. In Obrzut, J.E. & Hynd, G.W. (Eds.), *Neuropsychological foundations of learning disabilities.* San Diego: Academic Press, 1991, 79–97.

Siegel, L.S. IQ is irrelevant to the definition of learning disabilities. *Journal of Learning Disabilities,* 1989, *22*(8), 469–478, 486.

For a discussion of the formation and functions of the International Academy for Research in Learning Disabilities (IARLD), see:

Cruickshank, W.M. Learning disabilities: An international overview. *Paedoperisse,* 1987, *1*(1), 1–15.

The whole issue of *Paedoperisse* is devoted to discussions of the IARLD in various countries around the world. These include Great Britain, by Klaus Wedell; Canada, by David Kendall and Bernice Wong; Denmark, by Mogens A. Dalby; the Netherlands, by Luc M. Stevens; Czechoslovakia, by Z. Matějček & J. Sturma; Chile, by L. Bravo-Valdivieso; and the United States, by James D. McKinney & Lynne Feagans. All these writers are Fellows of IARLD.

2 The Nervous System and Learning

In modern psychology, it is now widely accepted that each kind of mental activity has a distinct psychological structure and is effected through the joint activity of discrete cortical zones.
A.R. Luria (1970)

No human being is constituted to know the truth . . . and even the best of men must be content with fragments, with partial glimpses, never the full fruition.
Sir William Osler (1906)

Most teachers and clinical psychologists are reluctant to assume the responsibility of learning neurology in addition to their many other duties. Whereas a disregard of neurological correlates is possible in teaching a child with a normally functioning brain, however, it may easily lead to misunderstanding and mishandling of the child with brain damage or some type of cerebral dysfunction. In fact, in the past, large numbers of children were misdiagnosed as "mentally retarded" because of unawareness of some type of sensory imperception, language deficit, or motor impairment that interfered with their learning. Had they been correctly understood and had a successful remedial program been established early, their lives might have taken a happier and more satisfactory direction.

Most LD children are not brain damaged, but if they have persistent difficulties in academic learning, it is likely that some area or areas of the brain are not functioning as well as they might, or that for some structural or chemical reason, or for some reason not yet understood, the neural processing of verbal or mathematical material cannot be done easily. Because it is frequently easier to understand minimal deviations in behavior by studying severe, pathological cases, the discussion in this chapter draws heavily on cases of brain damage because so much has been learned about its impairing effects on perception and learning.

Neurological Model of Behavior

The teacher, the parent, or anyone else working with a child with cerebral dysfunction can learn to use the neurological model of behavior profitably in educational planning. In simple form, it recognizes three processes in behavior: (1) sensory input (carried on by the sensory or afferent nerves, which conduct neural impulses from the various sense organs to the brain); (2) integration, recording, recognition, interpretation, storage, and retrieval of learned material (mediated primarily by the cerebral cortex and brainstem); and (3) neuromuscular–skeletal expressive behavior (effected by the motor or efferent nerves). In brief, all behavior includes input, integration, and output. If neural pathology in the sensory cortices and pathways (visual, auditory, tactile, or kinesthetic) obstructs or modifies the input, a potentially bright child may be mentally starved or frustrated for lack of mental stimulation. If neural pathology involves the cerebral cortex, the normal functions of mental integration and understanding are blocked, and if neural pathology occurs in the motor cortices or pathways, a potentially bright youngster may be obstructed in learning by difficulty in reciting, expressing, or establishing the motor match (Kephart, 1960/1971, 1966) so necessary to efficient learning. To understand these problems however, the clinical psychologist and the teacher must have at least a practical knowledge of the gross structure and function of the nervous system.

The study of the brain and nervous system is complex and detailed, and the reader who wishes to study in greater depth is referred to a good introductory text in neuroanatomy (e.g., Gardner, 1975; Nolte, 1988; Schmidt, 1978a,b). A good text in human neuropsychology will provide basic neurological knowledge as well as research findings on the relation between brain function and behavior (Kolb & Whishaw, 1990; Walsh, 1987). In this book, because we are stressing neuropsychology and its value in education, the sections on neurology are much briefer and less developed. But we hope they are adequate to provide a basic understanding of brain function for the educator and/or the psychologist unfamiliar with this material.

One can recognize three broad levels of knowledge about neuroanatomy and clinical neurology and neuropsychology: (1) the pediatric neurologist typically has detailed knowledge of neurology, moderate knowledge of neuropsychology, and little or no expertise in special education; (2) the clinical school neuropsychologist has moderate knowledge of neurology, detailed knowledge of neuropsychology, and moderate familiarity with methods in special education; and (3) the teacher should have a simplified but basic idea of brain function, some knowledge about the most common "molar" brain–behavior relationships, and profound knowledge of remedial procedures and teaching skills. Such a team will have an "expert" covering each of the three major professional areas of expertise, and the teacher will be able to understand the reports of the neurologist and neuropsychologist well enough to use their findings in constructing a remedial program for a LD student. The level of neurology described in this chapter is intended for the student in psychology or education or both who is being introduced to neurology and neuropsychology for the first time.

How Neuroanatomy Is Studied

The physiological study of the central nervous system (CNS) may use any of four main approaches (Kolb & Whishaw, 1990): (1) The *comparative* approach examines the various brains of organisms on the phylogenetic scale and notes the increasing structural complexity from simple wormlike animals to humans; (2) the *developmental* approach examines the increasing neurological complexity that accompanies normal growth of an individual; (3) the *cytoarchitectonic* approach examines the varying size, shape, and structure of different nerve cells (neurons) and their locations in the brain and spinal cord; (4) the *biochemical* approach is developing with new scanning techniques and is revealing new information about the electrochemical transmission of neural impulses in the brain. In this book we concentrate on the structure, function, and developmental pattern of the human brain and refer only in passing to comparative and biochemical information, not because they are unimportant but because they are beyond the scope of this book. Outside references in neurology are listed at the end of this chapter.

The Neuron

The various tissues and organs of the human body are composed of different types of somatic cells that make up tissues, bones, blood, muscles, and nerves. The nerve cell, or neuron, in large numbers makes up the nerves and, in part, the nerve tissue, but the neuron differs from the other somatic cells in two basic ways. First, unlike the other cells, which are tiny membranous spheroids, the neuron possesses in addition to the cell body a sort of "aerial" or "receiver," the *dendrites*, and a sort of "ground connection," the *axon*. The neuron differs, then, in structural design from the other body cells. Like them it has a cell body with a nucleus, but it also has delicate, threadlike appendages, the dendrites, and the axon, which act as conductors of the neural impulses.

The second basic difference is the neuron's inability to reproduce itself postnatally. It is common knowledge that somatic cells when they are damaged can divide and reproduce themselves, and in this way the damaged tissue eventually is replaced with new cells. For example, following a hemorrhage, new blood cells are produced to replace the blood loss within a few hours. If a bone is broken it will knit. If the skin is cut it will soon replace the damage with a new patch of skin made up of newly produced epithelial cells. Unfortunately, when neural cell bodies are damaged and destroyed, they usually are never replaced and the person suffering this nervous system insult must continue life with a permanently reduced number of nerve cells. For example, victims of poliomyelitis have usually suffered from the destruction of motor cells, which activate the muscles, and if enough of their motor cells are destroyed a type of muscular paralysis will result. Brain damage, whether inflicted by a penetrating head injury, infection, or concussion, will mean that the person so damaged will have to meet the world with fewer cerebral cells than he or she began life. Because the average human being possesses billions of nerve cells in the central nervous system,[1] we can afford to lose a fairly large number of neurons, provided they are not in narrowly localized cortical areas or are not crucially involved in highly specific kinds of behavior. Touwen has wisely advised us, "a brain lesion should not be considered as a static condition" and "it is well known from various animal species that several morphological compensatory mechanisms can be operative, often with striking differences between the infant and adult animal" (Touwen, 1981). And it is possible that similar mechanisms may be active in man (Prechtl, 1978).

In fact, some people who have suffered rather serious brain injuries have not been noticeably impaired mentally. Hebb and

[1] Estimates of the number of nerve cells in the human brain and central nervous system range from 10 billion (Wooldridge, 1963) to 12 billion (Herrick, 1926) to 50 billion in the neocortex (Rockel, Hiorns, & Powell, 1974), and up to 75 billion in larger brains (Whishaw, 1983 personal communication). Others have estimated 10^{12} neurons in the human brain, and "the number of possible interconnections among these neurons . . . is greater than the total number of atoms making up the entire universe!" (Thompson, Berger, & Berry, 1980, p. 3). These variations in estimates result from different methods of measurement, the complexity of the problem, and whether the investigator is including all or part of the central nervous system.

Penfield (1940) reported an early case in which behavior actually *improved* following the surgical removal of frontal lobe tissue, and a study by Weinstein and Teuber (1957) revealed that a number of brain-injured soldiers who suffered mental impairment at the time of their cerebral gunshot wounds had gained back normal IQs within a few years. Milner (1975) has reported postoperative improvement in full-scale IQ in patients surgically treated because of epileptic seizures. Some of these patients made marked postoperative gains over a long period.

Teachers and parents of children with cerebral deficits should be reminded of the rehabilitative and adaptive tendencies of the remaining healthy tissues of the human brain and nervous system. Although many of these children may have to live with some type of permanent perceptual or learning disability, many of them will profit from enriched educational experience almost as much as the brightest students, and most will gain to some extent.

Having drawn attention to some of the educational implications of the neuron's vulnerability, let us now return to consider its structure and function. The neuron has two basic functions, self-nutrition and transmission of the neural impulse or nerve current. It ingests nutrients from the bloodstream through its delicate cell membrane and gives off waste products, like any other living organism.

The classical view of synaptic conduction of neural impulses implies that they are received by the "branches" of the dendrites and then transmitted down the dendritic trunk, through the cell body, and on down the length of the axon to the end brush. The brushlike endings of the axon make a functional connection (synapse) with the dendritic brush endings of another neuron, or with several others, the conduction of neural energy usually being unidirectional from dendrites to axon within a neuron, and from axon endings to dendrites across the synapse. This transmission across the synapse does not include direct physical contact because while the tiny neural endings may touch or become entwined with one another, in the peripheral nervous system they are covered by an outer membranous layer, called the neurilemma, which keeps the end brushes from actual physical contact. In the central nervous system the synaptic gap is minimal (the space being about $100\,\text{Å}$, or 10^{-10} meter).

Anatomists since the time of Golgi's researches in the 1880s have recognized two main classes of neurons (Hirsch & Jacobson, 1975, p. 110). The first are the large and distinctive neurons in the different functional areas of the brain. These cells with their long axons have been called Class I neurons (Jacobson, 1970); they form the main neural tracts. The Class II type, have short axons, and, though they occur throughout the nervous system, they appear in large numbers in the cerebral cortex and are believed to be involved in modifiable behavior.

As well as being different in structure, they differ in their developmental patterns. The Class I, or large neurons, are usually formed first during the fetal growth of the brain, and the Class II, small neurons with short axons, develop later, some even post-natally. This pattern of neural development has special significance for the educator, the physiotherapist, and the occupational therapist, because it implies the possibility of environmental change in the structural growth and mature functioning of the nervous system.

The Class II neurons, because of their shorter axons, their presence in the human cortex, and their later ontogenetic development, appear to be well suited for processing information in the nervous system, and to be "responsive to environmental influences and thus responsible for the plastic or modifiable aspects of behavior" (Hirsch & Jacobson, 1975). It seems that these structural and developmental properties of the human nervous system may very well be a basic determinant in all learning and behavior change.

The transmission of some neural impulses is primarily chemical and that of others, largely electrical. In chemical transmission, different chemicals may be secreted across the synaptic cleft, some facilitating the passage of the neural impulse and others inhibiting or blocking it. The electrochemical changes at the synapse are highly complex, and the pattern of electrical conduction is more complicated than the classical view proposed. Schmidt (1978b) demonstrated that in the cortex, synaptic transmission sometimes may travel from an axon to another axon, and in some cases from dendrites to dendrites, and from dendrites to axon (Schmitt & Worden, 1979). McGeer, McGeer, and Innanen (1979) provided evidence of dendroaxonic transmission in the rat's brain, but in humans the whole picture is not yet clear. We do know that in the peripheral nervous system and probably in most of the human central nervous system, the conventional serial pattern of axon-to-dendrites transmission occurs, but with some of the axonless or short axon cells in some parts of the human brain there may be reciprocal synaptic arrangements (Dowling, 1979). For the school psychologist and the educator, all this discussion may seem confusing, but the intricate possibilities of the electrical and chemical processes of the human brain are beyond the limits of the present discussion. Regardless of the details of synaptic conduction, we know that neural impulses are conducted systematically from one part of the brain to another, and that these neural activities mediate ideas, memories, and all cognitive functions.

To integrate our broad knowledge of this system into a theory of learning, it is useful to know that (1) different synapses offer different levels of resistance to the passage of neural impulses; (2) chemicals are secreted by the axon, some of which facilitate the conduction of some neural impulses and some inhibit others; and (3) the dendrites may extinguish some weak impulses and conduct those above a certain threshold intensity. The brain and brainstem form a three-dimensional complex of millions of interconnecting nerve cells. These cells are tiny, varying in diameter from 4 to 5 µm (a micron, or µm, is one thousandth of a millimeter) up to 50 or even 100 µm (Gardner, 1975, Chap. 3), and provide an electrochemically active network with large numbers of cells and patterns of cells producing neural impulses (i.e., neural "firing") at different time intervals.

To develop a mental picture of what goes on in the brain, the interested reader would do well to read a book on electroencephalography—that is, the study of the electrical changes that occur in the brain and cerebral cortex. These changes are detected by a sensitive electronic device, the electroencephalogram (EEG), developed in Austria in 1929 by a psychiatrist, Dr. Hans Berger. Some of the cortical cells discharge spontaneously as slowly as 2 or 3 times per second, others at about 10 times per second, and some as fast as 12 to 16 times per second. During sleep the neural cells usually fire at a regular rate, but when the subject is awake and alert and there is a "sensory input" reaching the visual, auditory, or other sensory cortical areas, a speeded up and irregular pattern of neural firing is superimposed on the regular spontaneous pattern. For example, a subject undergoing EEG examination may show an even rise and fall of electrical energy with the eyes closed. With no visual input to the subject in a relaxed state, the brain may produce *alpha* waves, which have a frequency of about 10 times per second. Hebb (1966) has explained, "If he opens his eyes and attends to his surroundings, or if with eyes closed he is given a problem to solve, the *beta rhythm* appears: small, fast waves characteristic of the actively thinking subject."

The EEG has been a useful clinical technique for identifying highly localized brain lesions and for understanding epilepsy. The medically trained electroencephalographer knows the normal frequencies and intensities of electrical changes ("brain waves") in different parts of the cortex, and the presence of cerebral pathology may show as a marked increase in both frequency and amplitude (spike activity). In cases of diffuse brain pathology, or even moderately localized lesions, the EEG pattern may be generalized because it is picking up changes in a broad electrical field.

Some clinicians use a grading system of i, ii, and iii to indicate minimal, moderate, and severe pathology, and most of the cases described in this book are so designated. Also, the presence of abnormally slow waves (delta waves) is common in LD children and in children with attention deficit disorder (ADD). The measurements and their interpretation possess a rather marked subjective component, so that the school psychologist may need to view the EEG findings, when they are inconclusive, with healthy scientific skepticism. In some cases where localized pathology is clearly indicated, however, this information may be particularly useful, along with a large number of findings from a detailed battery of neuropsychological tests. A recent adaptation of the EEG with topographic mapping and a computerized display provides more elaborated and exact knowledge of damaged or dysfunctioning areas of the brain. The new methods of brain scanning are also improving the quality of knowledge about brain structure (e.g., computerized axial tomography or CT or CAT scan, and magnetic resonance imaging or MRI scan), and function (e.g., positron emission tomography or PET scan, and brain electrical activity mapping or BEAM), and how these structures and functions are related to specific cognitive tasks. These scanning techniques are explained later in this chapter.

Synaptic Theory of Learning and the Neural Trace

The presence of the synaptic gap in the nervous system was discovered during the 1890s and since that time imaginative educationists and psychologists have been hypothesizing about the function of the synapse in learning.

As early as 1913, E.L. Thorndike wrote at some length on "the physiology of the capacity to learn and of readiness" (Thorndike, 1913), but because of the limited knowledge of the brain–behavior relationship at that time, what he had to say was almost the pure hypothesizing of a brilliant mind. J.B. Watson also used the idea of varying synaptic resistance (Watson, 1919, 1924) to explain the varying pathways of neural impulses during the learning of habits. Drawing on his own work with monkeys and rats, Lashley (1950) attempted to account for the "engram" or permanent change that evidently must occur in the brain and nervous system when some new idea or skill is acquired. Obviously, there must be a change in the nervous system following learning that enables the subject to retrieve it and express it, and this change must have some degree of permanence.

These early investigators had no success in their search for the engram because they were looking for a neural trace that was both linear and localized. By 1950, Lashley had declared his failure in the search and at about that time theories of multineural systems began to replace the simple rigidity of localized, linear causality. Hebb (1949), with an innovative and useful theory of behavior, proposed the existence of cell assemblies and phase sequences in the brain, and though his theory could account for Lashley's findings of equipotentiality and mass action, it was completely speculative and too nonspecific to be testable (Thompson et al., 1980). Pribram, Lindsley, and others in the 1960s began to propose multiple-systems theories to account for memory and learning. These could include sensory systems, motor systems, the limbic system, and the hippocampus, as well as many smaller systems in both the cortex and brain stem. They also recognized the influence of environmental stimulation on neural growth, the effects of decremental and inhibitory neural processes on attention, and the nature and functions of neural coding (Pribram, 1971). But for the most part, the researches of these investigators, though valuable, are segmental, and many deal only with classical conditioning in animals. They tell us very little about the complexity and fluidity of human thought and learning, and how and where the latter is stored in the human CNS.

While the neurologists, biochemists, and physiologists are attempting to unravel the mystery of the neural trace, the psychologist and the teacher need only know that some change does take place in the brain when learning occurs and that this change may be more or less permanent. The degree of permanence seems to depend on certain chemical changes, on whether the learner *intends* to remember it for a short or a long time, whether the mental image is vivid and accompanied by strong and pleasant affective overtones, and whether the learned skill is reinforced with spaced practices.

Short-term memory, such as remembering a phone number long enough to dial it, may depend on a reverberating cerebral circuit that decays as soon as the need for its use terminates. Some fleeting perceptions, such as reading an exciting story, do stay with us, however, probably reinforced by cognitive associations and positive emotional responses. In old age, the neural and physiological processes (most likely synaptic changes) necessary to maintain the reverberating activity become weakened, and as a result the senile patient has difficulty recalling an experience once attention to it has ceased. Because the neural traces of earlier experiences are still there such a person can remember the events of his youth or successful middle life, but he may already have forgotten that his son visited him a half hour before.

Some children with poor short-term memory no doubt have inherited a predisposition for poor conceptual imagery. These children, like the senile patient, may forget very rapidly material that has been taught to them. To overcome this limitation, the teacher may check with the parents to make sure that the child's diet is rich in all the necessary vitamins, particularly those of the B complex. Studies have shown that temporary conditions of avitaminosis will produce a temporary condition of mental deficiency, but with adequate diet, the normal mental level may be regained within a few days (Gaddes, 1946; Guetzkow & Bowman, 1946). In recent years interest has increased in the relationship among mental development, learning, and nutrition. Social and nutritional factors appear to affect mental development independently and may also show a strong interaction effect (Scrimshaw & Gordon, 1968). For students interested in the importance of nutrition for learning, Hallahan and Cruickshank (1973, Chap. 2) produced an interesting review.

The endocrine glands also are important determiners of motivation and mental level. Although endocrinologists are reluctant to experiment with a child's glandular functions, they can achieve dramatic changes with thyroid and pituitary feeding in some cases. If the parents or teacher of a child with a learning disability suspect a glandular deficiency they should consult a competent endocrinologist who can test the child and administer medication if it is indicated.

Once the primary physical processes have been checked for possible deficit, then the teacher should attempt to teach the child so as to involve him or her positively with the material. There is physiological and psychological evidence to suggest that perceptions operating when the perceiver is happy and interested are more likely to be retained than those experienced during unhappiness and/or boredom. This would seem to be an example of psychosomatic processes in learning, and for this reason the teacher should avoid sarcasm or any disciplinary technique that is likely to condition the child to dislike the material being presented or any event likely to be associated negatively with it. Glasser (1969) wrote persuasively on this point: "If school failure does not exist, other handicaps can be more easily overcome." Although such an approach is purely behavioral, it is also supported by neurological and physiological evidence.[2]

[2] Readers particularly interested in this topic should read at more length books and papers on psychosomatic medicine and related problems.

In teaching a child with identifiable neural pathology, the teacher may learn from the school psychologist who is trained in neuropsychology, something of the intensity, size, and locus of the damage or dysfunction (see Chapter 3) and from this knowledge may better understand the child's strengths and weaknesses. The teacher's knowledge of cortical function and the child's aptitude pattern should provide a theoretical background with which to improvise new and specific remedial teaching techniques. This, in essence, is the model of educational neuropsychology.

Gross Structure and Functions of the Central Nervous System

The brain, brainstem, spinal cord, and peripheral nerves make up the nervous system. The chief integrating functions occur in the central nervous system, that is, the brain, brainstem, and spinal cord.

The cerebral hemispheres (Fig. 2.1) form a cranial shape something like that of a football helmet. The outer covering, or cortex, is gray and is about one-eighth inch thick. The main body of the cerebrum is white and is made up of supporting and interconnecting fibers. These cerebral hemispheres, including the cortex and supporting white layers, are from 1 to 2 inches thick. The surface is wrinkled and convoluted so that about two-thirds of the cortical surface line the fissures and about one-third of the cortical surface is open to view in an exposed human brain. Some biologists hypothesize that this design of the brain is related to human survival; to

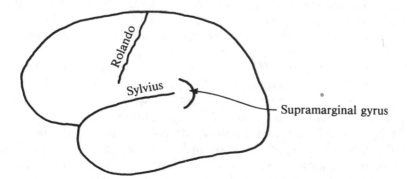

Figure 2.1. Left cerebral hemisphere showing the central sulcus, or fissure of Rolando; the lateral fissure, or fissure of Sylvius; and the supramarginal gyrus.

gain the same cortical surface and the same number of cortical cells, had the cortex been smooth, the human head would have had to be as large as a basketball. But by being accordioned into its present small space, the brain is kept relatively small—an insignificant target and so less liable to external trauma.

The cortex is made up vertically of about six layers of different types of cells, and as the different parts of the cortex are examined horizontally, different cell densities are found. For example, in the motor strip (Fig. 2.3) the fifth cortical layer is much thicker than in either the sensory or associational areas. This layer is richer in *pyramidal cells*, so called because their cell bodies are relatively large and so shaped as to suggest a pyramid. In the parietal areas are differently shaped cells, and in the occipital, temporal, and frontal lobes, different types of cells again. Although cortical cells have been observed to differ structurally both horizontally (across the layers) and vertically (from one layer to another) still very little is known about their various functions. The specific projection areas (vision, audition, somesthesis, and motor control) are well known, but most finer discriminations are still not fully understood. Neurologists tell us that most of the afferent pathways connect into the fourth layer, which is thickest in the sensory cortex and thinnest in the motor strip (see Netter, 1972, p. 73). The nerve fibers connecting the motor cortex with the spinal cord and muscles arise mainly in the fifth layer, and the cortex is composed chiefly of interconnecting neurons, which provide neural stimulation between millions of cerebral centers. Neurologists, conscious of the meager knowledge about the structure and function of the human brain, are hesitant to go beyond the evidence. Psychologists are less cautious. For example, Gardner (1968), an eminent neurologist, has written, "Actually, our knowledge of cortical structure is so fragmentary that any attempts to compare these units to man-made electronic feedback circuits are purely speculative." By contrast, Hebb, who was a psychologist, followed the lead of Lorente de Nó who, in the late 1930s, first proposed the idea of "loop" or "reverberating circuits." Hebb has emphasized this concept and developed it (Hebb, 1949, 1958/1966/1972) in the idea of the "cell assembly," that is, a circuit of cells reflecting a feedback mechanism and maintaining a reverberating energy within the brain, and the "phase sequence," or a sequentially related number of cell assemblies. Hebb supported his hypothesis, pointing out that "much of the CNS, but especially association cortex and certainly closely connected subcortical structures, is filled with paths that lead back into themselves as well as leading on to other paths" (1966). This concept, growing out of histological knowledge and neurophysiological observations, has been a most useful idea in attempts to rationalize brain–behavior relationships. Hebb warned, however, that like any theory it is a tentative answer or possible explanation, and should not be confused with established fact.

As long as the teacher can remember that the "reverberating circuit" is a useful idea to stimulate new ways of teaching a handicapped child and a productive way to stimulate imaginative teaching methods, then it will have served a useful purpose. However, we all must be ready to discard an hypothesis when a better one appears.

The Cerebral Cortex

Although the external appearance of the human cerebrum is convoluted so as to be completely covered with gyri (convex surfaces) and sulci (fissures or deep ridges), only two of the fissures need to be learned by the nonmedical student. These are the central sulcus (also called the fissure of Rolando) and the lateral fissure (also called the fissure of Sylvius). These two fissures divide the cerebral area into the frontal, parietal, occipital, and temporal lobes (see Figs. 2.1 and 2.2), and as we shall see in Chapter 3, each of these seems to be more or less involved in mediating particular behavioral functions.

The motor cortex, a strip about an inch wide immediately anterior to the fissure of Rolando (Fig. 2.3), controls muscular-expressive movements and is usually called the motor strip. The motor strip of the left hemisphere controls activity of the right arm, right leg, and nearly all muscular movements of the right half of the head and body. The right motor strip dominates the left musculature. Because the two motor strips are located in the frontal lobes, motor control is a known function of the posterior parts of the frontal lobes. Damage or dysfunction of either motor strip may result in some degree of paralysis on the contralateral side.

A strip of cells just posterior to the fissure of Rolando (see Figs. 2.2 and 2.3) registers sensations of touch. It is called the somesthetic strip (soma, body; esthesis, sensation). This is the area of the brain where tactile sensations are recorded and, like the motor strips, the somesthetic strips receive information from the opposite sides of the body. Damage or dysfunction in these areas may result in anesthetic areas of the skin, poor finger localization, or disturbed body-part identification while blindfolded, and this may have a deleterious effect on classroom learning, such as arithmetic, spelling, and any hand–eye coordination skill.

The motor and sensory strips, because of their close cortical proximity, function together. Any electrochemical activity in one

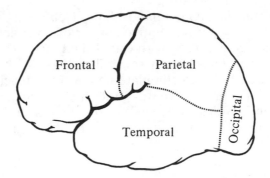

Figure 2.2. The cerebral lobes of the left hemisphere. (© 1984 William D. West)

strip is likely to arouse some reciprocal response in the other, and this integrated function is enhanced by the many sensory fibers that go to the motor strip and the many motor fibers that go from the sensory strip. The two strips are sometimes referred to as the *sensorimotor cortex* (Calanchini & Trout, 1971), and their synthesized functions provide the neural basis for kinesthesis (awareness of the body in space and its movements); temperature awareness; muscular movement and its relation to visual, auditory, and tactile feedback; and the growth of language and mental development. Integrative processes occur in all levels and areas of brain function, but those connected with sensorimotor integration are basic to all learning and mental function (Ayres, 1972a).

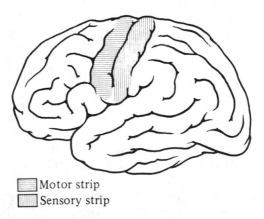

Motor strip
Sensory strip

Figure 2.3. The left hemisphere showing the location of the left motor strip and the left sensory or somesthetic strip. (© 1984 William D. West)

The back part of the brain houses the occipital lobes, which are centers of visual impressions. Because the optic nerves and tracts have to travel from the eyes at the front of the head to the occipital lobes at the back, any head injury has a greater chance of disturbing the visual processes. Visual-perceptual activities are basic to most classroom learning, making it important for the teacher to understand the structure and function of the optic neural mechanisms and to identify the various visual–perceptual abberations that are likely to occur.

The temporal lobes house the acoustic areas, and damage or dysfunction in these lobes may result in auditory imperception or distortion. Because language and speech development depend largely on exact phonetic auditory perception, temporal damage or dysfunction may result in some form of aphasia (disability of understanding or expressing language). The neuropsychological and educational problems of aphasia are discussed in Chapter 8.

The Brainstem and Corpus Callosum

The brain and spinal cord constitute the *central nervous system*, and the nerves outside this network—the cranial nerves connecting the sensory and motor systems of the head, the spinal nerves connecting the neuromuscular–skeletal systems, and the peripheral portions of the autonomic system—constitute the *peripheral nervous system*. Although both the central and peripheral nervous systems are involved in a child's learning, most of our discussion in this book, is concerned with a study of the structure and function of the central nervous system.

The brain includes the cerebrum, with its two hemispheres, and the brainstem joining it to the spinal cord (see Fig. 2.4). Below the cerebrum is the corpus callosum (the broad band of fibers joining the two cerebral hemispheres) and the thalamus (which includes sensory nuclei of both vision and hearing, as well as centers of the autonomic nervous system); the brainstem includes the midbrain, pons, cerebellum, and medulla oblongata (see Figs. 2.4 and 2.5).

The Corpus Callosum

The corpus callosum is a wide band of millions of neural fibers connecting the cortices of the two hemispheres (see Figs. 2.4 and 2.5). Although the Bible has advised, "Let not thy left hand know what thy right hand doeth" (Matthew 6:3), this is neurologically impossible in sensorimotor behavior because of the corpus callosum. The child who is taught to write with the right hand will be able to write with the left hand—rather badly, but without having to

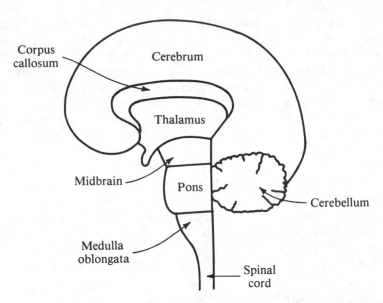

Figure 2.4. Medial view of the brain and brainstem in simplified and stylized form.

practice. The manual or hand area of the left motor strip connects through the corpus callosum to the manual area of the right motor strip, and training in one of these areas is carried automatically from one to the other. Psychologists have recognized this automatic neural transmission for years as "bilateral transfer."

Not only can the right-handed child write with the nondominant hand; he finds that he can also write with the right foot in wet sand at the beach, with the left foot, with a stick in his mouth, and all

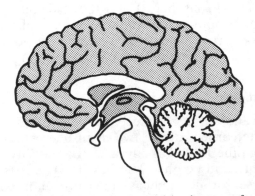

Figure 2.5. Medial view of the brain and brainstem after the brain has been cut through the midline.

with no previous practice. This type of evidence suggests that training that modifies a localized area of one hemisphere is not only carried to various parts of the opposite hemisphere (contralateral) through the corpus callosum, but to other parts of the same hemisphere (ipsilateral) through the subcortical white matter. For these reasons multisensory and multimotor-expressive teaching techniques have had great success because they increase the cerebral internuncial connections, thus promoting the possibility of wider cortical activity and better learning. The physiotherapist speaks of "reeducation" when he or she attempts to train healthy areas of the brain to circumvent a damaged area.

Normally the two hemispheres function together, but if through disease or trauma the corpus callosum is damaged or cut, various mental functions are impaired. Sperry (1964) and others have cut the corpus callosum by surgical section in animals to learn more about the specific functions of each hemisphere. Commissurotomics are carried out with human subjects to reduce the frequency of or to eliminate epileptic seizures; and following such surgical procedures these "split-brain" patients are often studied to provide information about brain–behavior relationships of each separated hemisphere (Zaidel, 1979). If all the direct interhemispheric connections are cut the subject behaves as if he possesses two independent brains (Sperry, 1974). If the subject is taught something through the right halves of each eye (by displaying the stimulus in the left visual field) to the right hemisphere, no bilateral transfer can take place and there is no memory of the learned material in the left hemisphere. The evidence from split-brain experiments and cases of disease or agenesis of the corpus callosum are discussed in greater detail in Chapter 6. Here, these few remarks will remind the reader of the important function of the corpus callosum in interhemispheric integration, in establishing cerebral dominance, and in normal competence in reading, writing, and arithmetic.

The Thalamus

The thalamus is a particularly complex area of the midpart of the brain located beneath the corpus callosum and immediately above the brainstem (see Fig. 2.4). Medical students may spend several months studying the structures and various functions of the thalamus, subthalamus, hypothalamus, and their related parts. The teacher and school psychologist may find it useful to know that it is an important *relay station* carrying impulses from the cerebellum (see Figs. 2.4 and 2.5), the reticular system, and certain neural ganglia to the cerebral cortex, chiefly the association areas. In fact, all the senses but smell are processed through the thalamus before they reach their respective specialized areas in the cortex. Lower on the phylogenetic scale, the thalamus appears to be the highest organ of perception, but in humans it acts as an organ of crude consciousness between the sensory tracts and the cortex. Because most of the sensory tracts pass through the lower level of the thalamus, a thalamic lesion may result in disturbances of visual, auditory, and tactile perception.

The hypothalamus is a complex area anterior to and slightly below the thalamus. Its exact role is not completely understood yet, but we do know that as "the physiological seat of emotion" it monitors many autonomic functions. It triggers "thermostat-like" mechanisms to control such functions as blood pressure, body heat, hunger, thirst, and sex, but its determination of such emotional states as anger and fear interests the student of human behavior. Some years ago, Masserman (1941) demonstrated immediate "sham rage" in the cat by controlled electrostimulation of the hypothalamus. Because hypothalamic lesions may cause abnormal anger or fear reactions, the hyperactive and/or emotionally explosive child may in some rare cases be suffering from a brainstem lesion affecting the normal functioning of the hypothalamus. Behavior, at least in part, seems to result from the reflexive and spontaneous stimulation of the hypothalamus and related structures and the inhibitory learned processes emanating from the cerebral cortex.

Not all antisocial behavior stems from organic pressures, of course. Many such cases are psychogenic, frequently resulting from a severe parental rejection pattern at home, but when a brain dysfunction accompanies explosive, disruptive behavior, as thorough a knowledge as possible of the brain lesion may help the therapist, care worker, or teacher to decide on a treatment method. It may include individual or group therapy, psychodrama, environmental control, social activities, counseling, drug therapy, or a combination of some or all these.

The Midbrain

Immediately below the thalamus is the midbrain, a stout column of the brainstem between the thalamus and the pons (see Fig. 2.4). Its chief behavioral function is the control of cranial reflexes, such as blinking, ducking the head to visual stimulation of quick movement in the peripheral visual fields, and the pupillary reflex. Auditory reflexes, such as the startle reflex or turning the head and eyes following a loud noise, also find their stimulation here. The corpora quadrigemina, a body of four protuberances situated on the posterior surface of the midbrain, mediates these reflexes. The two upper ones, the superior colliculi, are the vestigial remains of the optic lobes and, although occipital cortices register vision in humans, the superior colliculi act to integrate incoming impulses from the visual retinae; kinesthetic input from the muscles of the eyeballs and from muscles, tendons, and joints throughout the body; and the output of impulses along the efferent motor tracts that produce the visual reflexes necessary for visuomotor coordination. As can be seen, this is a complex and delicate energy system, and a lesion or locus of dysfunction anywhere in the system may produce variations and impairments of visual perception. The two lower protuberances of the corpora quadrigemina, the inferior colliculi, provide an integration of incoming auditory and kinesthetic impulses in basically the same way as the superior colliculi serve vision. Gellner (1959) suggested that a child who can copy words but cannot use them meaningfully may be suffering from a lesion between the inferior colliculi and the acoustic areas of the temporal lobes (the gyri of Heschl). Although purely speculative, this appears to be a more logical rationale than a "general lack of mental ability" or "mental retardation" and finds its diagnostic understanding in trying to pinpoint spatially specific neural dysfunctions in the "auditory circuits." Some children labeled mentally retarded, autistic, or dyslexic may be suffering from some disruption in visual or auditory perception because of a midbrain lesion. More exact knowledge about the locus of the lesion should lead to a better theory of the dysfunction, and this, in turn, should provide a more effective remedial educational treatment.

The Pons

Students of Latin will recognize pons as the word for "bridge," and in fact this enlarged section of the brainstem is a bridge for afferent fibers connecting the spinal cord with the cortex, for motor pathways from the motor cortex to the cerebellum, and for connections from the cerebellum to the spinal motor pathways. A tumor in the pontine area may develop in childhood and may result in visual–perceptual and visual–motor disturbances. Physical damage to the pons may result in disturbance of somesthesia if the sensory fibers are cut, and in paralysis if the motor tracts are damaged or severed.

The Cerebellum

As can be seen in Figs. 2.4 and 2.5, the cerebellum is a sort of simplified cerebrum attached to the brainstem at the level of the pons. In structure it has two hemispheres, a cortex of gray matter and a middle area (medulla) of nerve tissue that is both white and gray. Unlike the cerebrum, which has irregular convolutions and different types of cells in different cortical areas, the cerebellum is lined with more regular convolutions and the cortical cells are similar throughout the surface area. They include granule cells and Purkinje cells in large numbers, and both of these possess unusually thick and complex dendritic development. These cells are inter-related synaptically, permitting a "widespread discharge following relatively limited afferent input" (Gardner, 1968).

The cerebellum acts as a filter to smooth and coordinate mus-cular activity. Sensory neural stimulation reaches the cerebellum from the skin, the muscles, the tendons, the joints, the labyrinth in the nonauditory part of the ear (static and position sense), the eyes, the ears, and the cerebral cortex, and from the feedback of its own discharges to the cerebral cortex. Superior cerebellar func-tion permits the graceful movements of the ballet dancer or the smooth, quick, and coordinated responses of the swimmer, sprinter, basketball player, and other athletes.

Damage to the cerebellum may cause paralysis of the arm or leg on the same side (ipsilateral) as the lesion, unlike a lesion in the cerebral motor strip, which always results in paralysis or motor disturbance maximally on the opposite (contralateral) side. Cerebellar dysfunction in milder form may result in general motor clumsiness, which in its own way may impede classroom or intel-lectual learning. Where the clumsiness includes a visuomotor dis-ability even in a child of bright verbal intelligence, it frequently interferes with manual dexterity (apraxia), the perception of im-bedded figures, writing, and other fine-muscle performances. Brenner, Gillman, Zangwill, and Farrell (1967) matched 14 of these children in age, sex, handedness, verbal IQ, and home and school background with 14 children free of agnosic–apraxic dif-ficulties. The impaired group were significantly inferior on tests of spatial judgment, manual skill, spelling, arithmetic, and social adjustment. Such motor clumsiness may find its origin in dys-functions of the cerebellum, of one of the two cerebral motor strips, or of the efferent motor pathways, or in some imbalance in one or more of the sensory neural mechanisms. Little hard evidence relates cerebellar dysfunction directly to learning disabilities, but Dr. J. Valk, of the Netherlands, has reported interesting findings from his neuroradiological studies of children. He found ten boys with evidence of abnormal development of the cerebellum and accompanying disturbances of fine-motor control, which interfered with normal school progress (Valk, 1974).

Until recently the human cerebellum was recognized only for its importance as part of the motor system, although neuroanatomic evidence had been showing that neural tracts connected it to both the motor cortex and the association cortex. Impressed by the latter knowledge, Henrietta C. Leiner and her colleagues proposed the hypothesis that the human cerebellum can contribute to mental skills in much the same way as it contributes to motor skills. In 1986, she and her colleagues published the first of a series of papers (Leiner et al., 1986, 1989, 1991) in which they presented evidence obtained in various laboratories, showing that lateral cerebellar lesions can produce some cognitive deficits such as impaired anticipatory planning (Dow, 1988), mental imagery (Decety et al., 1990), and word processing (Petersen et al., 1988). They found evidence that the cerebellum may be involved in a wide range of cognitive functions, and structurally defective cerebella have been found in some autistic subjects (Courchesne et al., 1988). Leiner concludes in part (1991) ". . . the contributions of the cerebellum to human behavior are underestimated at present. Evidence is available that the human cerebellum is involved not only in autonomic and somatic motor function, and not only in sensory and emotional control, but also in mentation and in language." Similar reports from other researchers, recognizing the possible contributions of the cerebellum to higher cognitive functions, are beginning to appear (Ingvar, 1992; Schmahmann, 1991).

The cerebellum, as a primary structure in the brainstem, is necessary to all forms of normal behavior and possibly to creative artistic expression. Some pianists who compose or improvise report that the muscular feel of their hands and fingers on the keyboard is a part of their emotional response to the music, and that it helps in the creative process. And dancing and acting are examples of the merging of neuromuscular movement and artistic expression.

The Medulla Oblongata

The medulla oblongata, the lowest section of the brainstem, is in a sense in the middle of the central nervous system. The brain is above it and the spinal cord and most of the rest of the nervous system are below it. It has more interest for the neurologist than for the educator; consequently, little is said here, other than that it is the level at which many of the sensory and motor nerves cross over to the opposite side (neural decussation) and that, in collaboration with the pons, it is the neural center for the various vital organs (heart, lungs, and digestive system).

The Peripheral Nervous System

As already explained, the central nervous system includes the brain and spinal cord. The peripheral nervous system is made up of all nerves outside the central nervous system, both afferent

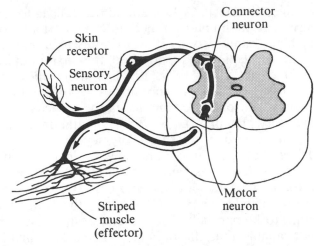

Figure 2.6. Cross-section of the spinal cord showing one sensory (afferent) neuron, to represent a spinal nerve; one connecting neuron within the spinal cord; and one motor (efferent) neuron. In reality, a sensory nerve is made up of a bundle of many neurons, all conducting impulses toward the brain. Similarly, a motor nerve includes a bundle of nerve fibers that all carry impulses away from the brain. (© 1980 William D. West)

(sensory) and efferent (motor). These are: (1) the cranial nerves; (2) the spinal nerves, with their sensory and motor connections; and (3) the autonomic nervous system, the neural subsystem that is intimately involved in motivation and emotion (see discussions of hypothalamic [later in this chapter] and frontal lobe function [Chapter 3]).

Twelve pairs of cranial nerves, attached to the brain and brainstem, have connections with cranial, spinal, and abdominal structures. The teacher is likely to be most interested in those mediating vision (cranial nerves II, III, IV, VI) and audition (VIII) and, if he or she suspects that a potentially bright child is impeded by visual or auditory maladjusted behavior, should refer the child for ophthalmological and/or audiological examination.

From the neck level (cervical level) to the lower extremity (sacral level) of the spinal cord there are 31 pairs of spinal nerves. Each nerve trunk includes sensory and motor nerves (Fig. 2.6); the sensory root joins the spinal cord on the posterior (dorsal) surface and the motor root joins it on the anterior (ventral) surface. The two roots then join inside the spinal foramen (hollow space inside the backbone designed to house and protect the delicate spinal cord) and pass out through an intervertebral cavity on the lateral surface of the backbone. These nerves are particularly interesting because they connect to all parts of the body, carrying sensory impulses of tactile and kinesthetic impressions to the brain and distributing motor impulses to the various body muscles. Possibly the sensory and motor nerves to the hands and arms are most important in classroom learning because writing, handedness, and cerebral dominance may be better understood with an awareness of peripheral sensory and motor nerve function.

In trying to understand a child with a learning disability, the teacher should attempt to discover, with the diagnostic help of the neurologist and the consulting help of the school psychologist, whether the child's neurological damage or dysfunction is *central* or *peripheral* or both. For example, a child may be mildly apraxic and have difficulty in writing and carrying out manual tasks. If the trouble is central it may be caused by a lesion in one or both cerebral sensory or motor strips, in the motor pathways connecting the motor strip with the cerebellum, in the cerebellum itself, or in the anterior (ventral) horns of the spinal cord. The neurologist may be able to supply the diagnostic knowledge of the locus and intensity of the lesion and the psychologist, supplied with this knowledge, should be able to help the teacher develop a remedial teaching program for the child. If the trouble is *peripheral*, then it may be located somewhere in the neural pathways of the arm and hand. Again, the neurologist and psychologist should supply this information to the teacher before the latter plans a specific remedial program. If the dysfunction is central, it is likely to distort perception or cognition or sensorimotor integration. If the dysfunction is peripheral, the impairment is more likely to affect sensory acuity or motor function, but not perceptual organization or mental imagery.

It seems highly likely that the problems of mixed laterality in some children who reverse numbers and letters occur because such children are *peripherally* left-handed and *cortically* or *centrally* right-handed. This concept is developed and examined in the discussion on handedness in Chapter 6.

Sensory Pathways

As already stated, neurologically all behavior includes sensory, cerebrally integrative, and motor processes. All perception and cognition depend on sensations of experience reaching the brain by the afferent or sensory nerves. If input is blocked then mental development may languish. If Annie Sullivan had failed to reach

Helen Keller's mind through touch, by circumventing her blindness and deafness, then Helen would almost certainly have remained intellectually starved and mediocre, instead of developing in the superior way that she did.

In the past, many teachers have labeled some children "mentally retarded" because they could not learn as rapidly or by the same teaching techniques as most other children. Some of these children have had superior minds but the sensory pathways have impaired perception in such a way as to disturb their learning. In such cases it is necessary to understand the nature of the disturbances and to develop a remedial teaching program to compensate for them.

Because visual, auditory, tactile, and kinesthetic imagery are essential to most learning, the sensory paths of these sense modes are examined briefly here. The discussion is simplified and abbreviated because the teacher needs only enough knowledge of neurological structure and function for meaningful communication with the school psychologist and the neurologist. The teacher will depend on them for exact and detailed clinical knowledge; it will be his or her responsibility to take the knowledge they supply and develop a specific learning program for the child. For problems so complex, a professional team approach should provide the best results. How this team may deal with these problems is proposed in the clinical addenda following most of the chapters.

Visual Pathways

The visual pathways extend from the retinae, along the optic nerves to the optic chiasma, through the superior colliculi, along the optic tracts to the lateral geniculate bodies, and finally along the optic radiation to the occipital cortices (see Fig. 2.7; also Netter, 1972, p. 63). Damage or dysfunction in parts of these pathways may produce particular types of visual field defects (see Kolb & Whishaw, 1990, p. 229), and brainstem, temporal, parietal, or occipital lobe dysfunction may result in visual–perceptual omissions, distortions, perseverations, rotations, misplacements, right–left reversals, and errors in judgment of size. Benton (1963b) has investigated these various types of impairments, and they are discussed in greater detail in Chapter 3.

Much research evidence supports "the doctrine that there are two visual pathways, the midbrain system (including the superior colliculi) answering the question 'where,' and the geniculocortical system (including the lateral geniculate bodies and the visual cortices) the question 'what'" (Barlow, 1980). With their midbrain structures animals can locate their prey rapidly; with their visual cortices they can recognize them. When the latter are ablated in

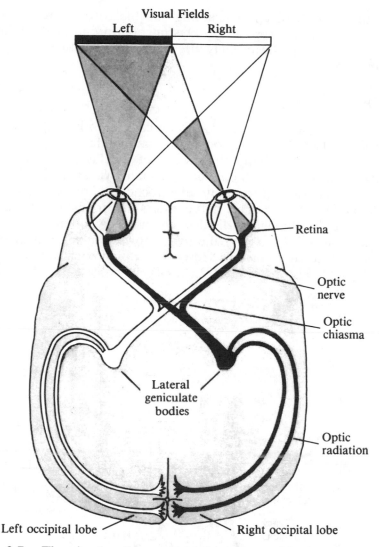

Figure 2.7. The visual pathways from the retinae of both eyes to both occipital lobes. Notice that stimuli in the left visual field are registered in the right occipital lobe. Similarly, stimulation in the right visual field feeds into the left occipital lobe. (© 1980 William D. West)

experimental animals, they cannot distinguish a carrot from a snake (Barlow, 1980) although they can focus on and locate the object. This two-process system also exists in humans. Barlow has called these two functions "the instrumental capacities of the visual system" and "the interpretive functions." If we extend these observations to the task of reading we can hypothesize that the midbrain structures are involved in scanning and the cortical areas in comprehension and interpretation. Dysfunction in one or the other of these two visual pathways may affect reading and other visual skills differentially.

Auditory Pathways

The auditory pathways run from both ears to both temporal lobes, specifically Heschl's gyrus, located in the middle and upper part of the temporal lobe lining the fissure of Sylvius (i.e., the supratemporal plane). From the inner ear, sound waves set up vibratory patterns that are converted into electrochemical or neural impulses in the auditory nerve. This nerve enters the brainstem at the level of the medulla oblongata, divides, and ascends on both sides to the inferior colliculi; from here the two pathways travel by way of the medial geniculate bodies to Heschl's gyrus in each temporal lobe (see Fig. 2.8; also Netter, 1972, p. 64).

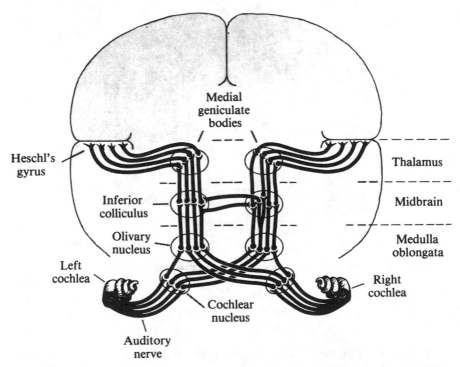

Figure 2.8. The auditory pathways from the inner ear to the cortical acoustic analyzers (Heschl's gyri). Notice that the cochlea of each ear connects more strongly to the opposite side of the brain. The reduced number of neurons indicates the pathways but not the number of nerve fibers to each side. (© 1980 William D. West)

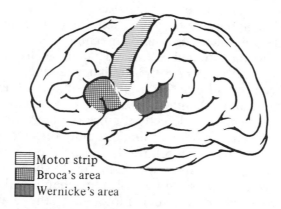

Figure 2.9. The language expressive and language receptive cortical areas of the left hemisphere. (© 1984 William D. West)

Although each ear is connected to both temporal lobes, the fibers are more strongly represented between each ear and the contralateral temporal lobe. Because the left hemisphere is nearly always dominant for language, it has been found that in most people the right ear is slightly more sensitive to verbal input, and the left ear is more sensitive to nonlinguistic material, such as melodies (Kimura, 1964) and social sounds (Spellacy, 1969).

Unilateral temporal lobe lesions, if severe, do not necessarily produce deafness in one ear because of the bilateral connections of the auditory nerves, but they may produce a level of auditory imperception for certain phonetic or nonlinguistic sounds. A child with this lesion sometimes measures within the normal range on an audiometer test because he can sense individual tones across the scale at normal intensities; but because of a lack of integrated function of the two temporal lobes he may be unable to attach meaning to what is heard. This is the basic pattern in Wernicke's aphasia (receptive aphasia) that usually results from a lesion in the left temporal lobe (Fig. 2.9), and it can be devastating when the teacher confuses it with mental impairment. Even worse is a diagnosis by the teacher of "failure to attend" or "unwilling to cooperate."

An example may make this clear. Some years ago a girl aged 9 was referred for neuropsychological evaluation because, the teacher's report stated, "she cannot spell at all and we cannot teach her to read." Such severe retardation suggested the possibility that the child was mentally defective. On arrival, however, she was well spoken and charming in manner. On the visual and tactile tests she measured "bright to superior." In fact, all her aptitudes were well above average except one, her auditory perception. Although her audiogram was in the normal range, she was unable to integrate phonetic sounds meaningfully.

Anyone who has studied a foreign language has had this experience. It is possible to *hear* the foreigner talking, but because of lack of experience and practice it is impossible to attach meanings to most of the sounds. Auditory *sensation* is normal in this example but auditory *perception* is defective. Once the teachers of this child understood the cause of her learning disability they stopped treating her as if she were mentally retarded, and on the recommendation of the psychologist (1) they spoke more slowly and enunciated more clearly when addressing her, (2) they abandoned phonics and taught her to spell by a visual–motor–kinesthetic method that showed some success immediately, and (3) they began teaching her to read by the same method.

Auditory imperception is almost impossible for the classroom teacher to detect, but when it occurs it can be ruinous. A suggested test battery in the Appendix may help the clinical psychologist to detect danger signs. The child suspected of such perceptual impairment should be sent first for audiological assessment to check the possibility of a peripheral hearing loss; once normal hearing is indicated, then psychological testing on a battery of tests of auditory perception may be carried out. Such a battery might measure recognition of nonverbal "social" sounds, tonal memory, nonsense phonetic sound discrimination, and sentence repetition.

Somesthetic and Tactile Pathways

The third sensory pathway relates to the somesthetic system and the sense of touch. Physical contact with the skin or hairs triggers nerve impulses in specialized neurons near the skin surface. These impulses travel along sensory nerves, enter the spinal cord through a posterior (dorsal) root, and ascend the cord and brainstem to the thalamus and somesthetic cortical strip just posterior to the fissure of Rolando in the contralateral hemisphere (see Figs. 2.3 and 2.6). Any lesion in any part of this pathway or in the somesthetic cortex itself may result in inability to recognize two-dimensional surface-texture patterns, such as Braille, or in misperception of one's own fingers. The practicing clinical neurologist may look for dysfunctions in (1) light touch, (2) pressure touch, (3) localization of touch (naming the place touched), (4) superficial pain (from a pin or needle), (5) pressure pain (deep pressure or squeezing), (6) skin temperature, (7) postural sensibility (awareness of bodily position in space), (8) passive movement (knowledge of the passive movement of a limb), (9) vibration, and (10) appreciation of form by touch alone (Brain, 1960). All these somesthetic functions are intimately involved with all learning that requires tactile sensitivity or kinesthetic awareness of body image, body movement, or manual recognition of three-dimensional forms. This last-named type of perception is of particular interest to the neurologist, the clinical neuropsychologist, and the special educator. Clinical tests require the blindfolded subject to palpate a three-dimensional object and match it with another one, also manually explored. Sometimes the subject may be asked to draw what he or she thinks the explored form looked like, once the blocks or objects are hidden and the blindfold is removed. This type of imagery and recognition depends on touch and kinesthesis and their cross-modal effectiveness with vision. This ability to recognize an object by touch alone (stereognosis) is believed to depend, at least in part, on the sensory strip as well as on greater areas of the parietal cortex and brainstem structures. Lesions in this area may result in defective finger localization, inferior directional sense, poor body image, and impaired academic work. In the classroom these skills include arithmetic, writing, spelling, and reading—in fact, all the "core" academic subjects. For this reason, calisthenics, the trampoline, and other techniques to exercise large body movements have been said to be related to improvement in reading and other academic subjects (Cratty, 1968; Kephart, 1971; Montessori, 1912, 1964).

Diagnosing the locus or extent of a lesion in the sensory pathways or cortices is, of course, the responsibility of the clinical neurologist, but with this knowledge, interpreted by the school psychologist, the teacher is much better equipped to plan an effective remedial program for the afflicted child.

Motor Pathways

Structurally the sensory and motor pathways are somewhat similar, but nerve impulses in them, of course, travel in opposite directions. As sensations travel to the somesthetic strip just posterior to the fissure of Rolando, motor impulses are initiated in the cortical motor strip just anterior to this fissure (see Fig. 2.3). Fibers from this area connect down through the brainstem to the pons, into and out of the cerebellum, and on down the anterior horns of the spinal cord to the various exits from the cord by way of the spinal nerves. In classroom learning the motor functions most essential to success are muscular control of the head and neck, including the eyes and speech muscles, and the hands in all types of fine-muscle manipulations. Abnormal eye movements may interfere with reading, and then the causes may be peripheral or central. If the lesion or dysfunction is central, possibly in the occipital lobes, the posterior part of the corpus callosum, in or near the superior colliculi, or the left angular gyrus, then the resulting dyslexia may be more resistant to remedial techniques and in any case will indicate different remedial measures. If the motor pathways are so affected as to cause manual clumsiness, the child may find academic learning, especially writing, spelling, drawing, and possibly reading and arithmetic, more difficult in spite of superior or above-average mental capacity.

Cerebral Blood Supply

The arteriovenous structure and the metabolic functions of the blood system of the nervous system are more the purview of the medical student than of the teacher or the psychologist. However, there are a few points relating to them that may help the teacher to understand a child's behavior. Those who wish a more detailed explanation are referred to Netter (1972, pp. 36–38), or to any good textbook on neurology. For those who wish brief but related knowledge of the topic, however, the following explanation may suffice.

The several million nerve cells in the brain and nervous system are interlaced with an extensive network of capillaries, the tiniest blood vessels. They carry blood and oxygen to the brain; in fact, "a significant part of the oxygen used by the body is for the metabolism of the brain" (Gardner, 1975). The brain cells use oxygen at a fast rate, and if, for any reason, this oxygen supply is cut off even for a few minutes, brain cells will die. Harvey (1950) found that abnormal electrical changes occurred in the brain of rhesus monkeys within 1 minute of closing off (occluding) the flow of blood in the middle cerebral artery. Almost as soon as the oxygen supply to the brain is reduced or cut off, deleterious mental changes may begin. If the blood supply is completely restored, normal physical and mental function will return, as long as complete lack of blood to the brain is not allowed to continue more than about 6 to 8 minutes (Kabat & Dennis, 1938; Kabat, Dennis, & Baker, 1941; Weinberger, Gibbon, & Gibbon, 1940).

Military personnel who have been placed in a decompression chamber and asked to carry out simple arithmetical calculations after the oxygen content has been significantly reduced have had first-hand experience of temporarily impaired mental functions accompanying reduced blood oxygen level. Harvey and Rasmussen

(1951) also found that occluding the middle cerebral artery of rhesus monkeys for up to 50 minutes could result in permanent neural damage, by showing paralysis in the arm and leg on the side opposite the occlusion (hemiparesis). This added time over that found by Kabat's and Weinberger's research occurred because their studies cut off the blood supply completely. Harvey's studies occluded only the middle cerebral artery so that some blood, but not enough, was permitted to flow into the central areas of the cortex through collateral blood vessels. The studies by Kabat, Weinberger, and Harvey provide an interesting conclusion for the clinical psychologist and the teacher. A child's brain needs adequate oxygen, and a partial supply can result in inferior mental functioning.

Ingvar and his colleagues in Sweden have been measuring cerebral blood flow in human subjects and studying its behavioral effects for more than 30 years (Lassen & Ingvar, 1961; Ingvar & Risberg, 1967). In their earlier studies they injected a mixture of an inert gamma-emitting radioactive gas and a saline solution into a carotid artery (the large artery on each side of the neck that supplies blood to the brain) and observed the movement of the radioactive solution through the brain on a detector sensitive to gamma rays. Such measures of regional cerebral blood flow give an *indirect* measure of neural activity in the regions of the brain in which the blood flow is measured (Ingvar, 1983). When the PET scan was introduced in the early 1980s, it became possible to make a *direct* estimate of the metabolic rate of glucose or oxygen in the tissues studied. More will be said in later chapters about neuropsychological studies of cerebral blood flow.

Normally the cerebral cortex is equipped with a fine net of interconnecting blood vessels that supply nourishment to all the cerebral cells. However, if a child is born with a brain in which an inadequate number of capillaries develops in one area of the cortex, then that area may suffer from an avascular growth anomaly, and mental or behavioral activities may be disturbed or impaired. For example, it is generally believed that damage to the left angular gyrus, a cortical convolution in the middle of the left parietal lobe, is intimately involved in determining normal function in reading and writing. This is known from studies on war victims with gunshot wounds localized in this area (Russell and Espir, 1961). We may hypothesize from this knowledge that children born with an avascular left parietal cortical area may suffer from developmental dyslexia unless other cortical areas can take over its normal integrating function. Frequently, these children show an abnormal EEG in this area, and in the posterior lobes, although the disturbance is usually minimal.

Although cerebral hemorrhages (strokes) usually occur in patients past middle age, children unfortunately are not free of them. A 6-year-old child, just prior to entering first grade, suddenly complained of a severe headache and became nauseated. She soon became unconscious and as a result was rushed to the hospital, where a neurosurgeon carried out brain surgery (craniotomy). He had preoperative knowledge of a sudden cerebral hemorrhage in the left hemisphere, and during the surgery he removed the large blood clot (hematoma) and stopped the bleeding. Had this mass of waste material been allowed to remain, its pressure probably would have cut off the oxygen supply to a large number of cortical cells and the anoxia would have resulted in permanent destruction of healthy neural tissue.

Immediately following the surgery this little girl's speech was seriously impaired, but she regained it well enough to enter grade 1 in November of the same year. She completed first grade by the following June, but she did experience considerable difficulty with reading because her left parietal lobe had been mildly and permanently affected by the hematoma.

Ten months after the "stroke" she measured a verbal IQ of 105 and a performance IQ of 101 on the Wechsler Intelligence Scale for Children. Her vocabulary was below average, but then for the first 2 or 3 months following the cerebrovascular accident (CVA) she had some difficulty understanding much of what was said to her (receptive aphasia) and this would be certain to retard her learning of new words. A year later, 23 months after the trauma, her IQ measures were about the same, but her vocabulary had improved markedly to a level average for a child of her age (8 years).

The left hemisphere damage resulted in a right visual field reduction, which complicated her reading and visual scanning in the classroom. In addition, the left temporal lobe had been affected, resulting in some mild auditory imperception by producing some loss in the right ear in the higher frequencies. By the time this girl reached grade 5, functional recovery of her brain was such that she could now read for pleasure and was particularly competent in arithmetic and art.

Damage to a young brain is more likely to be overcome in some cases because of the growth and relative plasticity of new tissue. Other cases of cerebral hemorrhage and arteriovenous malformations are described in later chapters. We remind the teacher that vascular accidents and anomalies do occur in children and some understanding of their perceptual and intellectual sequelae is neccessary before the teacher can plan an adequate remedial program for a child so afflicted.

The Autonomic Nervous System

In the discussions so far we have emphasized mostly the brain, thalamus, brainstem, and peripheral nerves and their relation to consciousness, cognition, perception, and learning. Most of the learning that takes place in the classroom demands attention and cognitive perception, hence it involves the cerebral cortex. Reflexive behavior may involve the cortex *after* the motor response has occurred, and in this sense it is involuntary and semiconscious.

Another segment of behavior that the teacher should understand is also purely automatic and occurs with no conscious intent on the part of the behaving person. For example, one's breathing, heartbeat, digestive functions, and other vegetative activities usually occur without voluntary control. They operate separately and autonomously because they are controlled by a subdivision of the central nervous system called the *autonomic nervous system*.

Neurological knowledge recognizes two subsystems of the autonomic nervous system, the *sympathetic nervous system*, which is usually activated when energy is expended at a level above normal, and the *parasympathetic nervous system*, which is usually activated when behavior is at a normal level and energy is being conserved. Students who wish to know more about the structure and functions of the various parts of the central nervous system may consult a good introductory text in neurology (e.g., Gardner, 1975).

By contrast with the neurologist, the psychologist is interested in the role of the autonomic nervous system in human motivation and emotion. It is this function that the teacher should study to better understand a child's behavior.

The conditions that throw the sympathetic nervous system into gear include fright, anger, exercise, pain, cold, infections, certain drugs, and lack of oxygen. The two causes most interesting to the psychologist are fear and anger. In psychosomatic medicine any physiological symptoms, such as dermatitis (skin eruption), asthma, such gastrointestinal disorders as ulcers and colitis, and many others, resulting from prolonged anxiety or resentment, are frequently referred to as "stress disorders." Because unhappy personal relationships with those close to us are a frequent type of stress stimulus, and because stress may be relieved by successfully manipulating the environment, it is important for the teacher to understand this neurochemical process, at least in basic function.

Many years ago, two medical researchers at the Mayo Clinic (Wolf & Wolff, 1942) reported an interesting and unusual case of peptic ulcer in which a patient's stomach lining could easily be observed. The patient, a man of 56, had swallowed scalding hot clam chowder as a child. Because scar tissue resulting from the burn blocked the esophagus, the tube leading from the throat to the stomach, it was impossible for the boy to eat in the normal way. From then on, he chewed his food, expectorated it into his hand, then inserted the chewed food directly into his stomach through a fistula or opening made surgically through the abdominal wall. This physical arrangement enabled medical scientists to observe the stomach walls through the fistula when the patient was relaxed and happy and when he was emotionally upset. They found that normally, when the man was secure and eating, the stomach lining became engorged with blood and strong digestive acids were secreted to break down the mass of food. The reader will recognize this as a physical state dominated by the parasympathetic nervous system. When he was angry or resentful, however, the same physical pattern occurred as the result of vagus nerve stimulation. This nerve connects from the medulla oblongata to the stomach and its stimulation results in the secretion of gastric juices. Because this secretion may occur when the stomach is empty, the harsh chemicals that nature intended should mix with food now irritate the delicate mucous linings of the empty stomach. This may result in perforation and hemorrhage, and the gastric acids may cause a peptic ulcer. If relieved of the anger and given milk or an alkaline diet, the patient's perforation may disappear.

When the man in Wolf's study suffered fear and anxiety the gastric secretion was inhibited and the rhythmic stomach contractions, normal during digestion of food, stopped. The stomach walls paled because the blood volume had moved to the extremities during sympathetic nervous system domination, and he now suffered from "nervous indigestion" with a mass of undigested food in his stomach.

A great deal of research has been done with animals to study experimental neurosis and the psychogenic production of gastric ulcers. Ulcers have been produced in rats (Sawrey & Sawrey, 1964, 1968; Sawrey & Weisz, 1956), dogs (Dykman and Gantt, 1960), cats (Masserman, 1950; Smart, 1965), and monkeys (Brady, 1958) by subjecting the animals to prolonged anxiety, frustration, and indecision. Because a teacher who is oblivious or indifferent to the feelings of pupils may create a classroom atmosphere conducive to sustained anger or fear, it is important that this whole physical and psychological mechanism be understood.

Sarcasm, intimidation, and overbearing behavior by the teacher may provide enough of a threat or irritant to the child to keep him in a mild "sympathetic" condition. This state will interfere with learning if it is so acute as to be disruptive to perception and reasoning. Parasympathetic behavior is pleasanter for the child and the teacher and is more conducive to the learning process.

How Brain Functions Are Observed

The detailed knowledge of brain functions still has so many gaps that it is premature to build a complete neurophysiological or neuropsychological theory of learning. That is our eventual goal, however, and as more sensitive and exact methods appear for observing gross and subtle brain functions, we will be better equipped to produce such a theory. Already, there is a useful body of neuropsychological knowledge, and every year new truths are coming to light. Although most of the research methods are in the area of expertise of the neurological researcher, the clinical psychologist and the special teacher should have some knowledge of how neuropsychological knowledge is amassed. Following are brief descriptions of some neurological or physiological methods and techniques for observing the brain–behavior relationship.

Cerebral Ablations. Many years ago, Lashley (1929) demonstrated the reliable relationship between brain damage in rats and resulting mental deficit. Halstead (1947) and Hebb (1939) were among the first to attempt the same type of study with human subjects. Cases of required brain surgery provide the neuropsychologist with one of the best sources of knowledge by supplying two independent bodies of data—the extent of tissue damage reported by the neurosurgeon and the extent of mental deficit measured by a comprehensive battery of neuropsychological tests.

Preoperative tests are carried out and compared with the test results of postoperative procedures. The neurosurgeon reports the locus, extent, and nature of the damage and these data are examined in a correlation study to discover relationships that provide a reasonable level of reliability. When healthy brain tissue is damaged or removed there is usually a decline in certain mental functions. However, when a benign tumor or encapsulated abscess is removed with little or no cortical damage, there may be a marked improvement in some or all mental functions.

Electroencephalogram (EEG). Electroencephalography, a method for recording the spontaneous electrical activity of the brain, is useful in locating a brain lesion (whether it is a neoplasm, traumatically injured tissue, or an epileptogenic focus), and it may provide information about the development of cerebral dominance for language and the determination of handedness. As we saw earlier in this chapter, alpha (α) waves (8–12 Hz) tend to appear when the brain is at rest and not involved in a mental task. Mental activity tends to suppress α activity and to replace it with beta (β) waves, which have faster frequencies and more irregular wave patterns (i.e., desynchronization). Some studies show greater α blocking over the left hemisphere during verbal tasks and over the right during nonverbal tasks (Goodman et al., 1980), suggesting left-hemisphere dominance for language. The same pattern of differential α activity in the two cerebral hemispheres can give information about cerebral dominance for handedness when a manual task is monitored.

Electroconvulsive Therapy (ECT). The ECT technique was introduced in the 1930s to treat psychotic behavior, and later, depression. It involves passing an electrical charge through the brain for about half a second. More recently, with neuropsychological knowledge of cerebral asymmetry, it has been used to determine the side of language dominance. Unilateral ECT to the left hemisphere is usually followed by confusion in verbal memory, word-finding, and other signs of mild aphasia (i.e., dysphasia) for a half hour to a full hour. Unilateral ECT to the right hemisphere is usually followed by temporary spatial and nonverbal deficits. A patient exhibiting these signs could be supposed to be left-hemisphere dominant for language. Bradshaw and Nettleton (1983) have suggested that this approach has the advantage of providing more time than the Wada test for observing and studying the changes in behavioral and cognitive signs.

Neurosonography. As the name implies, this investigative method makes use of the principles of sonar (sound navigation ranging). Formerly the technique was known as echoencephalography. Because of the new brain imaging methods (CT, MRI, and PET) introduced in the last 15 years, the use of neurosonography has been much reduced. However, it is still useful for exploring the brains of newborn babies with suspected brain pathology. A transducer unit is held over the fontanel (a normal opening in a newborn's skull that later closes with skull growth) and high-frequency sound waves are directed into the brain tissue. The sound waves are reflected back from abnormal tissue densities within the skull and any anomalies or irregularities are shown as blips on a scanning grid. Because it is a noninvasive technique, it is perfectly safe.

Radiological Brain Scanning. In the early 1960s, radionuclide brain scanning was introduced, but its images of the brain were primitive and the method carried some risk because of the radio-active material injected into the patient's arm. A radiation detector recorded areas of greater radioactivity in the damaged or patho-logical areas of the brain tissue as the injected liquid circulated through the brain. A major difficulty in this type of scanning was that it lost much of the available information because it was an attempt to portray a three-dimensional brain on a two-dimensional photographic plate. If the X-ray beam was picking up a tumor in the brain, it was also recording all brain tissue in front of and behind the tumor, and unless the lesion differed significantly in density from the background, it would not show clearly on the X-ray plate (Barnes & Lakshminarayanan, 1989; Hounsfield, 1973). This type of inefficient scanning was mostly abandoned when the CT scan was introduced.

Computerized Axial Tomography (CT). Introduced in the mid-1970s, CT scanning overcame the weakness of background inter-ference and revolutionized imaging of the brain with the clarity of its picture and the freedom from risk (Bigler, 1989). The CT scan provides an excellent picture of the *structure* of the brain because, unlike previous methods, it images a section or "slice" of the brain. With CT, in contrast to conventional radiography, X-rays do not pass through neighboring anatomy, but only through the section of interest (Barnes & Lakshminarayanan, 1989). The scan-ner produces a narrow beam of X-rays, allowing thousands of readings of transmissions through the head with one scan. The system rotates to scan one slice at a time and is repeated for 180 rotations. Thousands of readings may be taken by each detector during a complete scan; and the whole procedure may be com-pleted in a few seconds. This large body of data is digitized and analyzed by a computer that produces a clear X-ray picture of each slice of the subject's brain. These computer-analyzed X-ray transmission profiles are able to resolve gray and white matter, blood, and cerebrospinal fluid (Martin et al., 1991). Primarily a medical procedure, the CT scan has been useful in detecting abnormal brain structures in known dyslexics (Galaburda, 1983; Galaburda & Kemper, 1979) and other forms of LD.

Magnetic Resonance Imaging (MRI). The MRI type of brain scanning has a particular advantage over the CT scan in that it avoids the use of ionizing radiation and isotopes by depending on "the absorption and re-emission of radio frequency electro-magnetic energy by certain nuclei placed within strong magnetic fields" (Rosen & Brady, 1983). The ability of the atomic nuclei to absorb energy from radio waves is called nuclear magnetic resonance (Martin et al., 1991). The nuclei of certain atomic elements in human tissue react like tiny magnets. Because hydrogen makes up more than two-thirds of the body's atoms (Kinkel, 1987) the hydrogen proton is the nucleus most commonly used for imaging (Lee et al., 1989). When a patient is placed in a strong magnetic field, a small fraction of the body's nuclei align, but this number is enough to make imaging possible. This is a powerful imaging technique that can distinguish different body tissues because of their individual chemical compositions. Its images are superior in fine detail to that of the CT scan because its contrast resolution is finer. The MRI is used to reveal the structure and the functional state of the CNS (Martin et al., 1991). Where both CT and PET employ small levels of radiation that partially restrict examination of children younger than about 16 in many hospitals and clinics, MRI has no such risk and consequently may be used more freely for examining children.

Positron Emission Tomography (PET). The PET procedure involves injecting a radiopharmaceutical chemical in the arm, and produces numerous successive "slices" of the brain as the CT scan does, but the biochemistry and physics of the PET scan are different. The CT scan involves transmission of X-rays through the brain that provide information about its structure. The PET scan, by contrast, employs a positron-emitting substance (a radioisotope or "tracer"), thus enabling the researcher to measure physiological functions such as regional cerebral blood flow or glucose metabolism. Both measures estimate the degree of neuronal activity in different parts of the brain. Changes in neuronal activity reflect some form of behavioral or mental activity, so that the PET scanner can reveal both *structure* and *function* of the brain. For example, when a subject's left visual half-field is activated by a visual stimulus, the PET scan will show greater glucose consumption in the right visual striate cortex. Cognitive studies of verbal perceptions and reading with the PET technique have indicated the specific cerebral areas maximally activated with tasks of silent reading, oral reading, and verbal association (Petersen et al., 1988). The PET has also been used to compare brain functions of normal and dyslexic readers (Gross-Glenn et al., 1991).

Angiography. An angiogram is a medical technique in which a liquid containing material opaque to X-rays is injected into the carotid arteries and sequential X-ray pictures of the brain are taken as the liquid circulates in the cerebral arteriovenous system. It is primarily used for detecting arteriovenous malformations, aneurysms, and vascular lesions of the brain (Lawrence, 1992).

Although angiography is the best procedure for studying the intracranial vascular system, it has a drawback because it is invasive. To avoid this weakness, recent advances in MRI technology have been promising, but so far their images of intracranial blood vessels are not as clear as those of conventional angiography because the resolution of their pictures is not as fine. With further technical advances it should replace invasive angiography (Martin et al., 1991).

Cortical Electrostimulation. Penfield and Roberts (1959), Ojemann (1979, 1983), and others have discovered a great deal about the behavioral effects of electrostimulating specific cortical loci. These experiments are carried out during brain surgery with a conscious patient who is able to report the content of mental events or memories accompanying cortical stimulation. An interesting and nontechnical account of this procedure is given by Calvin and Ojemann (1980) Whereas this exciting and innovative technique makes it possible to manipulate the independent variable (the brain) and subsequently observe the dependent variables (behavior), one must be cautious in interpreting its manifestations.

Electrode Implantation in the Brain. We have mentioned the enterprising experiments with animals carried out by Delgado and others in which neuronal changes are recorded during perception and motor activity, and in which motor and emotional behavior may be manipulated. These techniques, which are pointing to closer control of the mind, may have advantages if they can assist learning (Delgado, Roberts, & Miller, 1954) but also may imply a social threat if they lead to coercive control of human behavior (Rosenzweig, Krech, Bennet, & Diamond, 1968). Many scientists, aware of the moral responsibilities of manipulating cerebral processes and behavior, have expressed such concern (Delgado, 1971). Regardless of the moral and social implications, it is useful to be aware of this neuropsychological knowledge because it may provide the theoretical basis for new methods of teaching and learning in the future.

Histological Studies. Autopsy studies of the human brain frequently provide valuable knowledge of the locus, extent, and nature of a lesion. If detailed records of the patient's behavior are available, then a neuropsychological correlation of two classes of events, observed at different times, is possible. It was this procedure that enabled Broca in 1861 to posit the possible cortical location of the motor speech area. Déjerine (Geschwind, 1962) in 1892 developed his explanation of dyslexia by this method.

More recently, Drake (1968) provided a beautifully detailed account of a learning disabled boy who died at age 12 and for
whom there are educational, psychological, psychiatric, social,
and neuropathological reports. Though not yet numerous, more
and more of these types of cases are finding their way into the
educational literature (Benson & Geschwind, 1969; Benton, 1964;
Galaburda, 1983; Rosen et al., 1986).

Use of Drugs and Chemicals. We have briefly referred in this
chapter to the chemical nature of the neural impulse and to
some experiments examining the interaction between brain biochemistry and behavior. One technique that is particularly useful is
the Wada Carotid Amytal Test (Wada & Rasmussen, 1960) in
which injections are made sequentially into the carotid artery on
the side of the neck. If made on the left side, the left hemisphere,
in a matter of seconds, becomes partially anesthetized or neurally
impaired, and flaccidity of the right arm and leg and temporary
aphasia result (when the left hemisphere is language dominant).
This is a useful technique for detecting cerebral dominance
for language.

Biofeedback Training. Biofeedback is a technique combining
knowledge of neural activity with principles of operant conditioning
in an attempt to modify behavior. Although the theoretical aim
is to formulate laws of neural information processing that may
help to understand brain–behavior relationships, until now "the
mechanisms underlying biofeedback's clinical efficacy are unclear"
(Hodes, 1989), and various explanations have been advanced.
Nevertheless the technique has had some success in treating
medical problems such as reducing pain, training in relaxation
for cerebral palsy and epilepsy victims, alleviating headache, and
sphincter training for incontinence. Methods of biofeedback training may include (1) the electromyograph (EMG), (2) the electroencephalogram (EEG), (3) the galvanic skin response (GSR), and
(4) the skin (surface) temperature measure, but the EMG has
been the most frequently used biofeedback approach for treating
hyperactivity (Lee, 1991). Of the behavior problems most amenable to biofeedback training the possible reduction of hyperactivity
in children with attention deficit disorder (ADHD or ADD/H) is
of particular interest to the educator. This procedure may involve
either the use of EMG biofeedback, in which information from the
EMG about the level of muscle tension is used to train the subject
to relax, or EEG biofeedback, in which the subject is trained
to increase specific brain waves in particular areas of the brain.
For example, Lubar and his colleagues have trained hyperactive

subjects to increase the sensorimotor rhythm (SMR)—that is, wave activity over the sensorimotor cortical strips, in the absence of excessive theta wave activity (slow waves), and they have had an encouraging success in training their subjects to increase beta wave activity (the small fast waves present in active thinking) and to decrease gross motor activity (Lubar & Lubar, 1984). Biofeedback is far from a completely reliable cure for behavioral problems, but when it has been successful in treating hyperactivity, it has sometimes allowed the physician to remove the previously required medication program. For the reader who desires further information on this topic, comprehensive reviews have been made by Hodes (1989) and Lee (1991).

Summary. The reader will recognize that some of the techniques above simply record the state of the brain and others manipulate it. Regardless of this, information may be gained about the structure and function of the brain, and many deficits can be identified. Behavior is then measured by a comprehensive battery of perceptual, cognitive, language, motor, and sensorimotor tests and any behavioral deviations are observed. These two sets of data are obtained from independent sources, and any reliable correlations between brain function and behavior add to our knowledge of the brain–behavior relationship. This is the essential pattern of human neuropsychology.

Neural Organization

Thus far we have examined physiological segments of living organisms, some small, such as nerve cells and synapses, and some larger functional units, such as arterial networks; but we have made only casual references to the total organization of the central nervous system and its control of human behavior.

In 1944, Herrick wrote, "Integration of bodily activities is a primordial essential; without it no living body can survive." This discussion will concentrate on the integrative functions of the brain and spinal cord, although the essential functional relations of other physiological subsystems (e.g., respiratory, circulatory, digestive, and endocrine systems) are recognized.

Functional Units

Luria (1973) tells us, "there are solid grounds for distinguishing *three principal functional units of the brain*." These are:

1. The activating reticular formation. Luria conceived of the brainstem (i.e., the midbrain, pons, and medulla oblongata) and the thalamus as working as a functional unit, the *first functional unit*, to maintain an animal's waking state. The chief function of this structure, which is organized like a nerve net, is to alert the various parts of the cortex to incoming signals. This is the chief function of the "ascending reticular system," and the "descending" fibers permit cortical control of the brainstem. This, then, is a physiological center for attention, for screening incoming messages, and for activating various cortical areas to maximize attention and mental efficiency. Dysfunction in this area may result in distractibility and hyperactivity (Lou et al., 1989).

The first function of the reticular formation is generalized arousal and the second, selective attention. Ojemann, a neurosurgeon, has found that part of the function of selective attention resides in the thalamus. By electrical stimulation of the thalamus during brain operations he can shift the patient's attention from his own internal, mental world of imagination to "what is coming in from the external world" (Calvin and Ojemann, 1980). These writers have suggested that autism might result from a dysfunction of brain structures that result in emphasis on "internal" attention, and failure to attend to external stimuli. This is an interesting proposal, but Calvin and Ojemann report that anatomical studies of the brains of autistic children show no structural abnormalities either in the striatum (basal ganglia) or thalamus, the specific areas believed to control selective attention. More recently, other investigators have found a defective cerebellum in some autistic patients (Courchesne et al., 1988).

2. The occipital, temporal, and parietal cortices. Although the nerve net of the reticular system works in accordance with the principal of nonspecific function and gradual change, the neural structure of the three cortices in the *second functional unit* isolates the three areas of neurons from one another so that each area receives discrete impulses. The occipital cortex mediates visual experience; the temporal, hearing; and the parietal, bodily sensation. Therefore, the primary purpose of this functional unit is *reception*, *analysis*, *interpretation* and *storage* of information. Lesions or dysfunctions in any of these cortical areas can result in a variety of impairments of academic learning, as we shall see when we examine specific case histories later in the book.

3. The frontal lobes. Whereas the second functional unit is located posterior to the fissure of Rolando (central sulcus), the *third functional unit* is anterior to it. As we have seen, the second unit mediates passive reaction to incoming information; the frontal lobes permit response to it through motor expression. Luria be-

lieved the frontal lobes were the centers for creating intentions, planning, and managing behavior in relation to one's perceptions and knowledge of the world.

Luria's concept of the vertical organization of all structures in the brain is a strong reminder that although the human cerebral cortex is necessary to our most abstract forms of thinking, the whole central nervous system contributes to it.

His concept of cortical function, based on prodigious clinical investigation, is in basic form, clear and easy to understand. In simple terms, Luria conceived of the human cortex as having primary, secondary, and tertiary zones, distinguished by their different functions.

Primary Projection Areas. The primary projection areas are (1) the primary visual areas of the occipital cortices, (2) the primary acoustic areas of the temporal cortices, and (3) the primary sensory areas of the parietal cortices. These zones are called "projection" areas because, although they are centers for the reception of incoming neural impulses, psychologically a person "projects" subjective experience to the outside world. Whereas the visual neural impulses stimulated by a writer's pen, as s/he writes, are recorded at the back of the brain in the occipital lobes, the writer has the experience that what is being written is about 12 in. in front of the eyes. Similarly, the sensation of holding the pen is recorded mostly in the left parietal area, but the writer's experience of gripping it is psychologically "projected" to the right hand.

The primary projection areas are so named because they are believed to record only the *elements* of experience and not organized forms of meaningful patterns. For example, the primary visual cortices record "flashes of light, tongues of flame and colored spots" (Luria, 1973). The acoustic cortices, lining the floors of the two fissures of Sylvius, record pure tone, such as "ringing, humming, clicking, rushing, chirping, buzzing, knocking or rumbling" (Penfield & Roberts, 1959), but not meaningful sounds, such as words or melodies, and the two sensory strips record pure tactile sensations.

Secondary Association Areas. The visual association areas (Brodmann's Areas 18 and 19, Fig. 2.10) are adjacent to the primary visual areas (Brodmann's Area 17). The auditory association areas occupy the lateral surfaces of the temporal lobes, contiguous to and just below the primary auditory projection area in Heschl's gyrus. Similarly, the secondary or association areas

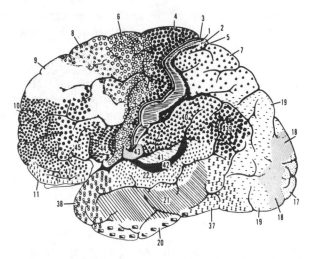

Figure 2.10. Cytoarchitectonic areas of the lateral aspect of the human brain. (According to Brodmann, *Vergleichende Lokalisationslehre der Grosshirnrinde*, Barth, 1909)

for touch are in the parietal areas bordering and close to the sensory strips.

The chief function of these secondary or association areas is to process incoming information and to give meaning to the input. Where the neural contacts to the primary areas are mainly from the sense organs by long-axon connections in the brainstem, by contrast, the neurons in the association areas have numerous short-axon connections transcortically. The primary areas thus receive the elements of sensation and the secondary areas, which contain thousands of neural traces built up through experience, analyze and integrate the incoming messages into meaningful, recognizable perceptions and experiences.

Experimental evidence from several sources supports this concept of primary and secondary cortical function. Electrostimulation of these two zones shows much greater spreading in the association areas, and by contrast the primary zones, when so stimulated, produce elemental visual or auditory experiences, as has already been described. Electrostimulation of the secondary visual cortices produces recognizable hallucinations of "flowers, animals and familiar persons" (Luria, 1973) and stimulating the secondary auditory cortices produces familiar voices and discernible sounds (Penfield & Roberts, 1959). This is a clear example of neural integration in which discrete neural stimuli are organized into a meaningful experience to which a person can respond.

Tertiary Cortical Zones. Tertiary cortical zones are the areas between the various sensory association cortical areas that permit an integrated multisensory experience. In humans, language is made possible by neural interconnections between the visual and the auditory association cortices, which are in the lower part of the left parietal lobe in most people. This neurally integrating area includes the angular and the supramarginal gyri (see Figs. 2.1 and 8.2), and it appears to have an essential function in language development, as discussed in Chapter 8. These areas are most developed in humans, appearing in only rudimentary form even in the higher apes. In fetal development this is one of the last areas in which dendrites appear, and sometimes it is slow to mature in childhood (Geschwind, 1965, Part II). These discoveries from developmental neurology suggest that both phylogenetically and ontogenetically these integrating neural structures are late to mature, and in cases of faulty development they seem to be highly vulnerable and at greater risk in attaining mature and normal function. In cases of defective growth one might expect problems in perception, cognition, and/or motor response, which are, in fact, essential causes of learning disabilities.

Ayres (1972a) developed an interesting theory and remediation program that has been used rather widely by occupational therapists. She contends that disordered sensory integration accounts for some aspects of learning disabilities and that remediation implies improving the neural integration of the child to increase the capacity of the brain to learn, rather than drilling specific academic skills.

Functional Units and Learning

The importance of sensorimotor integration to learning and normal behavior is supported by neurological and neuropsychological clinical studies. This integration is hierarchic in design, each smaller subsystem (e.g., a cell) requiring harmonious intraorganic integration, and each group of subsystems requiring an internal consonance free of stresses or occlusions.

Certainly a deficit in integration can produce learning problems at different levels. A lesion in any one of the primary cortical projection areas or in the neural pathways leading to them can produce a partial or distorted input, making it difficult for the contiguous association areas to integrate the elemental input into a meaningful cognitive pattern. This is an example of a visual or auditory or tactile perceptual deficit.

If the primary area is free of pathology but the association area is damaged, the process of sensory analysis and integration itself is impaired, and a perceptual deficit also results, but for different reasons.

If a lesion is localized in the motor strip or strips or the efferent nerves connecting to the muscles, the child may be partially immobilized. The child's intelligence level may be above average and perceptual understanding good, but expressive abilities (spoken speech, writing, general mobility) may be impaired. An intellectually bright child with cerebral palsy is such an example.

In all the examples above the lesions have been localized, so that normal integrative functioning of the whole central nervous system has been disturbed. If the brain pathology is more generalized, then a cognitive deficit is more likely to appear, and if it is diffuse, then some degree of mental retardation may result.

The majority of books on educational psychology urge the teacher to deal with the "whole child," but these same books cover only psychological and social aspects. If the teacher is to deal with the "whole child" then the best neurological, psychological, and educational knowledge must be integrated. The emphasis in this book is on the first of these three, but this does not imply a disregard of the other two. The interested teacher will need to relate the knowledge presented here with his or her own psychological and educational background. Books and courses covering these two areas are numerous; books and courses covering educational neuropsychology are almost nonexistant.

Clinical Addendum

What the Clinical Psychologist Can Do

This addendum, and those to follow subsequent chapters, presents in some detail a diagnostic approach that the clinical or school psychologist may use. It also describes how the teacher might use the information gained by the clinical neuropsychological approach. This procedure is proposed not as the only model but as a guide for school psychologists who wish to incorporate neurological knowledge into their diagnostic analyses and remedial prescriptions. Attempts to do so are not common, although increasing numbers of psychologists are expressing interest in using clinical neuropsychology in the study and treatment of learning disorders.

It is hoped that these clinical addenda will serve as a guide to relate neuropsychological test signs to better understanding of the LD child or adult, and to use this knowledge in preparing remedial programs. Inexperienced clinicians may follow this guide as a learning experience, if they so choose; experienced clinicians may wish to incorporate new material they may meet into their established clinical style.

A school psychologist who wishes to use neuropsychological knowledge in diagnostic reports will soon find that neither the neurologist nor the teacher is the appropriate person to integrate the neurological, psychological, and educational data on each LD child or adult. Each of these professional people has his or her own areas of expertise, and the essential functions of the clinical psychologist include diagnosis and therapy. Thus the school or clinical psychologist will likely have to collect the diagnostic data from the neurologist, from the teacher, and from his or her own test and interview results, and then attempt to put them together into a meaningful picture. The clinical psychologist will most likely emerge as the coordinator on this team, and this clinical procedure can soon become a smoothly running operation when each member has a clearly defined role.

At first there may be problems of interprofessional communication. Medical doctors sometimes approach discussions with teachers with caution, and many teachers are timid about approaching medical doctors about professional problems. In one isolated case, an authoritarian school principal, with strong feelings about territorial rights, wrote a note to a doctor telling her "to stay out of my school, and to keep your hands off what is none of your business." Such extreme views are not common, and teachers enjoy the opportunity to explain to the neurologist and to the psychologist the child's school problems. Periodic workshops on learning disabilities for medical, educational, and public health personnel have been popular and successful in breaking down much interprofessional isolationism.

Any clinical activity that promises competent help to learning disabled children will soon be inundated with referrals; hence a clearly defined admission policy is essential. All requests for our own program when it was initiated, whether they came from parents, teachers, or medical doctors, were referred first to a qualified neurologist for a complete neurological examination, including an EEG and a skull X-ray. After about the first three years of the plan, we dispensed with the skull X-ray because it produced no useful information in most cases. As a replacement for the skull X-ray, the neuroradiological examination (brain scan), described in this chapter, is a relatively new technique that has great promise for the study of children with learning disabilities (Valk, 1974).

Clinical Classifications

These classifications, first presented in Chapter 1, are examined here in more clinical detail, but with a view to relating them to problems of learning.

Brain Damaged

With at Least One Hard Sign. Some of these signs may be confirmed by neurosurgery, such as a subdural hematoma or a progressive lesion such as a cyst or tumor. Some may be identified behaviorally (e.g., hemiplegia) or by neuroradiological investigation (e.g., abnormal growth or atrophy of the cerebral structures). Some are identified at autopsy, and much can be learned by relating the recorded learning problems to the postmortem findings (Drake, 1968).

In many cases it may be difficult to decide whether a sign is "hard" or "soft." For example, a hyperreflexia on one side, if extremely strong, would be considered a "hard" sign by many neurologists, possibly most. The same sign, if weak, however, might be considered a "soft" sign. In practice, this definitional allocation depends on the neurologist's clinical experience and skill. In collaborative research projects involving neurologists and neuropsychologists where this procedure is required, reliability of report may be increased by having more than one neurologist make the assessments and diagnostic allocations. Such a study has been reported by Spreen, and the allocations of a number of signs have been made by the neurologist on the basis of whether the sign was "marked" or "slight" (Spreen, 1988, pp. 149–150).

Inferring brain damage or dysfunction completely on behavioral signs is done only by experienced neurologists, whose clinical criteria for selection may vary. Some may accept it on one hard sign (e.g., marked hemiplegia), or two or three moderate hard signs (e.g., grade ii EEG dysrhythmia, a mild ataxia or neuromuscular coordination, and an asymmetry of sensation in the hands). Obviously, brain dysfunction is a matter of degree, and diagnostic classifications result from clinical judgments. Signs that may contribute to a diagnosis of brain damage or dysfunction, when they are strong, may include ataxia, anosmia, nystagmus, dysarthria, choreiform or athetoid movements, marked tremor,

marked spasticity, hyperactive tendon reflexes, extreme incoordination, and unilateral simultagnosia. Neuropsychological behavior
signs that show in clinical testing can include marked asymmetry of
sensation in hands and/or face, marked asymmetry of finger tapping
between hands, and marked asymmetry of stereognosis between
hands. Some additional neuropsychological signs that may be observed by the teacher and the school psychologist include language
retardation, motor incoordination, visual perceptual deficits (e.g.,
rotations, reversals, inversions), defective body image, and poor
right–left directional sense. Because these latter signs may be
caused by developmental lag it is safer to use them only after the
neurological and sensorimotor signs have been established, and
only with children at least 9 years old.

Minimal Brain Dysfunction (MBD)

In Chapter 1 the MBD child was described briefly and symptomatically to help teachers better understand this frequently ill-
defined and confusing category. Here we will examine the problems
posed by this category and provide some suggestions that may be
useful to the school or clinical psychologist in the understanding
and treatment of children so classified.

At the outset, it is clear that the definition of MBD and the
understanding of its pathology, its etiology, and any characteristic
response pattern to its treatment (if such a pattern exists) are all
in a state of flux. The term "minimal brain dysfunction," first
formally recommended in 1962 by the Oxford International Study
Group on Child Neurology, was proposed in place of the term
"minimal brain damage" because it was believed by the members
of the group that brain damage should never be inferred from
behavioral signs alone (Strother, 1973). However, since 1962 the
recognition and treatment of MBD children have attracted the
attention of more nonmedically trained professionals, in particular
educators and school psychologists, and this has led to a greater
educational emphasis on the category. Strother (1973) tells us that
"authors who write from a medical orientation prefer the term
'minimal brain dysfunction' or its equivalent, whereas those who
write from an educational point of view tend to use the term
'specific learning disabilities' or its equivalent." As medical, neuropsychological, and educational researches reveal more knowledge
about MBD children, the present tendency to a divided view
should be replaced eventually by a common definition satisfactory
to all professionals. In the meantime it will fall to the lot of the
school psychologist to assess each LD child in depth and to decide
on the presence or absence of soft signs.

Rutter, Graham, and Yule (1970) have suggested three groups of soft signs:

1. Signs that reflect a developmental delay, such as speech and language retardation, motor incoordination, perceptual deficits in all sense modes, impaired right–left orientation, adventitious motor overflow, and extinction or suppression of double simultaneous tactile stimulation. We would add delayed or defective sequential perception and/or response. Any of these signs must be interpreted in relation to chronological and mental age.

2. Signs that may or may not result from pathological neurological factors, such as nystagmus, strabismus, and tremor. Causes other than neurological pathology may include muscular weakness, or toxic or drug effects.

3. Signs of slight abnormalities that are difficult to elicit, such as slight asymmetry of tonus or reflexes, just perceptible hemiparesis, minimal athetosis, or mild asymmetry of skull or limbs.

Other signs include (Clements, 1966; Tupper, 1987) EEG abnormalities without actual seizures, or possibly subclinical seizures that may be associated with fluctuations in behavior or intellectual function, and deviations in attention, activity level, impulse control, and affect. Clements listed 99 symptoms under 15 classes that the school psychologist may find useful.

The confusion in defining MBD stems from the common difficulty of identifying any borderline phenomenon appearing on a continuum reflecting an intense condition that gradually decreases until it is completely absent. Intense and localized brain damage in specific cortical or subcortical areas will produce predictable deficits in adult behavior with a high level of reliability (Luria, 1966, 1970, 1973; Reitan, 1959). Human subjects manifest a set of systematic brain–behavior relationships, as explained more fully in Chapter 3. Cases of traumatic brain damage provide a rich source of neuropsychological knowledge in which the neural pathology is known and the behavioral impairment is observed. In these cases the etiological factors and their psychological sequelae frequently are more clearly identified.

As we move along the continuum toward normal brain structure and function, however, we pass through a large number of children and adults who are not "brain damaged" and who, for no known reason, show many behavioral deficits similar to the brain-damaged patients, but in a much less intense way. These behavioral impairments (e.g., visual reversals, poor finger localization, asymmetry of finger tapping, and astereognosis) are the soft signs, and their presence suggests very strongly that the person's brain and central nervous system has some minimal areas of dysfunction, although a standard neurological examination may have turned up nothing.

Although brain damage cannot be diagnosed completely and always conclusively on behavioral data alone, Reitan (1964b), using only neuropsychological test results, has been among the first to predict the loci of localized brain lesions preoperatively in adults, and many of his students have learned the same clinical skill with some success.

Other clinical sources that are helping to complete the mosaic picture of the MBD child are the new scanning techniques described earlier. They are revealing areas of brain pathology previously missed by a standard neurological examination. A patient with a reading disability because of Déjerine's syndrome (alexia without agraphia; see Chapter 8 for a full account) was found on the CT scanner to have a lesion in the left posterior part of his brain (Staller et al., 1978), although the brain pathology was not evident in more common methods of investigation.

In the past, some authors (Schmitt, 1975) have dismissed the soft signs as indications of maturational lag, and thus completely unreliable and meaningless for both diagnosis and prognosis. Such conclusions have usually resulted from clinical observation only. One investigator who examined this problem experimentally and longitudinally was Hern (1984). Where most studies of the stability and persistence of soft signs have covered periods of a few weeks (MacMahon & Greenberg, 1977) or up to 4 years (Ackerman, Dykman, & Peters, 1977; Hertzig, 1982), Hern followed 123 learning disabled subjects for 14 years, from elementary school age into adulthood. She also compared these 123 adults neurologically with 46 normal learners who were matched for age and socioeconomic status. Using a regression analysis procedure Hern found a significant relationship among 19 neurological measures at time 1 (subjects' ages between 8 and 12 years) and time 2 (the same subjects 14 years later). An R^2 of .53 was found, which corresponds to a correlation coefficient of .73. The difference in incidence from middle childhood to adulthood showed a reduction in signs among subjects with the greatest number at time 1 and changes in both directions for those in the midrange. Hern's findings did not support the thesis that LD children suffer from temporary maturational lag that will be overcome with time. On the contrary, she found that most LD children "do not seem to improve in their performance on a neurological examination and many show additional and different signs in adulthood that were not seen in childhood" (Hern, 1984). In addition, she found that LD adults showed more neurological soft signs than a matched control group of normal learners.

What is the school psychologist to do about so-called MBD children in the face of this evidence? First, it seems advisable not to infer cerebral dysfunction conclusively from behavioral data alone, or to state this inference in a report. Then too, it should not be inferred that because the child shows a number of soft signs that he or she must be hyperactive or learning disabled.

If the child does have a serious learning problem and a large number of soft signs, however, the neurologically trained school psychologist may profit from hypothesizing what might be occurring in the child's nervous system, although the psychologist never mentions this to the parents or includes it in any formal communication. Such a practice is congruent with the idea of the unity of nature and with a possible later revelation of subtle brain dysfunctions in cases with only soft neurological signs. It has the advantage of encouraging more detailed consideration of the child's case, albeit speculative; of increasing or widening the scope of logically possible diagnostic hypotheses; and of improving the probability of hitting on fruitful diagnostic knowledge. Such an approach avoids damaging the child by labeling but stimulates in-depth consideration of a case that, at this stage in our knowledge, can be only partial at best.

The school psychologist who wishes further discussion on this important classification is referred to the scholarly and logical defense of the term MBD by Denckla (1978), who is a neurologist engaged in the study and assessment of learning disabled children.

In summary, the MBD classification may be useful for the physician, research psychologist, and school psychologist, although because of incomplete knowledge about its etiology at the present its definition may vary with the discipline in which it is stated. Nevertheless, it appears to be a neurologically and behaviorally recognizable group, where private speculation by the psychologist may lead to more fruitful understanding and treatment.

Learning Disabled with No Hard or Soft Signs

These include children of normal intelligence and good health, who are usually described as having a specific learning disability or a developmental learning disability with no known cause. Orton (1928) was one of the first to study and describe the reading disabled child, although he named the defect strephosymbolia, which meant a twisted perception of the written symbols. We now know that dyslexia can result from a perceptual deficit, a language disability, or a problem in sensorimotor integration. Ayres (1972a) has written ably on the last-named type. On a battery of neuro-psychological tests, a person in this category may have average or better scores on intelligence, on all the perceptual tests, and in motor response, but may have great difficulty in sequencing, in cross-modal tasks, in phonetic blending, or in any skill demanding an integration of input and output neural functions. Though all the causes of learning problems are not known, a disturbance in sensorimotor integration seems to be present in a number of them. Genetic defects may account for some others.

The school psychologist may select these children on the basis of teacher's reports, if they are obvious, or by psychometric means, such as a learning quotient (Myklebust, 1967a) or a multiple regression formula (Rutter, Graham, & Yule, 1970), as discussed in Chapter 1.

Normal Controls

It is advisable for any school psychologist to collect scores of normal children on any tests he or she uses, to avoid relying completely on collections of normative data from different populations. Some collections of normative data are available (Gaddes & Crockett, 1975; Gaddes, 1988; Klonoff, 1971; Knights, 1966; Knights & Ogilvie, 1967; Spreen & Gaddes, 1969; Trites, 1977), but these should be used with caution unless the two populations being compared appear to be reasonably similar.

Once a child or adult is accepted for diagnostic study (in our laboratory all children in Group 1 [brain damaged] are accepted automatically, and selected children in Groups 2 [MBD] and 3 [LD]), he or she is subjected to a test battery (see Appendix), which takes between five and six hours to administer. The tests are selected to measure visual, auditory, and tactile perception; verbal and spatial–constructional intelligence (WISC); motor speed; sensorimotor integration; serial order competence; attention and concentration; short- and long-term memory; and language development.

Patterns of deficits in a child's neurological data are compared with deficits on the neuropsychological tests and from the teacher's reports of the child's classroom difficulties. Group studies are carried out to examine the possibility of reliable correlations between these two sets of variables, as part of the research function of the clinical or school psychologist in this setting.

The psychological and educational data are studied in the light of whether the cerebral abnormality is general and diffuse, regional (left or right, frontal or posterior), or highly localized; whether it is developmental (that is, has existed since birth) or traumatic (acquired by postnatal injury); and whether, if it is traumatic, it is recent or long-standing.

After conferring with the parents and the child's teacher, the psychologist then writes a remedial prescription, stressing the child's strengths and weaknesses, listing the types of academic activities and skills with which he or she will likely have difficulty, and suggesting how these difficulties may be circumvented.

This report should be free of jargon, in clear, plain language that the parents and teacher can understand easily, and should include an overall diagnostic conceptual picture of the child that should help the teacher to perceive the child more accurately. It should also include a number of concrete remedial suggestions that the teacher can try.

What the Teacher Can Do

The teacher will usually have a more detailed knowledge of the child's social behavior than the school psychologist, but all signs of subtle deficits, such as phonetic auditory imperception, should be supplied to the teacher by the clinical or school psychologist.

The teacher may study the psychologist's report and build up conceptual knowledge of the child's perceptual, cognitive, or motor deficits. With this knowledge in mind he or she should then select from his or her own professional repertoire the remedial approach that seems best suited to the child's needs.

A baseline should be measured before the remedial program is begun and any progress or lack of it reported to the psychologist, who may act not as an expert authority but as a consultant to help the teacher. If the child is making good progress, it is likely that the remedial approach is valid. If no progress is made, the psychologist should decide in conference with the teacher whether more diagnostic procedures should be carried out, whether the teaching methods should be monitored and altered, or whether there are etiological factors not yet detected.

In Chapter 3, we discuss in detail current neuropsychological knowledge and its possibility for understanding learning. Following this discussion the Clinical Addendum at the end of Chapter 3 offers more specific suggestions about diagnosis and remediation.

Suggested Readings in Neuropsychology

Bradshaw, J.L. and Nettleton, N.C. *Human cerebral asymmetry*. Englewood Cliffs: Prentice-Hall, 1983.

Bryden, M.P. *Laterality: Functional asymmetry in the intact brain*. New York: Academic Press, 1982.

Filskov, S.B. & Boll, T.J. *Handbook of clinical neuropsychology*. New York: John Wiley, 1981.

Heilman, K.M. & Valenstein, E. *Clinical neuropsychology*. New York: Oxford University Press, 1979.

Hynd, G.W. & Willis, W.G. *Pediatric neuropsychology*. New York: Grune & Stratton, 1988.

Hynd, G.W. & Obrzut, J.E. (Eds.). *Neuropsychological assessment and the school-age child: issues and procedures*. New York: Grune & Stratton, 1981.

Kolb, B. & Whishaw, I.Q. *Fundamentals of human neuropsychology*, 3rd ed. San Francisco: W.H. Freeman, 1990.

Obrzut, J.E. & Hynd, G.W. (Eds.). *Child neuropsychology: Theory and research, Vol. I*. New York: Academic Press, 1986.

Obrzut, J.E. & Hynd, G.W. (Eds.). *Child neuropsychology: Clinical practice, Vol. 2*. New York: Academic Press, 1986.

Obrzut, J.E. & Hynd, G.W. (Eds.). *Neuropsychological foundations of learning disabilities*. New York: Academic Press, 1991.

Reynolds, C.R. & Fletcher-Janzen, E. (Eds.). *Handbook of clinical child neuropsychology*. New York: Plenum, 1989.

Rourke, B.P., Bakker, D.J., Fisk, J.L. & Strang, J.D. *Child neuropsychology*. New York: Guilford, 1983.

Spreen, O., Tupper, D., Risser, A., Tuokko, H. & Edgell, D. *Human developmental neuropsychology*, 2nd ed. New York: Oxford University Press, in press.

Tupper, D.E. *Soft neurological signs*. Orlando, FL: Grune & Stratton, 1987.

3 Using Neuropsychological Knowledge in Understanding Learning Disorders

All nervous centers have then in the first instance one essential function, that of "intelligent" action. They feel, prefer one thing to another, and have "ends." Like all other organs, however, they evolve from ancestor to descendant, and their evolution takes two directions, the lower centers passing downwards into more unhesitating automatism, and the higher ones upwards into larger intellectuality.

William James (1890)

In this chapter the current status of our knowledge of the brain–behavior relationship will be examined within the context of problems of cognitive function and classroom learning. This particularly interesting and promising area of exploration still has many gray areas. Current neuropsychological knowledge does not yet include the particular functions (if they exist) of most segmental parts of the cerebrum, thalamus, and brainstem, but it does possess knowledge of some of the gross relationships of the brain and behavior, and this knowledge has relevance for the clinical psychologist and the classroom teacher. This attempt to relate neurological, psychological, and educational knowledge is a radical one and is still in its infancy. Since 1963, many professional meetings have been held in the United States, Canada, Europe, and the southern hemisphere to discuss learning disorders, and most of these have included neurologists as major invited speakers. These meetings have been sponsored by medical schools, associations of ophthalmology and pediatrics, and other medical specialties, as well as schools of education. This is a healthy sign, because physicians, psychologists, and educators are now likely to progress more rapidly in understanding learning disorders by pooling their knowledge and professional experience.

What follows is an attempt to synthesize current knowledge from researchers in neurology, neurophysiology, neuropsychology, and education. The student of neuropsychology should understand at the outset that the brain operates as a dynamic unitary organ when the behavioral function seems to draw on all or most of the cerebral mechanisms. At the same time it also implies a maximal processing function of one or more localized cortical areas for certain types of behavior. For example, if Broca's area (see Fig. 2.9) at the base of the third frontal convolution of the left cerebral hemisphere is damaged seriously the person may not be able to speak. Such patients may hear what is said to them and may understand its meaning, but because one of the important centers in the motor-speech function is damaged their expressive speech may be impaired. By contrast, Teuber and Weinstein (1956) found a form of behavior that seems to require normal functioning of all cortical areas. This is the ability to perceive a hidden-figure task, or to see a geometric figure hidden in a camouflaged background. Patients with left-hemisphere, right-hemisphere, bilateral, frontal, nonfrontal, parietal, nonparietal, temporal, nontemporal, occipital, and nonoccipital lesions did almost equally poorly on this test, suggesting a rather generalized cortical function to mediate successful perception of this type.

More than a hundred years ago the famous French neurologist, Flourens (1794–1867), hypothesized that "one point excited in the nervous system excites all the others; one point enervated enervates them all; there is a community of reaction, of alteration, of energy . . ." (Boring, 1957). This unitary function of the brain he named "action commune." The localized functions of the brain he called "action propre." It is interesting that neuropsychological evidence currently appearing still tends to support Flourens's early insights, although with more precise knowledge.

At our present level of neuropsychological knowledge there is value in studying the brain as a whole and recognizing the behavioral effects that accompany both specific and localized brain lesions. Kurt Goldstein, an eminent German neurologist who studied the mental effects of brain injuries in German soldiers in World War I, developed a holistic theory not only of brain function, but of total behavior. In comparing the atomistic study of parts and the holistic approach, he favored starting with an examination of the whole organism, then dissecting, but always keeping the total function at the center of interest.

Riese, explaining Goldstein's work, has written,

Goldstein denied neither the significance of structures nor the possibility of cerebral localization. He only wanted to relegate both within their own limits. He was searching for a constructive formula of those functions which are accessible to cerebral representation and localization. . . . Cerebral activity, he said, is always a total one, but always with ever-changing regional accents. . . . (Riese, 1968)

In brief, this means that the brain functions as a whole, but many specific behaviors impose more demands on different cerebral parts. Consequently when a lesion occurs in a particular cerebral locus, behavior that draws heavily on the normal functioning of that area or areas joined by that locus may suffer. However, this does not mean that that form of behavior is determined exclusively by the particular locus under study. Hughlings Jackson, the eminent British neurologist, realized this 100 years ago and his theoretical insight was re-expressed by Weisenburg and McBride (1935/1964) when they wrote, "the aphasic symptoms are the result of the activity of the uninjured parts of the brain, for dead tissues cannot produce kinetic phenomena."

Thus, knowing the locus of a brain lesion may help us predict a particular behavioral deficit, and vice versa, but this does not necessarily support an exclusively localizationist or structural view of brain function and behavior. Knowledge of generalized or localized cortical dysfunction can provide the diagnosing clinical psychologist with different types of information that can help the special teacher to design an effective remedial program.

Adult and Child Neuropsychology

Just as child behavior differs from adult behavior in quality, complexity, and abstractness, so too, do brain–behavior relationships differ from child to adult. But how they differ is only partially understood because developmental neuropsychology is still a new science; a few clinical studies appeared following World War II (Strauss & Lehtinen, 1947; Strauss & Kephart, 1955; Cruickshank, Bice, Wallen, & Lynch, 1957), but most research in this area has appeared since about 1960.

Adult neuropsychology preceded child studies by more than a century, both because adult patients were more numerous and hence more available and because they were more easily understood. No problems in human neuropsychology are simple, but at least the adult brain and its correlations with behavior are reasonably stable after about midadolescence. By contrast, the brain of a child grows very rapidly to about age 9 then slows its rate of growth (see Fig. 3.1), and the cognitive and behavioral functions dependent on this cerebral growth show comparably rapid development. While adult norms of brain and cognitive

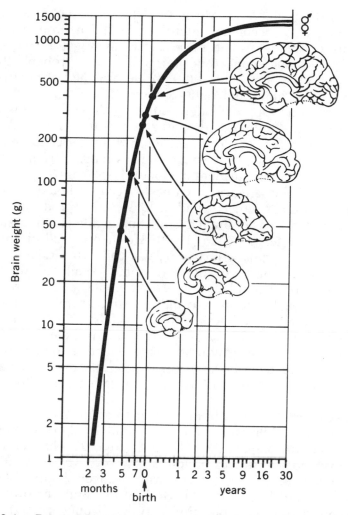

Figure 3.1. Pre- and postnatal growth of the human brain. (From Lemire, R.J., Loeser, J.D., Leech, R.W., & Alvord, E.C., *Normal and Abnormal Development of the Human Nervous System*. Harper & Row, 1975. Adapted from Larroche, J.C., in Falkner, F. (ed.), *Human Development*. Philadelphia: W.B. Saunders, 1966. With permission of the authors and the publishers.)

functions are relatively stable, those same measures in children change from year to year.

To understand the degree and quality of mental impairment associated with cerebral damage or dysfunction, it is essential to be able to compare the performance of normal subjects with that of brain-damaged subjects. One of the first researchers to draw attention to this need was Hebb (1942a), but his collections of normative data related only to brain-damaged adult patients

(Hebb, 1942b; Hebb & Morton, 1943). By the late 1940s a few people were becoming interested in the neuropsychological problems of children, but these early investigators made only clinical studies and supplied no normative data. Probably the first person to do this was Benton (1959); he provided normative data on finger localization and right–left orientation on sizeable samples of children (approximately 40 at each year) aged 6 to 9 years inclusive. Another investigator at that time was Wake, who provided normative data for finger localization for children at each year from age 6 to 12, with group samples ranging from 52 to 126. His data can be found in Benton's book (1959, p. 69).

Most books and studies of clinical neuropsychology, however, included only adult subjects, and in 1959 Reitan produced the first summary of test signs of brain dysfunction in adults as measured by the Halstead battery (Reitan, 1959). He then turned his attention to producing a comparable battery for children (Reitan, 1964a), which enabled him to examine in some detail the differences between children and adults. In 1974 he published what was up to that time probably the most comprehensive examination of child neuropsychological findings using the Halstead–Reitan battery (Reitan & Davison, 1974; 7 of the 12 chapters examine neuropsychological studies of children). These, and findings by other researchers, are described in appropriate places throughout the book, but a few of these differences and similarities follow:

1. Because the human brain is near to adult size by age 9, and some cognitive skills are at or near adult levels of competence, "the attempt to compare the patterns . . . of older children with . . . neuropsychological studies of adults may very well be fruitful, but this does not seem to be the case with younger children" (Rourke & Gates, 1981). Reitan (1974), Boll (1974), and our own experience support this. The transition between "younger" and "older" children appears to be about age 10 for many cognitive and behavioral skills. "For example, adult levels of auditory phonetic discrimination for nonsense syllables are reached by age 10, visual–manual reaction times do not improve significantly after age 11, and most basic language skills reach an adult level by age 13" (Gaddes, 1983). But the child of elementary school age is still increasing cognitive and behavioral skills by emerging from a sensorimotor–concrete–operational pattern to a level of intellectual abstract conceptualizing at about a mental age of 11 (Piaget, 1952).

2. Unilateral brain damage or dysfunction will impair the contralateral sensory and motor functions similarly in adults and children of all ages (Reitan, 1974).

3. However, lateralized brain lesions show some differences in their effects on cognitive abilities. Unilateral brain damage or dysfunction in adults in most cases will result in a pattern of left-hemisphere language impairment and right-hemisphere nonverbal impairment, but this relationship is not as clear in very young children and preadolescents. The reasons are not completely understood, but organic and psychological immaturity and the plastic adaptive qualities of the developing brain appear to be essentially involved.

Some early research, using behavioral criteria to select left- and right-hemisphere damaged child subjects (Reed & Reitan, 1969), and others using EEG selection techniques (Pennington, Galliani, & Voegele, 1965) failed to find the typical adult pattern, but most studies in the past 30 years of both normal and brain-dysfunctioning children have supported a cerebral asymmetry for cognitive functions and an asymmetrical deficit behavioral pattern related to it.

In the past, most selections of unilaterally damaged child patients had to be made on the basis of either behavioral or EEG signs, both of which methods will produce an unknown number of false positives. Where detailed neurosurgical information is available in young children the condition of exclusive unilateral dysfunction can be more firmly established, and the typical adult pattern of verbal impairment with left-hemisphere dysfunction and spatial–constructional deficit with right-hemisphere dysfunction can be observed in most cases. Such a case from our own files (Vera Brown, pages 364–366) of a 6-year-old child with left temporal surgery, showed an immediate problem with all verbal skills and superior ability in the graphic arts. This split did not show itself in the VIQ–PIQ pattern as explained on page 364; but this case is a good example of how children may differ qualitatively from adults.

In a study of 65 children with unilateral hemispheric brain lesions occurring after speech acquisition any time between ages 2 and 14, of 34 subjects with left-hemisphere lesions, 25 (or 73%) had an initial aphasic speech disturbance. Of 31 subjects with right-hemisphere lesions, only 4 (or 13%) showed any initial aphasia, and 2 of these 4 were left-handed (Woods & Teuber, 1978). These data seem to support the concept of early linguistic superiority of the left hemisphere in most children. Dennis and Whitaker (1976) in a study of three 9- and 10-year-old children who had suffered surgical removal of one half-brain prior to the beginning of speech, concluded that the right brain by itself is deficient in understanding auditory language, but phonemic and semantic abilities are developed by both hemispheres within the normal range.

Making inferences about brain function with children younger than about 10 years is much more difficult than with similarly injured adults, because there is "a far larger number of potentially interfering and confounding factors than . . . with adults" (Boll, 1974, pp. 91–92). More will be said about the development of cerebral asymmetry in Chapter 6.

Neuropsychological Tests

In a school system it is usual for the school psychologist or person responsible for selecting and administering diagnostic tests to assume responsibility for examining and evaluating the validity, reliability, and appropriateness of the tests to be used. This type of judgment depends on theoretical knowledge of test construction and administration, and, normally, teachers and many educational administrators are not trained to this level of knowledge and must depend on the decisions of the school psychologist.

For this reason, those responsible for testing programs will need to know how neuropsychological test batteries have been validated. Teachers too may be interested in reading this section, although, because their expertise and responsibility are principally pedagogical, they usually are not required to make responsible decisions pertaining to test selection.

A within-child model of diagnosis implies systematic examination of a child's cognitive skills, psychological structures, social environment, and attitudes to and perceptions of that environment. Such a study can include casual social observation; controlled social observation; reports by parents, teachers, medical practitioners, speech pathologists, and other professionals; and batteries of psychological tests.

In this section the use of neuropsychological tests in educational diagnosis is examined. The use of any types of psychological tests implies some basic rules:

1. The tests used should possess a reasonable measure of validity. That is, they must make a reasonable measure of what they claim to measure. The reader will discover that neuropsychological tests may have differing levels of efficiency depending on whether they are used to localize a brain lesion or to predict a learning disability. Measures of concurrent validity are usually higher than those used for prediction.

2. Tests should be reliable or show a high level of consistency in their measurement over time.

3. The battery should be appropriate. Many psychoeducational batteries are too limited. In the past a common battery was a Wechsler (WISC-R), a Bender–Gestalt, and maybe a draw-a-person or a Frostig test. Such a battery would take about 2 hours to administer, and this would seem to indicate a generous portion of the psychologist's time and a liberal amount of test findings. The school administrator, untrained in the problems of psychometrics, might misguidedly feel satisfied that his or her district was supplying an above-average caliber of diagnostic services. For the child with a minimal or moderate auditory imperception, however, such a battery would miss the crucial causal factor in his or her learning problem. Because the information from this battery is not likely to help the teacher solve the child's subtle auditory learning deficit, it is a waste of time and money, and the school administrator should be aware of this. Unless the test battery is designed to tap all or most of the possible problem areas it will be inefficient and expensive. If it taps most of the problem areas it will be expensive and time consuming, but it will most likely produce some useful diagnostic knowledge.

4. Some test batteries are redundant and hence too long. It is not difficult to find cases of children who, because of a persistent learning disability, have been tested and retested during their school experience. Frequently the child's file, which is usually thick, will contain several Wechsler tests done at different times and 10 or 12 educational achievement tests. There may be five or six in reading and several in arithmetic and spelling. A résumé of all these findings may produce very little information other than that the child is of average intelligence and cannot read, write, or do arithmetic very well. The teacher already knows this, but because of the redundancy and narrowness of the tests, little of use is gained from this expensive exercise. Again, the school administrator should be aware of this problem.

5. In our view, a neuropsychological test battery provides a more thorough and more systematic examination of a child's perceptual, cognitive, and motor abilities, and with its use there is less chance of missing the causal factor or factors of the child's learning problems.

Reitan validated his tests empirically during the 1950s (Reitan, 1955b, 1958, 1959), and in a series of original experiments (Reitan, 1964b) he showed that, when supplied with 112 adult patients with five categories of medically known brain damage [(1) left frontal lesion, (2) left posterior, (3) right frontal, (4) right posterior, and (5) diffuse brain damage], he could localize the damage correctly in 88 cases (78.6%), and very closely in another 15 cases (making a total of 92%). When asked to test 100 patients of whom 50 were medically diagnosed as brain damaged and 50 were normal, Reitan independently picked 96% of the brain-damaged patients correctly. All these studies were blind; that is, they took place without prior knowledge of the medical diagnosis. In these experiments Reitan showed that his test battery had a high level of empirical validity in detecting cerebral dysfunctions.

From 1960 to 1970, this method of neuropsychological identification of brain dysfunctions became more refined and more widely used (Reitan, 1966b) and it is now becoming known in educational circles (Hynd & Obrzut, 1981; Rourke, Bakker, Fisk, & Strang, 1983). Some writers on learning disabilities have claimed that no valid psychological tests yet exist to detect either brain dysfunctions or learning disabilities (Coles, 1978), but such writers must be unaware of the 40-year-old work of Benton, Reitan and many other research neuropsychologists (A. Smith, 1975; Teuber, 1964; Teuber, Battersby, & Bender, 1960) or they fail to relate it to the diagnostic problems facing the special educator.

To summarize, the neurologist and/or neurosurgeon can gain medical knowledge of the locus of a brain lesion by using radiological and other techniques and sometimes by direct observation during brain surgery. The neuropsychologist may predict the locus of the brain lesion by observing the pattern of cognitive and behavioral deficits as shown on a battery of neuropsychological tests and, by correlating these findings with the medical data, can recognize certain reliable brain–behavior relationships.

Once a body of principles (i.e., reliable human brain structure–function relationships validated empirically) has been established, then neurological inferences may be made with the neuropsychological test data alone. For years, neurologists have been localizing brain lesions prior to brain surgery on the basis of behavioral data. For example, the location of visual field defects (such as right or left, half fields, quarter fields) can tell the neurosurgeon prior to surgery where, in the optic nerves or tracts or occipital lobes, a brain lesion is most likely to be found and where he or she should explore (Kolb & Whishaw, 1990, p. 229; Manter & Gatz, 1961, p. 85).

Because most learning disabled children with cerebral dysfunctions never come to surgery, it soon became evident to clinical neuropsychologists that neuropsychological knowledge and assessment procedures would be an invaluable diagnostic method for better understanding the possible causal patterns of their learning problems. Reitan, as we have shown, in the early 1960s began to recommend a neuropsychological method to educators (Reitan,

1966a) and many of his students have incorporated it into their learning theories (Doehring, 1968) and promoted its use in special education (Gaddes, 1966b, 1968, 1969a, 1975, 1978; Knights, 1970, 1973; Rourke, 1975, 1981, 1985). The research of Satz and many other neuropsychologists has shown that sensorimotor and perceptual deficits, as measured by neuropsychological tests, are closely correlated with academic learning disabilities (Matthews & Folk, 1964; Matthews & Kløve, 1967), and that in young children they are reliable predictors of future learning disabilities (de Hirsch, Jansky, & Langford, 1966; Eaves, Kendall, & Crichton, 1972; Satz, Taylor, Friel, & Fletcher, 1978; Spreen, 1978).

The locus of lesion (left or right, frontal or posterior), whether it is focal or diffuse, whether, if it is a tumor, it is intrinsic (i.e., within the brain tissue) or extrinsic (sitting on the cortex), whether it is progressive (e.g., a tumor) or is subsiding (e.g., aftereffects of a stroke or hemorrhage), all these qualities will affect cognitive functioning differently. To relate these variables with any acceptable degree of reliability requires several years of training in neuropsychological assessment. If the school psychologist without this level of competence, or the educator or speech pathologist or other professional person, uses neuropsychological tests for screening learning disabled children, this is a justifiable procedure, but it should not be described as a "neuropsychological assessment," and any reference to brain dysfunctions should be carefully avoided. It becomes a neuropsychological assessment in a primary sense only when it is related to empirically derived medical data or draws on the tested clinical experience of a highly trained clinical neuropsychologist. If educators and others will be careful in their use of these test techniques they will avoid devastating and logical criticisms of the misuse of tests (Coles, 1978).

Arthur L. Benton, at the Medical School, University of Iowa, and Otfried Spreen, of the University of Victoria, have developed an interesting battery of tests to tap various neurosensory functions. In addition, Spreen and Benton have produced a detailed Aphasia Screening Test that has already been translated and standardized in a number of foreign languages, and normative data are available for children (Gaddes & Crockett, 1975) and for adults (Spreen & Benton, 1969/1977).

Following Hebb's early work at McGill University and the Montreal Neurological Institute, Brenda Milner and Laughlin Taylor and their colleagues developed a battery of tests designed to assess neurosurgical patients before and after brain surgery, but many of these tests are also useful for assessing nonmedical subjects with various types of cerebral dysfunctions (Taylor, 1979).

No attempt will be made to recognize all the researchers who have produced neuropsychological test batteries, but this list may be useful: Benton, 1962a, 1963b, 1967, 1969a,b,c, 1972; Benton et al., 1983; Kløve, 1963; Knights, 1971, 1973; Lezak, 1983; Milberg et al., 1986; Reitan, 1955b, 1956, 1959; Reitan & Davison, 1974; Rourke, Bakker, Fisk, & Strang, 1983; A. Smith, 1975; Spreen, 1969; Spreen & Benton, 1969/1977; Spreen & Strauss, 1991; and Taylor, 1979. The work in our own laboratory draws heavily on the Halstead–Reitan and Spreen–Benton batteries (see Appendix).

Cerebral Laterality and Behavior

As already explained, the brain is divided by the longitudinal fissure into the left and right hemispheres, and although these two halves appear histologically almost similar, or as "mirror mates," they are dominant for different types of behavior (particularly intellectual and cognitive behaviors) and equipotential, although contralateral, for most sensory and motor functions. A simple example of differential lateral control is the dominance of the left hemisphere for language in most people (even most left-handers) and the dominance of the right hemisphere for visual–spatial perception. An adult with a left-hemisphere lesion will usually obtain significantly lower scores on the Wechsler verbal tests than on the performance tests; a subject with a right-hemisphere lesion will usually show the reverse pattern, with lower performance scores (Reitan, 1955a). B. Milner (1968), a neuropsychologist at the Montreal Neurological Institute, demonstrated this laterality effect with an interesting study, in which she showed that patients with left temporal lobe lesions manifested demonstrable impairment of verbal memory but performed normally in remembering and recognizing faces in a delayed matching task. The right temporal lesion patients, by contrast, had great difficulty in remembering the same set of faces in a collection of photographs, although they showed no impairment on tests of verbal recognition and recall. Fedio and Mirsky (1969) showed the same laterality pattern with children aged 6 to 14, with unilateral epileptiform discharges localized in the left or right temporal lobe.

In the classroom a left-hemisphere lesion is more likely to impair performance in language, reading, writing, and verbal conceptualizing. By contrast, a right-hemisphere dysfunction is more likely to affect academic subjects drawing on spatial imagery, such as arithmetic, art, geometry, map reading, drafting, industrial arts, and sewing. Although a teacher will not use this type of evidence to localize a cerebral lesion (the neurologist will attempt that), if he or she is supplied with the knowledge of the locus and intensity of the lesion, the teacher can make sounder predictions about the child's potential ability and, with experience, may develop a more effective remedial program.

This recent neuropsychological insight of laterality of cerebral function and specific behavioral dominance has grown out of many researches, but one of the most interesting and definitive techniques used to examine this problem is the Wada Amytal Test. In the late 1940s, Dr. Juhn Wada, a research neurosurgeon, during studies on epileptic seizure mechanisms, injected sodium amytal and metrazol into the carotid arteries of human subjects. The left carotid artery runs up the left side of the neck and supplies blood to the left cerebral hemisphere; the right internal carotid artery does the same for the right hemisphere. Wada discovered that if the patient's left carotid artery was injected with amytal the subject usually became aphasic within a few seconds as a result of the effects of the drug in the cerebral blood stream. For several minutes, while the inhibiting effects of the drug were affecting the left cortical hemisphere, such patients, if they were completely left-hemisphere dominant for speech, were unable to speak, to understand what was said to them, to read, or to write. The patients might, however, be able to carry out nonverbal tests with pictures or cartoons successfully. Following right carotid amytal injection most patients may retain their speech and language functions but lose their visual–spatial perceptual competence temporarily (B. Milner, 1966).

In other studies, B. Milner (1966) carried out research with Wada's test to investigate short-term memory effects, temporary dysphasia, temporary facial agnosia, and retrograde amnesia, but so far this research technique has not been directed at classroom learning problems, except indirectly.

Visual–perceptual functions show a cortical laterality, and so too do auditory functions. The dichotic listening technique was introduced by Broadbent in England in 1954, and includes the simultaneous stimulation of both ears with different auditory messages. When the stimuli are verbal and balanced for initial consonant and equal length (e.g., "six" and "sin"), it is interesting that most people hear the word fed into the right ear, and tend to suppress the word stimulating the left ear. Kimura (1961a,b) was the first to relate the technique to cerebral asymmetry of function. Prior to this study, Broadbent had thought that the functional imbalance was caused by successive perceptual activity of the two ears. Kimura concluded from her study that both temporal lobes were essential to perception of verbal material, but that the left temporal lobe was more important. Because it is known that the auditory pathways from each ear are physically more strongly represented in the contralateral temporal lobe, Kimura reasoned that right-ear perceptual preferences occurred in most dichotically stimulated subjects because the left hemisphere is dominant for speech in most people. Although dichotic listening is not directly useful to the teacher of the child with a learning disorder, it has real value for the clinical psychologist in providing information on the hemispheric asymmetry and possible language dominance of the child (Strauss, Gaddes, & Wada, 1987). The clinician may need to supply this information to the neurosurgeon who is considering the possibility of removing temporal lobe epileptogenic foci; even when surgery is not considered, it may provide useful evidence on the cerebral dominance of a child who reverses letters in spelling or digits in compound numbers.

During the 1960s there had been occasional reports of contradictory findings but these were not satisfactorily explained because they were not clearly understood at that time. With the 1970s came findings revealing that lateral function was not rigidly tied to verbal and nonverbal processing, but that the brain reacted dynamically in terms of age (Bakker, Teunissen, & Bosch, 1976), sex (Buffery, 1976), stimulus complexity (Umilta, Bagnara, & Simion, 1978), and stimulus modality (A.E. Davis & Wada, 1977). These ideas are discussed at more length in Chapter 6.

Frontal Lobes

Cortically the frontal lobes include the brain tissue anterior to the fissure of Rolando and above the front parts of the temporal lobes. Below the outer layers of the cortex is the white neural tissue, which provides hundreds of thousands of interconnections to various areas of the opposite cerebral hemisphere (contralateral) and to various areas of the same hemisphere (ipsilateral). These numerous connections are believed to permit the variability and flexibility characteristic of rapid mental calculation, active imagination, and abstract conceptualizing.

The limbic system is located underneath and on the inside surfaces (the mesial surfaces) of the frontal and temporal lobes. This is a complex network of brain structures (cingulate gyrus, hippocampus, amygdala, uncus, etc.) that may be concerned with self-preservation (feeding behavior) and race preservation (sexual behavior; MacLean, 1959). It has also been thought to be involved in both emotional and intellectual functions, but its areas of behavioral control are not yet fully understood (Kolb & Whishaw, 1990).

The cortical motor strip, immediately anterior to the fissure of Rolando, is functionally the most clearly defined part of the frontal lobes. The left motor strip controls the voluntary muscular action of the right side of the body and vice versa. Figure 2.9 illustrates the motor speech area (Broca's area) and the left motor strip. A severe lesion in Broca's area may produce mutism, and a mild electrical dysrhythmia may result in an articulation problem (dysarthria). If the child is right-handed and has a mild dysrhythmia in the manual area of the left motor strip, he or she may have trouble writing and drawing because of a resulting manual clumsiness. Sometimes this type of interference in a child's learning is confused with mental dullness, when, in fact, his or her intellectual potential may be normal or above average. Muscularly awkward children may be mentally bright but impaired in classroom learning because so much of it requires motor-expressive activities. The teacher should try to decide whether the child's dysfunction is maximally sensory (input), intellectual (integration), or motor (output), or a fairly evenly distributed combination of two or three of these. If the dysfunction is in one motor strip, it is almost certain to show itself in motor impairment on the contralateral side of the body.

If, however, the lesion or dysfunction is in the frontal cortices anterior to the motor strips, it is more difficult to identify the behavioral effects related to these areas. In the past, a common belief has been that the frontal lobes are the seat of our highest intellectual processes, but neuropsychological research since Hebb's early work with Wilder Penfield (Hebb, 1939, 1945) and subsequent researchers (Luria, 1966, 1973; Teuber, 1959, 1964) have shown this simplistic interpretation to be unfounded. Teuber concluded that the "belief in the crucial dependence of higher intellectual functions on the integrity of the frontal lobes may have historical rather than logical reasons" (Teuber, 1959).

Numerous researchers during the past 30 years have revealed that damage or dysfunction in various parts of the frontal lobes can result in a wide variety of symptoms. These may include loss of fine motor movements, loss of muscular strength, poor movement control, poor voluntary eye gaze, impaired expressive speech, reduced behavioral spontaneity, reduced reasoning and strategy planning, perseveration in a test situation, failure to follow rules, poor associative learning, impaired recent memory, poor ability to estimate the frequency of a test stimulus within a specified period, impaired memory to direct oneself to follow specific test rules, poor delayed response, impaired spatial orientation, impaired social behavior, reduced olfactory discrimination, and altered sexual behavior (Kolb & Whishaw, 1990, p. 470).

In fact, individual cases have been reported in which patients with bilateral frontal damage have performed almost normally. Historically one of the most celebrated was the case of Phineas P. Gage, a young Vermont railway worker, who in 1848 suffered a bilateral frontal lobe injury in a blasting accident. A pointed crow bar, flung by the concussion, entered the left side of his face, passed through and upward, and emerged from the top of his head slightly to the right of the median line. On recovering from his head injury, he traveled with a road show and earned a good living for himself and his manager, although he suffered an explosive temper and other marked personality changes (Kolb & Whishaw, 1990, pp. 483–484).

Teuber (1959) reported the case of a man with a bilateral frontal pistol wound who "attacked one of the classical tests of concept formation [a modified Weigl card sorting test] with immediate and correct analysis of the three principles (color, form and number) built into the test." In our own research we have studied a man of bright mind and superior administrative abilities who suffered damage to his right frontal lobe. For several years he was a successful personnel manager in an industrial firm employing 2000 workers. Unfortunately, at age 52 he developed a large benign tumor in his right frontal lobe that was removed surgically. Although he still measured a verbal IQ in the superior range on the Wechsler Adult Intelligence Scale and talked fluently about all topics having to do with his work, it was necessary for management to retire him because of lost ability for subtle judgment, and for understanding of fine nuances of meaning in evaluating and handling social group situations.

B. Milner (1963) reported an interesting study suggesting that the dorsolateral parts of the frontal lobes are more important than other cortical areas for abstract tasks requiring mental flexibility and rapid *shift* to a new conceptual principle. Lesions in this area were more devastating to this task than those in any other cortical lobe or even the orbitofrontal (the parts of the frontal lobes at the extreme forward part of the brain and the undersides immediately above and behind the eyes) and temporal lobes together.

Occipital Lobes

In the posterior part of the brain are the occipital lobes (see Fig. 2.2), which are the cortical centers for visual experience. Area 17 in each occipital lobe is the primary visual sensory center, but the cortical areas immediately anterior to this are believed to be the visual association centers that provide "meaning" to what one sees. However, before discussing the evident relationship between the cerebral optic mechanisms and visual experience, it will be well to study the design of the cerebral visual neural pathways.

Figure 2.7 shows that the left occipital lobe is connected, by a circuitous route, to the left side of each retina. Similarly, the right occipital lobe is connected to the right side of each retina, and by this design the connections from the eyes contradict the usual contralateral connections of the sensory and motor tracts. That is to say, both eyes are connected to both occipital lobes; the usual contralateral design between hemisphere and the body does not hold. Light waves entering the eye stimulate a photochemical reaction in the retinal cells, the rods and cones. This process triggers neural impulses that travel along the optic nerves to the optic chiasma, which is located just in front of the pituitary gland. Here there is a partial decussation or crossing over of the nerve fibers so that fibers from only the nasal side of each retina cross to the other side. From the optic chiasma this new organization of nerve fibers connect to the lateral geniculate body, a sort of "junction box" in the thalamus. Here the optic fibers sweep forward and downward and then loop back along the outside area of the temporal lobes (the optic radiation) to the linings of the calcarine fissure, a part of the longitudinal fissure in the occipital lobes. It seems likely that the broad distribution of the optic pathways through every cerebral lobe is related to the sensitivity of many visual tasks to damage in any area (e.g., a figure–ground test; Teuber and Weinstein, 1956; Cruikshank, Bice, Wallen, & Lynch, 1957). The student who wishes a more detailed description of the structure and function of the visual mechanisms may see other sources (Netter, 1972, p. 63).

Although the visual pathways are clearly defined and micro-electrode studies in the occipital cortices have revealed a good deal about the point-to-point stimulation from retinae to visual cortex, overall cerebral function has been identified in more recent neuropsychological research.

The laterality effect of the right hemisphere, possibly the right temporal lobe, in visual–spatial perception has been mentioned. Kløve and Reitan (1958) studied 36 adult patients who were unable to copy a Greek cross without distorting the spatial configuration (see Fig. 3.2). Their results showed that the patients who had difficulty copying the Greek cross also did poorly on the performance tests of the Wechsler–Bellevue scale, tests that also demand visual–spatial–manual skills. Dysphasic patients did poorly on the Wechsler verbal tests, and a third group of patients with both difficulties had low scores on both parts of the Wechsler. The consistent inferiority of right-hemisphere lesion cases in visual–spatial tasks (Benton, 1963b; Kløve, 1959; Reitan, 1955a) implies

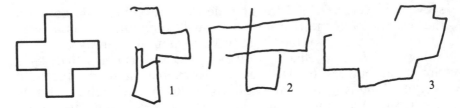

Figure 3.2. Attempts by three patients to copy the Greek cross (at left) in which the spatial configuration was distorted. (From Kløve & Reitan, *American Medical Association Archives of Neurology and Psychiatry*, 1958, *80*, 708–713. With permission of the authors and publishers. Copyright 1958, American Medical Association.)

that the occipital lobes may have a stronger functional relationship with the right side of the brain in most subjects, especially the parietal and temporal lobes, when a person is looking at nonverbal stimuli such as a map, studying a mechanical diagram, viewing a blueprint of a house plan, doing geometry, and attempting routine arithmetical calculations. The last-named task possesses a strong visual–spatial component; it requires one to write digits vertically to add; to write digits in a horizontal and vertical relationship to subtract, multiply, and divide; and to scan horizontally left and right from a decimal point. These procedures may be relatively simple for the average child or adult, but they may be difficult or almost impossible for the bright youngster with a right-hemisphere dysfunction.

An example should make this clear. A 17-year-old boy, whom we followed for 14 years, suffered, during birth, damage that affected the sensorimotor strips and the parietal cortex of his right hemisphere. As a result he has always had mild weakness of the left hand and foot. In addition, the permanent damage to the right temporal lobe is so severe that it evidently impairs his visual–spatial perception so that he cannot copy a simple Greek cross (Fig. 3.3). Artwork has always been painful for him, although because his left hemisphere is both intact and superior, he has always done well in reading, social studies, science, language, and verbal arts. Algebra has not caused him too much trouble, but geometry, because it is spatial, has been impossible. This boy, when first seen, was counseled away from spatial activities and toward verbal ones. As a result he completed high school, took a typing course, and is successfully employed as a clerical worker in a government office. His initial Wechsler IQs were performance, 69 and verbal, 110. Over the years these measures have shown marked stability, and as a young man in his late 20s, he still is unable to recognize or interpret geometric figures.

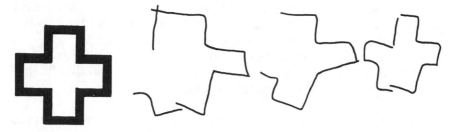

Figure 3.3. Three attempts to copy the Greek cross at left by a 17-year-old boy with a congenital right-hemisphere medial lesion. Notice the difficulty with the left side of the figure and the lack of continuity of lines.

This and many other cases suggest that our traditional school system, with its emphasis on reading and language skills, favors the child with a superior left hemisphere. A poor right hemisphere, as in the case above, may be a frustration, but it may not be a major academic handicap if a suitable remedial program is designed to meet it.

In Chapter 2, reference was made to Benton's (1963b, p. 5ff) categories of visual–perceptual errors common in a task of visual memory. Because it is important that clinical psychologists and teachers be aware of these, a brief description of them follows.

Omissions and Additions. When a person studies a geometric pattern for 10 seconds and then attempts to draw it from memory, he or she may omit one of the figures or part of one. Patients who have shown this difficulty have frequently had posterior cerebral dysrhythmias, suggesting that registration centers in the occipital and parietal lobes or some part of the optic mechanisms may be dysfunctioning or structurally lacking. In such a case it is possible that certain parts of the design are never accurately perceived and that the pattern finally reaching the occipital cortices has gaps, blind spots, or scotoma. Damage to the primary visual cortex may produce the same results. Obviously, the child can remember only what is impressed on his or her visual cortex and, if this lacks parts of the original pattern, reproduction will be inaccurate. The neurologist describes the process of memory as "neural storage." If the brain is healthy and whole it is well equipped to store a memory accurately with its transient electrical phase sequence and protein changes in the neural cell bodies; but if it is damaged or dysfunctioning, these electrochemical processes are less efficient.

Visual scanning may be difficult either peripherally (ocular muscle weakness) or centrally with a frontal lobe lesion (Karpov, Luria, & Yarbuss, 1968). Efficient scanning is necessary for accurate perception, memory, and reproduction, and if the clinical psychologist detects this trouble he or she should help the teacher devise suitable remedial measures to assist the child.

A child with defective perception and memory, who is trying hard to succeed and hence overcompensates, may add details that were not present in the original stimulus.

Distortions. A figure may be reproduced inaccurately by simple substitution (e.g., of a pentagon for a hexagon). Again this may result from dysfunction of the posterior part of the brain (usually some part of the parieto-temporo-occipital area) or the frontal lobes. As usual, there is a greater incidence of right-hemisphere lesions. When the cerebral dysfunction is disruptive enough, the child cannot copy the simple figure, even with unlimited time (see Fig. 3.3).

Perseverations. K. Goldstein (1939, 1942), in his study of head-injured veterans of World War I, described their tendencies of mental rigidity and perseveration. This symptom may result from the patient's simplified perception and memory and increased stereotypy of response because of his impaired cortex.

Rotations. That a subject will view a design and reproduce it in a rotated position is intriguing but so far inexplicable. For example, on the Benton test, where one is required to draw from memory a geometric design after viewing it for 10 seconds, a subject may draw the design accurately except that it is rotated to the right or left 45°, 90°, or 180°. Occasionally rotations of less than 45° may occur, which can happen with either memory reproductions or copying.

One of the most interesting cases of this in our own laboratory was a 15-year-old girl who suffered a cerebral hemorrhage in the deep tissues of the right occipital lobe. A neurosurgeon evacuated the large blood clot (intracerebral hematoma) with a small incision in the posterior part of the right parietal lobe. He was careful not to cut tissue in the occipital cortex because this might have resulted in "central blindness," showing itself in a dysfunction of the right halves of the two retinae, and a resulting left visual field reduction or some degree of blindness. Surgery was carried out but within a week another craniotomy was necessary to clean out the same right occipital–parietal area. This second treatment was successful and 4 weeks later the girl was ready for testing. A large and detailed battery of tests was carried out, among which was the Benton Visual Retention Test. She was able to remember the general shape and detail of 8 of the 10 diagrams, but there was a consistent tendency to rotate her drawings about 30° clockwise. This rotational tendency necessitated scoring those patterns as mistakes. This gave her a correct score of 4 out of 10 with 6 rotations. Six weeks later she was tested again and the rotational responses had disappeared and her correct score was now 6.

Three years later she developed seizures from complications following her brain surgery and, when tested on the Benton Visual Retention Test, she now had a correct score of 7, but two rotations had reappeared. On Benton's Embedded Figures Test, on the first testing a month after her surgery she showed great difficulty keeping her pencil on the dotted lines. She tended to draw her line to the right of the actual dotted line she meant to copy. This also seemed somewhat similar to her rotational tendency in a clockwise direction on the Benton Visual Retention Test, and with the normal rehabilitation of her brain following surgery this visual–motor impairment disappeared within 6 weeks on both tests.

This case provides evidence that is particularly interesting in the consideration of visual rotational responses. Why did this girl rotate the diagrams when tested soon after her surgically imposed brain damage? Also, why did she consistently rotate the figures to the right and outline figures with the pencil to the right of the dotted lines she was attempting to copy? Why had this visual–motor impairment disappeared on the next testing, which was 9 weeks after the second craniotomy?

Hypothetical answers can be proposed that may help the clinical psychologist and the special teacher to consider this problem more fully. It is possible that in this case, because the right occipital lobe was not functioning normally and this resulted in a reduced left visual field, there may have been an unconscious attempt to compensate for this imbalance and the girl distorted her perceptions so that the left side of the figures seemed, in retrospect, to be higher. Likewise, because the left occipital lobe was normal and operating with greater energy than the right, possibly the incoming images actually were tilted slightly to the right. Also, the swelling of brain tissue that frequently follows brain surgery may result in visual rotations; when the swelling disappears the rotations may also. Regardless of the cause, it is interesting to know that within 6 weeks her brain rehabilitated itself well enough to return her perception of horizontal to normality. When the seizure problem developed later with an epileptogenic focus in the right temporal lobe, the rotational tendency returned, but not seriously.

Visual rotations can also appear in an adult following a penetrating head injury. A man referred for neuropsychological evaluation had suffered a very severe head injury in which the left side of his skull was crushed. The frontal, temporal, and parietal lobes on the left side were all damaged, with the greatest injury in the left frontal lobe and temporal pole. A right temporal–parietal burr hole was made, indicating that there may have been some damage from pressure on the right side of the brain. On the Wechsler Block Design Test, which requires the subject to build a mosaic design while looking at the pattern, he rotated pattern 3, 90°, pattern 6, 180°, and pattern 10, 45°. All rotations were clockwise.

If a child is having difficulty with reading, map drawing, arithmetic, geometry, or any other spatial academic task, the possibility of visual rotation should be checked. The clinical psychologist may use a matching test, a copying test (e.g., Bender–Gestalt, Benton, Graham–Kendall), a visual retention test (Benton), the Block Design Test on the Wechsler, or any other suitable test in his or her repertoire. The teacher may notice the tendency in the child's artwork, printing, or writing of numbers, and if it appears serious, the child should be referred for neurological and psychological evaluation.

Visual Scanning. It must be remembered that visual perception probably never depends exclusively on the occipital cortices but includes a transcortically integrated function of these areas and other parts of the cerebral cortex and brainstem. A common neurological view, as already described, considers the occipital lobes (Area 17) as centers of visual sensation, but the parietal cortices bordering Area 17 as necessary to visual understanding and meaning. A study of a patient with a right parieto-occipital lesion (Karpov, Luria, & Yarbuss, 1968) showed that he still possessed normal active searching movements, but he lacked ability to synthesize what he saw. When presented with a detailed picture, Repin's "Unexpected Return," depicting the return of a prisoner to his family after many years of imprisonment, the patient, although previously familiar with this picture, which is famous in Russia, was unable to relate the parts. He commented: "This is a rather well known picture but I don't remember it. I don't remember its contents, as though I never paid attention to it before.... I think a father is returning home to his family after being away ... his children are sitting ... he himself ... the woman, probably the mother ... on the wall there are pictures, icons...." From this patient's report it can be seen that he was able to perceive individual objects but was unable to integrate these meaningfully. This is a sort of partial visual agnosia, and the patient was helped when the clinician asked specific questions, such as "How old is each person? How is he dressed?"

This case has relevance for the psychologist because some understanding of the more severe pathological cases, such as the one just described, will aid the clinical or school psychologist in a better diagnostic evaluation and the special teacher in a better remedial plan. The special teacher will rarely have a student with severe neuropathology, but children with minimal occipito-parietal dysrhythmias occur in some classrooms. Such children may have difficulty in producing meaningful stories about pictures, although the sensitive psychologist would need to experiment to discover whether this reflected a visual perceptive or linguistic deficit. Remedial measures with these children can include practice in looking at discrete objects, then two objects together with helpful questions from the teacher, cross-modal reinforcement with visual–tactile and visual–auditory associations, and finally increased multiple stimuli.

Temporal Lobes

The lateral cortical surfaces of the temporal lobes, as can be seen in Fig. 2.2, include the lateral surfaces of the cerebrum below the level of the fissure of Sylvius. The posterior boundaries, both between the parietal and between the occipital lobes, are arbitrary and are based on a localization of special functions. The surfaces are roughly similar in location to the ear protectors in a football helmet. A comparative neurological study of subprimates and primates, including humans, reveals that the temporal lobes do not occur in subprimates. The fissure of Sylvius, and its inner vertical surface (the temporal operculum), is just beginning to appear in small animals, such as the shrew and marmoset; it is more invaginated in monkeys; and is most deeply developed and differentiated in humans (Sanides, 1975).

On the undersurfaces of the temporal lobes, the inside or mesial surface next to the brainstem, are a number of different structures, known collectively as the *limbic system*. These include the hippocampus, amygdala, and uncus, (see Fig. 3.4). B. Milner (1954) reported that until her study of the functions of the temporal lobes in humans, completed in 1952, there were no such studies in the scientific literature. Whereas temporal function in subhuman animals had been studied, humans had been neglected.

Among the important behavioral functions dependent on normal temporal lobe function are auditory sensation, auditory and visual perception, long-term memory, and emotional response to perceptual experiences.

The acoustic areas of the auditory cortices are in Heschl's gyrus, or the superior temporal gyrus on the floor of the fissure of Sylvius.

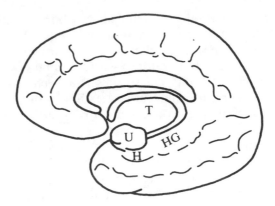

Figure 3.4. A simplified medial view of the human brain showing the location of the uncus (U), hippocampus (H), hippocampal gyrus (HG), and thalamus (T).

Connections from each ear go to both auditory cortices (see Fig. 2.8) so that unilateral temporal lobe damage does not cause deafness in either ear, and normal function of both ears provides the subject with cues for auditory localization. Because hearing is essential to the normal development of speech and because in most subjects the left hemisphere is dominant for language, normal temporal lobe function and left-hemisphere action are necessary for a child's learning to speak, read, and write normally. When the left hemisphere is damaged or dysfunctions, there may be impairment in the child's language development (aphasia), and when there is inferior temporal lobe function on one or both sides, he or she may suffer from some degree of auditory imperception or agnosia. Such disorders are often confused with mental retardation by the inexperienced clinical psychologist or special teacher. Aphasia is discussed at greater length in Chapter 8.

   B. Milner (1967) reported an interesting study in which 38 patients with temporal lobe lesions were given the Seashore Measures of Musical Talents. In all 38 patients the left hemisphere was dominant for speech; 22 had left-side lesions, and 16 right. The Seashore test includes six subtest measures of pitch, loudness, rhythm, time, timbre, and tonal memory (Seashore, Lewis, & Saetveit, 1960). That the right hemisphere is more involved in the perception of nonverbal material (Kimura, 1964; Spellacy, 1969) was supported by the left-hemisphere lesion cases' showing no change preoperatively and postoperatively for such stimuli when sections of the left temporal lobe were surgically excised. All pre- and postoperative changes occurred only in the right-hemisphere lesion cases and the most marked impairment was in the perception of timbre changes and the memory of sequential tonal patterns. Subsequent research suggests that this may result because the right hemisphere is specialized for analyzing harmonic information (i.e., the number and complexity of overtones) rather than general ability for the perception of music (Sidtis, 1980). Also, hemispheric specialization should not be considered as an immutable single dominant function; by increasing the complexity of the stimulus and the strategies of the perceiver, it is possible to produce a right-ear advantage for tones and a left-ear advantage for words on the first trials, but with continued trials, the expected ear advantages will emerge (Sidtis & Bryden, 1978). Because each ear is physically represented more strongly on the opposite side of the brain than on the same side, and a sound delivered to one ear alone excites more neural activity on the opposite side than in the same side (Rosenzweig, 1961), the right ear, in most children, is slightly more sensitive to verbal material and the left ear to nonverbal material (Kimura, 1964; Spellacy, 1969), as mentioned in the discussion of cerebral laterality effects.

Although both temporal lobes are involved in auditory perception, the left one is more concerned with verbal learning and the right with storage of nonverbal information regardless of the modality of presentation. Left temporal lesion cases have been found to be relatively poorer in verbal associative learning (Meyer & Yates, 1955) and for story recall (B. Milner, 1958). By contrast, right temporal lesion cases have shown disturbances in pictorial comprehension (B. Milner, 1958).

B. Milner (1958) has also found that left temporal lobe lesions affect verbal memory, whereas right temporal lesions affect memory for nonverbal material. Although the temporal lobes are important in mediating memory, other parts of the cerebrum are involved. More will be said about this subject in Chapter 8.

In summary, unilateral temporal lesions of the left hemisphere may result in difficulties of verbal recall and the understanding and retention of verbally expressed ideas (receptive aphasia). In dichotic listening experiments with normal subjects, it is usual for more words to be recognized by the right ear (contralateral) than by the left (ipsilateral), because most people are left-hemisphere dominant for language (Kimura, 1961a,b). However, this normal pattern is disrupted in cases of unilateral temporal lobe damage; in these cases better dichotic perception for speech stimuli may occur in the ipsilateral ear (Berlin, Lowe-Bell, Cullen, Thompson, & Stafford, 1972) when both ears are stimulated at normal and similar intensities. When the ipsilateral ear is stimulated below threshold, then the contralateral ear may approach normal function (Berlin, Lowe-Bell, Jannetta, & Kline, 1972).

Right temporal lesions are usually accompanied by impairment of spatial perception and imagery and the comprehension of pictorial material. Children with temporal lobe seizures tend to be more impaired than normals in stereoscopic vision (Webb & Berman, 1973). Whereas unilateral temporal lesions result in relatively mild or moderate memory deficits, bilateral damage to the hippocampal areas produces severe and generalized loss of recent memory.

Epilepsy and Brain Function

Because epilepsy is a disorder of youth (80% of epilepsy cases commence before age 18, Wada, 1978), it is important for teachers and parents to have some understanding of its nature and its treatment.

The human cerebral cortex is made up of an intricate three-dimensional network of billions of nerve cells, each having the capacity of self-firing several times per second. In the normal brain an integrated rhythmical pattern is produced, each cell generating a neural impulse in a smoothly timed sequence so that the impulses feed into other cells and other circuits in such a way that normal rhythmic patterns can be detected on the EEG. Sensory inputs, whether visual, auditory, or tactile, show themselves as volleys of electrochemical or neural impulses traveling to the brain along the optic, auditory, or cutaneous nerve pathways. Light waves impinging on the retinae stimulate the retinal cells, which in turn trigger neural impulses in the optic nerves, leading to the occipital lobes. Sound waves vibrating the eardrums in turn stimulate the sensitive hair cells of the inner ear (organ of Corti), which also trigger neural impulses in the auditory nerves, leading to the acoustic areas in the temporal lobes. Similarly, all sensory input is converted into irregular patterns of neural impulses, which are superimposed on the regular rhythmic patterns of spontaneous self-firing in the brain.

Sometimes, however, because of injury, infection, pressure resulting from a tumor or any abnormal growth, lack of oxygen, or high fever, an area of the gray matter may discharge volleys of impulses irregularly. Such an area may develop into a self-discharging electrochemical unit, or *epileptogenic focus*. Penfield has described this phenomenon: "In such an area or focus, excess electrical energy is formed and so, from time to time, unruly mass discharges may be released" (Penfield & Roberts, 1959). Such an explosive discharge may produce an epileptic seizure or fit and may be large or small depending on the extent and intensity of discharge. If it is minimal (petit mal) the patient's eyes may turn up involuntarily for a few seconds, resulting in brief inattention, but there is no loss of consciousness except possibly for a second or two. Such small seizure conditions may interfere with a child's concentration and productivity in school and may be undetected by a teacher with no knowledge of these conditions.

Because of the minimal signs of petit mal, they are often ignored or misinterpreted by teachers and classmates. Because the child so afflicted may appear to others as inattentive, disinterested, and mildly incompetent, he may be the butt of jokes from other children and the focus of adverse criticism from the teacher. Even some medical doctors have been known to fail in recognizing the condition and have referred the child for psychological assessment and treatment because of incorrigible and disruptive behavior, when, in fact, a thorough medical examination by a competent neurologist should have been the first step.

Grand mal attacks are more intense, they involve a loss of consciousness, and possess a typical behavioral pattern. Many victims of grand mal epilepsy experience an *aura*, which warns them of the imminence of the attack and enables them to sit down or lie down in a relatively safe place. Some patients have no aura and hence no warning. The nature of the aura differs in patients and may include brief mutism, involuntary motor movements, a "strange" feeling probably emanating from organic changes, some type of hallucination, or localized pain. Several children we have seen have complained of "feelings like needles" in the upper middle part of the abdomen just prior to a grand mal seizure. "The convulsion proper may begin with a loud cry, but this is more absent that present. Consciousness is lost either immediately after the aura or at the very beginning of the attack" (Brain, 1960).

With loss of consciousness the patient falls to the ground and goes into a muscularly rigid state (tonic phase), during which the jaws are clenched and breathing ceases for a few seconds or usually not more than half a minute. This stage is followed by rhythmic contractions of the muscles (clonic phase) during which the patient may bite his tongue, foam at the mouth, and fling his arms and legs out. During this period he may injure himself, but gradually the jerking movements grow weaker and finally cease. Following the seizure he may remain unconscious for up to half an hour, and on regaining consciousness may be fatigued and may sleep for several hours.

As in petit mal, grand mal produces the same social problems for the child or adult so afflicted, but they may be more intense. Sometimes teachers and others are fearful about the possibility of a grand mal seizure, and they imply rejection of the child either directly or indirectly. Sometimes even parents will not fully accept their epileptic child, which will certainly affect the child seriously and adversely. The physician should explain the condition fully to the parents and stress that it "is not contagious, and that there is no reason why the child should not mix with others. . . . Children with epilepsy should go to school. It is important that the principal and teacher know of the problem so that they can take appropriate steps in the event of a seizure" (Robb, 1981, p. 64). Persons with epilepsy will have numerous questions about schooling, occupational training, and social behavior (jobs? marriage? etc.). A well-informed counselor should be consulted so that the epileptic patient will not limit his opportunities unnecessarily.[2]

Various authorities have attempted to classify the epilepsies but because of their variability of etiology and description this is a difficult task. Many introductory books include the categories of petit mal, grand mal, psychomotor, and Jacksonian epilepsy. The last-named, first described by Hughlings Jackson, the famous nineteenth-century British neurologist, consists of a twitching of one side of the face or of a finger or arm on one side of the body. The motor activity gradually spreads in intensity and extent to include the whole side of the body. Interesting discussions of the epilepsies for classroom teachers have been made by Folsom (1968), Haslam (1975), and Jan, Ziegler, and Erba (1983).

Although these classifications may be expedient in the clinic, a classification having more useful information for the neuropsychologist may be in terms of whether the epilepsy is (1) *generalized* or (2) *focal*, as suggested by Hess (1966). In cases where a chain reaction of neural overexcitability spreads to include most or all parts of the brain there may be no brain lesion and hence no mental deficit when the patient is free of seizures. As is well known, many mentally superior professional people have suffered grand mal seizures. Julius Caesar, Lord Byron, Swinburne, Dostoevsky, and Guy de Maupassant are known to have suffered from epileptic attacks. Some forms of epilepsy are believed to originate in the brainstem or central parts of the brain (centrencephalic epilepsy), possibly in the subcortical, mesial, and basal surfaces of the frontal lobes (Hess, 1966). The generalized symptoms may result from the deep location of the point of origin and its spreading effect as it travels to the cerebral cortices.

---

[2] The U.S. Department of Health and Human Services has produced an excellent monograph for counselors: P. Robb, *Epilepsy, a manual for health workers*. Bethesda, MD: NIH Publication No. 82-2350. September 1981.

Focal epilepsy, by contrast, is stimulated by a lesion or epileptogenic focus on or near the cerebral cortex, which may be congenital (e.g., a cerebral growth anomaly) or a tumor or a scar resulting from actual brain tissue damage. Birth injuries, cerebral infections (e.g., encephalitis), or severe trauma followed by permanent neural destruction may produce various types of *posttraumatic epilepsy*. War and traffic head injuries have accounted for thousands of these cases, and "by far the most common form of focal epilepsy in the adult is temporal epilepsy" (Hess, 1966). A study of school-age children (aged 6 to 14) with either temporal lobe or centrencephalic epilepsy showed the expected verbal–spatial split in those children with unilateral temporal lobe disease. The split was not evident in the children with centrencephalic epilepsy, presumably because they possessed bilateral disturbances. However, they had difficulty in tasks demanding sustained attention (Fedio & Mirsky, 1969), possibly because of electrical disturbances in the brainstem.

Some examples may make this clear. For experimental purposes epileptogenic lesions have been surgically imposed on monkeys (Seino & Wada, 1964) and following the imposition of the brain lesion the animals were found to be inferior to normal monkeys in learning a spatial delayed and a delayed alternation problem. In humans, focal epilepsies have been shown to be related to inferior performance on tasks that regularly depend on the normal functioning of the cortical area locating the lesion.

A 40-year-old man seen in our laboratory had fallen down a flight of stairs and suffered a severe injury to the right side of his head. Neurological examination indicated a massive right-sided hematoma (large mass of blood resulting from a brain hemorrhage) and a craniotomy was carried out in order to evacuate the blood clot and free the brain from the abnormally increased cerebral pressure. Brain surgery revealed that the right temporal lobe was severely lacerated, and this extended back almost to the occipital lobe. Within a few months post-traumatic epileptic seizures began, although this man had no history of convulsions at any time prior to his head injury. The EEG revealed a moderate to severe dysrhythmia in the right fronto-temporal region, which resulted in two types of seizures: generalized convulsions that rendered the patient unconscious (grand mal) and a focal type of seizure involving the face and throat. Anticonvulsant medicines had reduced the grand mal attacks to about two a year, but he was bothered by the minor spasms affecting the right face and sometimes the left arm and leg.

A detailed battery of neuropsychological tests revealed that this man obtained a verbal IQ on the Wechsler Adult Intelligence Scale

(WAIS) of 108 but a performance IQ of 91. He had great difficulty with the tests requiring visual–spatial perception. Adaptive behavior in terms of inductive and deductive reasoning was impaired, and visual perception of figure and ground was below average. Auditory perception was normal, which suggested that the healthy left temporal lobe maintained normal function or that the acoustic area of the right temporal lobe was spared. Three-dimensional construction of a model with blocks was slow and included minor errors, suggesting mild right parietal involvement (Benton, 1968). This man's most marked mental symptom following his injury was his faulty short-term memory, which was a constant handicap. At work he would forget to carry out some duty he had been asked to do, and unless he wrote everything down and referred to the list frequently, he was constantly in trouble both at work and in his personal life. He still possessed bright-average verbal intelligence that resulted in considerable insight into his condition. This type of case is a reminder that certain seizure cases and those with a combination of above-normal, normal, and subnormal behaviors are difficult for most people to accept. These fluctuations of normality create much more tension than do the consistent shortcomings of the mentally retarded child: Others know what to expect from him or her (Ross & Ross, 1976/1982).

Although it is known that individuals with idiopathic epilepsy (i.e., epilepsy without known causes) may be mentally superior, as already mentioned, two neuropsychologists at the University of Wisconsin Medical Center, Kløve and Matthews, have made several interesting studies of large numbers of epileptic patients of different etiologies. Prior to their studies, most investigations had concluded that "the IQ's of institutionalized epileptics are generally lower than those found in non-institutionalized epileptics, and that the IQ's of non-institutionalized are comparable to those in the normal population" (Kløve & Matthews, 1966). Their study did not support this conclusion, chiefly because along with the Wechsler test (WAIS) they used the Halstead battery of tests, which is more sensitive than are standard intelligence tests to behavioral changes resulting from brain damage (Reitan, 1956). Halstead based his theory of testing on investigating "biological intelligence" (i.e., behavior depending more on adaptive abilities and sensorimotor functions) rather than "psychometric intelligence" (i.e., behavior heavily loaded with verbal learning and long-term memory). Measures of the former show greater deficits following cerebral organic damage; measures of the latter show greater resistance to brain damage, possibly because of the greater degree of overlearning. Consequently, Kløve and Matthews found that when they compared four matched groups—(1) a control group, (2) a group of verified brain-damaged patients without epilepsy, (3) a brain-damaged group with epilepsy, and (4) a group of patients with epilepsy of unknown etiology—the controls, as would be expected, were significantly superior to the other three groups on most measures. Group 4, the idiopathic group, was next, and the two brain-damaged groups were poorest. Of these two, the brain-damaged group with epilepsy was slightly better than the brain-damaged group without epilepsy, but the differences were not significant. This study, with sizable groups ($N = 51$ in each of the four groups) suggests that epilepsy in the majority of cases impairs most intellectual and sensorimotor functions, but when it is accompanied by verified brain damage, impairment is worse. In another study, Matthews and Kløve (1967) found no differences between the test performances of controls and patients with psychomotor epilepsy of unknown etiology (i.e., automatic behavior for which the patient is usually amnesic). These patients performed at significantly better levels than did patients with major motor seizures of unknown etiology. However, a teacher, ignorant of the nature of psychomotor epilepsy, might reasonably misinterpret a child's mental confusion that typically accompanies this form as inattention, stupidity, or incorrigibility. It is important that all teachers familiarize themselves with the various types of epilepsy so as not to misunderstand the behavior of children so afflicted.

In summary, it seems that epileptic patients of unknown etiology (idiopathic) may or may not suffer mental deficits.

Seizure conditions without any brain damage frequently do not impair learning except temporarily at the time of the seizure. Therefore an abnormal EEG by itself cannot necessarily be regarded as evidence of a disturbance causing learning disorders. In fact many epileptics with grossly abnormal EEGs are highly intelligent and have no particular learning problems . . . the evidence suggests that epilepsy is one manifestation of cerebral dysfunction, which, when no tissue damage occurs, may not impair learning at all, except temporarily. When epilepsy occurs with evident brain damage, the location and extent of the lesion, rather than the seizures, are chiefly responsible for the impairment of learning and behavior. (Gaddes, 1972)

Patients with post-traumatic epilepsy are most likely to suffer behavioral impairments in relation to the locus of the cerebral lesion. Most of these involve temporal lobe lesions or dysfunctions, and as a consequence the behavioral and mental effects are usually related to defective temporal lobe function.

Parietal Lobes

The parietal lobes, like the temporal lobes, appear to be essential cortical processsing areas for a great variety of distinctive behavioral functions, and lesions in these areas may produce a number of specific sensory and cognitive deficits.

Each parietal lobe is cortically bounded as follows: anterior boundary, fissure of Rolando, or central sulcus; superior boundary, longitudinal fissure; inferior boundary, fissure of Sylvius; and posterior boundary, the occipital lobe. Arbitrary boundaries between these natural borders are indicated graphically by dotted lines in Fig. 2.2. Just posterior to the fissure of Rolando is the postcentral gyrus that is known as the *somesthetic strip* (see Fig. 2.3) and is the primary receiving area for tactile sensations from all parts of the body. Because the tactile sense is the first sensory modality to develop prenatally (about the 49th prenatal day) compared with the vestibular (90–120 days), visual (180 days or earlier), and the auditory (210 days or earlier) (Gottlieb, 1971), its longer history appears to provide it with special value in sensorimotor remedial procedures, as we will see later in the book. Just as the motor strip or precentral gyrus is located on the anterior or frontal boundary of the fissure of Rolando and is contralaterally and inversely vertically related to motor functions in the body from head 'to feet, so the somesthetic strip in the anterior parietal lobe is similarly contralaterally and vertically connected to the tactile receptors throughout the body.

If the left hand is stimulated by a fine nylon hair (esthesiometer) it is usually maximally recorded in the right somesthetic strip, but a lesion in this area may reduce, obliterate, or distort the tactile input. The somesthetic strips are the primary projection or sensory areas of the two parietal lobes, and their normal function is essential to competent neuromuscular coordination and control. The remaining part of the parietal lobe has important integrative functions. It is involved in blending sensory information from a number of modalities into a single percept, and in coding the spatial location of sensory information. A third major integrative function is the formation of abstract concepts such as those involved in reading and arithmetic. It also forms the spatial coordinates that are the bases for one's "directional sense."

Books by neuropsychologists (Kolb & Whishaw, 1990; Luria, 1973; Walsh, 1987) provide detailed discussions of the neural structures and psychological functions mediated by these cortical areas. They are interconnected with the frontal, temporal, and occipital lobes, and to various subcortical centers, including the thalamus, the striatum, the midbrain, and the spinal cord. These neural connections with all the primary and association cortical areas and brainstem centers make possible a delicate integration of spatial imagery with all other sensory experiences, verbal and nonverbal memory, and language and motor functions.

Disorders of Tactile Recognition

The thumb, index finger, other digits, and the hand are all represented in the two sensory and motor strips (Fig. 2.3). This provides the experiencing subject with the ability to recognize form by touch alone. For example, if sandpaper figures are placed under a screen, the child may feel or palpate them and form a mental image from this source alone. This ability to recognize two-dimensional objects by touch alone is known as *stereognosis* and may include two-dimensional stereognostic recognition, such as reading Braille or figures outlined by differences in surface texture, (see Fig. 3.5) or three-dimensional stereognosis, such as re-

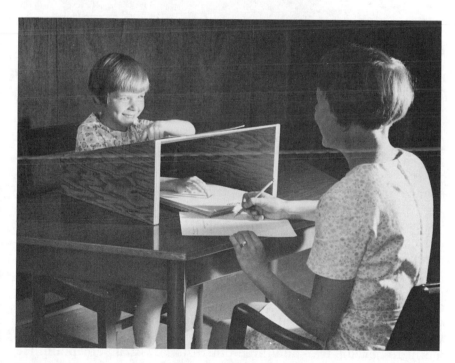

Figure 3.5. Stereognosis Test. The child is palpating a sandpaper figure under a screen with her right hand, and then points to a similar shape in an array of line drawings, with her left hand. This is a cross-modal test (from tactile to visual) that measures two-dimensional tactile perception.

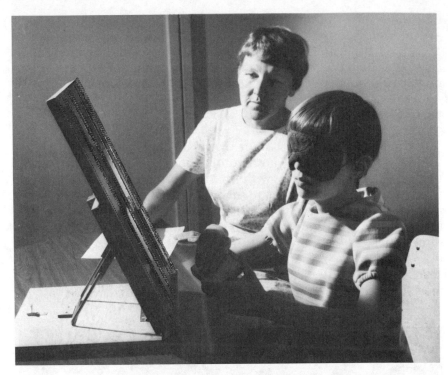

Figure 3.6.   An 11-year-old girl attempting the Tactual Performance Test from the Halstead–Reitan battery. This test makes a measure of three-dimensional stereognosis or haptic recognition and imagery. (From "A neuropsychological approach to learning disabilities" by W.H. Gaddes, 1968, *Journal of Learning Disabilities*, *1*, 523–534. Copyright 1968 by PRO-ED, Inc. Reprinted with permission.)

cognizing blocks by touch and replacing them in a form board (see Fig. 3.6). The latter type is also called *haptic recognition*. When lesions occur in the somesthetic strip and the parietal cortices adjacent to them, the person may experience difficulties in tactile recognition in the contralateral hand. With bilateral parietal lesions, stereognostic deficit may be experienced in both hands.

Stereognosis is an important sensory and perceptual source for all types of learning. The infant explores the world first by touch with both hands and mouth. By repetitive synchronization with the visual and auditory correlates of an object, the infant gradually learns to develop two- and three-dimensional visual perception. He learns to recognize his mother by the feel of her arms and face against him, the sound of her voice, and the visual topography of her face and figure. No doubt, olfaction and other senses reinforce this recognition, but it seems certain that touch, vision, and hearing are the major sense modes in learning. As the child grows, he learns to recognize books, dogs, chairs, tables, spoons, tricycles, and hundreds of other objects by feel, appearance, and sound, when sound is involved. Unconsciously he begins to use stereognostic knowledge independently or almost separately, when he hops on a tricycle and puts his hands on the handlebars and feet on the pedals without looking. We may learn to play the piano or finger a violin without visual cues. Later, as an adult driving a car, a driver will manipulate many hand and foot controls without taking his eyes off the road and will learn to recognize a dime and a quarter in his pocket by palpating them. Dressing will become a complicated but largely automated daily routine mainly dependent on stereognosis.

It is interesting that many elderly people, when their brains begin to deteriorate, gradually lose their ability to dress themselves. Presumably because of parietal lobe degeneration they have lost normal spatial imagery related to their own body-image and their perceived form and location of their clothes. This phenomenon is known as "dressing apraxia."

In the classroom, the child with a parietal lesion may have trouble with stereognosis and hence have difficulty in learning to spell, write, read, or do any academic skill drawing on reading and writing. Such a child, if mentally bright, may show superiority in discussions, oral composition, and dramatics, and because of this brightness may learn to spell and read through a visual–auditory match. Such a learning process makes less use of the tactile and kinesthetic input.

Such a case is rare, however. It is much more common to find the child with impaired visual perception or auditory perception, or both, but with average or better than average tactile imagery and recognition (stereognosis). This type of child will often have muscular clumsiness resulting in a "visual–motor disability" (e.g., difficulty copying spelling words from a book or chalkboard, hitting a nail with a hammer). To teach this child it is usually better to subordinate the visual and auditory experiences to the tactile. This type of child may be taught to spell by a technique emphasizing tactile–motor input (e.g., using a tactile alphabet, writing in damp sand with the index finger, writing spelling words in finger paints, with a felt pen, on a typewriter or computer keyboard). For many years, the Montessori system has stressed a multisensorimotor approach in learning to spell, read, and write, and no doubt gains much of its success because tactile recognition is grosser and more primitive than both visual and auditory perception and arises earlier in the child's developmental history. Most teachers of special education have discovered over the years that teaching a child with learning disabilities frequently succeeds when tactile emphasis is coupled with visual and auditory recognition. Ideally, the child's body image should include a smoothly synthesized input pattern of visual, auditory, and tactile stimuli.

Parietal dysfunction may result in graphesthesia (i.e., inability to recognize numbers traced with a stylus on the fingertips or palms of the hands), poor judgment of weights; inability to localize the point of tactile stimulation; finger localization (Benton, 1959; Benton et al. 1983); confusion in recognizing two-point simultaneous stimulation; and a number of specialized sensations to touch and pain that usually may be more interesting and valuable to the diagnosing neurologist than to either the clinical psychologist or the special educator. The neurologist draws heavily on almost pure sensory functions to localize lesions and diagnose neurological dysfunction. The special educator, by contrast, is not primarily concerned with pure sensory data (e.g., can the child hear pure tones at certain intensities? What is the child's threshold of auditory sensation? What is his or her tactile threshold?) but with learning disabilities for specific types of academic material. The neuropsychologist, although interested in both of these areas, is primarily concerned with perceptual, cognitive, and motor functions and how they are related both to neurological structure and function and to behavioral and cognitive impairment. For example, the neurologist may be able to state that a child has a left parietal lesion; the psychologist can say that the child has impairments in directional sense, finger localization, stereognosis in the right hand, and poor body image; and the teacher knows that the child is a poor speller and reader. The remedial learning program should be constructed around the data supplied both by the teacher and the psychologist, to avoid remedial programs based largely on trial and error and to develop instructional techniques based on both neuropsychological and educational data.

Neuropsychological Theories of Tactile Recognition

The classical view of astereognosis is that it is a form of tactile agnosia. According to this theory, perception requires two successive processes: first, primary registration of simple elements of sensation or tactile awareness, and second, integration of these elements into meaningful whole patterns that may be related to past experience and that are essential to perception and recognition. In the parietal lobe, sensation was supposed to have taken place in the postcentral gyrus or somesthetic strip and perception to have taken place in the "association areas" of the middle and posterior parietal lobes. As Teuber (1965) has pointed out, "The classical doctrine of agnosia was simple and eminently teachable," but recent research has thrown genuine doubt on this simple and structural view.

When the subject is unable to be sure if he has been touched on the hand, or his tactile threshold varies very unevenly across his hands or from finger to finger, then astereognosis may be suspected because of such a severe sensory defect. One cannot interpret when one cannot be aware. If a child possesses normal tactile sensation and still is impaired in perceiving differences in surface, roughness, texture, size, form, and pattern, then the classical view of astereognosis is untenable. Such cases, although rare, suggest that the processes of sensation and perception are separated and that different cerebral structures mediate them. Semmes (1965) investigated this possibility but found no support for the view that the "tactual association area" mediates shape discrimination selectively. She found that lesions in the parietal lobes did produce impairment in this perceptual ability, but so too did cortical lesions that spared the parietal lobes and the motor strips. In addition, Semmes carried out an ingenious search for a nontactual factor in subjects with tactile sensory defect. As a result, she found no significant correlation between astereognosis and hand-grip strength, finger tapping, intelligence as measured by the Army General Classification Test, ability to categorize on a sorting test, and dysphasia. She also found no correlations between spatial orientation and roughness, texture, and size discrimination, but she found a high correlation between spatial orientation as measured by route finding on a map and shape discrimination, and this relation held whether the maps were explored visually or tactually. From this evidence Semmes concluded that visual and tactual orientation are both related to stereognosis. When she examined the association between visual–spatial orientation in subjects with no tactile sensory defect, and also in subjects with a sensory defect of both hands, an interesting finding emerged. Those with sensory defect of the *left* hand only showed difficulty in stereognostic recognition, but those with a *right* hand defect were no different from those with no sensory defect of either hand. Because the right hemisphere is more involved in spatial perception, it seems logical that this functional asymmetry between the two hands should show itself, and it is interesting to know that this spatial function includes shape discrimination (stereognosis) as well as visual–spatial orientation. Semmes concluded that:

> The spatial factor (i.e., directionality in space) might enter into all performances which require appreciation of spatial arrangements, regardless of the modality transmitting the information. It is possible that this factor might be more important in tactual

than in visual form perception, however, since in the case of objects palpated, the spatial arrangement of the elements (and hence the form) must usually be reconstructed from a temporal series of partial impressions, rather than being simultaneously given as in vision. (Semmes, 1965)

Interestingly almost all auditory perception is sequential and has to be decoded in the brain as it is received, as in listening to a melody or in understanding oral speech. This process requires a normal serial order function of the brain, but more will be said about sequencing in Chapter 4. Nevertheless, whereas most visual perception usually involves scanning stimuli that are "simultaneously given," as in looking at an object or a map, some visual perceptual processes require successful serial order cerebral functioning, as in reading, walking, and driving a car. Luria (1973) described in considerable detail the holistic and simultaneous spatial sensations of visual perceptions and the temporal sequential neural input of verbal–auditory speech. This description led to a popular and simplified model among some professionals that described the left hemisphere as mediating sequential processes and the right hemisphere as subserving holistic perceptions. Das and his colleagues (Das, Kirby, & Jarman, 1979) developed this idea with a model of simultaneous and successive cognitive processes.

Disorders of Spatial Imagery

We have seen from Semmes's research, described above, that stereognostic perception, particularly shape and pattern recognition, seems to be strongly related to spatial orientation. Although much of spatial perception includes vision and is discussed earlier in this chapter, many nonvisual functions believed to depend on the parietal lobes are also involved. Benton (1969a), in discussing disorders of spatial orientation, listed these: (1) inability to localize objects in space; (2) inability to estimate the size of objects; (3) inability to judge the distance of objects from the observer; (4) impaired memory for the location of objects and places in recalling the spatial position of furniture in a room after leaving it; (5) inability to trace a path or follow a route from one place to another, as from one's hospital room to the physiotherapy room, or on a map from New York to one's home or to a named city; (6) reading and counting disability to the degree that reading and counting require comprehension of a spatiotemporal directional stimulus sequence; (7) incapacity to relate spatially separated objects or events to each other; (8) visuoconstructive disability as indicated by impairment in viewing a model and constructing an identical one when supplied with all the blocks (Benton, 1969b); and (9) disorders of the body schema, such as defective identification of the right and left body parts and impaired finger localization. These functions fall into two broad categories, those concerned with body awareness or *personal space*, and those having to do with perception of objects in space, *extrapersonal space*, although they are functionally related and appear to feed into one another. Parietal lobe lesions may disturb the body image and hence impair some or all of the spatial functions listed above.

Gerstmann's Syndrome

Between 1924 and 1930, Josef Gerstmann published several papers in which he related focal disease in the dominant parietal–occipital region (in the left hemisphere in most subjects) to a constellation of four behavioral deficits, namely right–left disorientation, bilateral finger agnosia (somesthetic inability to indicate accurately which fingers have been touched by an experimenter), agraphia (inability to write), and acalculia (inability to carry out arithmetical calculations). Although there appears to be a tendency for these four deficits to occur together in patients with left parietal disease, they sometimes appear in isolation or in partial groupings. This inconsistency led Benton (1961) to question the validity of the Gerstmann syndrome. He tested the hypothesis that if the four deficits comprised a natural constellation then they should show stronger associations among themselves than with symptoms outside the syndrome. In comparing them with constructional praxis, reading, and visual memory, he did not find that they clustered any more than other combinations. From this evidence he concluded that the Gerstmann syndrome was an artifact of selective perception. Nevertheless, the four behavioral deficits described by Gerstmann do seem related to left parietal dysfunction, and the syndrome is a firmly established concept in clinical neurology. Whether or not the Gerstmann syndrome is exclusive of other disabilities, it is a useful descriptive label because these symptoms so frequently occur with parietal pathology, particularly when it occurs in the language-dominant hemisphere.

Visual Defects

In discussing the occipital lobes earlier in this chapter, descriptions of cases with visual defects resulting from lesions in the parieto-occipital areas were presented. Parietal lesions themselves may produce various visual defects for at least two reasons. First, the posterior parietal cortices bordering on the occipital lobes are intimately involved with vision. Second, the optic radiations, as they bend back from the lateral geniculate bodies, connect through the subcortical white matter of the temporal and parietal lobes and terminate in the upper and lower lips of the calcarine fissure. Although the optic radiations do not lie in the parietal cortical tissue, they do occupy the white matter immediately below the angular gyrus on each side, and considerable evidence suggests that lesions in the left angular gyrus result in dyslexia (Benson & Geschwind, 1969; Russell & Espir, 1961), and unilateral parietal disease may result in agnosia and neglect of one-half of the extrapersonal space. For example, such a patient, if asked to make a freehand drawing of a daisy, may draw petals on only one side, neglecting them on the side contralateral to his or her parietal damage or dysfunction. Other visual defects that may result from parietal pathology are central or cortical blindness, hemianopia (possessing only half visual fields), difficulty in color naming, visual agnosia for objects, facial agnosia (common in senile patients, who may have difficulty recognizing members of their own families), loss of three-dimensional or stereoscopic vision, dyslexia (discussed in Chapter 8), inability to retrieve memories of visual images, and many others.

Warrington, James, and Kinsbourne (1966) found that drawings by adult patients with known brain pathology were impaired by unilateral lesions on either side, but each side showed different types of errors. Left-hemisphere lesion cases tended to widen all angles (e.g., in drawing a cube) and to put fewer details in a freehand drawing (e.g., of a house). The right-hemisphere lesion cases tended to reduce all angles, to show more asymmetry in their drawings, and to "doodle" or build up complex geometrical figures (Warrington, James, & Kinsbourne, 1966). Right parietal damage may impair the visual perception of fragmented figures, figure–ground discrimination, recognizing common objects when re-produced larger than life size, and recognizing an object in an unconventional view (e.g., photograph of a pail inside view and from above into its interior; Warrington & Taylor, 1973).

Apraxia

The inability to carry out specific neuromuscular acts at will is called *apraxia* and it appears to result from abnormal parietal function. *Ideational apraxia* is the inability to demonstrate how to use a common object, such as a hammer or toothbrush, when it is placed before the subject. The ideational motor patterns necessary to such demonstrations evidently draw markedly on the parietal lobes. *Ideomotor apraxia*, by contrast, is the inability to perform an intransitive gesture, such as saluting, waving goodbye, or pretending to comb one's hair with an imaginary comb. DeRenzi, Pieczuro, and Vignolo (1968) in Italy found ideational apraxia to be associated with left-hemisphere lesions, usually parietal. The reader will realize that ideomotor functions are essential to carrying out voluntary behavioral acts. Miming, for example, demands this function, so that one might conclude that superior parietal function, among other cerebral superiorities, is essential to a successful career in acting. A common need is *dressing praxis*, or the tactile and kinesthetic awareness essential to putting on one's clothes. Small children are usually unable to dress without help until about age 4 or 5, as every parent and kindergarten teacher knows, not because they lack the physical strength, but because they lack the necessary ideomotor images. In senility, with the breakdown of parietal cortical cells, old people also may suffer from *dressing apraxia* and need help as they did as small children.

Integrating Function of the Parietal Lobes

In Chapter 2, the "tertiary cortical zones" were described as:

> the zones of the posterior regions of the brain that lie at the boundary between the occipital, temporal and postcentral regions of the hemisphere, where the cortical areas for visual, auditory, vestibular, cutaneous and proprioceptive sensation overlap. (Luria, 1973)

The reader will realize that the parietal lobes are the center of all this cortical organization. The transcortical connections of millions of short axons provide the physiological bases for an analysis and synthesis within a sensory projection area (e.g., within the visual or auditory cortex) and an integration between these areas (e.g., cross-modal function). Many writers have considered the angular gyrus and the immediate cortical areas vital in mediating these intersensory functions (Benson & Geschwind, 1969; Déjerine, 1892; Geschwind, 1965), lesions of these areas do not produce disturbances specific to vision, audition, or tactile sensation but do disrupt the integrated reception and analysis of information. Probably the most common behaviors disrupted in this way are reading, writing, and all forms of perception involving spatial imagery. Neuropsychological studies of adult patients with parietal damage, compared to patients with lesions in the frontal or temporal cortices, show them to be impaired on all cross-modal matching tasks, even though each sense mode by itself was functioning normally (Butters & Brody, 1968). These same investigators concluded that auditory–visual cross-modal tasks depended more on the left parietal lobe, and more is said about this in Chapters 8 and 9 in discussing the neurological bases of reading and writing. Nonverbal spatial reversible operations (e.g., "You are to make your stick pattern look to you like mine looks to me") appear to draw more on the right parietal lobe. The "left may be more crucial than the right for cross-modal associations while the right plays a slightly more dominant role than the left in the performance of spatial rotations" (Butters, Barton, & Brody, 1970).

In summary, the anterior portion of the parietal lobes, immediately posterior to the sensory strips, is primarily involved with somatic sensation and perception. The posterior portion is specialized for integrating and analyzing sensory input from the somatic, visual, and auditory areas of the cerebral cortex. In addition to integrating information, it is involved in cognition—that is, in understanding and giving meaning to sensory input. The posterior portion of the parietal lobes is also involved in giving sensory events a spatial location, and in controlling and guiding the body and its parts relative to the immediate extrapersonal space. It also seems to be involved in mediating abstract concepts that are required in reading and mathematics, as well as in the mental manipulation of spatial coordinates (e.g., drawing an object from another person's perspective). Because of this complex integrative and interpretive role, lesions in the posterior portions of the parietal lobes may significantly influence performance on tests of cognitive ability. "Relative to other cortical regions, the loss of the posterior parietal area probably has the most debilitating effects on a person's intellectual life, especially if he or she loses the ability to understand abstract concepts" (Kolb & Whishaw, 1990, p. 420).

Environment, Learning, and the Brain

So far we have examined cases of brain damage or dysfunction and how these pathological processes can result in deficits in behavior. This influence is from *brain to behavior*. But the brain–behavior relationships *are not unidirectional*; they imply a two-way process. Although the influence of brain changes affects behavior potently and immediately, environmental influences can affect structural and functional changes in the brain, although many of these may be minimal and subtle and take considerable time.

Probably the quickest environmental alteration in the brain and CNS occurs in classical conditioning. Pavlov working with animals

(1928) and J.B. Watson working with children (1919) showed that fear can be established in two or three associations with a loud noise. The exact nature of the neurological change was not clear, but the involuntary fear response that followed the cue, after a few treatments, seemed to be evidence that a change had taken place in the CNS and that it was persisting.

More recent research with animals shows that environmental stimulation can result in increased growth of brain structures, and conversely, prolonged environmental deprivation can modify and reduce cerebral growth. In one such experiment (Rosenzweig, 1966), litters of rats were divided at the time of weaning (about 25 days postnatally) and kept either in an enriched or an impoverished environment. In the enriched situation the animals were housed in groups of 10 to 12 to a large cage that had ladders, activity wheels, boxes, and platforms. The rats in this group were given free play and formal training sessions. These animals enjoyed stimulation from their cagemates, their supervised training, and their complex environment. Each of these rats had a littermate assigned to the impoverished condition, where the animals were in solitary confinement in small cages with solid walls. No training or stimulation was given these animals and they were deprived of social contact with any other animals. After 80 days the animals were sacrificed and their brains examined. The 130 littermate pairs showed that overall, the cortex of the enriched rats weighed 4% more than the cortex of the impoverished rats ($p < .001$) and was also thicker. Also, enzymes that facilitate the production of neurotransmitters at the synapse were more plentiful in the brains of the enriched rats. "An enriched environment after weaning, increases, respectively, the number of dendritic spines and the dendritic branching of cells in the rat cortex" (Berlucchi & Buchtel, 1975). "This type of evidence suggests that rather than being fixed and pre-determined, neural mechanisms are responsive to and capable of being shaped by a variety of external factors" (U. Kirk, 1983a).

Let us now move up from rats to monkeys for an example of how experience can modify the brain's wiring. From the retinal cells (rods and cones) in the primate brain to the visual cortex, neural impulses travel along a tract of six synaptically connected neurons. In these optic pathways, impulses come from stimulation of either the left eye or the right. The slightly different views of the world from each eye are not merged until after the impulses reach the sixth-order nerve cell in layer IVc of the visual cortex (Calvin & Ojemann, 1980). Cells in the layers above, the outer cortical layers, contain neural cells sensitive to input from *both* eyes, and it is in these layers that convergence takes place and stereoscopic vision is made possible. Calvin and Ojemann (p. 122) describe an experimental situation in which a frosted contact lens is alternated daily from one eye to the other in an infant monkey, thus making normal binocular vision impossible. The cortical cells that are wired to respond to both eyes never get a chance to react normally; instead they become habituated to one eye or the other. If in the monkey's adolescence or young adulthood (about 9 months of age) the contact lens is discontinued, the ability for both eyes together to stimulate the cortical cells is almost completely lost, permanently. Evidently the early months postnatally are critical to ensure normal and optimal environmental modifying of the brain's wiring.

Although radical experiments are possible with subhuman animals, they are not with human subjects. However, "studies of . . . a number of species will provide some basis for tentative extrapolation of the curves of phylogenetic development through chimpanzee to man" (Hebb & Thompson, 1954). Such extrapolation has obviously led to the infant stimulation programs practiced in children's hospitals and recommended to young parents. This area of investigation provides some of the neurological knowledge on which to develop theoretical models of learning for the normal child and adult, and rehabilitation procedures for those suffering from various types of CNS damage and/or dysfunction.

Summary

This chapter, in retrospect, may seem paradoxical. We set out to stress the unitary action of the brain and then supply evidence for lobular and hemispheric specialization, *but the reader will understand that brain function is both holistic and localized.* Although Flourens in the first half of the nineteenth century believed in the unitary activity of the brain, after 1850 belief increased in specific cerebral localization. This view was reinforced by the continued influence of phrenology; Broca's celebrated discovery in 1861 of the relation between mutism, or expressive aphasia, and a lesion in the third frontal convolution of the left hemisphere; the improvement of the microscope, and the consequent increased knowledge of nerves and neural connections; and the discovery by Hughlings Jackson in the 1860s of the relation between unilateral cerebral disease and one-sided convulsive movements on the contralateral side of the body. In 1870 Fritsch and Hitzig electrostimulated the cerebral hemispheres of dogs and learned a great deal about the behavioral relationships of the motor strips. This led to many similar studies in other animals, including monkeys and later, humans, and by 1900 the projection areas of the cortex were known, that is, the motor strips, somesthetic strips, acoustic areas, and visual centers of the occipital lobes (Tizard, 1959).

In psychology and physiology from about 1890 to 1930, Pavlov's reflexology, J.B. Watson's behaviorism, and E.L. Thorndike's connectionism dominated North American psychological thought. This approach conceived of nervous action as *linear* and mechanistic (the telephone model) and it tended to favor a localization view in neuropsychology. As is well known in the history of psychology, however, the imaginative researches of the Gestaltists and the brilliant work of Karl Lashley during the 1920s were among the major influences in support of unitary function of the brain. Lashley's work spoke forcefully against a segmental cerebral function. Although he started his studies under Watson about 1914 and hence believed that the linear reflex arc was the unit of all behavior, Lashley's researches after 1917, when he first met Franz, led him to the belief that behavior might be controlled by widely separate cerebral loci and prompted him to produce his theory of cortical *equipotentiality* and *mass action*. Although *projection function* (i.e., the action of the three sensory and one motor cortical areas) is localized, even it shows some within-area variability in the rat. For example, even in the motor strip the same center at one moment may stimulate a finger, at another time another finger, and at yet another time the shoulder. He concluded that *projection function* is localized, although not rigidly, but *correlation function* (i.e., the neural action of the remaining association cortices) is not.

Judson Herrick (1944) wrote:

> Integration of bodily activities is a primordial essential; without it no living body can survive. . . . No local activity of sensorimotor type can be carried on by well-insulated autonomous reflex arcs as these have been conventionally described. *There are no such reflex arcs in the amphibian nervous system.* There are reflexes, because of a pathway of preferential discharge, but there is a spreading effect, and accompanying the response there is also excitation of much nervous tissue not involved in the overt action.

Hebb (1949) was one of the first psychologists to see the efficacy of accepting both concepts, Herrick's "pathway of preferential discharge" (a kind of connectionism) and the field action of the cell assembly. Geschwind (1965) more recently has proposed the concept of the "cerebral disconnexion syndrome" in explaining aphasia, apraxia, dyslexia, and agraphia. Essentially this is a more recent version of earlier connectionist models, in which destruction of transcortical or subcortical pathways joining two functional centers in the cortex produces an isolation of those centers or impairs the normal interaction between them. Coulter, a pediatric neurologist, uses this same concept to explain learning disabilities in children. He proposes that "functional hypoconnection of cerebral cortical regions important for cognitive growth could result from relative underdevelopment of specific cerebral association fiber pathway systems necessary for learning. Hypoconnection could reflect decreased myelination, axodendritic underdevelopment, synaptic dysfunction or neurotransmitter abnormalities" (Coulter, 1981). In simple language, this means that a lesion in one cerebral locus may incapacitate two or more other centers remote from it, even though the tissues of those centers themselves may be healthy and undamaged. In spite of this complex and dynamically variable action of the brain, a lesion in some specific loci tend to have a reliable result.

Diffuse left-hemisphere dysfunction is likely to impair verbal abilities and cause them to be inferior to visual–spatial and constructive functions. However, localized left-hemisphere lesions, depending on their location, may have little or no effect on verbal skills. A 12-year-old boy seen in our laboratory had the front third of his left temporal lobe removed surgically, and postoperatively he obtained a WISC verbal IQ of 116 and a performance IQ of 97 even with left-hemisphere language dominance. Because no language areas of the left hemisphere were seriously affected by the surgery, he retained much of his preoperative verbal superiority, but because he had to learn to write and manipulate objects with his left hand following a postoperative hemiparesis on the right side (partial paralysis of the right hand), his slowness on coding and object assembly pulled down his performance IQ. This is a good case to caution us against making quick or superficial diagnoses from knowing the site of the lesion. The verbal–spatial–left–right dichotomy usually holds in adults and older children, but a focal lesion requires more knowledge before statements can be made about probable behavior. Similarly the neuropsychologist cannot deduce the side of the lesion *only* on the basis of a verbal–performance imbalance on the WISC.

Although parietal lobe lesions usually impair the subject's directionality, this does not always hold. In our laboratory we have encountered two adult patients with space-occupying parietal lesions who both pre- and postoperatively obtained perfect scores on Benton's Right–Left Orientation Test. Such seeming contradictions require more knowledge of the exact locus of tissue damage and the quality of performance on the test.

Another patient, aged 20, following the surgical removal of her right parietal, temporal, and occipital lobes, was still able to do simple route-finding problems and locate major cities on a map of North America, although her spatial–perceptual abilities were impaired. Her WAIS performance IQ was only 77, although she could still obtain a nearly superior verbal IQ of 117.

The two cases above, though contradicting what we would expect using the classical model of brain function as a basis of prediction, are useful as a caution against quick and simplistic diagnoses. In both cases, more knowledge accounted for the seeming paradoxical behavior, in the form of localized lesions that spared essential neural pathways and compensatory learning strategies acquired by the patients.

Clinical Addendum

What the Clinical Psychologist Can Do

Using a detailed battery of neuropsychological tests has the advantage that it provides numerous measures of sensory, cognitive, motor, sensorimotor, and serial order behaviors. The psychologist familiar with such a battery soon learns to read the test profile and to hypothesize that the cerebral area of dysfunction is likely to be central or peripheral, cortical or subcortical, and diffuse, regional, or highly localized. He or she proposes a diagnostic hypothesis from this knowledge of specific brain–behavior relationships.

Let us look first at an adult case of traumatic head injury. This young man had successfully completed the freshman year of university and so it seems safe to conclude that, pretraumatically, he did not suffer from a severe learning disability.

Clinical Case Findings

Male; age 21 years; tests administered 3 months posttraumatically.
Wechsler Adult Intelligence Scale: Verbal IQ, 95; range of verbal subtest scores, 8–11; performance IQ, 59; range of performance subtest scores, 4–5.
Halstead Aphasia Screening Test: Verbal responses, average to above average; drawings, inferior.

Visual Perception: Visual–motor tasks, poor; imbedded figures, weak.
Nonverbal sound recognition and phonetic discrimination, poor; oral
    repetition of sentences, normal.
Stereognosis: Right hand, near normal; left hand, inferior.
Finger localization: Right hand, one error; left hand, three errors.
Right–left orientation: Very poor, many reversals.
Finger tapping: Right hand, slow; left hand, inferior.
Discussion: The test data suggest that this young man suffered a very
    severe head injury, with bilateral dysfunctions but maximal impair-
    ment in the right hemisphere.

These tests were administered 3 months after the injury, and that
he still showed so much perceptual and motor impairment tells us
the injury was very severe.

Even so, there are some hopeful signs. That he could score in
the normal range (although in the low side of that range) in spatial
inductive and deductive reasoning (Halstead Category Test), in
common arithmetical problems (Wechsler arithmetic) and abstract
verbal conceptualizing (Wechsler similarities) strongly suggests that
large areas of healthy cortical tissue were spared. In addition, the
above-average performance on the Weschsler Comprehension
subtest provides some evidence of retained integrative mental
functions.

The signs of impairment are many. The consistent relative
inferiority on the Wechsler performance scores, the visual perception tests, and the many inferior scores on the left hand are typical
of right-hemisphere damage and resulting dysfunction. The left
hemisphere did not escape completely, however, because his
verbal IQ of 95 is much lower than measures made when he was in
elementary school (Grade 3 IQ, 112; Grade 6 IQ, 115). Also, his
inability to do serial order tasks (Wechsler Digit Span and Digit
Symbol; Seashore Tonal Memory; Reitan Trail-Making Test)
strongly suggests left-hemisphere damage and/or dysfunction. Also,
both hands were below average in their performances on the
Benton Stereognosis Test, Benton finger localization, Benton
Right–Left Orientation Test, finger tapping, and hand-grip strength.

Medical History

The deductions about brain damage so far in this case have been
made purely from the psychometric data. Let us see how this
record is complemented by the medical history. The neurologist
reported: "This young man was in an automobile accident in which
he suffered a depressed skull fracture in the left frontal area. He
was brought in to the hospital in a completely comatose state and

was completely unresponsive even to painful stimuli (pinpricks in his hands and feet). His arms and legs showed a neuromuscular rigidity (hypertonicity) that indicated bilateral brain damage. He was unconscious for almost 3 weeks, and when he first regained consciousness he was mentally confused." His speech was slurred and still was when he was tested 3 months later. He was hospitalized more than 2 months, and when he was finally able to walk, his gait was unsteady and poorly coordinated. His EEG showed generalized bilateral disturbance with greater dysrhythmia in the left frontal and right parieto-temporal–occipital areas.

Combining the information from both the medical and neuro-psychological data, it seems almost certain that the severe impact to his head on the left frontal side of his skull had a *contre-coup* effect in which the concussion traveled through to his right hemisphere, where most of the damage occurred. The left frontal damage seems to be related to his slurred speech (Broca's area) and his problems with sequencing, and the right-hemisphere damage is most likely correlated with his poor visual–spatial–constructional skills.

Follow-up

This young man was clinically followed for 6 years with periodic test measurements and is still contacted intermittently in connection with his occupational placement. On the Wechsler he showed a pattern of improvement listed in Table 3.1.

On the last Wechsler (WAIS) administered, 6 years and 1 month posttraumatically, his above-average scores were:

Arithmetic	15
Comprehension	14
Vocabulary	13

Table 3.1. WAIS Results

Posttraumatic testing times	Verbal IQ	Performance IQ
3 months after trauma	95	59
8 months after trauma	106	89
15 months after trauma	102	91
2 years and 4 months	100	94
6 years and 1 month	112	90
Mean IQs	103	84.6

Information	12
Similarities	12
Block design	12
Verbal IQ	112
Performance IQ	90

All other subtests were below average, presumably from the permanent brain damage. However, the general test profile shows him to be verbally mentally bright.

He still suffers from minimal balance problems, although he has learned to water-ski again, something that he enjoyed prior to the accident. His speech is permanently slurred and this has proved a handicap in job interviews because it has sometimes been mistaken for mental retardation and/or drunkeness. This young man took several years to adjust his vocational aims from a professional level to a type of work he could enjoy and at which he could be successful. He could handle his first job as a filing clerk because of his above-average verbal intelligence, but he disliked the tedious routine and the confinement of an office. Preferring outdoor work, he took a professional gardening course, and eventually he was hired as a gardener by a city parks board. He has subsequently married and made a good adjustment to his injury.

A Cautionary Note to the School Psychologist

In this chapter the major part of the discussion has focused on cases of brain damage or localized cerebral dysfunction, because an introduction to organically based LD students is easier to understand with these types of cases. Although these are selected because of their pedagogical usefulness, the reader will remember that they occur in only a minority of cases (probably 2% to 3% of the elementary school population). Such cases fit our category 1 (see Table 1.1). The subjects in the second category (MBD) may have CNS lesions or dysfunctions, but as we have seen, it is frequently difficult or impossible to be sure. Category 3 has subjects with no evidence of brain dysfunctions, and they include most of the LD children seen in a large elementary school. Thus, although most LD children have no clear evidence of specific brain lesions, they may exhibit subtle perceptual or motor deficits that suggest possible cerebral dysfunctions, and to analyze a minimal learning problem it is often useful to understand more severe cases of impaired cognitive processing. As we have observed before, the school psychologist with competent knowledge of

normal brain function and dysfunction is likely to be better prepared to propose realistic hypotheses for remediation. But we must
be reminded that conclusive brain lesions occur in a minority of
LD cases, and the school psychologist should guard against looking
for brain damage or neural pathology in every case of academic
underachievement.

What the Teacher Can Do

The case of traumatic brain damage in an adult described above
is likely to be of more interest and use to the teacher in a
high school, a college, or an adult rehabilitation center. We have
chosen adult cases to examine first because they do not have the
complicating developmental changes that are typical in childhood.
Even so, many of the same remedial measures used with children
are useful with traumatically brain-damaged adults because their
cognitive skills may have been temporarily repressed and con-
strained at a childish level.

In the case of our young man, there were several positive indications for the remedial teachers and therapists. Chief among these
were (1) his cheery personality and his cooperative acceptance of
direction (frequently right-hemisphere lesion cases react euphori-
cally); (2) his above-average verbal intelligence; and (3) his
supportive family.

The program of remediation included speech therapy; exercises to improve visual discrimination, visual–motor speed, and
accuracy; phonetic discrimination and oral verbal memory; tactile–
kinesthetic (or haptic) recognition; large- and small-muscle activities to enhance his sensorimotor integration; and reading and
writing. Specific remedial activities have not been listed because
they should be selected in each case by the therapist and/or
remedial teacher, but the areas needing attention were indicated
by the neuropsychological test battery. Also, the teachers and
therapists were provided with the medical and neuropsychological
findings, and the expected pattern of competent and deficit behaviors. This information supplied a better basis for their continuing program evaluation of the case and the possible prognosis.
His increase in verbal IQ from 95 to 112 six years later suggests
that the activation of his brain and neuromuscular system may
have had some restorative value.

4 Perceptual Disorders

. . . the input is never into a quiescent or static system, but always into a system which is already actively excited and organized. In the intact organism, behavior is the result of interaction of this background of excitation with input from any designated stimulus. Only when we can state the general characteristics of this background of excitation, can we understand the effects of a given input.

Karl S. Lashley, *The Hixon Symposium* (1948)

The education of children with perceptual handicaps . . . is the most technical of all aspects of teaching. It cannot be taken for granted that any teacher can teach these children on the basis of the usual teacher preparation or special education teacher preparation programs. Teachers of children with perceptual developmental problems must be skilled diagnostic and educational technologists as well as excellent teachers.

William M. Cruickshank (1975)

Teachers characteristically have directed their pupils to "pay attention" or "settle down and concentrate" when they wished to communicate a new idea or concept. The simplistic implication is that if the pupils pay attention to the teacher's statements (that is, open up their receptive apparatus in some unexplained way), that learning will take place. Unfortunately the process of learning is not that simple.

Since the beginning of the gradual integration of neurological, psychological, and educational knowledge in the early 1960s, it has become useful for both psychologists and teachers to use the neurological model of behavior for diagnostic understanding. As described in Chapter 2, in this model there are three areas of neurophysiological functions: (1) sensory nerve function, (2) cerebral or brain function, and (3) motor nerve function. The first of these includes the afferent nerves leading from the sense organs (chiefly the eyes, ears, and touch receptors in the skin) to the brain. Once the various nerve patterns reach the brain they are decoded, integrated, and reorganized; some are stored, others are retrieved from the brain's data bank. Finally, they are encoded into the nerve pattern to travel down the motor nerves to the muscles, tendons, and skeletal connections. Observed behavior is actually the neuromuscular activity resulting from the expression of the nerve patterns traveling along the motor or efferent nerves to the effectors. The behavioral correlates of these neural events are (1) sensation, (2) cognition, and (3) response. Although this mechanistic view of behavior is useful for diagnostic trouble shooting, it must be remembered that all behavior is holistic and involves all three areas interacting and operating simultaneously. More will be said about this subject later in the chapter.

Sensation

It may be useful for the special educator to have a clear and workable though simplistic concept of sensation, in contrast to perception. Sensation may be thought of as the sensory awareness of simple elements of experience in the "distance senses" of seeing and hearing and the "skin senses" of touch, warmth, cold, and pain. Examples of these stimuli are spots of light on a screen, a tone on an audiometer, or the pressure of a fine nylon hair on a finger. In such experiences the subject has only to report when he or she has the sensation of the light, or the tone, or the physical pressure. These stimuli can be started at a weak level of intensity below the threshold of sensitivity (i.e., subliminally) and increased systematically to a level where the subject will report first being aware of the stimulus. In such a situation, known as the study of psychophysics, a known physical intensity is related to a reported subjective experience. In neuropsychology this can be a useful technique for inferring the presence and locus of a brain lesion.

Hebb (1958/1966/1972) has described the neurological substrate of sensation as involving the activation of receptors "and the resulting activity of afferent paths up to and including the corresponding cortical sensory area" (1966). He viewed sensation as a "one-stage" process that is little affected by learning, if at all. It implies a simple neural process from the sense organ to its appropriate projection area in the cortex, with minimal stimulation of association cortical area. The automatic perception of figure and ground appears to be nativistic and a sensorily determined unity, mediated by the inherited structural and functional characteristics of the nervous system (Hebb, 1949). Two examples may make this clear. Newborn infants appear to fixate an object held above them, and perception can be elicited by varying its brightness, color, or movement. Fantz originated an ingenious experimental method for observing this process:

> The infant's eyes are observed through a $\frac{1}{4}$ inch hole in the center of the chamber ceiling. To provide an objective criterion of fixation, the stimulus and lighting conditions are adjusted so that tiny images of the targets are clearly visible to the observer, mirrored from the surface of the infant's eyes. (Fantz, 1961)

Fantz inferred that when the reflection of a target is directly over the center of the pupil, the infant is looking at that target.

Our second example circumvents the lack of verbal report from infants by referring to clinical reports of initial vision in adults following surgical operation for the removal of cataracts existing since birth. These cases are not numerous and frequently are incompletely reported, but Hebb (1949) described several, in particular one examined by Senden (1932). Evidently these patients, immediately after the bandages are removed from their eyes, can see an object or simple geometric design, such as a square, but they cannot learn to name it without several weeks of repetition. In other words, they can sense a figure against a background but they cannot perceive and remember small distinguishing features until many repetitions have occurred. This may give the teacher of the dyslexic child some insight into the problem and generate more tolerance for the child who has no difficulty in pointing to letters and words, but who cannot remember their meaning in spite of frequent remedial drill.

These types of research and clinical findings may be interesting to the teacher, but their practical value is indirect. What is useful is to know whether or not the child with the learning problem is free of any sensory deficit. For example, a dyslexic child may perform normally on the ophthalmologist's tests of visual acuity, and in fact usually does; but one can only infer from this that his reading problem does not stem from visual dysfunctions as measured by the usual visual tests. Because the child's problem is not in the visual tracts, one can presume that it is primarily central or neuropsychological, genetic or social. It is not a problem of sensation, then, but of perception.

Less frequent is the child who shows normal hearing on an audiometric test but is unable to perceive phonetic differences. One girl seen in our laboratory showed nearly normal auditory sensation and high nonverbal intelligence but was "deaf" to almost all words, even her own name. Again, this was a problem of almost normal sensation with auditory imperception.

Perception

By contrast with sensation, perception implies recognition, discrimination, and understanding of what one is aware. Where, in our definition of sensation, the subject had only to report awareness of a spot of light or a tone, in perception he must now recognize the form of an object, such as a chair; a graphic symbol, such as a letter or word; or a stream of speech sounds as meaningful language. To learn to recognize an object and to identify it meaningfully is the product of repeated experiences and motor responses to the environment. The child must be sensorily and emotionally aware of an object, must store an image of this object in the form of a neural engram somewhere in the brain, and must react to the object and retain a memory of one's reaction to it. Then, when next confronted with it, he compares the immediate sensation of the object with the active memory of it; in this way the child can recognize it and decide how to deal with it in relation to its immediate environment and to one's own wishes at the time.

Sensation and perception, though functionally interacting, differ in that sensation implies simpler and more direct neural circuits between sense organ and brain (e.g., between the eye and area 17, the primary visual receptive area in the occipital lobes). Behavior resulting from sensation is simpler, more reflexive, and more predictable. Because it narrowly involves one of the senses, such behavior is said to be dominated by sensory control (e.g., the cataract patients described above could see a square immediately after they gained their sight for the first time, but they had no understanding of its description or use). By contrast, perception, although initiated by sensation, implies more complex neural circuits from the sense organ through various parts of the brain to the secondary and tertiary, or association areas of the human cortex. Hebb (1966) described this as "higher behavior, dependent on mediating processes (ideas, thinking)." For example, the cataract patients after several weeks of seeing a square, repeating its name, drawing it, feeling a square block, and writing its name, gradually developed a mental concept of "squareness," presumably because most or all areas of the brain were excited in addition to the simple sensory circuit between the eye and area 17. This elaborated sensory awareness, which includes cognitive and emotional response, is perception. Perception includes sensory awareness plus some degree of understanding.

By contrast with the rigidity and invariance of response in sensation, in perception "the same stimulus can produce different perceptions and different stimuli the same perception" (Hebb,

1966). It is common knowledge that the same Rorschach card will produce various descriptions from a number of viewers and that a movie or play will arouse in different members of the audience reactions ranging from disapproval to enthusiastic admiration.

It is important that teachers have clear and distinguishable concepts of sensation and perception so as not to fall into the trap of thinking that the dyslexic child who performs normally on a visual acuity test is free of all visual difficulties. Frequently teachers, deceived by this seeming paradox, have concluded, "It can't be his vision because his eyes are okay," and they have tried to look elsewhere for causes, or they have abandoned the search as insoluble. An eye chart will not reveal perceptual rotations nor an audiometer, a phonetic imperception. Accurate information about the child's modes of perception is essential to the diagnosis of his learning problem.

Lateral Asymmetries in Perception

We have already seen that brain damage and/or dysfunction in the left hemisphere usually impairs verbal skills, and dysfunction in the right hemisphere, visual–spatial competence. In this section we look at research studies designed to examine the hemispheric differences in subjects with *normal* brains, when they are confronted with visual stimuli or subjected to auditory excitation. In other words, we shall look at the innate perceptual tendencies of the normal brain.

Before we examine experiments in visual perception we should recall that the left half of each retina connects into the left occipital lobe, and the two right halves to the right occipital lobe (Fig. 2.7). Thus if the left halves of the retinae are stimulated, only the left cerebral hemisphere is affected, and by stimulating only the right retinal halves there results only right-hemisphere processing of the neural input. If the two hemispheres possess innate tendencies to treat verbal and spatial material differently, as the lesion studies suggest, then it should show itself in controlled experiments with normal brains. A visual stimulus in the left visual field—that is, to the left of the midline—will excite points in the right half of each retina because the incoming light rays cross in the lens. Similarly, objects in the right visual field will impinge on the left half of each retina (Fig. 2.7).

To study this process a subject is seated before a white screen with a fixation point or X at its center. The subject is asked to fixate the X and report what he sees as visual stimuli are flashed on the screen in either the left or the right field for short periods, usually between 100 and 200 milliseconds (one-tenth to one-fifth of a second).

In the 1950s, it was discovered that when stimuli were presented rapidly on a tachistoscope (a device for presenting very rapid visual stimuli under highly controlled conditions) to either the left or the right visual field, verbal material was usually reported more accurately from the right visual field (Heron, 1957; Mishkin & Forgays, 1952). At that time this finding was interpreted completely in terms of learned scanning habits acquired through reading. However, Dr. Doreen Kimura, a Canadian psychologist then at McGill University, first proposed that this asymmetry was caused, at least in part, by the more dominant participation of the left hemisphere in the processing of words and letters (Kimura, 1961b), and this neuropsychological interpretation, added to what was already known of perceptual learning, resulted in a great body of research into perceptual asymmetries (Dimond & Beaumont, 1974; Kimura, 1959, 1961a,b, 1966, 1969, 1973a; Kimura & Durnford, 1974; Kinsbourne & Smith, 1974).

This discovery of the possible relation of cerebral dominance and perceptual asymmetry in the right and left visual fields and the right and left ears was a major accomplishment in acquiring neuropsychological knowledge. The interested student might like to read Kimura's early paper (1959), in which she tried to explain the right visual superiority only in terms of increased facility in reading. Kimura sensed that some other force was at work, because she concluded that the neural feedback model of learned eye movements "cannot be the complete explanation" (Kimura, 1959). However, within two years she had concluded from her dichotic listening studies and her work with temporal lobe lesion cases that the crossed auditory pathways are more effective than the uncrossed (Kimura, 1961a).

To understand this conclusion, the student must be reminded that each ear connects to both temporal lobes, but the crossed neural pathway or the connections to the contralateral hemisphere are more strongly represented than those to the ipsilateral temporal lobe (Fig. 2.8). Kimura (1961b) wisely extended her conclusions from the auditory to the visual sense mode. "If the relation suggested here between the identification of verbal stimuli and the hemisphere at which they arrive is correct, one might expect a similar effect with visually presented verbal material." Once the importance of cerebral dominance, as well as learning, was invoked to explain perceptual differences for verbal and nonverbal visual and auditory stimuli, many of the previously- unexplained discrepancies could be understood.

In further studies, Kimura (1966) showed a superior right-hemisphere function or left visual field superiority for spatial material. She provided not only an excellent summary of her work in left visual field superiority for dot enumeration and right field superiority for letter identification, but she reported (Kimura & Durnford, 1974) better left field recognition of geometric forms; sex differences for spatial localization, with males showing a significant left field effect; better binocular depth perception in the left field but no differences for monocular depth perception; and slightly better identification of line slant in the left visual field.

The student new to these ideas must realize that functional hemispheric asymmetries are not rigidly and exclusively determined by verbal and nonverbal input. As we have shown in Chapter 3, other variables are also at work, such as attention (Kinsbourne, 1975c), expectancy (Spellacy & Blumstein, 1970), level of intellectual complexity or difficulty (Buffery, 1976), age of the child (Bakker, Teunissen, & Bosch, 1976), stimulus complexity (Umilta, Bagnara, & Simion, 1978), and stimulus modality (Davis & Wada, 1977). These ideas are explored again in Chapter 6 and throughout the book.

Visual Agnosia

Because it is frequently easier to understand behavioral imperfections within the normal range by examining the grossly abnormal, we will look briefly at a severe and somewhat rare clinical example of impaired or distorted visual perception. Although not all neurologists agree on a definition of the visual agnosias, they are disorders of perceptual recognition caused by dysfunctions of higher cerebral nervous activity.

Benson and Greenberg (1969) have reported the rare case of a man with normal visual fields but severely impaired form recognition. At age 25, this young man suffered permanent and diffuse brain damage as the result of inhaling carbon monoxide fumes from a leaking connection in an army shower room. Prior to this accident he had been physically normal and healthy. Following his brain injury he could name colors and appeared to follow moving visual stimuli, but he could not recognize by vision alone familiar objects placed before him. He was able to walk along hospital corridors and avoid furniture, although his movements were jerky and awkward. His understanding of spoken speech was normal and his tactile form recognition (stereognosis) was unimpaired. Visually he was unable to recognize large letters or numbers on a blackboard, although he could name them if he watched them being drawn slowly. This ability suggests that he was using proprioceptive cues rather than visual ones to perceive the form of the letter.

His recent and long-term memory, his speech (both comprehension and spoken), and his ability to repeat sentences were all normally intact. Although he could name colors, he was unable to identify objects, pictures of objects, body parts, letters, numbers, or geometric figures on visual confrontation. He could, however, identify objects by touch, smell, or sound. He was totally unable to copy letters or simple figures, a condition that is partially similar to a severe case of developmental agraphia.

He was unable to select his doctor or family members from a group until they spoke, and he identified his own image in a mirror as his doctor's face. This case illustrates highly selective visual–perceptual impairment, the inability to recognize forms of familiar objects and letters. Because this ability was normal prior to the brain injury, we can conclude that the association cortical areas essential to visual form recognition were most likely permanently destroyed.

This case of visual agnosia reminds us rather forcibly that brain damage or dysfunction can impair the ability for normal visual recognition of common objects, persons, and letters. The last named will interest the remedial teacher because it proposes a possible primary cause of dyslexia. However, not all cases of visual object agnosia are dyslexic, nor are all dyslexics suffering from some form of visual–perceptual impairment.

Levine (1978) has reported a particularly interesting case of a woman who, in her late 50s, developed a brain tumor in the lower posterior subcortical part of her brain. The tumor, a space-occupying progressive type, pressed on the right occipital lobe with such force as to displace it laterally to the right and down onto the cerebellum to produce an awkward gait. To remove the tumor, the surgeon was forced to cut into the occipital lobe at both its upper (by the falx) and lower (by the tentorium) extremities. Following this surgery, the woman was unable to recognize by sight her own relatives, her doctors, and hospital ward personnel. However, her speech was fluent, her comprehension of language excellent, and her reading competent with large print.

It seems likely that in the Benson and Greenberg case, because the damage was diffuse, the patient suffered bilateral occipital damage, so that both visual reading and object recognition were impaired. In contrast, Levine's case suffered severe damage to the right occipital lobe as a result of surgery, which produced visual object agnosia. Because the left hemisphere was spared, reading, speech, and language were intact.

Visual agnosias can also impair recognition of drawings and pictures of common objects, ability to name colors of common objects (e.g., What is the color of a banana?), and to distinguish hues in a color spectrum although the retinal cells are normal. Kolb and Whishaw provide a useful summary of the visual agnosias (1990, pp. 236–241) for the reader who wishes more information on this interesting syndrome.

Auditory Imperception

We have referred briefly to two cases of auditory imperception, in Chapter 2 and previously in this chapter, but because this process is essential to normal academic learning, we examine the consequences of its dysfunction more thoroughly here.

First, the teacher and the diagnostician must be clear in understanding that auditory imperception may result from neural damage or dysfunction in (1) the peripheral auditory nervous system, resulting in deafness or some degree of hearing loss; and/or (2) the central auditory tracts in the brain and auditory cortex, resulting in some type of auditory agnosia.

Because subtle forms of hearing loss are often missed and are nearly always at least a partial source of a learning disability, it is imperative that at the outset a competent audiometric test be carried out. If the child is obviously hard of hearing, a technical aid may compensate for the difficulty, and if the child's brain functions are normal he should be able to learn at a normal or nearly normal level. In this case the physiological deficit is *peripheral*, not *central*, so that the correction of sensory input will provide the child with a normal learning situation. The teacher, once advised of the presence and nature of the hearing loss, should be able to obtain suggestions for management of the case from the speech therapist or school psychologist.

Although cases of sensorial or peripheral deafness are more common, cases of *central* deafness, when they occur, are more devastating in disruption of learning. These are the cases of auditory agnosia for speech, nonverbal sounds, and music, and they include inability to recognize or decode auditory stimuli, although hearing may be intact (Frederiks, 1969a). Whereas neurologists and audiologists may provide a more elaborate and definitive classification, the teacher and clinician may find it more practical and expedient to concentrate only on aspects of auditory perception and imperception that are strongly related to classroom learning. These are (1) speech perception and language, the deficit being known as receptive aphasia; (2) perception of nonverbal environmental sounds, such as a fire bell, whistle, handclapping, the deficit being known as auditory agnosia; and (3) perception and enjoyment of music, the deficit being known as amusia.

At this point auditory imperception for speech will not be discussed, because sensory aphasia is examined in Chapter 8. Neurologically, however, it is interesting that this deficit appears to result from a brain lesion or dysfunction in Wernicke's area of the dominant hemisphere (Luria, 1966).

By contrast, it appears possible that nonverbal sound recognition may depend more on the nondominant hemisphere, although as symbolic processes are drawn on for more subtle understanding and apperception, it seems certain that both hemispheres are increasingly involved, especially the first and second convolutions of both temporal lobes (Frederiks, 1969a). In fact, all or most tasks of auditory perception of so-called nonverbal stimuli include some degree of verbal mediation. The Spreen–Benton Sound Recognition Test (Spreen & Strauss, 1991, p. 313) requires the child to name the source of the sound after listening to a tape of a cat meowing, a church bell ringing, people clapping, etc. For an aphasic child, a multiple-choice form is used that allows the child to avoid the word-finding task by pointing to a picture in an array. Even in this form of the test, which is designed to minimize the language aspects of the situation, there is symbolic content that is likely to include some degree of verbal activity. Music is a nonverbal auditory stimulus, and what clinical evidence exists suggests that a motor amusia (inability to sing and imitate a tune) may result from a right frontal lesion, in roughly the mirror position of Broca's area. Receptive amusia (inability to recognize a tune or appreciate music) appears to include the temporal lobes bilaterally (Wertheim, 1969). For a person to sing a song with words, both hemispheres contribute. Wada (Wada, Clarke & Hamm, 1975) demonstrates this condition neatly in a simple clinical test. After he injects sodium amytal into the patient's left carotid artery, he asks the patient to sing "Happy Birthday." If the patient is left-hemisphere dominant for language, as most people are, he will be able to hum the tune but not produce the words. When the same patient after right-side amytal injection is asked to sing the same song, he will recite the words of "Happy Birthday" in a monotone, unable to produce the tune. Wada has found this asymmetrical pattern in the majority of the patients he sees.

A survey of the literature of auditory imperception shows that most, if not all, patients also have some signs of receptive aphasia, or difficulty in understanding spoken speech. However, rarely a case occurs wherein the patient cannot recognize simple environmental sounds but has no problems either in understanding or expressing language. Such a case was reported by Spreen, Benton, and Fincham (1965).

   This was a 65-year-old man who had suffered a right-hemisphere stroke resulting in impairment of his left arm and left leg (left hemiparesis). The hemiparesis gradually disappeared during the following 6 months, to be followed by left-sided clonic seizures. His right side was not affected during these seizures, indicating that he was suffering from a unilateral lesion in the right half of his brain. The seizures were successfully managed by administering anticonvulsive medication. During the next 2 years he was hospitalized from time to time because of frontal headaches, emotional personality changes, difficulty in walking, and a mild left visual field defect. An EEG showed abnormal activity chiefly over the right temporal area.

   On neuropsychological testing his overall intelligence was in the lower scores of the normal range, but he had most difficulty with visual–spatial tasks, performances usually impaired by right-hemisphere dysfunction. Finger localization was normal for the right hand but inferior for the left, although detailed language testing revealed no signs of aphasia. His worst performance was in sound recognition; he was unable to recognize a machine gun, knocking on wood, a door banging, handclapping (applause), and water running. Although he was tested several times during the 18 months prior to his death, he persisted in showing this severe deficit in auditory recognition. Nevertheless he could do arithmetic relatively well and he showed no disturbances in reading, writing, or carrying on normal conversation.

   At autopsy a large area of deteriorated tissue was found in the right frontal, temporal, and parietal lobes. The left hemisphere and the corpus callosum were normal and healthy.

   The evidence provided by this case, as well as those studies of right temporal lesion cases being inferior in tonal memory (B. Milner, 1962) and in dichotic recognition of melodies and tonal qualities (Kimura, 1964; Spellacy, 1970; Spellacy & Blumstein, 1970), suggests that nonverbal sounds are processed mainly by the right cerebral hemisphere, but as they involve greater verbal mediation both hemispheres become increasingly activated.

Sequencing

The neurological mechanisms underlying serial order behavior are only just beginning to be understood. An early experiment with monkeys (Kimble & Pribram, 1963) suggested the left hemisphere (specifying the left hippocampal area) as dominant in the control of serial order processing. Lashley wrote in 1948 that the study of language and the evidence that the brain readies or prepares the words in a sentence just prior to their expression suggest that "some scanning mechanism must be at play in regulating their temporal sequence" (Lashley, 1951). However, he admitted that he had no answer about the nature of this selective mechanism or its location in the central nervous system. In our own laboratory we have produced a mechanism to present moving lights sequentially to study its usefulness in detecting brain damage in human patients (Gaddes, 1966a, 1969b, 1988). In an early study (Gaddes & Tymchuk, 1967) we found that left hemisphere lesion cases were inferior to right hemisphere lesion cases in remembering the sequentially presented light patterns. As well, frontal lesion cases performed worse than those with posterior lesions. This study suggested the left frontal cerebral areas as being important in controlling serial order functions on this test.

A study on split-brain patients (D. Zaidel & Sperry, 1973) required the subject to palpate two or three three-dimensional nonsense figures and some familiar household objects, and then to reproduce from memory the objects in correct order. "The left hemisphere was found consistently to be superior to the right in patients with complete section of the forebrain commissures, regardless of stimulus type or sequence length, and in agreement with the general association between language and temporal order." Such a finding leads one to wonder whether the left hemisphere is usually dominant for language because it genetically is supplied with the scanning mechanism that regulates temporal ordering. If it is, then the left hemisphere is better equipped, but not exclusively so, to provide meaningful order to language perception and expression than the right hemisphere. However, this is not to say that the right hemisphere is illiterate, because some findings have shown it to have some limited language functions (Gazzaniga & Hillyard, 1971; E. Zaidel, 1973).

No doubt the researches of psychologists into this phenomenon (Bryden, 1960a, 1967; Epstein, 1963; Gottschalk, 1962, 1965; P.M. Milner, 1961) interested professional educators, because the mention of serial order functions, both perceptual and motor, increased in books on remedial education (Johnson & Myklebust, 1967; Kephart, 1960/1971, 1964; Myers & Hammill, 1990; Valett, 1973) as a recommended corrective procedure, but with no proposed empirical justification. Because all behavior occurs in a temporal continuum, and because serial order can easily be identified in classroom learning, tasks such as reading, spelling, and adding, it is logical to believe, a priori, that facility in sequencing skills is essential to academic learning.

The chief reason that little rational support has been given to promoting remedial sequencing drills for LD children is that very little research pertinent to this question has been carried out until recently. In the late 1950s, as the result of the interest and stimulation of D.O. Hebb, a number of graduate students and researchers at McGill University (Bryden, 1960a, 1962, 1966, 1967; Gottschalk, 1962, 1965; Heron, 1957; Kimura, 1959; P.M. Milner, 1961) carried out a number of valuable studies into the logical and orderly arrangement of thought and action, which Lashley (1951) described as "the most complex type of behavior that I know."

A few educational references have provided research evidence for, or attempted to investigate the relationship between, sequencing ability and academic achievement. Chalfant and Scheffelin (1969), in an able review of research findings relative to cognitive dysfunctions in children, discussed sequencing in auditory perception; however, no comparable discussion occurs for the visual or haptic sense modes, although these are implied under "visual scanning and tracking" and tactile recognition of "movement patterns."

Other researchers who have studied the significance of sequential processes in academic learning include Das, Kirby, and Jarman (1979), Denckla (1979), Leong (1975, 1976), Mattis (1978), and Senf (1969). It is noteworthy that the first test battery of children's intelligence and cognitive achievement to use neuropsychological knowledge in its design, the Kaufman Assessment Battery for Children (K-ABC), appeared as recently as 1983. Drawing on the the original work of Luria (1966, 1970, 1973) and his followers, Das, Kirby, and Jarman (1979) and others, the Kaufmans included three sequential subtests in their battery of 16 subtests. They included the sequential processing function of the brain in the rationale of their test battery, along with simultaneous (gestalt–spatial) processing, and they also have provided a discussion of remedial teaching programs that have enlisted the neuropsychological strengths of the child (i.e., analytical–sequential or holistic–simultaneous) rather than stressing traditional drilling of simple auditory or visual-processing, motor, or psycholinguistic skills (Kaufman & Kaufman, 1983, Chapter 7).

Probably the first comprehensive study of temporal order perception and reading was made by Bakker (1972) in the Netherlands. He investigated the visual, auditory, and haptic serial order perception of normal and learning disturbed children aged 7–11, inclusive. Bakker defined his terms carefully; for him succession implied the presentation of two identical stimuli (e.g., tones or light flashes) with a time interval between. By contrast, temporal order (or sequencing) implied the ordered succession of stimuli that were different so that they could be identified singly (e.g., tones of different pitch). Bakker has recognized two types of response to serial order stimuli: (1) imitation and (2) explication. Repeating digits forward is an example of imitation, because the subject can merely echo the sound pattern with little cognitive awareness of the numbers. Repeating digits in reverse order is an example of explication, because the subject must recognize the position of each digit and indicate the serial order of each number. It would seem that, neuropsychologically, imitation is mediated largely unconsciously, whereas explication demands selective attention and memory, and presumably a larger cortical function.

Bakker's research, completed in the late 1960s, led him to conclude that *verbal* sequential tests discriminate between good and poor readers, and that *nonverbal* sequential tests do not. His nonverbal tests, however, which required the child to look at series of pictures, were not timed. The Dynamic Visual Retention Test (DVRT) (Gaddes, 1966a), because it is designed to present patterns of lights at various speeds with light exposures and between-light intervals as short as 100 milliseconds (one-tenth of a second), provided the opportunity to test the possibility that *speed of sequencing* was an important causal factor in reading retardation.

Consequently, two pilot studies, one with eight severely reading retarded children and the second with eight adult dyslexics, showed that when these subjects were matched for Wechsler performance IQ with normal readers, that as the light sequences were speeded up, the dyslexics in both groups were inferior. In the child study, the LD and control children performed significantly differently on the DVRT ($p < .001$) a test ostensibly designed to be a *nonverbal* visual sequential task (Gaddes, 1982). A tachistoscopic sequential presentation of single letters at slow and fast speeds, although a *verbal* sequential test, did not discriminate between the good and poor readers. The same basic findings were obtained in the adult study.

These findings were contrary to Bakker's general conclusion, and there are reasons for the differences. Although the DVRT appears to be a *nonverbal* test (i.e., series of lights on a screen), the child is asked to count the lights to help him or her identify the changed light in the second sequence. Also, the rapid speed of presentation (100 msec) subjects the child to cerebral processing functions unlike the slower viewing tasks of Bakker's research (1 minute or no limit).

The knowledge of sequencing has progressed since the late 1950s from a fixed idea about the cerebral locus of the sequential scanner to a much more dynamic view. In 1963 Efron wrote, "temporal analysis of sequences, interval and simultaneity is performed in the left hemisphere in right-handed *S*s, as well as in the majority of left-handed ones" (Efron, 1963). By the early 1970s a synthesis of numerous sequential studies from lesion cases, dichotic listening and tachistoscopic half-field studies, carotid amytal injections, electrophysiological studies, split-brain experiments, comprehensive batteries of neuropsychological tests, and longitudinal studies of aphasic patients, traumatically brain-damaged persons, and those with developmental learning disabilities was taking place. Bakker (1972) produced an improved concept of sequential cerebral function. Where most of the researchers of the 1960s had thought the scanning center had a fixed location in the brain, Bakker concluded that it could be either left- or right-brained depending on whether the stimulus was verbal or nonverbal. Research findings during the 1970s enable us to conclude:

1. Visual sequential perception is sensitive to brain dysfunction anywhere in the brain.
2. It is a discrete ability and, although associated with normal perception and memory, it possesses its own functional integrity and can be independent under certain conditions. For example, a child presented with the letters T, X, A serially at a very fast speed on a tachistoscope may report all three letters correctly, but in the wrong order. This response seems to indicate that the child's perception and memory are normal but cerebral ordering is defective.
3. It is task specific, varying with the degree of verbal or nonverbal quality, the level of difficulty of the task, and/or the sense mode involved.
4. There is no fixed cerebral locus for sequencing. Both hemispheres and possibly the cerebellum (Ingvar, 1992), are involved, depending more or less on the nature of the sequential task, the experience and training of the subject, and his or her intentions and planned strategies.

What has all this to do with LD children? It should help the clinical or school psychologist to improve his or her diagnostic understanding of the child. In cases where the loci of cerebral dysfunction are known, it should help to conceptualize the delicate, dynamic, and adaptive pattern of cerebral serial order functioning. Its relation to remediation is not clear yet, although one study (Gaddes & Spellacy, 1977) compared seven nonverbal and verbal sequential tasks with success in reading, spelling, and arithmetic and showed, by correlational analysis, a stronger relation between the verbal sequential tasks and academic success than between the nonverbal sequential tests. Measures of sequential skills were made in grade 2 and grade 5 to provide information on developmental changes. The first multivariate analysis of the grade 2 data showed a significant relationship between success in reading and the ability to recognize differences in sequential light patterns at a slow speed. The evidence from this study suggested that "verbal serial order tasks for grade 2 students are only a little more strongly related to academic success than nonverbal sequential skills when speed is introduced in the presentation of the latter" (Gaddes, 1982).

Reading in grade 2 showed the highest correlation with the DVRT[1] at the slow speed. Reading in grade 5 showed three steps that produced significant multiple correlations. These were with the Visual Expressive Test,[1] the Auditory Expressive Test,[1] and the DVRT at the slow speed. These findings suggest a shift from an emphasis on slow visual decoding at the grade 2 level to a more integrated auditory and visual processing (see Fig. 4.1).

Spelling showed different patterns of involvement with nonverbal sequential skills (Fig. 4.2). A multiple regression step-up analysis of grade 2 data showed significant correlations with the DVRT at the slow speed, the Visual Expressive Test, the Auditory Expressive Test, and the DVRT at the fast speed.

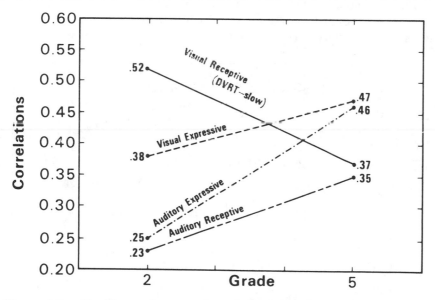

Figure 4.1. Reading and sequencing. Progressive changes in correlations between reading and various sequencing processes from grade 2 to grade 5. (From Gaddes, 1982; with permission of Syracuse University Press.)

[1] For a description of the five nonverbal sequential tests, see Appendix, page 486.

Analysis of the grade 5 spelling data showed that children in this age range prefer the DVRT at the fast speed. Because their visual scanning skills have improved since grade 2, the fast speed is more satisfying and less tedious for most of them, as is any task administered at a speed well below the level of comfortable achievement. Significant correlations were found between success in spelling and achievement on the DVRT at the fast speed, the Auditory Expressive Test, and the DVRT at the slow speed. These correlations were considerably lower than those for reading, and one reason is likely the failure of the nonverbal tests used in this study to tap the kinesthetic–sequential motor skills so essential to writing and spelling.

When testing arithmetic achievement it is important to examine both oral skills and written ability, because they appear to draw on different patterns of cognitive skills and neuropsychological processes. In this study we were interested in learning how nonverbal sequential skills related to competence in both oral and written arithmetic.

Oral arithmetic at the grade 2 level produced significant correlations (see Figs. 4.3 and 4.4) with three of the tests, the DVRT at the slow speed (.43), the Auditory Receptive Test (.34), and the DVRT at the fast speed (.23). Written arithmetic at this grade level showed only one significant correlation and it was with the

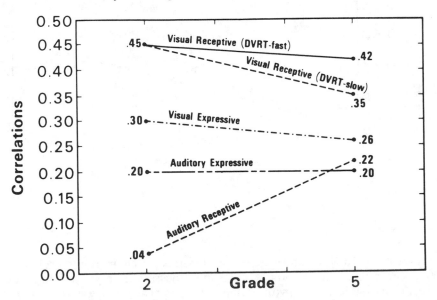

Figure 4.2. Spelling and sequencing. Progressive changes in correlations between spelling and various sequencing processes from grade 2 to grade 5. (From Gaddes, 1982; with permission of Syracuse University Press.)

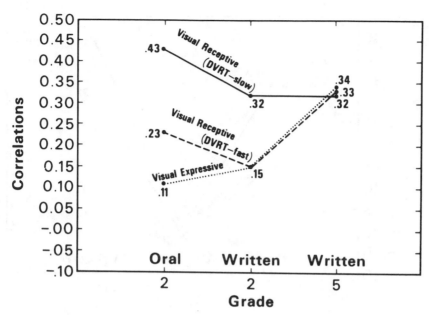

Figure 4.3. Arithmetic and visual sequencing. Progressive changes in correlations between oral and written arithmetic and visual sequencing processes from grade 2 to grade 5. (From Gaddes, 1982; with permission of Syracuse University Press.)

DVRT at the slow speed (.32). These findings suggest that the 7-year-old in our schools may be primarily concerned with the spatial aspects of numbers and "possibly oral arithmetic frees the child to give his attention more to number concepts, and hence the stronger relation of both auditory and visual sequential processes" (Gaddes, 1982).

A multiple regression step-up analysis of the grade 5 arithmetic data showed significant correlations with the Auditory Receptive Test (.44), the DVRT at the slow speed (.32), and the Auditory Expressive Test (.32). "The evident ascendancy of the auditory sequential skills may mean that the older child conceptualizes arithmetic more in oral and subvocal language, and has now automatized many of the visual–motor skills required in reading and writing" (Gaddes, 1982).

This evidence suggests that remedial drills probably should include verbal material first, because it is more strongly related to academic skills, and then nonverbal sequential drills should be introduced. If this is true, it would not agree with Ayres' thesis (Ayres, 1972a) that one should develop the brain's ability to learn rather than teach specific skills. However, our evidence derives

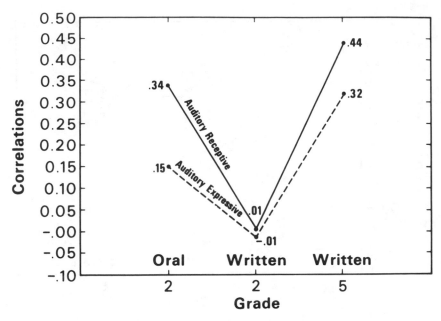

Figure 4.4. Arithmetic and auditory sequencing. Progressive changes in correlations between oral and written arithmetic and auditory sequencing processes from grade 2 to grade 5. (From Gaddes, 1982; with permission of Syracuse University Press.)

only from correlational data and hence we cannot infer causal relations about remediation.

Summary

This discussion of the neurological evidence of the LD child's perceptual functions and dysfunctions should improve the reader's understanding of the breadth and subtlety of problems that prevent normal learning. It is invaluable for the clinician and teacher to have a delineated conceptual view of the scope of these problems. Behavior is viewed holistically, but for purposes of study, sensation, perception, attention, lateral perceptual asymmetries, and sequencing have all been examined separately.

Clinical Addendum

In this section we look at two cases with evidence of fairly clearly defined regional cerebral dysfunction, one with left-hemisphere dysfunction and one with right-hemisphere impairment. Both children had suffered these deficits since birth so that their mental and psychological development had been shaped by these abnormal neurophysiological conditions. One of these children is described briefly in Chapter 3, but here we examine this case in more detail.

These two cases have several advantages for the teacher and the psychologist in their attempts to integrate neurological information and behavioral data. They each show clear laterality effects, they were each seen initially at about the same age (12 and 13 years), they each showed interesting perceptual problems, and they were followed for more than 10 years.

Case I: Left-Hemisphere Dysfunction

Sam was referred by a neurologist to the neuropsychological laboratory when he was 12 years old because of poor academic school performance and a history of epileptic seizures. Sam was the second oldest of three children and his prenatal and birth history were normal. At the age of 6 weeks, however, he developed meningitis and apparently convulsed at that time. He was quite ill but made a good recovery and remained well until age 6 years, when he developed the second convulsion. On this occasion this was a right-sided seizure (his right arm and right leg were activated in involuntary clonic movements). In a few moments the seizure involved both sides of the body, which suggested that the epileptogenic focus was in the left hemisphere and stimulated the right side of the body; the cerebral electrical storm gradually spread bilaterally throughout the brain, and the seizure became generalized. Two EEGs carried out previously supported this diagnosis by showing severe dysrhythmia in the central temporal area of the left hemisphere. An EEG done just prior to our seeing Sam showed continued presence of a grade iii spike activity in the left frontotemporal area.

At age 7 years, Sam was placed on anticonvulsive medication, which was largely successful. At age 7, he suffered a minor episode in which the right side of his mouth drooped and his right hand twitched.

His development appeared to be normal except for his language. He was even tempered and cooperative, but he spoke very little. He had great difficulty saying anything until after age 2, and even when we saw him at age 12, he answered only when spoken to, and then very meagerly.

The psychometrician wrote, "He is extremely uncommunicative but not surly, simply withdrawn." He enjoyed the performance part of the Wechsler (WISC) and even smiled occasionally during completion of the Block Design Test. On the verbal tests, however, he had trouble. He had a peculiar habit of cupping one hand over his mouth when he was speaking, as if he were embarrassed to have any one see him talk. On the Vocabulary test he used a minimum of speech and when asked, "Go on, tell me more," he usually remained mute. He never said, "I don't know" or "I can't," he just sat waiting passively for the tester to make the next move. He did not appear to have any articulation problems; the little he did say was pronounced correctly.

On the initial Wechsler (WISC) he measured a verbal IQ of 87 and a performance IQ of 110. On the verbal tests he scored in the average range on Arithmetic and above average on repeating digits back, but on all subtests using words he did very badly.

On the performance tests his achievement was at a very superior level on the Block Design subtest (spatial imagery), and he obtained high scores on Picture Completion (identifying small errors or omissions in line drawings) and Object Assembly (a jigsaw puzzle task). His visual memory and tactile perception were good, but he had difficulty with the auditory–perception tests for both language and nonverbal stimuli.

His sensorimotor skills, manual reaction times, finger tapping, finger localization, and right–left orientation were all intact. His hand-grip strength was weak in both hands; this finding is frequent in cases with neurological damage or dysfunction somewhere in the central nervous system.

The Psychologist's Role

This boy, because of his poor verbal abilities, had never done well at school and in fact had been kept in a slow learners' class for the first 6 years of his school life. The test findings showed that whereas he had a definite impairment in spoken speech, his word recognition on a reading test was normal for his age, as was his written arithmetic. He was also quite superior in tasks involving spatial imagery, spatial analysis and construction, and visual perception for detail.

It was quite clear that this boy considered himself intellectually inferior and suffered strong feelings of personal inadequacy and social isolation. It was explained to him that although he did not talk much, he should be aware that he was quite superior in the kinds of skills that led to mechanical work, construction, architecture, and engineering.

From a neuropsychological view, Sam was a classic example of left-hemisphere dysfunction, as indicated by his poor verbal skills and his strong right-hemisphere (spatial–constructional) abilities.

A letter to the boy's school principal described the history of meningitis, mentioned the left-hemisphere dysfunction as related to his weak verbal skills, but stressed his superior spatial abilities and his average performance in arithmetical deductive reasoning. The letter said in part, "He should do very well reading maps in geography, interpreting blueprints and mechanical drawings, and doing geometry when he reaches that stage. In these areas he is a bright boy." This was an attempt to alter the image of Sam, which likely had developed because of the verbal emphasis of most school programs, and to draw attention to specific areas his teachers might explore if they had not already detected them. The letter ended with a request for a normal placement for Sam: "May I suggest that I think that a boy as potentially bright as this, may profit from placement in a regular class, with daily remedial assistance in reading and spelling."

The School

The principal and Sam's teacher were interested enough in the reports and suggestions that they visited the laboratory to discuss further the management of Sam's case. On the basis of the evidence, they decided to move him into a regular class and teach him reading and spelling with an emphasis on visual–motor aspects rather than phonics. He read silently better than aloud because of his motor–speech difficulties, and so his teacher decided to stress silent reading.

When Sam returned the next year for evaluation the Wechsler (WISC) showed a phenomenal improvement in his performance scores. His verbal IQ measured only 80, but his performance IQ was now 132, better than 99% of other children his age. He also showed a little improvement in the Information, Digit Span, and Similarities subtests, but his overall verbal abilities were still below average. It seems reasonable to conclude that, because the school authorities moved Sam into a normal class, began to think of him in different terms, and to use remedial measures based on his strengths, he became at least partially emancipated from his former feelings of inferiority and alienation.

By the time Sam reached grade 9 he elected an "occupational program" that stressed drafting, mechanics, and industrial arts. He completed this program and on graduation entered an apprenticeship in automechanics.

A number of interesting points emerge from Sam's case and are worthy of note. First, there was clear evidence of electrical dysfunction in his left temporal lobe near the Sylvian fissure. Because this disturbance was strong enough to produce epileptic seizures and appeared to involve Wernicke's area (see Fig. 2.9) at least in part, this would lead us to examine his phonetic auditory perception. In fact, on our first administration of the Halstead Speech Perception Test, he had real problems discriminating nonsense phonemes (e.g., weech and weej), and his error score out of 60 phonemes placed him more than one standard deviation below the average score of normal 12-year-olds. It seemed reasonable to assume that this auditory imperception was related to his retarded speech development, his poor spelling, and his slow reading. Also, the three EEGs administered intermittently during his first 12 years of life all showed a grade iii disturbance in the left Sylvian area, and suggested strongly that a permanent lesion, existed in Sam's left temporal lobe. Although this speculation should not excuse his teachers from trying to teach him to speak, read, and write, it could reduce their feelings of frustration if his verbal progress was unusually slow. Herein lies one of the greatest values of neurological knowledge in understanding and managing learning disabled children: *the better opportunity for prediction.*

The next year, when Sam was 13, we retested him on the Meikle Consonant Perception Test. This purely auditory perception test requires the child to answer "same" or "different" to two nonsense phonemes and a few words, presented on a tape recorder. This time, Sam's score placed him more than two standard deviations below the average score for normal 13-year-olds and enhanced our tentative prediction a year earlier that Sam had a chronic temporal lesion that would always interfere with his reception and expression of oral language.

When he returned at age 20 for a recheck, the left temporal disturbance still showed itself, but Sam had gained considerable success in his drafting and mechanical courses as a substitute for his weak academic achievement, and though still quiet and nonaggressive, he was developing signs of adult assurance in his apprentice training.

Case II: Right-Hemisphere Dysfunction

Until Will was 13 years old, when we first saw him, no one had ever attempted to relate his neurological impairment (a mild left hemiparesis) and his learning problems at school. Because they did not impair his verbal abilities, Will did reasonably well in the core academic subjects except when spatial skills were required. As a consequence, he was frustrated and anxious, wondering whether he were really stupid. His parents also were confused, and they became somewhat defensive and hostile toward the school for not helping their only son more.

Will's birth was about 2 months premature and he was in an incubator for 7 weeks. When he began to stand at about 18 months, it was noticed that he could not put his left foot flat on the floor. A diagnosis of mild cerebral palsy was made, with spasticity in the left arm, leg, and face.

An EEG carried out when he was 13 years old showed a minimal dysrhythmia in the right occipital, parietal, and motor strip areas. Hand grip was normal in the right hand and inferior in the left.

The Psychologist's Role

The Wechsler (WISC) showed a verbal IQ of 110 and a performance IQ of 69. He was severely impaired on the Block Design, Picture Completion, and Maze Tests. He could not draw the Benton geometric diagrams from memory except very poorly, and his attempts to copy a Greek cross were sketchy, incomplete, and uneven (see Fig. 3.3). Although his visual and tactile perception were poor, his auditory perception and memory for both verbal and nonverbal material were superior.

His impaired spatial skills had made art, paper construction, map reading, and interpretation of diagrams in arithmetic and science a real punishment. Will reported, "I hated all art work from grade 1. If the teacher showed us how to fold a paper, the others could do it, but mine was never right." Arithmetic was also difficult because of the many spatial demands in the first few grades (vertical columns in adding, reading right and left from the decimal, diagonal columns in multidigit multiplying and long division).

Following the testing, Will's father, who had brought him for testing very reluctantly and somewhat defensively, was counseled. The relation between Will's left hand and foot weakness with the right half of his brain was explained, and the further relation of this and spatial imagery. Will's success in reading, language, social studies, and science (only the reading parts, not the maps or diagrams) was explained in terms of his superior left hemisphere. This simplistic model was something the father could understand and welcomed, in that it objectified Will's learning problems and removed the confusion, frustration, and feelings of possible guilt. He left the laboratory expressing his gratitude and offering to bring Will back any time.

Two years later we saw Will again, at which time he measured a verbal IQ of 106 and a performance IQ of 71, still the same verbal–spatial split, because Will's right hemisphere was chronically damaged and hence his spatial skills permanently restricted. The degree of his impairment could be revealed only by longitudinal observations over a period of time.

At 15, Will was still severely handicapped in any task requiring spatial imagery, visual perception for small detail, visual–manual integration, visual figure–ground perception, and visual memory. Also, his hand-grip strength was very weak in both hands, and the sensory and motor functions of his left hand were inferior. His auditory phonetic discrimination was still good and his immediate verbal memory as measured by the Spreen–Benton Sentence Repetition Test, almost superior. Fortunately, Will was right-handed, and because his left hemisphere was above average in processing verbal material, he had no problems in spelling.

During later adolescence, Will was seen twice very briefly, but his relative verbal superiority and spatial inferiority still showed itself. At 23 he was tested more fully, and his Wechsler (WAIS) verbal IQ measured 110 and his performance IQ only 68. It was interesting that on the Information Test purely verbal questions were answered well, but when direction, distance, or measurement were involved he "had no idea." When asked the distance between Chicago and New York, he said, "Oh, 2000 miles. I have no idea." When asked where China was located, he hesitated a long time and then said, "Oh, in the south half of the hemisphere." He had no concept of the population of Canada, nor of the number of seats in the legislature. However, he was able to answer all the pure verbal questions from history or literature.

He still had great difficulty on the Block Design Test, being unable to do even the simple patterns without a demonstration first, and in some cases even then he could not analyze the design spatially and construct it. On the Benton Visual Retention Test (visual memory and visual–motor skill) he performed at the level of a borderline mental defective. On the Halstead Finger Tapping Test he did well above average with the right hand, but increasingly poorly with each trial with his left.

It was clearly evident that Will's lateralized pattern of competence and failure was still with him into adulthood.

The School

Will was in grade 7 when we first saw him. He did well in English and the verbal aspects of all subjects where reading and writing were required. His achievement in arithmetic was extremely poor, but it seemed certain that much of this failure stemmed from his lack of confidence and his spatial difficulties. Consequently, Will's father was advised to encourage oral arithmetic and to watch for difficulties when he was confronted with geometry in a later grade. Although Will was not told of this possible future learning problem (because our prediction might have been wrong), we asked Will's father to advise any of his teachers to contact the university lab if they ran into a problem they could not solve. Two years later, when Will was in grade 9, we received a call from his mathematics teacher, who sounded desperate. He complained that although Will seemed like a normally bright boy, he was hopeless in geometry. He could neither interpret nor draw a simple geometric figure, although he could handle algebra. This made no sense, said the teacher, until it was explained in terms of left- and right-hemisphere function. "Very interesting," said the teacher, "but what am I to do? One half of the grade 9 mathematics course includes introductory geometry, and the other half algebra." In conference with the junior high school principal they decided to redraft Will's program. He took English, Latin, and French and avoided geometry from then on. As a result, he graduated from high school with a plan to be a high school language teacher, but when faced with 5 years of university studies he decided against it. Instead, he attended a business college and learned typing, filing, and bookkeeping. Because of his cheery personality he is a typist–receptionist in a public library, where he is fairly free of spatial problems. As a result he is now successfully employed.

Summary Comment

The two cases of Sam and Will point up some important considerations for the educational management of children with *unilateral* brain dysfunction.

1. Because most elementary school programs stress the teaching of verbal skills, most teachers teach more to the left hemisphere than the right. For the child who is bilaterally normal this is no problem.

2. The child who suffers left-hemisphere dysfunction is frequently treated unfairly by the school system. His skill in drawing,

construction, sewing, map drawing, and singing are frequently more or less ignored because problems in reading, writing, and spelling are so apparent. Although Sam was globally superior intellectually to Will, he never was able to complete high school in the present system and had to be assisted, at age 20, by a government agency for the handicapped to help him find placement in an apprenticeship.

3. By contrast, the child who suffers right-hemisphere impairment is frequently treated normally because he can usually handle the verbally loaded core subjects. That he cannot draw, sing, or read maps is not considered serious as long as he can pass in reading, writing, and arithmetic. This means that the *present school system tends to discriminate unfairly against the child with unilateral left-hemisphere dysfunction* and to favor the right-hemisphere lesion child because he usually has a better chance to satisfy the demands of the system.

4. To counter this injustice, the school psychologist can draw attention to the child's left- and right-hemisphere skills, attaching importance to all of them. Eventually, with this type of input more teachers will learn to respect the poor reader with a performance IQ of 148. From this information they may also derive new insights in how to teach reading to such a child.

5. Both cases presented here suggest that learning impairments resulting from chronic brain lesions are likely to be permanent. This does not mean that remediation should not be attempted, but dramatic positive results cannot be expected in most cases at age 12 or 13 and older.

6. Early detection of brain dysfunctions and learning disorders should lead to more successful remediation because of the greater plasticity of the young brain.

7. At present, some school systems may neglect and/or fail to meet the educational needs of children with aphasia, subtle sequencing problems, or spatial difficulties resulting from unilateral brain damage or dysfunction. Increased knowledge of the neuropsychology of learning disabilities should better prepare school psychologists to understand these children and to assist teachers to help them. With this increased understanding and better-directed remediation the school system can learn to treat these children with greater competence and justice.

5 Sensory and Motor Pathways and Learning

Movement is in fact the basis for the development of personality. The child, who is constructing himself, must always be moving. Not only in those large movements which have an external aim, such as sweeping a room . . . but also when the child merely sees, or thinks, or reasons; or when he understands something in relation to these thoughts and sensations—always he must be moving. . . . [This idea] will unlock for you the secret of the child's development.

Maria Montessori (1912).

In Chapters 3 and 4, a review was made of research evidence providing knowledge of various cerebral cortical activities and their possible behavioral correlates. When damage or dysfunction occurs in the cortical layers or the neural connections between various cortical areas, it usually impairs the specific sensory, intellectual, or neuromuscular behaviors maximally dependent on these loci.

In this chapter we examine the possible behavioral deficits or learning disorders that may result from cortical lesions in the somatosensory and motor strips, in the sensory or motor pathways of the peripheral nervous system, or in the interconnecting pathways in the cerebrum linking these two major systems. Defective tactile form perception is known as *astereognosis*; defective motor accuracy and control is called *apraxia*.

The Sensory and Motor Systems

The afferent neural pathways that mediate proprioception (awareness of the body in space and internal bodily states) and stereognosis (awareness of extrapersonal or environmental objects by touch alone) are depicted in Fig. 5.1. As explained in Chapter 2, impulses from the cutaneous receptors travel along sensory neurons to the spinal cord, where they enter through dorsal roots (see Fig. 2.6) and then extend vertically to the medulla oblongata,

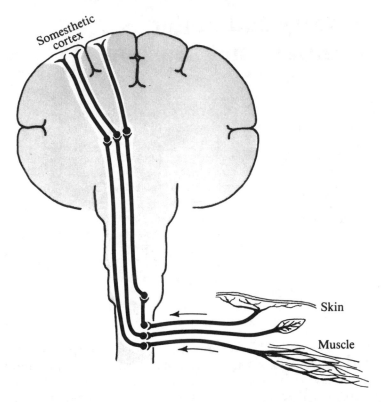

Figure 5.1. Simplified diagram of the sensory (afferent) pathways from skin and muscle to the sensory or somesthetic cortex. Notice the contralateral connections. (© 1980 William D. West)

where most of them cross over to the opposite side (neural decussation); they then continue vertically to the thalamus and finally to the somesthetic strip on that side. Proprioception and stereognosis involve much more complicated spinal and lateral pathways, but Fig. 5.1 provides the reader with simplified and grossly accurate information about the sensory pathways that supply information about the hand movements in writing, spelling, drawing; fingering a musical instrument; or any other fine manual activity involved in academic learning.

Figure 5.2 is a simplified representation of the efferent or motor neural pathways from the motor cortex to the neuromuscular system. Impulses originating in the motor strip travel down the efferent pathways to the medulla oblongata, where they cross over to the other side (neural decussation); they then enter the cerebellum, then out to the pons, down the anterior or ventral horns of the spinal cord, out through a ventral root (see Fig. 2.6 on p. 66), and along motor neurons of the peripheral nervous system

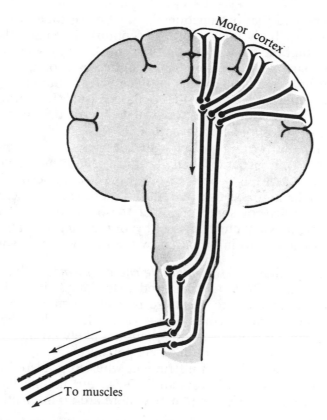

Figure 5.2. Simplified diagram of the motor (efferent) pathways from the motor cortex in the left hemisphere to the muscles of the right arm and hand. (© 1980 William D. West)

to muscle tissue. The cerebellum acts as a sort of "filter" to provide smooth and accurate action of muscle groups. Dysfunctions in the cerebellum, the sensory or motor pathways, or the sensory or motor areas of the cerebrum may result in awkward motor behavior that may interfere with normal learning. For example, a mentally bright cerebral palsied young adult may be unemployable because of severe spasticity of the speech and hand muscle systems and involuntary movements (athetosis) of the head and hands. Other examples are *apraxia*, the inability to imagine a motor act and carry it out, and *ataxia*, an incoordination of neuromuscular action. These impairments and their relation to learning are discussed later in this chapter.

Although it is convenient to think structurally of afferent nerves (*ad fero*, to carry toward), interconnecting cerebral nerve networks, and efferent nerves (*ex fero*, to carry away from), the teacher must keep in mind that all these structural systems work as one and that dysfunctions in any one of them may impair stereognosis or body image (proprioception). Even so, there are techniques that the clinical or school psychologist may use to try to isolate the part of the system giving the greatest trouble.

An example may make this problem clear. Suppose a child obtains an inferior score on the Benton Visual Retention Test, where he is required to draw a series of geometric designs following a 10-second exposure of each design. Is this child's performance poor because he cannot perceive the designs, cannot remember them, or has he a motor disability (apraxia) and cannot control the pencil well enough? Is it because of areas of skin anesthesia in his fingers and hands, because of reduced stereognostic help in his drawings, because of some or all of these, or because of some other problem completely missed by our examination? We can tease out some of this information by the following procedure:

1. Suppose that on the *multiple-choice form* of the Benton Visual Retention Test, administered a few days after the usual drawing administration to minimize possible memory effects, this child obtained a high score. This score tells us that the child's perception and memory of the diagrams are likely normal, and that the trouble may be motor rather than perceptual.

2. The esthesiometer, an instrument wherein graded fine nylon hairs are applied to the fingers and hands, tells us that the child's tactile sensitivity is normal and hence there are no insensitive areas of the skin.

3. The Halstead Finger Tapping Test reveals normal tapping speed for the child's nondominant hand, but severely slowed tapping speed in his dominant hand, thus strengthening the tentative diagnosis in (1) above that this child suffers from a manual–motor disability. Remedial drills, in this case, would stress activities to improve motor skills and muscular integration. The teacher could feel reasonably confident that the child's visual–spatial perception of geometric designs was within normal limits, but his motor expressive abilities were more impaired.

Sensorimotor Integration

The idea that normal behavior includes well-balanced sensory integration (a smooth blending of visual, auditory, tactile, and kinesthetic input), and that this collective pattern of neural energy must be integrated with the complex pattern of outgoing motor impulses, has been recognized at least since the discovery of the Bell-Magendie law in about 1820. Bell, in Great Britain, and

Magendie in France, working independently, demonstrated the separate locations and functions of the sensory and motor nerves in the spinal cord. In 1900–1901 Pavlov, the famous Russian physiologist, working on the process of digestion and the sensorimotor mechanisms that produce salivation, controlled the biological (or unconditioned) stimulus and the learned (or conditioned) stimulus, and he discovered a principle of behavior control (the conditioned reflex). This concept was taken up by psychologists and extended to social behavior (the conditioned response) and it became the theoretical basis for the then new and influential school of Behaviorism (J.B. Watson, 1919). Sir Charles S. Sherrington in Britain, in his classic work, *The Integrative Action of the Nervous System* (1906), described the *simple reflex*, the basic input-output unit of behavior, and he explained that it was part of the whole nervous system "because all parts of the nervous system are connected together" (Sherrington, 1906) and he admitted that "it is probably a purely abstract conception" and 'is a convenient, if not a probable, fiction." Years later Herrick (1944), taking the same view of spreading activities in the nervous system, denied the very existence of reflex arcs in the amphibian nervous system (see Chapter 3).

John B. Watson, the founder of the school of behaviorism, was satisfied to be more restrictive in his concept of the reflex arc. To him it was purely linear, being "an actual chain of nerve cells (and their fibers) running from each sense organ to the central nervous system (the brain and spinal cord) and out from the central nervous system to the muscles and glands" (Watson, 1924). This simplistic and linearly mechanistic view of sensorimotor neural conduction, the "classical view" of reflexes, was perpetuated by psychologists for many years after neurologists knew it to be inaccurate. We now know that all the input mechanisms of the amphibian are controlled by the central nervous system (CNS) via feedback loops. Just as the "response" of a furnace (production of warm air) controls the thermostat and turns the furnace off, thus cooling the air until it again triggers the thermostat to reactivate the furnace, so too, many control mechanisms operate in the human body to maintain a number of homeostatic processes within normal ranges. These are examples of the simple feedback loop, and the nervous system is equipped with a large number of them. In walking, the efferent control of the foot and leg swinging through the air provides ongoing and rapidly changing information to the brain about the sensory awareness of the foot and leg in space. In other words, the input or perceptual content is constantly monitored by the changing motor activity or efferent control. The same process is true of reading; the muscular eye movements across the page provide judgment about the speed with which one can attend and comprehend the material on the printed page. Should there be even a slight deficiency in the speed or accuracy of neural conduction in any part of the input, integrative, or output mechanisms in the CNS, a child may have difficulty in learning to read.

Not only are the sensory and motor functions necessary to perception and learning, but they must be integrated in a well-balanced and smoothly running energy system. Many years ago, P. Weiss (1941) demonstrated the continuous though uncoordinated motor activity of muscle tissue when that balance is interrupted. He surgically removed an animal's limb and kept it alive in a pool of nutrient fluids maintained at body temperature. Because all normal sensory input was removed, only the motor twitching, resulting from the incessant neural firing of live tissue, remained. Hebb concluded from this evidence that "sensory activity is essential to the regulation of central firing but not essential to initiating it" (Habb, 1949). In this case there were no afferent fibers but only efferent ones, and hence no sensory control, but only internal spontaneous stimulation. Lashley's expression of this basic neurophysiological knowledge appears in the quotation prefatory to Chapter 4: input is always into an actively excited system.

Sensorimotor integration may be examined with a visual–manual and an auditory–manual reaction time test. The child is asked to press a telegrapher's key as quickly as possible when a light appears or an auditory tone sounds in headphones. Reaction time has been investigated for the past 100 years, but interest in its relation to cerebral dysfunction came later, dating from World War I. Controlled studies with matched groups of normal and brain-damaged adults have shown the brain-damaged group to be slower with both simple and choice reaction time tasks to a visual stimulus (Blackburn & Benton, 1955) and much greater variability of response (Benton & Blackburn, 1957).

Up to this point we have discussed single motor performances and brain functions, but much behavior includes several motor activities occurring simultaneously (e.g., walking and talking). If the brain is required to mediate two concurrent motor performances, the degree of interference of one performance by the other, or the degree of independence of the two motor skills, will depend on which parts of the brain are controlling the two performances, and how near or far apart these areas are transcortically. If a subject is carrying out two activities simultaneously that are programmed by the same cerebral hemisphere, these motor acts will tend to be inferior to two acts each mediated by separate hemispheres. For example, when adult subjects are asked to speak and balance a dowel rod on the right and then on the left index finger, more interference in speech occurs in right-sided balancing than left (Kinsbourne & Cook, 1971). Finger tapping is also decreased more in the right hand than the left with concurrent verbal tasks (reciting a nursery rhyme, reading words silently, and solving anagrams silently). The pattern of difference between the hands is more pronounced for familial dextral (right-handed) subjects than familial sinistral (left-handed) subjects, and the difference increases with the complexity of the verbal task (Kee, Bathurst, & Hellige, 1983). This effect occurs also in kindergarten children (Kinsbourne & McMurray, 1975), although more exacting verbal tasks must be used with adults because of their better automatizing of finger-tapping skills. Kinsbourne and McMurray (1975) have suggested that "the present methodology appears to offer a simple and convenient way of ascertaining the lateralization of the control of expressive speech in children (and probably also of other forms of vocalization)."

Clumsy Children

A common classroom example of poor sensorimotor integration is the "clumsy child." These are the children who "in comparison with normal children of the same age . . . are characterized by a reduced ability to coordinate body posture and movement, and/or by problems in the execution of fine, perception-guided, movements" (Vaessen & Kalverboer, 1990). They may have difficulties writing, hopping, drawing, doing handcrafts, throwing or catching a ball, and maintaining normal bodily balance. Though clumsiness is difficult to define, the uncoordinated child or adult is easily recognized by teachers, dance instructors, and parade-ground drill sergeants. Identifiable CNS damage or dysfunction is known as the cause in some cases (e.g., cerebral palsy), but most of these children, who make up 5% to 10% of elementary-school classes (Schoemaker & Kalverboer, 1990), have no clear evidence of neural damage or dysfunction. In fact, the causes are not known and one can only speculate at best (MBD? diabetes? some chemical or nutritional cause? etc.). Because sensorimotor integration requires perfect neural timing and normal muscular response, Kalverboer (1975) has proposed that clumsy children show less than optimal neurological status. Most investigators find more boys than girls afflicted, and one study in the Netherlands found twice as many boys as girls categorized as "clumsy" (van Dellen et al., 1990). These same researchers proposed a two-step procedure for identifying these children and for measuring primary-school populations with teachers' ratings on a motor observation scale. This procedure will select the 5% to 10% sample of the target children suspected of clumsiness, and will lead to the next step, subjecting this sample to the Test of Motor Impairment (Stott, Moyes, & Henderson, 1984).

Because poor sensorimotor integration can interfere with learning, many of these children have problems that need to be analyzed and remediated. Not all clumsy children are poor students, however (some have high verbal IQs), and they may learn to compensate by avoiding athletics and gaining recognition in some other activity in which they can excel. And superior athletic ability does not guarantee academic success or verbal competence (witness televised interviews with top athletes, some of whom are articulate and fluent, but many of whom are verbally inept). Remedial treatment will have to be designed with the knowledge of each child's cognitive and behavioral strengths, but most clumsy children appear to benefit from teaching methods that stress physical movement (Ayres, 1975; Barsch, 1966; Cratty, 1967, 1970; Frostig & Maslow, 1970; Kephart, 1960, 1966; Montessori, 1912, 1964, 1965; Schoemaker & Kalverboer, 1990).

Basic Research in Tactile Perception

An esthesiometer is an instrument designed to stimulate the skin in a graded way to enable the experimenter to measure the threshold of pressure sensitivity. This type of measure may be done singly, providing information about pressure sensitivity and/or the ability to localize the source of pressure. Likewise, two points on the skin may be stimulated simultaneously to provide information about two-point discrimination or extinction or obscuration of one stimulus during a double stimulation.

Because tactile and manual proprioception seem to be intimately involved in learning to write and spell, and more tenuously in learning to read, it is interesting that controlled studies of linear tactile perception of direction have shown that in normal subjects it is slightly more accurate on the left hand than on the right hand of right-handed subjects (Benton, Levin, & Varney, 1973). These findings support the results of studies of subjects with unilateral right-hemisphere lesions; it was found that many of these subjects show bilateral impairment, but that patients with left-hemisphere disease may show a deficit only in the right hand (Carmon & Benton, 1969; Fontenot & Benton, 1971). For the child with normal brain functions the left- and right-hand differences are so small that the teacher can normally ignore them. If it is known, however, that the right-handed child has identifiable left- or right-hemisphere dysfunction, the possibility can be expected of some manual awkwardness or inferiority that may show itself in errors of copying from the blackboard, frequent misspellings, untidy writing, or poor spacing and scanning.

The diagnostician soon becomes aware that two-dimensional tactile recognition (such as reading Braille letters or palpating sandpaper letters on a flat surface) is a different process than haptic or proprioceptive recognition of a three-dimensional object (e.g., putting one's fingers and hands around all sides of a block or other object; see Fig. 3.6). The first requires maximal stimulation of the skin receptors in the fingertips, and the second includes not only that but much greater proprioceptive involvement of the muscles of the fingers, hand, and arm. Because the second perceptual task implicates many more muscle patterns in its three-dimensional activity, it is reasonable to infer that different patterns of cortical neurons are activated, and probably more of them. Many years ago this difference between tactile and haptic functions was demonstrated by showing that discrimination of passive movement (e.g., stroking the hand) was not affected by anesthetizing the overlying skin and muscles (Goldscheider, 1898). In this same experiment it was shown that when a strong faradic current was passed through the joints (the receptors for proprioception are the muscles, tendons, and joints) the thresholds for detection of movement were increased. This same phenomenon has been demonstrated more recently without pharmacological blocking. Levin (1973) showed that when fingertip tactile sensitivity is changed by a covering with a foam-rubber pad, no difference occurs in the efficiency of a proprioceptive task requiring precise manipulation of a button within a specified range of distance. This was true for both younger (age 19.9 years) and older (age 56.7 years) subjects. This information suggests that body-image and proprioceptive defects will be more seriously impairing than poor finger tactile sensitivity in learning manual–motor classroom skills. In other words, restricted sensory deficits (in this case, tactile sensitivity in the fingers) are probably not as important to learning as perceptual organization (in this case, somesthesis and stereognosis).

Basic Research in Motor Functions

Electrostimulation of the motor strip in animals was first done a little more than 100 years ago. These types of experiments demonstrated the contralateral connections of motor tracts, as well as localized functional areas in the motor strips themselves. It has been found (Hunter & Jasper, 1949) that by stimulating various parts of a cat's thalamus a number of excitatory and inhibitory types of behavior may be produced. One of the most interesting of these is the "arrest reaction," in which the animal can be made to stop and "freeze" in midaction, whether eating, walking, or pursuing a mouse. A more dramatic example of the arrest reaction was produced by Delgado when he stopped a charging bull by remote-control electrostimulation of its brain (Delgado, 1971). These examples remind the diagnostician and the special teacher that motor acts, both excitatory and inhibitory, are controlled by delicate electrochemical changes in a complex neural circuit originating in the sensorimotor strips of the cortex and ending in the neuromuscular system of the effectors. Any slight dysfunction in any part of the circuit may interfere with the afferent integrating processes of the brain and so result in a disturbance of the body image or ideomotor patterns necessary to initiating motor responses. Such dysfunctions may show themselves as apraxias, body-image deficits, and forms of motor aphasia (i.e., problems in expressive oral speech).

The Apraxias

A person "is apraxic when he is unable to act, although the systems through which he carries out his actions are intact (i.e., when there is neither paralysis, ataxia, nor abnormal movements), and he presents no marked intellectual disturbance" (De Ajuriaguerra & Tissot, 1969). A 10-year-old girl seen in our laboratory was unable to touch her fingertips behind her back, although the action was demonstrated several times for her. To please the tester, she eventually placed her hands on her hips. This girl walked and talked normally, but because of a biparietal dysfunction her spatial abilities were severely impaired, and she was unable to imagine or produce the ideomotor patterns necessary to guide her fingertips kinesthetically into the correct position. One child, who watches the dancing teacher demonstrate a series of steps, may imitate the whole movement correctly and rhythmically after one demonstration. Another child may want to see it repeated three or four times and have his or her own feet guided through the dance step before managing it slowly but successfully. The first child is quick to acquire the cortical–muscular pattern; the second lacks this aptitude, although neither child is paralyzed, ataxic, palsied, nor mentally retarded. Every drill sergeant is plagued with clumsy recruits, whom he relegates to the "awkward squad." These are the individuals who need more repetitions to acquire the cortical engrams and their correlative symbolic spatial patterns necessary to the required motor act. These adults in the awkward squad no doubt were the clumsy children in their youth.

Just as a computer needs a ready-made program to produce a solution or response, the human nervous system requires a repertoire of ideomotor programs on which it can draw. Sometimes the apraxic person may have difficulty carrying out an intransitive act related to his or her own body (e.g., salute, blow a kiss, pretend to clean his teeth or comb his hair). Sometimes such a person may be awkward in dealing with objects in the environment (i.e., carrying out a transitive act), such as hammering a nail, batting a ball, writing with a pencil, or constructing a model. Preschool children who cannot put on a coat demonstrate a type of "dressing apraxia," but as their nervous systems develop they reach a level of neural maturity where they can produce the necessary symbolic patterns. By age 6, most children, if they have been taught, can put on a coat because they have acquired the sequence of complex cortical and neuromuscular processes necessary to the act. In old age, senility may cause a breakdown in cortical and central nervous system structures, so that old persons may regress to a dressing apraxia and cannot put on their clothes without direction or assistance.

Body-Image Deficits

The clinical investigation of a body image or body schema began in about 1890, and so historically it is a relatively recent concept in neuropsychology. The first theories stressed "coenesthesis" or the coordinated input of kinesthetic or muscular sensations. This view, however, ignored the *spatial* aspects of the body image, and it was Head and Holmes (1911) in England who first presented a theory attempting to account for the temporal and spatial aspects of the awareness of one's body in space. They proposed that the body schema was a function of comparing the position or posture at any moment with the preceding one, and this comparison was supposed to be preconscious. In this view, a person is continuously building a schema that is constantly changing; therefore Head and Holmes named it a "plastic schema." In the past it has been believed that disturbances in the body schema are correlated with defects in right–left orientation and finger agnosia, but one report (Poeck & Orgass, 1971) has failed to find supporting evidence for this claim. In fact, the evidence found by Poeck and Orgass throws doubt on the usefulness of the concept of body schema itself because measures of its presence and/or nature are contaminated by both verbal and nonverbal factors. In spite of the methodological problems of measuring or detecting the proprioceptive awareness of one's own body in space, most researchers, teachers, psychotherapists, actors, and athletes find it a very real concept, essential to the learning and performances of their profession. A normal body schema has been described as "the peripheral, schematically conscious, structured, plastically bordered spatial perception of one's own body, constructed from previous and current (especially somesthetic) sensory information" (Frederiks, 1969b). To understand the types of minimal impairments frequent in some LD children, it may help to look briefly at the clinically pathological extremes resulting from moderate to severe brain damage and/or dysfunction. These include loss of perception of one-half or one part of the body. When this experience is conscious, the experience may be similar to that of an amputee, though without an amputation. When the hemiasomatognosia is nonconscious, the patient simply ignores one-half or one part of his body and behaves as if it did not exist. Sometimes a patient, because of brain dysfunctions, is unaware of his limb paralysis and cannot be persuaded of its existence even through logical demonstration. Others are unable to localize the parts of their bodies touched by the examiner, or to name them. A finger localization test can be used to investigate this (Benton et al., 1983, p. 84) and to relate it to academic performance in the classroom (Satz et al. 1978). The phantom-limb phenomenon, when it results from cortical damage or dysfunction, is an obvious perversion of the body image, as is the uncommon tendency of some patients to perceive the size of their body parts inaccurately. Later in the chapter we look at performances on tests of finger identification, right–left orientation, and other tactile and motor responses and their relationships to successful or disabled classroom learning.

Cortical Electrostimulation

Electrostimulation of the cerebral cortex was first attempted by Fritsch and Hitzig in Germany in 1870. They exposed the brain of a dog under light anesthetic and touched areas of the motor strip with an electrode delivering minimal electric current. This electro-stimulation produced motor responses in the contralateral legs. By the 1920s, the famous German neurosurgeon Otfrid Foerster was treating cases of traumatic epilepsy in human subjects (many of these were war injuries) by excising the epileptogenic scar tissue. He was also using the technique of cortical electrostimulation to explore the brains of his patients prior to the actual surgery.

In 1928, Wilder Penfield went to the University of Breslau to study with Foerster, who was professor of neurology and neurosurgery and president of the prestigious German Society of Neurology and Psychiatry (Penfield, 1977). On his return to Montreal, Penfield established the Montreal Neurological Institute, where he refined the technique, and during the 1930s and 1940s "cortical mapping" became an established diagnostic procedure for the surgical treatment of epilepsy and the incidental study of brain function (Penfield & Roberts, 1959).

During brain surgery the patient remained conscious, all probable pain being controlled by local anesthesia. An electrode applied to the cortical sensory strip (postcentral gyrus) was charged with a weak electrical current. The voltage strength would gradually be increased until the patient reported the presence of a bodily sensation. This was taken to be the threshold strength for sensory functions for that patient, and it provided a guide for the stimulus strength of the motor strip (precentral gyrus) to activate an involuntary motor activity (e.g., movement of the fingers or hands). Usually the stimulus strength to activate motor activity was greater, sometimes twice that of the sensory threshold strength. Stimulations in different cortical areas may produce inhibition of specific movements, temporary paralysis during the stimulation, or activation of activity that the patient cannot resist. Interference with the motor speech areas may cause temporary interruption with naming a series of objects, counting, reading, and writing. This impressive and imaginative clinical research may help the clinician and the special teacher to conceptualize and better understand problems of stammering, stuttering, articulation, word finding, spelling, writing, and sequential motor speech.

Since the 1950s, cortical mapping has been adopted by numerous neurosurgeons in other centers. A few, like Penfield, have used it to increase our knowledge of brain function. One of these, George Ojemann, at the University of Washington in Seattle, has collaborated with a professional team of neurophysiologists (Calvin & Ojemann, 1980) and neuropsychologists (Ojemann & Whitaker, 1978; Ojemann & Mateer, 1979), and he and his colleagues have produced a valuable collection of papers for the clinical neuropsychologist and student of the human brain.

Sensorimotor Functions and Learning

The myelination of cortical cells in the sensory and motor strips and the occipital lobes is most advanced at birth (Flechsig, 1927), which may explain why the infant during the first few months of life explores the world largely through his tactual sense mode. He finds the object by sight but explores it by touch with hands and mouth. This knowledge has led some educators to propose that the child's tactile sense is the most primitive, and historically most practiced; hence it is the one to use as a basis for remedial teaching when that is indicated. Infants learn about the three-dimensional environment by integrating what they see with what they can touch and move.

Many professional educators have made use of this observation in both their theories and practices, but one of the earliest and most influential in this century was Maria Montessori, an internationally recognized Italian scholar. It is notable that her first strong academic interests were in mathematics, and this led to technical training in engineering, then in biology, and finally in medicine. She became the first woman to complete a medical degree in Italy (1896), and it was this background that was to alert her to the importance of the biological bases of behavior and learning in her long career as an influential educator. After several years of practical experience in medical practice and treatment of mentally impaired children, she returned to the university to prepare herself for educating the normal and subnormal. She studied philosophy, psychology, pediatric neurology, and the theories and methods of Itard and Seguin, both of whom had devoted their lives to the treatment and education of the retarded. With her training in rigorous scientific principles, physiology, neurology, psychology, philosophy, and the special education of the mentally retarded, and her strong humanistic drive to help children, both normal and impaired, she was one of the best prepared educators of her time. So convinced was she that the teacher must consider the child completely, in terms of his physical and mental inheritance, that she never made the error of viewing the child only in behavioral terms but emphasized that the child's intellect was intimately bound up with his body, particularly with the nervous and muscular systems. Although Montessori's methods were developed prior to modern neuropsychological knowledge, she was convinced of their value. She believed that "the hand is the instrument of the brain" and that the education of the child demanded activation and interaction of these two. She talked about the sensorial foundations of intellectual life and recommended sensorial, mainly tactile and visual, contact with objects in the initial stages of learning about them. To teach the abstract concept of "triangularity," she would give the child a triangular block that he could handle and fit into a form board. When this skill was mastered, the child was then shown printed cards with silhouettes of triangles (with the inside spaces filled in). When the child could recognize these as triangles he was shown line drawings of triangles; finally the child was taught the verbal abstraction of the concept, the description of a triangle (i.e., a plane figure enclosed by three straight lines). In other words, what he first experienced tactually, and then visually, he now was able "to see" mentally (Standing, 1962). Like Piaget, Montessori proposed a developmental pattern in which the child at first learned about the environment unconsciously, simply by being moved about in it, but later, conscious learning occurred through repeated manipulation and tactile and motor exploration of environmental objects. By this time the hand had truly become the instrument of the brain, and it was through this manual activity that the child enriched his experience and developed himself (Montessori, 1965; Standing, 1962). We introduce Montessori in this chapter to remind ourselves that successful remedial teaching practices have always made use of tactile and visual–manual activities, and that their value has been recognized in many developmental theories.

Piaget, in his theory of child development, proposed the sensorimotor period as the first stage of growth ranging from birth to about 2 years of age (Piaget, 1952); this sensorimotor interaction provided the child with increasing information about the world. Some of the child's responses are automatic or reflexive (or unconscious in Montessori's theory) and some provide variable patterns of interacting.

> Sensorimotor space begins to evolve right from the child's birth, and together with perception and motor activity it undergoes considerable development up until the appearance of speech and symbolic images. . . . This sensorimotor space is superimposed upon various pre-existing spaces such as the postural, etc., though it is by no means a simple reflection or repetition of them. (Piaget & Inhelder, 1956)

As students of Piaget know, he developed a highly detailed theory of visual perception and its relation to haptic experience. Like Montessori, he drew attention to the perceptual and conceptual processes in cognition, but he proposed a more refined and sequential analysis of the small child's responses to perceptual or sensorimotor space. All understanding of the physical environment includes both sensory awareness and imaginary recall of objects in their absence, and perception in its complete sense means an interaction of these two processes. Where these two provide a smooth reciprocal function, perception occurs with a sense of familiarity, ease, and confidence. Where these two do not, as in viewing a formless, abstract painting, the perceptual response may bring a sense of incomprehension, frustration, and insecurity. Piaget expressed this cognitive process thus: "It [perception] completes perceptual knowledge by reference to objects not actually perceived" (Piaget & Inhelder, 1956).

The first exhaustive developmental observation of a child's haptic perception, it seems, was carried out by Piaget. He discovered, in studying the child from 2 to 7 years, an unfolding and self-revealing pattern. Below age 2 years 6 months, experimentation with hidden figures is limited. From then up to $3\frac{1}{2}$ or 4 years, the child can recognize haptically familiar objects (such as a ball, scissors, or spoon) but not geometric euclidean figures (such as a square, circle, or triangle). This interesting finding suggests that haptic recognition (i.e., three-dimensional stereognosis) is not only easier but developmentally earlier than two-dimensional stereognosis of very thin abstract forms. In this same connection, clinical neuropsychologists and speech therapists are aware that aphasic patients with word-finding problems may be unable to name pictures of objects (i.e., two-dimensional ones) but may be much more successful when these objects are handed to them to examine (i.e., three-dimensional ones). More is said about the understanding and treatment of aphasia in Chapter 8.

At the preschool age of $3\frac{1}{2}$ to 4 years, Piaget found the beginnings of haptic recognition of shapes, but "curiously enough, the shapes first recognized are not eucliden but topological" (Piaget & Inhelder, 1956). He found that the child at this stage could distinguish open from closed forms (e.g., O and C) but could not distinguish a square from a circle because both are closed, and straight lines and angles are still not identified. The poor haptic recognition in the early years is correlated with relatively passive tactile exploration, which frequently provides only chance discoveries.

As children mature, their tactile–kinesthetic exploration becomes more vigorous and searching so that, by $5\frac{1}{2}$ to 6 years, they begin to identify abstract forms, with much hesitation, such as the rhombus and trapezium. Between ages 6 and 7 the child becomes much more methodical in such tactile–kinesthetic exploration and now can discriminate among complex forms, such as a semicircle, a diamond, and a star. It is at this age that we begin to study children in the Victoria laboratory, and we find that they can replace the blocks in a six-block version of the Seguin formboard, although with great variability in performance (Spreen & Gaddes, 1969).

Although the theories of both Montessori and Piaget were developed before modern neuropsychological knowledge, both theories either stressed or implied the importance of the biological bases of behavior, the presence of mediating organic processes, and the necessity for adapting to the environment. Whereas they recognized the important presence of underlying physiological processes, however, their primary interest was behavioral phenomena, which is the proper province of the teacher and school psychologist.

To become aware of the neurological correlates of tactile perception, we must go to the research neuropsychologist. It is interesting that when Luria described the topic of "tactile perception" he first described the brain structures mediating it. When explaining "disturbances of tactile synthesis," Luria (1966) wrote, "These disturbances (i.e., tactile agnosia or astereognosis) may arise from lesions of the parietal areas of the cerebral cortex, areas constituting the cortical portion of the cutaneo-kinesthetic analyzer. . . ."By this "analyzer" he meant the sensory strip just posterior to the fissure of Rolando and the adjacent parietal cortex. He reported damage to these cortical areas resulting in disturbed body image, poor finger localization, impaired cutaneous localization, inaccurate perception of the direction of a line drawn on the skin, and astereognosis, even though in some cases tactile awareness was intact. Luria has written at some length not only on disorders of tactile perception, but also on visual imperceptions and the many varieties of visual–motor disorders. Any remedial teacher would do well to study this material, which is supplied with many graphic examples (Luria, 1966, pp. 134–153).

Many educators have recommended a perceptual–motor or motor emphasis or a sensorimotor integration model for learning (Ayres, 1968, 1972a, 1975; Barsch, 1965, 1966; Cratty, 1967, 1968; Cruickshank, 1975; Fernald, 1943; Freidus, 1964, 1966; Getman, 1966; Kephart, 1960/1971, 1966, 1975; Kirk, 1966; Strauss & Lehtinen, 1947; Valett, 1973), and with the assessment batteries included in some of these (e.g., Ayres, Cratty) the teacher will become prepared with more comprehensive understanding of the functions of somesthesis and its role in classroom learning.

Neuropsychological Findings

Having presented a neuropsychological model of the sensorimotor structures and functions in learning, the next step is to relate test findings of these behavioral processes to success and failure in academic learning.

In the 1950s, Ralph Reitan was a leader in developing neuropsychological tests for use in localizing brain lesions. This was a useful new procedure because the current brain scans had not yet appeared. By the 1960s, he began to expand his knowledge and

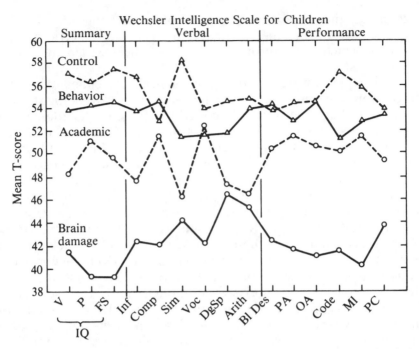

Figure 5.3. Graphic presentation of mean performances on the Wechsler Intelligence Scale for Children for a control group, a brain-damaged group, and minimal brain-damaged groups with academic deficiencies and school behavior problems. (From Reitan & Boll, 1973. With permission from the authors and the New York Academy of Sciences.)

assessment techniques to the study of LD children. In one study (Reitan & Boll, 1973), he subjected four groups of children (mean age 7.3–7.5 years) to a large battery of intellectual, educational, and neuropsychological tests and compared their group differences (Fig. 5.3). The groups included 25 normal controls (none had ever failed a grade in school or been referred for acadcmic or behavioral problems), 25 who were brain damaged, 25 who were referred for academic and learning difficulties but not behavior problems, and 19 who were referred for school behavioral difficulties. In any school population it is almost certain that all of these types of children are represented and must be dealt with by teachers.

Reitan and Boll found that on the Wechsler (WISC) the brain-damaged group consistently performed more poorly than the other three groups and, of these three, the group with academic deficiencies (that is, the LD group) was the poorest. This same order of performance—the controls best, the behavior disorder group next, then the learning disabled, and finally the brain-damaged group worst—also held for academic measures (reading, spelling, and arithmetic as measured by the Wide Range Achievement Test), visual–spatial skills, motor functions, tactile perception, and incidental memory. The control and "behavior" groups were very close and their scores on most tests were, for the most part, not statistically significantly different. Although such a study concerns itself with group performance levels on various skills and hence tells us nothing specific about a particular child, it does suggest the strong possibility of subtle cerebral dysfunctions in some LD children. Certainly, the group test results show such a child to be closer in behavior to the known brain-damaged subjects than either the normal control or the child with behavior problems. It is quite possible that the child with poor social control is a product of family pressures or other psychosocial forces, whereas the child refractory to normal learning and motivational procedures may be suffering from chronic intrinsic conflicts stemming from organic dysfunctions. Reitan and Boll's study, combined with our own clinical experience, has led us to the view that many or most of the LD children are suffering from the same kind of sensorimotor, perceptual, and cognitive disabilities as the brain-damaged child, although to a lesser degree, regardless of the absence of conclusive evidence on a standard neurological examination.

Table 5.1 summarizes the findings of a computer survey of the files of 154 children referred to our laboratory because of moderate to severe learning disorders. These children ranged in age from 8 to 15, and about 70% were boys and 30% girls. They were selected by computer from our files in Category 3 (see Table 1.1), that is, *LD children with no clear neurological signs.*

Examining the data summarized in Table 5.1 (see page 196) reveals that (1) Although the neurologists found no clear-cut neurological findings of abnormality, most of these children performed at a level below average on most of the sensorimotor tests listed here, in the same way that children with known brain dysfunctions do. (2) Although most of the LD children were inferior on sensorimotor tasks, a few of them achieved normal scores in a few instances. (3) Though the numbers of subjects in some age groups were small, especially for the girls, this tended to make the ranges greater (e.g., from 0 to 100%), but even so the average performances were inferior except on the Tactual Perception Test. It is useful to observe that the Esthesiometer Test and Dynamometer (hand grip) were failed by the greatest mumber of LD boys and girls. These tests are also sensitive indicators of CNS damage or dysfunction.

Table 5.1. Percentages of LD Children, Aged 8–15, Scoring Below One Standard Deviation on a Number of Sensorimotor Tests

Test	N	Dominant Hand <−1 SD (%)	Nondominant Hand <−1 SD (%)	Both Hands <−1 SD (%)	Range (%)
Esthesiometer	20 boys and girls	95.0	85.0		87.5–100
Stereognosis	80 boys	46.4	44.6		20.0–96.0
	25 girls	40.9	59.1		0.0–100
Tactual perception	44 boys			31.3	19.2–66.4
	15 girls			25.9	0.0–100
Hand grip	61 boys	65.6			90.0–93.3
	21 girls	61.9			75.0–100
Finger tapping	19 boys and girls	63.0			60.0–100
Visual–manual R.T.[a]	56 boys	57.1	57.1	57.1	50.0–100
	26 girls	46.1	38.5	42.3	25.0–100
R-L orientation	83 boys			51.8	18.2–100
	22 girls			45.4	0.0–100

[a] The complete name is "Visual–Manual Reaction Time Test." (The child presses a key as soon as he sees a light.)

In summary, then, we can conclude that inferiority in a sensory, and/or a motor, and/or a sensorimotor integration task is a sensitive indicator of CNS dysfunction and a reliable correlate of learning disorders.

Clinical Addendum

Two Cases of Parietal Dysfunctions

Because "the parietal lobe not only integrates sensory and spatial information to allow accurate movements in space, but also functions to direct or guide movements in the immediate vicinity of the body" (Kolb & Whishaw, 1990) we have included two cases in this discussion that include serious parietal dysfunctions and accompanying sensorimotor problems. Kolb and Whishaw are careful to state that "the parietal lobe is not considered to be the *only* motor command system, but rather one of several" (p. 421).

Case 1

Some years ago a neurologist referred to us a 6-year-old boy who had a problem of poor coordination and hyperactive behavior. His mother reported that he was easy to raise, he walked early, and he developed speech at the normal time. The parents, both young (the father was 24 and the mother 20 at the time of Mark's birth), reported that they noticed the hyperactivity by Mark's second birthday. In school his poor coordination showed itself in an inability to draw, cut with scissors, and carry out normal manual activities. In addition he was distractible, excitable, and easily frustrated. The neurological examination revealed one minimal and one major finding: involuntary movements of his hands and feet, and a grade iii dysrhythmia in the left cerebral motor region, respectively. Because Mark was right-handed this had a seriously disturbing effect on his writing and manual skills.

Our test examination showed Mark to be an alert, likable boy. Throughout the 5 hours of testing he showed no signs of distractibility, because in the testing laboratory he was on a one-to-one situation. There were no clear signs of "hyperactivity" so that these reported behaviors seemed to be more related to situational and psychological factors than to organic ones.

On the Wechsler (WISC) he measured a verbal IQ of 118 and a performance IQ of 105. He had superior scores on the Vocabulary, Digit Span, and Similarities subtests but had only average scores on Picture Arrangement and Coding, because of his moderate apraxia. On the Benton Visual Retention Test he neglected the peripheral figures in the right visual field, which suggested that the left-hemisphere disturbance, although centered in the left motor strip, must also have affected the left visual tracts minimally. Other than the minimal right visual field neglect, his visual perception was intact, as were also his auditory and tactile recognition. He showed inferior scores with his right hand relative to his left on visual–manual reaction time, finger tapping, and hand-grip strength. The parents reported that in running or climbing he showed slight awkwardness in his right arm and leg.

In the report to Mark's teacher it was stressed that he was a bright, eager little boy whose reported hyperactivity was likely to be related more to situational frustrations than to any perceptual problem. Because the school knew that Mark had been referred to a neurologist, this report made it clear that "there is no conclusive evidence of brain damage, but because of a slight unevenness of electrical function in the left side of his brain, he will likely always have a certain awkwardness of manipulation in his right hand. This means that he may be slow in writing and carrying out many manual tasks requiring speed and fine precision."

A year later, on recall, we found that Mark's learning problems had largely disappeared. His teachers realized his potential brightness and the specific nature of his manual apraxia, and they allowed for this in their dealing with him. His "hyperactivity" disappeared and was replaced by an image of alert, energetic interest in learning.

A follow-up interview, when Mark was in Grade 9, showed him to be a bright, well-adjusted adolescent, with A grades in mathematics and science. His handwriting was still slow and awkward, but he had learned to live with it and to compensate for it successfully.

Case 2

Donald is one of the most extreme cases of "spatial disorientation" in a child that one is likely to see in 30 years of teaching. He was first referred for testing by a pediatric neurologist when he was 10 years old, because of seizures (both petit and grand mal) and severe learning disabilities.

Donald's mother reported no unusual health history with him until age 5, when he developed a brain infection (encephalitis), followed first by staring spells and later by occasional grand mal seizures. Anticonvulsive medication was prescribed with fairly heavy doses to control the frequency of the seizures. Donald's EEGs showed bilateral spike activity in the left frontal and parietal lobes and in the right parieto-temporal areas. At age 7, Donald showed a WISC verbal IQ of 91 and a performance IQ of 86. His spoken language was normal but he could neither read nor write, and he had great difficulty with spatial (e.g., Block Design on the WISC) and sequential–visual–motor tasks (e.g., Coding on the WISC). Donald not only suffered from a poor sense of direction, but he also showed awkward coordination in hopping and skipping. The evidence from the EEGs suggested strongly that there were bilateral dysfunctions in the motor and sensory strips as well as some areas of both parietal lobes.

At age 10, Donald measured a WISC verbal IQ of 74 and a performance IQ of 52. His poorer mental measures seem to have stemmed from the heavy medication program. Although he tried to cooperate in the testing situation, he yawned continually and usually fell asleep on arriving home from school in the afternoon. Because learning is related to the degree of "motivated activity" (Montessori, 1965), the drug-imposed reduction of Donald's activity seemed to result in an impoverished school experience. Although detailed remedial exercises were proposed, Donald made little or no progress for the next 2 years, either because his teachers gave him inappropriate instruction or because he was unable to profit from it on account of his imposed lethargy.

Observation during testing focused on Donald's ability to perceive visual forms and to draw them or react to them spatially. He was able to copy a square and a triangle reasonably well, although he hesitated to do this at first. After drawing them he was able to name them correctly. It was interesting to observe that whereas his speech was normal, his vocabulary was very limited because of his learning problem. When shown a Greek cross, he made a vertical line and was unable to do anything more. Even when urged to continue, he was unable to scan it, analyze it, and draw it. Evidently he had not yet acquired the necessary cortical engrams or the ideomotor images (Fig. 5.4).

In stereognosis he had great difficulty in recognizing forms with his left hand, although performance with the right hand was a little better. This response supports the hypothesis that although there was pathology in both hemispheres, it was more pronounced in the right. His inferior spatial imagery correlated with this supposition, and his normal expressive speech supported normal or nearly normal functions in the motor–speech tracts of the left hemisphere.

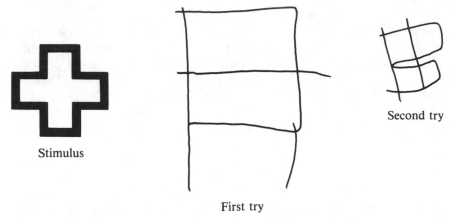

Stimulus

First try

Second try

Figure 5.4.   Donald's attempts to copy a Greek cross (age 11 years 3 months).

Donald's auditory–linguistic abilities were among his best. When we saw him a year later at age 11, he was able to recite the complete alphabet correctly, but he could not remember the visual form of some of the letters, and his visual scanning was so chaotic that there was no semblance of straight lines (Fig. 5.5).

Motor activities requiring spatial scanning were impossible. He could not imitate a sequential pattern of tapping a series of blocks, no matter how many times or how slowly the tapping sequence was repeated. Hopscotch was impossible for him and he was unable to touch his fingers behind his back, although this was demonstrated several times. Nevertheless, he was neither paralyzed nor ataxic, and he walked normally.

Donald's mother reported he had fluctuating success in dressing himself. Sometimes he suffered from severe dressing apraxia and at other times there seemed to be little or no problem. Such fluctuations in behavior suggest biochemical changes (possibly dietary or transitory blood chemistry imbalances).

His spatial disorientation in extrapersonal space had been chronic since his encephalitis. He got lost in his own house and had difficulty finding the bathroom or his own belongings in his bedroom. When sent for something in the back yard he sometimes could not find the kitchen door to return to the house. In three test sessions in our laboratory (totaling about 18 hours) over a period of 18 months, he never learned to find his way from the testing room to the hall where his mother was waiting, although all the other children we have seen (more than 2000 up to that time) learned this route on their first visit.

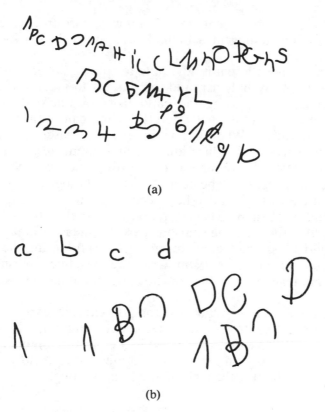

(a)

(b)

Figure 5.5. (a) Donald's spontaneous writing of the alphabet and numbers (age 11 years, 3 months), and (b) his copying of four letters that had been written and named for him.

What Donald's Teachers Might Do

A teacher confronted with a child as severely impaired as Donald will have a monumental task, and will need as much help as possible in the form of professional information and suggestions. Donald's teachers faced two basic problems: (1) the mental lethargy and reduced attention resulting from the heavy medication program and (2) the chronic visual–motor–spatial deficits resulting from the bilateral parietal brain dysfunctions.

Let us look at the first of these. If Donald were hospitalized and taken off his anticonvulsive medication, his IQ might have been higher. However, in his case, because the parents were afraid that severe seizures would cause more brain damage, this was not tried, and his teachers had to struggle to teach him with his drug-imposed mental sluggishness. This is frequently the cruel dilemma of the epileptic child; the advantage of being seizure-free is often at the cost of functioning at a mental level much below his or her potential.

In cases such as these it is advisable for the pediatric neurologist, teacher, school psychologist, and the parents to meet to clarify the possible risks of removing the child from or markedly reducing medication dosage to a level where the child can profit more from remedial education. When this is done, then "baseline" measures on psychological and educational achievement tests should be carried out after the reduction of the drug dosage and prior to the remedial program. The teacher or psychologist, in obtaining baseline measures, should take special care to wait long enough after withdrawal of medication to be sure there are no residual drug effects; otherwise the spurious baseline measures may operate to the child's disadvantage. Intermittent testing during the months ahead will permit comparison with the baseline measures and inform the teacher whether or not the remedial measures are effective.

The second problem relates to Donald's chronic learning deficits. Before attempting to devise a remedial program, all available evidence will be assembled to provide a conceptual model of what is likely to be going on when Donald views the world or tries to acquire ideas about it through reading and writing.

Diagnosis

The diagnostic paradigm used in all our analyses of individual cases is based on the neurological model of sensory input, cerebral integration, and motor output, as described in the preceding discussions in this book.

Sensory and Perceptual Functions

Visual Perception. The teacher will want to know answers to the following questions. Does Donald perceive his environment visually in such a chaotic way that it is virtually impossible to teach him to read or write, or is his visual perception normal, but his visual memory defective? Likewise, are both these functions reasonably normal, but his visual–motor abilities so defective that he is unable to reproduce drawings or to write in an average way for a boy his age? On the Benton Visual Retention Test, which required him to copy 10 geometric diagrams, he obtained zero scores at ages 9 years 11 months and 10 years 5 months; he was unable to draw any of the designs although the average child of this age can draw from memory (a more difficult task than copying) four designs at age 9 and five designs at age 10 (Benton, 1963b, p. 46). On the third testing, when Donald was 11 years 3 months old, he completed one of the designs successfully. This was Card 3, which was fairly detailed; it included two linked circles at the center of the card with a small square in the right peripheral area. Some parts of the other cards were drawn correctly, but no part marks are allowed. To compare this with his verbal memory of the designs, the multiple-choice form of the Benton Visual Retention Test was administered twice, and both times he remembered 2 of the 10 designs he had seen on the initial viewing. This evidence suggests that his visual memory when free of drawing or motor demands was accurate, although inferior for his age. When asked to draw something, Donald's scanning and visual spacing was so impaired that he was unable to draw what he could remember.

This hypothesis was also supported by the evidence from drawing and writing. When asked to draw a square and a triangle, he could do this satisfactorily, although he required a great deal of urging and encouragement to do it. Evidently, the scanning required to draw these basic figures was simple enough to permit him to draw them. The Greek cross, however, which analytically is made up of five squares of equal size, was beyond his abilities to translate into accurate motor patterns. At age 9 years 11 months he drew one vertical line; at age 11 years 13 months he made two more complicated attempts, but neither resembled a Greek cross (Fig. 5.4). It is interesting that he did perceive the analytical fact that the cross was made up of rectangular spaces, but his severely impaired spatial orientation made it impossible for him to scan the figure mentally and to arrange the arms in their correct spatial relationships.

Figure 5.5 shows his writing of letters and numbers. At first he was asked to write the alphabet and the numbers from 1 to 10 from memory. Scrutiny of his writing shows that his auditory–linguistic knowledge was completely accurate, but his visual–graphic transposition produced many errors. The letter A lacks the crossbar, as it does everywhere on that sheet. On B, he remembered only the top eliptical form and neglected the bottom one. C and D are satisfactory. E is reversed and lacks the crossbar, as did A. F also lacks the crossbar. G is correct except that it is reversed *and* inverted. H and I are acceptable. J is reversed. K lacks the vertical line. L, M, N, and O are recognizable. P and Q are linked because of his poor spacing, and Q lacks closure. R is a lower-case letter, and S is acceptable. T lacks the left half of the top crossbar, and U, which is rotated, is joined to it. V is rotated and resembles U rather than V. He needed two tries at W, the second being successful but inverted. X and Y are recognizable and Z lacks the top crossbar. When we look at the numbers, they are all there, but in some cases badly deformed: 1, 2, 3, 4, 6, 7, 9, and 10 are recognizable; 5 has an extra inverted 6 on it, which suggests he wrote it over the 6, unable to space it separately. He needed another three tries on 6, but it is notable that he was aware of the reversal and inversions on the first two tries and corrected himself successfully on the third try. Figure 5.5b gives us some useful information about his abilities to copy. The psychometrician wrote the four *lower-case* letters, a, b, c, and d on the sheet and asked Donald to copy them. Because most of the visual–graphic–motor patterns that he had mastered were capital, or upper case, letters, he wrote the four letters in that form. Again, however, he neglected the crossbar on A on all three tries and reversed C. B and D are satisfactory. This information tells us that he was able to *read* lower-case letters, but because of his severe spatial disorientation he did not have confidence that he could copy what he saw. Instead, he transcribed the *concept* of what he read into a *motor pattern* with which he had some familiarity.

We tested his visual discrimination of "larger than" and "farther and closer" and found these completely successful for common environmental objects.

In summary, the test evidence suggests that Donald's perception had some degree of accuracy and that it could be helped by mnemonic devices, and his visual–perceptual attention improved by multisensorimotor exercises. The exact nature of these is described later under remediation.

Auditory Perception. Donald's phonetic discrimination was in the normal range, as was his verbal memory in repeating sentences on the Spreen–Benton Sentence Repetition Test. Dichotic listening suggested that he was markedly left-hemisphere dominant for language, which was fortunate in that neurological examinations had indicated his left hemisphere to be less affected than his right. His speech abilities appeared normal in ordinary conversation, in his ability to recite the alphabet and numbers, in naming objects he could not draw, and in sentence repetition. Because oral speech was one of his relative strengths, it was exploited in his remediation program.

Stereognosis (Tactile Form Recognition). Because of his biparietal disturbance, Donald's tactile recognition was not good in either hand, but it was better with his right hand because of the relative superiority of his left cerebral hemisphere. Because he was strongly right-handed this was fortunate and permitted his spatial orientation to be encouraged through a manual–spatial set of exercises.

Intellectual Abilities

Intelligence quotients cannot be used in their usual way to indicate the native intelligence of a child on a heavy medication program, but the subtest scores are useful if viewed qualitatively in light of the pharmacological influences. In our four test sessions, Donald obtained verbal IQs of 91, 74, 63, and 58, and performance IQs of 86, 48, 44, and 45. The diminishing verbal IQs reflect the debilitating effects of the drug program along with an educational program in a small rural school that was willing but unprepared to deal with such a difficult and complex learning problem. Because of his nearly normal speech skills his WISC vocabulary conceptual abilities measured almost in the normal range. However, arithmetic was inferior because of his spatial deficits, and general information, comprehension of common problems, and memory for digits were extremely poor because of his inability to read and learn normally. All the WISC performance tests were inferior because of their heavy spatial loadings. This information suggests that a major part of Donald's learning should occur through conversation and discussion, and that reading, writing, and spelling should be assisted through multisensorimotor–spatial reinforcement.

Motor Skills and Sensorimotor Integration

Donald's finger tapping was neuromuscularly fluent but slow, presumably because of the drugs. Reaction times to a light and to a tone were his best measures, in this group of tests, although they were slow and hence below average for his age. Donald's hand grip in his right hand was better than in his left, but still below average, and his finger localization was inferior on both hands. His performance on the Benton Right–Left Orientation Test was defective, showing poor directional identification of his own body parts and of objects in extrapersonal space. Because all these skills are believed to draw heavily on parietal function, the poor scores on these sensorimotor tests are not surprising. At the same time, they are not discouraging because his neuromuscular integration appears to be normal and this is a good basis for motor learning.

Remediation: What to Do to Help Donald

Because Donald was a happy, reasonably well-adjusted youngster, the primary therapeutic responsibility was to help him circumvent his specific learning disabilities, once the depressing effects of the medication program could be reduced. Obviously when a child manifests chronic emotional symptoms stemming, at least in part, from the frustrations he suffers from learning problems, then the teacher must devise ways of minimizing the effects of the perceptual and/or motor deficiencies but also must try to help the child to resolve these feelings and attitudes and to develop better self-acceptance. In Donald's case, it seemed that a remedial program to help the first aspect of the problem could have no other effect on his self-esteem but to improve it. Basically, however, his learning problems were not maximally "emotional"; Donald was cheery and well adjusted with his peers, his teacher, and his family.

Donald's remedial program included the following cognitive and behavioral procedures:

1. Attention: Medical readjustment of his medication program to maximize attention.
2. Visual processes.
    a. Visual memory. Donald was shown nonverbal stimuli (actual common objects first, then line drawings of objects) in increasing numbers and asked to report on or describe them. This report was requested immediately following the removal of the stimuli, then after 5 seconds, after 10 seconds, etc. Following this, the same procedure was done with geometric figures, then single letters, words, phrases, and short sentences. Any remedial teacher will have a repertoire of exercises to improve visual memory. The inexperienced teacher has many sources to draw on (Cruickshank, 1961, 1977; Myers & Hammill, 1990; Rosner, 1979; Valett, 1973).
    b. Visual–motor skills. A large variety of hand–eye co-ordination exercises were carried out *after* Donald had practiced the motor skill with his eyes closed. This was to eliminate the disturbing effects of his visual–spatial deficits in the early stages of learning. At this stage his drawing of simple objects was severely impaired (Fig. 5.6).
3. Auditory processes. Although his conversational speech was unimpaired, Donald was given practice in talking, memorizing and reciting poetry, and taking part in classroom plays. This practice not only provided language development for him but gave him an opportunity to gain success in one of his behavioral strengths. Use of a tape recorder assisted him in learning to spell and to read.
4. Validation of remedial measures. A case as difficult as this needs constant monitoring and evaluation to discover whether the methods are appropriate and what progress, if any, is resulting.

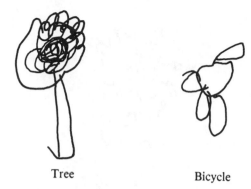

Tree   Bicycle

Figure 5.6. Donald's attempts to draw two common objects (age 11 years 3 months).

Donald's teacher will need to be supplied with a great variety of remedial suggestions and the patience and interest to continually measure possible progress.

Progress Report on Donald

Figure 5.7 shows the marked improvement in Donald's writing after only 8 months of training in a special center for severely learning disabled children. He entered this special school at age $11\frac{1}{2}$. He was taught to read by a modified Gillingham method because his auditory language was good. Essentially the procedure made use of phonics coupled with multisensory stimulation. By the end of his second year he read at a Grade 5 level, slowly, but accurately for the most part. His progress in both reading and spelling was rapid.

His writing within 2 years progressed from chaotic inaccuracy (Fig. 5.5) to legible and well-spaced writing (Fig. 5.7). Three sentences were dictated, and other than one visually misspelled word (tier), a lack of periods, and a capitalized first word in the third sentence, they are written neatly and intelligibly. He was taught to write using dark-lined paper and with his eyes closed or averted. This made use of a strong tactile–auditory match and avoided the disturbing effects of his poor visual perception and memory. Initially grid paper was tried but was visually more confusing than lined paper, so it was abandoned in favor of heavy lined paper, which worked successfully.

Donald's arithmetic was still very weak. At age 13 he could add and count, but other skills were unreliable. No doubt the strong

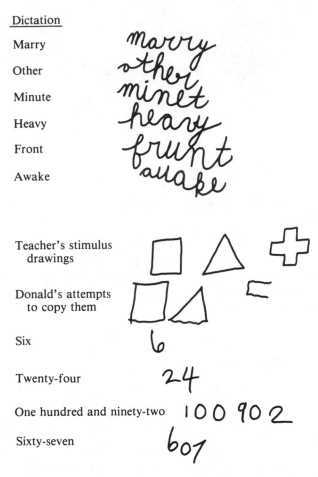

Figure 5.7. Donald's writing and drawing after 8 months of intensive remedial teaching (age 12 years 10 months).

spatial component in elementary written arithmetic has been a serious impediment. Figure 5.7 shows how his good auditory memory and impaired visual scanning produced "logical errors" in writing to dictation multidigit numbers with internal zeros. He later learned to write such numbers correctly with the aid of skilled remedial teaching.

Because his oral speech is fluent and competent, Donald's written English is reasonably good. Once he learned to space his letters and write on lines, he showed an ability to compose short stories and write them at about a Grade 5 level. His spelling includes "phonetically correct errors" (e.g., minet and frunt)

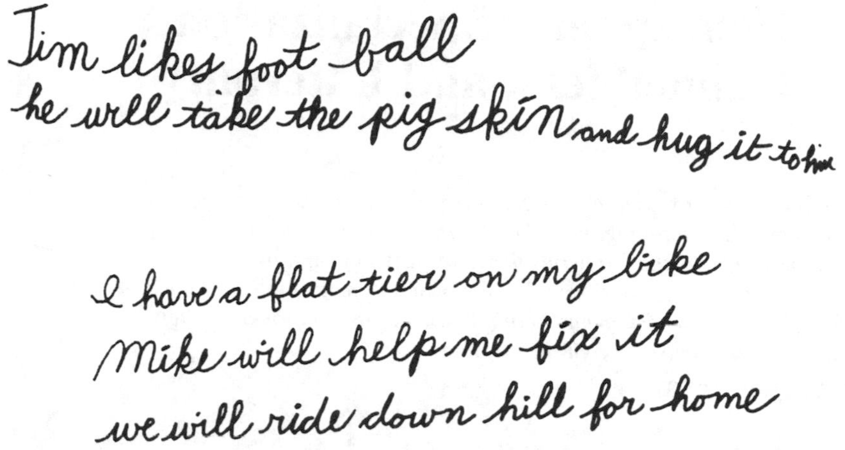

Jim likes foot-ball
he will take the pig skin and hug it to him

I have a flat tier on my bike
Mike will help me fix it
we will ride down hill for home

Figure 5.8. Donald's writing to dictation after 17 months of intensive remedial teaching (age 13 years 8 months).

because of his good auditory memory but weak visual memory (see Fig. 5.7).

His spatial orientation has improved with training since he embarked on the special remediation program. When he first arrived at the school he was continually lost unless someone accompanied him to the washroom, gymnasium, crafts building, or dining area, because each of these was in a separate building. Because Donald's biparietal damage made it difficult for him to produce mental schemata of the buildings and school campus, his teachers helped him to develop proximal cues in the environment. After a few weeks he was able to walk independently on the campus, until the first snowfall! That morning he was found completely confused about 100 yards away from the school. He has since been taught a number of routes by walking with him from A to B, where Donald hid a bag of peanuts or chocolate. He was then accompanied back to A and left free to find his way back to B. The reinforcement of the hidden reward, plus the sensorimotor action of hiding it, plus verbalizing the cues as he walked the route, all seemed to have combined to help Donald learn some common routes on the campus of his school, around his home, and in the small town where he lives.

By age 13 he could read and write at about a Grade 5 level, could manage Grade 2 arithmetic, and had learned to overcome his spatial-orientation deficit to a marked degree. He was well motivated to learn and he continued to show progress, particularly in the language arts.

6 Hemispheric Specialization, Handedness, and Laterality

The main theme to emerge from the foregoing facts is that there appear to be two modes of thinking, verbal and non-verbal, represented rather separately in right and left hemispheres respectively, and that our educational system, as well as science in general, tends to neglect the non-verbal form of intellect. What it comes down to is that modern society discriminates against the right hemisphere.

R.W. Sperry (1973)

Until recently it was thought, perhaps simplistically, that a right-handed person was necessarily left-hemisphere dominant for language, and similarly a left-handed person was right-hemisphere dominant for language. Now it is known, from neuropsychological researches over the last 40 years, that this is not so and that the whole question of the relation between handedness and hemispheric specialization is highly complex and variable within certain limits. Before we examine the relationship between cerebral function and handedness, however, let us look at these two behavioral processes separately.

Cerebral Dominance

More than 30 years ago a conference was held at Johns Hopkins University School of Medicine at which the topic "Interhemispheric Relations and Cerebral Dominance" was discussed. A number of eminent neurologists and neuropsychologists were invited to present papers on their research, and these papers and their discussions were subsequently published (Mountcastle, 1962). During the 3 days of the conference 11 scholarly presentations were made and valuable discussions followed these papers, but because the members of the group could not agree on a definition of cerebral dominance, none was given. Although this important neurological and behavioral phenomenon was named in the title of the book, nowhere in the subject index did the term appear.

Such is the difficulty of describing what happens in the brain tissue when an area of the cerebral structures seems to dominate or control some particular form of behavior. Although unable to explain how the brain provides selective control, we can describe it behaviorally, and some of its neuropsychological relationships.

Following discoveries by Dax in France in 1836, Broca in 1861, and others at that time that aphasia was a result of disease of the left hemisphere, the belief developed that the left hemisphere in most people was dominant, because it seemed to influence and direct language functions. So absorbed were neurologists in attempting to identify the "leading" or "major" hemisphere that the "minor" hemisphere was considered subordinate and vaguely inferior in function. In fact, only recently has scientific attention been directed to study the "nondominant" hemisphere; as a result, evidence has appeared to suggest it possesses its own dominance, particularly for nonverbal functions (Benton, 1965), although it is not exclusively nonverbal (Gazzaniga & Hillyard, 1971; Kinsbourne, 1975a; E. Zaidel, 1973). We now know that the two hemispheres work together, possessing a reciprocal and interacting variety of hemispheric specialized functions.

A child born with a defective left temporal lobe, particularly if the defect affects Wernicke's area, may have a shift of the language functions to the right hemisphere, and will learn language with the normally "minor" hemisphere. The child may still be right-handed if the left frontal lobe and motor strip are healthy and operative. This means that the two hemispheres share control of different behavioral functions in different ways, depending on the locus of the healthiest cerebral tissue.

When damage to the left hemisphere occurs early in life (e.g., following a severe epileptic seizure during the first year), language dominance may, or may not, shift completely to the right hemisphere, or it may shift partially (i.e., represented bilaterally in both hemispheres). Where it does shift completely, the right hemisphere can adapt to mediate language at a workable level, though not necessarily to complete normality (Dennis, 1980). Teuber (1974) first suggested the hypothesis that in those cases of language shift, it was possible that the nonverbal spatial and constructional skills, normally associated with the right hemisphere, might suffer by being crowded out of their normal space. Teuber did not live to test his "crowding hypothesis," but more recently it has been tested by Strauss, Satz, & Wada (1990). They studied 27 young adults, all of whom had suffered their first left-hemisphere seizure before the age of 18 months. Of these subjects (18 women, 9 men) carotid amytal testing showed that language dominance in 14 had remained in the left hemisphere even though it had been damaged by the early seizures, 6 in the right hemisphere, and 7 bilateral. On a comprehensive battery of verbal and nonverbal tests (visuospatial, right–left identification of body parts, embedded figures, and mental rotation of two-dimensional figures), it was found that the performance of the 14 left-hemisphere dominant subjects on the verbal tests suffered only moderately, and their nonverbal skills were spared. But the performance of the "shifted" subjects on the nonverbal tests was more severely impaired. There was a tendency for those with a complete shift of language to the right hemisphere to be more impaired on nonverbal tests than those with only partial shift (i.e., bilateral speech). This observation led to the conclusion that "there is a hint in the data suggesting that the degree of deficit on tests of nonverbal ability is related to the extent of language transfer" (Strauss et al., 1990).

Because of sex differences in brain structure and development (Kolb & Whishaw, 1990), the possibility that there might be gender differences in the cognitive results of early left-hemisphere damage led Strauss, Wada, and Hunter (1992) to study 24 young adults, who had all suffered early left-hemisphere damage and who had had their language dominance determined by the sodium amytal test, as in the previous study. In brief, they found that men in their sample showed more generalized impairment than the women, particularly in tests of language, learning, and memory, regardless of whether their language dominance was in the left or right hemisphere. By contrast, the women with left-hemisphere language dominance suffered only linguistic impairment depending on the locus and severity of the left-hemisphere damage (i.e., a lesion effect) and their nonverbal abilities were completely spared. Those with right-hemisphere language dominance showed low scores in both verbal and nonverbal tasks. Luria described this dynamic cerebral function thus: "The dominance of one hemisphere in relation to speech functions proved not to be so absolute as was supposed, and research showed that the degree of dominance varied considerably from subject to subject and from function to function" (Luria, 1966).

Cerebral language dominance has also been studied in a few cases of hemidecortication that was carried out in early infancy. This surgical procedure, which involves removing a complete cerebral hemisphere to terminate or alleviate intractable and frequent seizures, is rarely done, so that these cases are not numerous. Seizure conditions are usually treated with anticonvulsive drugs, but when these fail in early infancy, sometimes surgical removal of the offending hemisphere is carried out. When these cases are available for study, they provide the opportunity to discover the nature of all cognitive acquisitions, including language, developed with only one hemisphere instead of two. Dennis and Whitaker (1976) reported on three children, all between 9 and 10 years of age, and who had surgical hemidecortication before the age of five months. Those possessing only a left half-brain were better in syntactic comprehension and association of spoken speech. Those with only a right half-brain were better in understanding and making associations to visual stimuli (Dennis & Kohn, 1975; Dennis & Whitaker, 1976). More will be said about the linguistic deficits of these patients in Chapter 8. Here they are useful in providing information to elaborate the normal pattern of hemispheric specialization.

Before we look at the functional relationships between the cerebral hemispheres and language and handedness, let us define our terms.

Definition of Cerebral Dominance

We have already commented briefly on the difficulty of explaining cerebral dominance, and if we cannot explain it, it will be difficult to define. Operationally we know *what* happens (at least in gross terms) when one area of the cortex is maximally involved with a contralateral motor function, but we do not know completely *how* all this happens. We know that the pyramidal or motor tracts from one side cross over, mostly at the medullar level (see Fig. 5.2), but the physiological controls that direct the neural energy in the appropriate amounts and to the precise peripheral locations are not yet understood. A. Meyer, drawing on the writings of Hécaen (1969), Subirana (1969), and Clarke and Dewhurst (1972), has written "The underlying structural and physiological substrates of dominance are so far unknown" (A. Meyer, 1974).

Because at this stage in our knowledge we cannot define cerebral dominance completely, let us list what we do know about the functional relationships among cortical activity and speech, brain, and handedness.

1. Cerebral dominance, until about 35 years ago, usually referred to the language mediation of the left hemisphere, along with a silent or "minor" right hemisphere. More recently neuropsychological research has produced a concept of bilateral function with each hemisphere specialized for different forms of information processing. The left hemisphere in most people is more efficient in processing serial order perceptions, verbal cognitions, and motor responses (Geschwind, 1975; Kimura, 1976; Mateer & Kimura, 1976), and for logical, sequential analysis. Because spoken and

written language fit this analytic–temporal sequential mode of processing, it tends to be regulated by the left hemisphere.

The right hemisphere in most subjects is better suited to process spatial and holistic material that is recognized instantly rather than sequentially. The perception of spatial relationships, whether visual, auditory, or tactile, depends largely on this type of cerebral processing. Because spatial–perceptual–constructional tasks fit this type of processing, they tend to be regulated by the right hemisphere.

But because most perceptions include both linguistic and spatial aspects, any ongoing cognitive process will include bilateral functions that vary in relative emphasis from moment to moment. Throughout the following discussion, when we use the term "cerebral dominance" we mean "hemispheric specialization" of *either* hemisphere. In each instance, it will be indicated whether the dominance (i.e., specialization) relates to language, spatial, perceptual, or other cognitive or behavioral functions, and whether it is a left, right, or bilateral cerebral process.

2. Cerebral dominance for speech is central, unconscious, and beyond the ordinary control of the subject.

3. There seems to be an association between handedness and speech lateralization, but it is not yet fully understood. In almost all right-handed and more than half of the left-handed subjects, cerebral dominance for speech is in the left hemisphere.

4. Right-handers usually show little or no evidence of bilateral language dominance. About 95% of them are left-hemisphere dominant for language, and about 5% are right-hemisphere dominant. By contrast, left-handers are more variable. About 61% are left-hemisphere language dominant, about 20% are bilaterally controlled, and about 19% are right-hemisphere dominant for language (Segalowitz & Bryden, 1983). It should be understood, however, that all these figures are *estimates* and that individual studies show marked variability in their estimates. For example, in a recent study of five patients showing bilateral speech representation as determined by the Wada sodium amytal speech test (Strauss & Wada, 1983), four of the patients (or 80%) were right-handed. This type of evidence is a continued reminder that all estimates made by different researchers using different selection criteria, and studying groups of subjects with varying types of cerebral dysfunctions, cannot be accepted as final, nor as a basis for uneqivocal interpretation of the brain–behavior patterns of single cases.

5. Although handedness for writing and fine manual–motor movements develops with a preference for the right hand in most children, it can be changed. A left-handed child can be trained to

write with the right hand, and right-handed subjects who have lost
their right hands by amputation or accident have learned to write
successfully with the left. This suggests a basic difference from
speech in that the lateral preference for handedness may be peripherally imposed, is conscious, and is within the ordinary control
of the subject (Subirana, 1958).

6. The behavioral manifestations of dominance are at both the
cerebral and effectoral levels.

Phenomena considered to reflect cerebral asymmetry directly have
been traditionally classed as "cerebral dominance" phenomena,
while phenomena which appear to be only indirectly related to
cerebral asymmetry of function have been classed as "lateral
dominance" phenomena. More specifically, cerebral dominance has
been generally used to refer to asymmetry of functions primarily
resident in the cerebral hemispheres, e.g., language and perceptual
functions. Lateral dominance, on the other hand, has referred to
peripheral asymmetry of function manifested by lateral preferences
at the effector level, e.g., handedness and footedness. (Higenbottam, 1971)

The term "cerebral dominance" can imply the involuntary domination of brain functions that the subject cannot perceive. The term
"lateral preference" can imply the voluntary choice of hand or foot
action that the subject can perceive.

Determinants of Dominance

Physiological Determinants

Structural Asymmetries. Since 1861, following Broca's statement
of left-hemisphere dominance for speech, numerous researchers
have sought structural differences between the two hemispheres to
account for the prodigious disparities in function. Some investigators have found differences in volume and length of the carotid
arteries on each side, in the weight and complexity of the two
hemispheres, in the varying number of Betz cells, and in the
asymmetries of the two temporal lobes. Although many researchers
have found differences, which usually favored the left hemisphere,
some found none, and even the differences that were discovered
were so small (Von Bonin, 1962) as to be "unable to answer how
to correlate these small differences with the astonishing disparities
in function in the two sides of the brain" (Subirana, 1969). Since
1968, belief in the structural differences has been increased by the
finding of Geschwind and Levitsky (1968) that of 100 adult brains
studied histologically, the planum temporale was larger on the left

in 65%, on the right in 11%, and equal in 24%. Wada has studied not only the brains of adults, but also the brains of neonates and fetuses. He reported that "the left temporal planum was larger than the right in the majority of both the adult and the infant brains" (Wada, Clarke, & Hamm, 1975). Wada's data showed a larger left planum in both adults and infants in roughly 90% of the cases. Geschwind and Levitsky had reported left planum superiority in only 65% of the cases, but when they added the 24% of the cases showing equality between the hemispheres, they had a group with a left planum temporale either equal to or larger than the right homologous area in 89% of their cases. In a study of only 10 brains by Von Economo and Horn (1930) reported by Wada, a similar pattern of 90% of cases showing an equal or larger left planum was found. Witelson and Pallie (1973) studied the brains of 14 infants and 16 adults and reported "that the left-sided area was statistically significantly larger in the neonate, as in the adults."

The findings from these studies indicate that structural asymmetries begin to show themselves and become measurable by the 29th week of gestation. This imbalance shows an equal or larger planum temporale on the left side at birth in about 90% of the cases and suggests that the temporal asymmetry precedes speech and language development, a conclusion impossible from the earlier studies of only adult brains. In this regard Witelson and Pallie (1973) concluded, "it is suggested that this neonatal asymmetry indicates that the infant is born with a pre-programmed biological capacity to process speech sounds."

The relationship between planum asymmetry and functional lateralization, however, is not a simple one. Amytal studies show that about 88% to 95% of the population have left-hemisphere speech dominance, yet the left planum temporale is larger than the right in about 70% on the average. In some samples this measure is as low as 55%. Obviously there is a discrepancy here. Witelson (1983) has provided a detailed and useful critique of the problems relating to this issue that the clinical neuropsychologist will find valuable. Although there appears to be a possible relation between planum asymmetry and language dominance, it is not yet clear, and full understanding will have to await further research.

Other possible structural asymmetries were reported by Yakovlev and Rakic and described by Benson and Geschwind (1968). They found that in most fetal and newborn brains, the pyramidal tract (the motor nerve fibers connecting from the motor cortex to the muscles) from the left hemisphere began to cross to the right side of the spinal cord *before* the motor fibers from the right hemisphere. Not only was the neural decussation from left to right earlier, but the *size* of the pyramidal tract on the right side of the cord was larger. Kertesz and Geschwind made the same finding about the initial decussation of the left pyramidal tract in the human adult (Benson & Geschwind, 1968), and these authors concluded that "the demonstration of a larger pyramidal tract in the right cord suggests that hand preference may depend upon increased innervation available to one side of the cord, which leads to finer digital control on that side."

Later, Geschwind (1979a) reported a difference in the angle of the Sylvian fissure in right- and left-handed people (the fissure on the right was angled up more sharply in 67% of right-handers) and in the width of the frontal lobes (the right frontal lobe was wider in 70% of right-handers). Left-handed people tended to show little difference in these measures. Ratcliff, Dila, Taylor, and Milner (1980) studied 59 patients with amytal to establish the side of speech dominance and also used carotid angiograms to examine the asymmetry of the angle of the posterior Sylvian branches of the cerebral blood vessels. Their findings were basically similar to those reported by Geschwind (1979a)—that for right-handers the angle is higher and wider on the right and a little lower and more acute on the left. They found that the left-handers were more atypical for both Sylvian angle and side of speech dominance. These writers concluded that the "measure of the posterior Sylvian asymmetry is related to cerebral dominance for speech in the sense that it is present in association with left-hemisphere speech but significantly less marked in the presence of atypical speech repre-sentation" (Ratcliff, Dila, Taylor, & Milner, 1980). To account for the lack of complete agreement among cerebral language laterality, Sylvian angle, and handedness, they invoked a model of inheritance of both handedness and cerebral language dominance proposed by Annett (1972). According to Annett's theory, hand preference is determined by two factors: (1) a genetic predisposition in favor of right-hand superiority, which is present in the majority of the population, and (2) chance, which affects the minority who for some reason have not inherited the genetic tendency to shift. "The majority of the population, in whom the shift factor is present, will be biased in favor of right handedness, left hemisphere speech, and a narrower left Sylvian arch. The minority, lacking the shift factor, will be unbiased with respect to all three variables which will be randomly and independently determined" (Ratcliff, Dila, Taylor, & Milner, 1980). This is an interesting theory that makes use of genetics and chance and accounts for the observable facts.

In another study, McRae, Branch, and Milner (1968) reported a longer left occipital horn in the ventricular system in right-handed people, and a longer right occipital horn in about half the cases of left-handers. The behavioral significance of this difference is not yet known, but it may be part of the process of revealing many more anatomical asymmetries that at some time may show themselves to be functionally related to handedness, cerebral dominance, and other behavioral and functional asymmetries.

Possible genetic determinants of cerebral dominance have been studied using handedness as the indicator, but because correlation between the hand and contralateral hemisphere is not perfect, findings from such studies have not been conclusive. Theories growing out of these kinds of studies range from denial of innate factors to emphasis on them. Although the causes are masked, some data suggest that genetic factors are involved. Subirana (1969) reported that 46% of offspring from 31 pairs of homozygotic left-handed parents were also left-handed, whereas only 2.1% of children from two right-handed parents were left-handed. The proportion rose to 17.3% when one parent was left-handed. These findings, which may be genetically determined, do not, of course, rule out environmental influences.

An interesting theory linking handedness, cerebral dominance, and genetic factors is that of Annett (1964). She proposed that handedness is genetically determined by a dominant (D) gene pattern and a recessive (r) one. Dominant homozygotes (DD), that is, children who have inherited dominant handedness genes from both parents, are consistently right-handed, with language dominance in the left hemisphere. Recessive homozygotes (rr), that is, children who have inherited recessive handedness genes from both parents, are consistently left-handed, with language dominance in the right hemisphere. Genetically these children are "pure" right-handed and "pure" left-handed, respectively, and except when they suffer traumatic brain damage they have no unusual learning problems. The heterozygotes (Dr), that is, children who have inherited a dominant handedness gene pattern from one parent and a recessive one from the other, are usually right-handed and left-hemisphere dominant for language, but they may usc cither hand for skilled abilities and they can develop speech in either hemisphere.

Annett makes the interesting proposal that if genetic determination were the only cause of handedness, then the distribution of "pure" right-handed, hybrid right-handed, and "pure" left-handed people would reveal a binomial distribution. In every 100 subjects ($8^2 + (2 \times 8 \times 2) + 2^2$) there would be 64 ($DD$) pure right-handed, 32 (Dr) right- or left-handed, and 4 (rr) pure left-handed ones. Genetic determiners are not the sole cause, however, because cerebral dysfunctions and social learning are organic and functional influences that may intrude unsystematically on the effects of genetic programming. These variables then may cause shifts in normal language dominance in cases of early unilateral brain damage or dysfunction and/or deliberate training of a child to write with the hand opposite to his or her natural preference.

This model has the advantage that it explains why most left-handed people are less consistent (i.e., they show more mixed handedness, footedness, and eyedness) than most right-handed subjects. However, some left-handed people are consistent. By this theory, the inconsistent left-handed subjects are heterozygotes (*Dr*) and the consistent ones recessive homozygotes (*rr*). Traumatic damage to the central or peripheral nervous system may result in the use of the alternate hemisphere or limb, but only heterozygotes, according to Annett's theory, can shift dominance to compensate for injuries. Homozygotes injured in the dominant hemisphere will be unskilful with either hand and may be subject to speech disorders. "Although there is some indirect support for this position, the mechanisms still remain obscure" (Satz, 1972).

It is clear from this discussion that although there may be conclusive genetic determiners of handedness, an individual child may vary from his or her inherited predisposition if traumatic injury or forcible training intervene to disrupt the theoretical binomial distribution proposed by Annett, which is reasonably close to her findings in a study of 1226 subjects (Annett, 1970b). Satz (1972), in a theoretical discussion of pathological left-handed patients, has shown that half of manifest left-handed subjects have signs of brain dysfunction, particularly mental retardation and/or epilepsy.

Coren and Porac (1977) surveyed more than 5000 years of artworks, scoring instances of unimanual tool or weapon use in 1180 photographs and reproductions of drawings, paintings, and sculpture. They covered the period from 15,000 B.C. to 1950 A.D. in seven geographic regions (e.g., Central Europe, Mediterranean Europe, Africa, etc.) and found that 92.6% were right-handed with no trend toward increasing right-handedness, and no differences among regions. These researchers concluded: "Thus, as far as the historical record takes us, man appears to have always been right-handed" (Coren & Porac, 1977).

A more speculative but still useful approach is through historical ethology that draws on probable genetic mechanisms and environmental influences, rather than emphasizing one or other of these etiological determiners exclusively. Using the assumption that humans have always been right-handed, at least since recorded history, Calvin (1983) proposes "a fanciful reconstruction of events" to account for left-brain–right-handed writing and general right-handedness. He suggests that when humans began to write, about 5000 years ago, they first chiseled symbols into hard rock, but because of right-handedness, there was a tendency to chisel from the easier side of the tablet (the right side) to the more awkward side (the left). The right-to-left sequence of ancient written languages, such as Hebrew, has sometimes been explained in this way. Later, when ink or dyes were first used to write on skins or papyrus, writing was assumed to have switched to a left-to-right sequence to avoid smearing the ink.

But this fantasy is based on the assumption of the right-handedness of the majority of the population, and we have to wonder how this preference developed.

Some manual skills, as Calvin describes, can be done with both hands (e.g., clubbing), but throwing a rock is necessarily one-handed. Present surveys show that about 90% of the population throw a ball right-handed. To account for this imbalance, Calvin looks to the phenomenon of maternal heartbeat. He proposes (1983), as have others before him (Huheey, 1977; Salk, 1973; Wyeth, 1880, quoted in Harris, 1980), that because the mother's heartbeat is loudest on the left side, and because it has a soothing effect on the infant's behavior, a mother usually carries her infant on her left arm. This common custom, supported historically by surveys of hundreds of pictures of madonnas and their children, may have resulted from imprinting (Salk, 1973). Calvin suggests that millions of years ago women were the chief hunters for food, and so they soon learned to throw rocks to kill small animals at a distance. Modern studies of the great apes show the females to be better hunters and more competent in handling tools. Women in some primitive cultures are still active hunters, and maternal left-armedness obviously left the right arm free to throw. After many centuries, the better hunters survived (natural selection) and tended to increase the proportion of right-handed genes in the population. However, a minority always preferred to use the left hand for throwing and to hold a child with the right arm.

It is also likely that the left hemisphere was always programmed for better sequential perceptual analysis and more precise motor response. If so, it could account for the more accurate throwing of prehistoric woman and the better left-brain–right-hand pattern in most writers.

Brain Damage and/or Cerebral Dysfunction. The use of the Wada Amytal Test and the Dichotic Listening Test for determining hemispheric language dominance, has demonstrated that most right-handed people have speech represented in the left hemisphere and they rarely have bilateral speech. Some years ago Milner, Branch, and Rasmussen (1964), using the Wada test, showed that of 48 right-handed adults, 90% were left-hemisphere dominant for language, none was bilateral, and 10% had language represented in the right hemisphere. A group of 44 adults with no history of known brain injury but who were either left-handed or ambidextrous was found to be left-hemisphere dominant for language in 64% of the cases, bilateral in 16%, and right-hemisphere dominant in 20%. In a study of 27 left-handed and ambidextrous subjects who did have a history of early left-hemisphere damage, the investigators found speech in the left in 22% of the cases, bilateral speech in 11%, and right-hemisphere speech in 67%. These data reveal two important findings: (1) Early left-hemisphere brain injury will shift language to the right hemisphere in a large number of cases (in the Milner, Branch, and Rasmussen study cited above there was a shift in the most deviant sample, from a norm of 90% left-hemisphere dominance to only 22%, or a shift to some degree of right-hemisphere processing of 68% of the cases); and (2) even in spite of early left-hemisphere damage, 22% of the cases retained their language dominance in the injured hemisphere. Why this is so is not yet clear, although it may be because the speech areas have been spared, or it may be that homozygotes and heterozygotes react differently to brain damage (Annett, 1964). Whatever the cause, in large numbers of LD children it is evident that a shift from the language-dominant hemisphere has not occurred. Examples of some of these are included in the Clinical Addendum at the end of this chapter.

Handedness and Cerebral Blood Flow. Using skin temperature over the ophthalmic branches of the internal carotid arteries as indexes of blood flow to the two sides of the head, Dabbs and Choo (1980) found that cerebral asymmetry as indicated by side of blood flow is related to handedness. "It has been found that among right-handed subjects the right side of the brain has more blood flow, higher blood pressure, a wider frontal lobe, and more protrusion of frontal bone" (Dabbs & Choo, 1980). Their findings indicate that more blood goes to the nonverbal side of the head, and suggest that spatial mental functions involve slightly more blood flow than verbal functions. These researchers also studied two types of left-handers, those with upright handwriting posture, and those with inverted or "hooked" handwriting posture. The "hooked" group, like the right handers, showed more right-sided blood flow, and the "upright" group involved slightly more on the left side. Although these differences are small, they are quite reliable and seem to be part of the related pattern of cerebral asymmetry and handedness.

Training

Environmental influences can change handedness, as has been demonstrated many times. Right-handed subjects who have lost their right hands traumatically have learned to write with their left. A Norwegian friend reported that all children in his school in Norway during the 1930s wrote with their right hands, because no one was allowed to write with the left hand in those days. Benson and Geschwind (1968) reported that Déjerine in France in 1912 commented that he had never met anyone who wrote with the left hand. It may be that left-handed writing was accepted to a greater degree in North American than in European schools at that time.

Although a parent or teacher can shift handedness by training, it seems improbable, if not impossible, that cerebral dominance for speech can be shifted in this way. As we have already seen, even early left-hemisphere damage will not shift speech dominance in a large number of cases, even though the child would seem to gain markedly should the shift take place. Some writers have suggested that writing with the right hand by a left-handed person may shift speech dominance to the left hemisphere, but there is no neuropsychological evidence that this has ever taken place. This is not to say that it should not be tried, if there is strong behavioral or other evidence that the child should write with the right hand. The child's improvement in learning, when it occurs, would seem to be caused not by a shift in cerebral dominance, but by an improvement in the neural communication between the right hand and the cortical language centers, be they in either hemisphere or in both hemispheres.

Behavioral Manifestations of Cerebral Dominance

Language

Because about 90% of humans have left-hemisphere dominance for speech and language functions, whether they are right- or left-handed, a teacher can expect most pupils to have left-brain language dominance. However, it must be remembered that though most people are left-hemisphere dominant for language, they are not exclusively. The right hemisphere may also contribute, though to a lesser extent, to language functions. If the child is right-handed then he or she is nearly always left-brained for speech, but not always. Very rarely a right-handed child may be *right*-brained for language, and unless the teacher is advised of this unusual cerebral-linguistic pattern, the child's poor academic achievement, if it results from this conflict, may be credited to laziness, inattention, or some other undesirable sign that may be secondary to the cerebral condition. Such cases are rare, but two from our files are described in the Clinical Addendum at the end of this chapter, one in which a boy suffered from a subtle learning problem and one in which a girl was a good student.

At present, the most reliable technique for detecting cerebral language dominance combines a neurological investigating technique (the Wada Amytal Test) and a neuropsychological assessment technique (the Dichotic Listening Test). This clinical combination may not be available to most teachers, but any serious school or clinical psychologist can acquire a dichotic tape and add the technique to his or her repertoire of clinical skills.

However, the clinical or school psychologist with no previous experience with the dichotic technique must guard against accepting without question its indication of cerebral language laterality. The Wada Carotid Amytal Test, a reliable indicator of cerebral speech dominance, shows that about 90% of the adult population are left-hemisphere language dominant and about 10% are right dominant (Milner, Branch, & Rasmussen, 1964). But studies employing injection of amytal always include patients with some type of cerebral pathology or dysfunction; because it is an invasive technique, the amytal test is rarely used on normal subjects. Studies of normal subjects with the dichotic listening technique often show about 70% to 75% right ear advantage (REA), and if the test is being used as an indicator of cerebral laterality of language, there is an obvious discrepancy between known language dominance and that suggested by the dichotic procedure.

Nevertheless, there are some redeeming features in this picture. The dichotic technique shows a high level of agreement with amytal findings in the same subjects being examined for medical reasons. In our laboratory we have studied 90 epileptic patients, all of whom had both the amytal and dichotic tests. Although these patients were referred for medical reasons the findings enabled us to test the validity of the dichotic listening test for detecting cerebral language dominance. We did not find the two tests to agree completely, but agreement (right ear advantage or REA–left cerebral speech, and vice versa) did occur in 83% of the cases (Strauss, Gaddes, & Wada, 1987). Using a different method of report, Geffen and her colleagues (Geffen et al., 1978) stated that they accurately classified 97% of their cases. These levels of accuracy of prediction are high enough for the neuropsychologist to use the dichotic listening test, in a large neuropsychological battery, with a reasonable level of confidence.

How can the neuropsychologist guard against making erroneous conclusions on single cases?

1. The subject's ear dominance scores (i.e., difference score, R − L)[1] can be compared with the group findings of a number of subjects on the same test, evaluated in reference to a statistical probability criterion before inferences are made. Wexler, Halwes, and Heninger (1981) propose using a χ^2 statistical significance criterion to increase the diagnostic accuracy of single cases.

2. A test of substantial length should be used because the REA may be increased by presenting more pairs before recall or by using words rather than digits (Bryden, 1964). Many tests use 40 groups of 3 pairs of words (i.e., a total of 120 words).

3. The test should be administered *at least twice* to check on the reliability of the results. Wexler, Halwes, and Heninger (1981) found with their 33 subjects a test−retest correlation (Pearson *r*) of .91. If the R − L score is consistently high on both administrations the clinician, without the availability of the amytal test for cross-validation of the results, nor the time to calculate a validity measure based on statistical probability, may infer, with a strong degree of probability, that the language dominance of the subject is in the left hemisphere. If, however, the R − L difference score is close to zero, then no conclusive diagnosis can be made without a cross-validating check, but the subject can be suspected of bilateral language dominance or mixed left or mixed right cerebral laterality.

4. The clinician, in using dichotic data alone for detecting cerebral language dominance, should accept it as a *suggestion*, not a conclusive indication, of probable brain function. It should be kept in mind that ear preferences may or may not change with age (Bryden & Allard, 1981), with sex (Bryden, 1970), with the frequency of use and concreteness of words (Dodwell, 1964), with the syntactic meaning of groups of words (Gray & Wedderburn, 1960), with the meaningfulness and emotional arousal of different words (Emmerich et al., 1965), and with the spatial direction of the auditory stimulus (Pierson, Bradshaw, & Nettleton, 1983). However, if difference scores are consistently high on successive administrations, and they can be related to behavioral and medical

---

[1] The difference score is some form of R − L (i.e., the number of stimuli identified correctly by the right ear minus the number identified by the left ear). Some researchers prefer not to use raw difference scores (i.e., R − L), but to calculate a laterality quotient (e.g., R − L/R + L), or in addition, a total errors score (i.e., the number of pairs minus the number correct, n − (R + L)). These types of scores imply a *degree* of cerebral language laterality depending on the size of the difference score. Some researchers have argued that because of causal factors other than hemispheric asymmetry (e.g., input asymmetry and attentional variables), the degree of laterality is not indicated by dichotic scores, and that it is important to recognize *only* REA, LEA, or RE = LE. A proponent of this view, Clark (1981), scored LEA as 1; RE = LE as 2; and REA as 3. This type of scoring ignores the possibility of degree and indicates only the side or neutrality of ear preference. A huge literature in dichotic research has accumulated since 1961, and the reader can find various scoring procedures and their respective rationales.

data (when available), the dichotic procedure can be a useful added technique to the armamentarium of the clinician. But the careful clinician must guard against simplistic interpretations of dichotic experiments, because "not all behavioral asymmetries are necessarily related to the differing functions of the two hemispheres" (Bryden, 1982).

Hand Preference

The clinical methods described above are reasonably reliable for detecting cerebral dominance, but they may not be immediately available to the classroom teacher. One method that is available may be used casually as a peripheral but not conclusive indicator; that is, hand movements during speech. Kimura has carried out some imaginative and interesting research in which she showed that right-handed subjects who were left-brained for language tend to make many more free hand movements (e.g., any hand or finger movement that is free of their body) with their right hands while speaking (Kimura, 1973b) than with their left. Self-touching movements in these same subjects (e.g., scratching, running fingers through the hair) was greater in the left hand. When left-handed subjects were examined (Kimura, 1973c), free hand movements were greater for the left hand, but the differences between the two hands were not as great as for the right-handed subjects. Related to this knowledge are some interesting findings reported by Moscovitch (1980). He found that Kimura's findings hold only when the speaker is discussing nonemotional material, but when he or she becomes emotionally moved by the subject matter so that his facial expression reflects his feelings, there is no contralateral hand preference for activity. Because the right hemisphere is usually more involved with emotion, it seems that the greater bilateral involvement obliterates the hand preference activity. Presumably the left-hemisphere activity (language) is canceled out by the right-hemisphere activity (emotional expression).

Kimura maintained strict controls to avoid observer biases, which would not be normally possible for a classroom teacher, and for this reason this method for identifying cerebral dominance in the classroom is not strongly recommended except as an interesting peripheral observation to help the teacher conceptualize what may be occurring in the LD child's central nervous system. If the child is right-handed, makes the majority of free hand movements with the right hand during speech, and has most or all lateral preferences on the right, then any serious learning problem, if one exists, is likely to result from causes other than cerebral–manual conflict. In contrast, if the child is right-handed, makes about equal numbers of free hand movements during speech, and shows signs of considerable mixed laterality and serious learning problems, then the possibility of cerebral–manual conflict should be followed up with a referral to a school psychologist with the competencies to investigate it. The same type of referral should be made for the left-handed LD child with mixed laterality.

Left-Handedness

Most mothers recognize the usual indifference to handedness in their infants and small children. During the second year of life most children are as likely to use their push-spoon in either hand, but if the mother consistently offers it to the child's right hand, he or she will usually become habituated to hold it with the right hand.

However, some children from the very start are highly resistant to training that discourages their left-handedness, and many of these cases are probably the genetic left-handed children, those who are right-brained for language and naturally superior with their left hands. There is also the possibility that they are left-handed because of brain damage or cortical dysfunction somewhere in the left hemisphere, a condition that may have existed since birth or early infancy. Many years ago, Gordon (1920) recognized two categories of left-handed people: those he called "natural" and those he called "pathological." Hécaen and de Ajuriaguerra (1964) have reported Subirana's finding "that the percentage of right- or left-sidedness of children from a high social level is different from that of orphans placed in an institution," and Mayet, as early as 1902, "remarked upon this frequency (of left-handers) in idiots and in epileptics." In 1952, Hordijk found, in a study of 4307 school children, 15 times as many epileptics in left-handed families as in those who were clearly right-handed. A large number of studies have shown that left-handedness "probably exists to about twice the extent in the markedly retarded as in normal subjects" (Hordijk, 1952), although this difference cannot be completely attributed to left-hemisphere pathology. Being less competent with the right hand because of left cortical inferiority, the retarded child may also be less able to profit from social experiences.

Satz (1972), in a noteworthy study of pathological left-handedness, recognized the higher probability of left-handedness in brain-damaged samples (an increase from 8% among normals to 17% in brain damaged); the high probability ($p = .81$) of left-hemisphere lesions, regardless of pathological or natural left-handedness; the greater chance of pathological left-handedness following early brain injury; the greater chance of right-hemisphere dominance for language following early left-brain damage; the lack of shift of language dominance in patients with no evidence of early left-brain injury; and the difference between pathological left-handedness, which is the result of injury, and natural left-handedness, which presumably is the result of genetic and cultural determinants. Satz also made the important observation that occasionally there are cases of pathological right-handedness, but these are rare and likely to be ignored in a right-handed world. Only careful genetic and neuropsychological examination would reveal such a case, but a teacher who suspects this possibility should seek competent diagnostic help.

Whether left-handedness decreases with age or is constant throughout childhood is still questionable. In 1964 Hécaen and de Ajuriaguerra wrote:

> Among 10,000 children tested, Ballard (cited by Bloéde) found 4.1 percent left-handed in a group 4 to 14 years of age as against only 2.7 percent in a group 8 to 14 years of age. Likewise, Johnson, in a dynamometric test of 57 children $5\frac{1}{2}$ to 13 years old, found a left-handed superiority in 16 of them, but a year later control tests showed only a single case of superiority of the left hand. Heinlein's studies, carried out in a more systematic way, also confirm this decrease of left-handedness with age.

At the same time, Annett (1964) remarked that "the well-documented decline in the incidence of left handedness with increasing age is accounted for by supposing that the dominant gene increases its control during growth." However, it is interesting that when she put this idea to the test (Annett, 1970a) she found that the distributions of hand preference and relative manual speed were unchanged in children aged $3\frac{1}{2}$–8 and 9–15 years. Boys in the younger group showed clear left-handedness in 6.1% of the cases, and in the older group in 6.0%. Girls in these two age groups showed frequencies of 1.9% and 4.4%, respectively, a tendency in the reverse direction and also numerically different from the boys. However, she did find that mixed and left preferences were more frequent in boys than girls.

What does this seemingly conflicting evidence tell us?

1. Any results in an experiment are a function of the type of tests used. In Johnson's study, hand-grip strength, as measured by a dynamometer, is a gross muscular function and improves as finer muscular skills are acquired. However, it should be remembered that although 5- and 6-year-old children tend to prefer their stronger hand, they may shift to their other hand for writing when

they enter school if they discover that using the other hand improves the quality of their handwriting.

2. Ballard's study included 10,000 children, whereas Annett's included 219, but we are not told the nature of Ballard's tests. It is possible that some of them included tests of strength rather than fine neuromuscular coordination. Annett's tasks are described, and all required manual dexterity and specific neuromuscular control. Annett's evidence strongly suggests that:

a. Hand preference is established at least by age $3\frac{1}{2}$ years.
b. Proportions of right-, mixed-, and left-handed subjects among boys and men remain constant.
c. Girls show a little variation but the cause of these differences is not clear.
d. Consistently left-handed children in her sample showed superiority in vocabulary and those with mixed handedness were more variable.
e. There was an excess of mixed-handed children among those of lower IQ.

Many early researchers (Hécaen & Sauget, 1971; Milner, Branch, & Rasmussen, 1966; Satz, Achenbach, & Fennell, 1967) consistently found a greater tendency to bilateral language dominance in left-handed subjects compared with left-hemisphere dominance in most right-handed subjects. However, the relationship of cerebral dominance and language development is examined in more depth in Chapter 8.

Levy (1974) made an interesting discovery in the understanding of left-handed subjects. She observed a right-handed writer, T.N., who wrote with his hand inverted in the manner common to many left-handed people. Although he had always written with his right hand, he was ambilateral for some manual activities and left-handed for throwing a ball. Levy investigated three groups, right-handers (Group R), left-handers who wrote normally (group L-N), and left-handers who wrote with the hand inverted (group L-I), and found evidence strongly suggesting that the L-I group members were ipsilateral for their left language dominance and left-handedness, whereas the L-N group members were not. This evidence appears to be in basic agreement with the hemispheric blood-flow patterns and handwriting posture reported above (Dabbs & Choo, 1980).

Mirror Writing

It is generally agreed that mirror writing (that is, writing whole words, phrases, or sentences from right to left with all letters

reversed and in correct sequence) occurs in all or most cases
in left-handed individuals (Benson, 1970; Benson & Geschwind,
1968; Hécaen & de Ajuriaguerra, 1964). This seems to occur
because the human body is symmetrical, but only in the vertical
plane. For this reason the small child may have difficulty learning
left from right. However, Benson (1970) pointed out that because
"there is no symmetry in the horizontal plane" the small child has
little or no difficulty learning up and down on his own body,
because the differences are obvious.

It is evident that it is easier to draw a line from left to right with
one's right hand and from right to left with one's left hand. One
moves out from the midline because it is easier to pull a pen than
push it. Hécaen and de Ajuriaguerra (1964) recognized that "the
left-handed child has to push his pen instead of pulling it," and because his centrifugal movements are easier and more harmonious
than his centripetal movements (those moving toward the center),
the left-handed child can more easily write from right to left.
Requiring him to write from left to right immediately imposes
neuromuscularly awkward demands.

Although the explanation above may account for the neuromuscular aspects of mirror writing, it does not explain the cognitive
process involved. How is it that only a few left-handers produce
mirror writing but most do not? A study reported by Hécaen and
de Ajuriaguerra (1964) suggests that this ability is a function of age
and maturity of the central nervous system, and that dyslexics
(those with CNS dysfunctions) are less able to do it. Positively
stated, this evidence suggests that the mirror writer is free of brain
lesions and can conceptualize spatially in reverse in a flexible,
mature, and reliable way. Harris (1980) pointed out that Leonardo
da Vinci and Lewis Carroll, both mentally superior, were accomplished mirror writers, "but there is no evidence that [either of
them] was ever *confused* about spatial direction, or that their
practice of mirror writing was anything but strictly controlled"
(Harris, 1980, p. 61).

Herron (1980) combines our knowledge of upright or "noninverted" left handwriting position, inverted position, and mirror
writing. When the left hand in the noninverted position writes
from right to left, mirror writing is produced. The inverted left
hand will produce mirror writing *upside down*, but the letters will
be in the normal left-to-right sequence (Herron, 1980, p. 244).

Few cases have been reported in the literature, but Benson
(1970) described an $8\frac{1}{2}$-year-old boy who was *strongly left-handed*
and whose immediate family had four sinistrals. On entering
school he was a mirror writer, but this trait disappeared completely
by the end of first grade. He did, however, possess a develop-

mental dyslexia, although he had normal intelligence. This case indicates the independence of mirror writing and developmental dyslexia in some cases but does not necessarily indicate freedom from brain dysfunctions.

Although reversing letters is common in 6- and 7-year-olds, and this is mirror writing at a single-letter level, cursive mirror writing is not common. Its cause is not known, but Benson (1970) believes the various theories can be reduced to three major hypotheses:

1. An early theory posited the existence of two writing centers, one in the language-dominant left hemisphere and the other in the right. If the right hemisphere is dominant, then mirror writing, according to this theory, will result. However, the facts do not support this theory, because Annett's consistent left-handers should all be mirror writers initially if this were true.

2. Bilateral differential cortical visual imagery has been a more popular theory. According to this view, two separate visual images are formed with the right-hemisphere image a mirror reversal of the left. In most cases, because the left hemisphere is dominant, the right-hemisphere image is suppressed; but if the right hemisphere is dominant, mirror writing will occur. Benson's objection to this theory, on the grounds that mirror writers should also copy drawings reversed, seems questionable for two reasons. First, mirror writers act spontaneously when they are producing the sinistrad (reversed) form; if asked to copy writing or printing they can do it, although awkwardly. Second, drawings of common objects normally have no "correct" direction, as do letters and sequences of letters. Also, the fact that strongly left-handed children when forced to write with the right hand, are consistently slower and less proficient in their handwriting than normal right-handers, suggests they are slowed by the frustrations of having to adapt to the more complex cerebral circuits and the normally suppressed visual image. Orton was the first to propose this theory, which was based on extensive studies of the writing of left-handers (Orton, 1937, pp. 99–110).

3. Benson prefers the theory of mirrored motor patterns in the two hands. According to this view, mirror writing is normal for left-handers but is usually suppressed because the output is socially meaningless and hence not reinforced.

It seems likely that both visual imagery and motor patterns are involved because mirror writing disappears with age. Moreover, "masked left-handers" (i.e., a child who from the beginning preferred to write with the left hand but was forced to write with the right hand) can frequently improve their handwriting if shifted to the left hand even as late as age 11 (Orton, 1937) or 15. Two cases of ambidextrous individuals reported by Orton (1937, pp. 106, 108), whose best writing was sinistrad (in the right-to-left direction) with the right hand, appear to flout the mirror motor theory and be supported by the hemispheric visual imagery theory. Both subjects were older (11 and 21) and both were mentally bright.

The teacher faced with the problem of poor handwriting and frequent spelling errors should obtain the following information before deciding on a remedial program:

1. A detailed measure of handedness on a well-constructed inventory (examples are given at the end of this chapter).
2. Manual–motor tests of both hands.
3. Examples of writing with both hands.
4. A comparison of the child's drawings of simple forms, such as a square, triangle, star, or cross, from copy and with his or her eyes closed after studying the figure for a few moments. This last test will give some information on whether the visual–motor relation is disturbed and whether motor skill is better when the visual input is withheld.
5. Measures of writing speed and legibility from standardized handwriting tests.
6. A comparison of the child's cursive writing with his or her printing. Cursive writing tends to help mirror writers overcome their problem, but not always (Durbrow, 1963). Grace Fernald, in her training school, encouraged the child to write a word cursively and without interruption. This approach is based on a belief that *whole* cortical and muscular patterns are being established in the CNS.
7. Evidence of the child's language cerebral dominance.

Handwriting is not a simple learning task. It is not just essentially related to cerebral dominance; many other functions must be sequentially integrated with handwriting, such as visual scanning, right–left orientation, sequencing, motor development, spatial imagery, visual–motor coordination, visual form recognition, visual form memory, and all or most of the complexities of speech and language development.

Interhemispheric Functions

Throughout this chapter we have been examining the lateral asymmetries both in the internal processes of the central nervous system and in the external manifestations of human behavior. In such a discussion there is a real temptation to refer to "left-hemisphere abilities" and "right-hemisphere skills" as if these functions were completely independent. Of course, they are not, and in any normal, healthy brain whatever occurs in one hemisphere is affected by the other, this influence being mediated largely through the corpus callosum. Kinsbourne (1974, Chap. XIII) described the possible competitive, compensatory, and collaborative effects of the homologous areas of the two hemispheres where one hemisphere is maximally involved in behavior (e.g., speech) and where both hemispheres are equally involved (e.g., auditory localization).

Since the early 1950s, neuropsychologists have recognized that the two cerebral hemispheres mediate different functions, and this concept has been well established by unilateral lesion studies (Reitan, 1955a), and more recently by blood-flow studies (Risberg, Halsey, Wills, & Wilson, 1975) and positron emission tomography (i.e., PET scan; Gur et al., 1983). These findings over a 30-year period indicate that in most adults the left hemisphere is more competent in handling verbal and linguistic tasks, and the right hemisphere is better with visual–spatial–constructional and other nonverbal skills. This concept of hemispheric specialization has appealed to many psychologists and educators, but like all new ideas that at first appear clearly defined, it may be interpreted by enthusiastic clinicians and applied workers simplistically and with little understanding.

Let us look at this problem first with adult subjects. Bryden, Hécaen, and DeAgostini (1983) (Table 6.1) examined 270 adult patients with unilateral brain lesions; 140 left-handers and 130 right-handers. From the neuropsychological test results, each patient was classified as aphasic or not, or showing a visual–spatial disorder or not. If the left–right hemispheric specialization pattern,

Table 6.1. Association between Aphasia and Spatial Disorders in Patients with Unilateral Brain Lesions[a]

	Left-handed				Right-handed			
	Left lesion		Right lesion		Left lesion		Right lesion	
	Aphasia	Spatial	Aphasia	Spatial	Aphasia	Spatial	Aphasia	Spatial
Men	35.6%	6.8%	9.7%	31.7%	39.5%	7.0%	0	63.3%
Women	39.3%	3.6%	8.3%	33.3%	37.0%	14.8%	6.6%	30.0%

[a] Number of subjects: Men: right-handed = 73; left-handed = 100; total = 173
Women: right-handed = 57; left-handed = 40; total = 97
After Bryden, Hécaen, & DeAgostini, 1983. With permission.

described above, is valid in all cases, then we can expect to find all the left lesion cases impaired in language and the right lesion cases visually–spatially impaired. But this is not what Bryden and his colleagues found. Some of their major findings follow:

1. Of the 173 men in the study, 21% showed *both* language and spatial deficits; 23% of the 97 women showed both deficits. These findings could suggest that in some cases the same hemisphere can be superior for both verbal and nonverbal processing (Bryden, 1973), or that more than one-fifth of this sample had bilateral control of both language and spatial skills and that damage to either hemisphere could affect both abilities. Obviously these findings do not support the simplistic view of this concept that is so prevalent in the popular press and in some educational publications.

2. Of the 73 right-handed men, left lesions produced aphasia alone in 39.5% of the sample, and right-sided lesions produced spatial problems in 63.3%. No deficits of either type were found in 37%, no doubt because the locus of cerebral dysfunction was outside the language centers of the left hemisphere, and/or anterior to the temporo-parietal areas of the right hemisphere. However, the interesting findings in the left lesion group are the 7% who suffered only spatial problems.

3. Of the 100 left-handed men, left-sided lesions produced aphasia alone in 35.6% of the sample, and spatial problems in 6.8%. Right-sided lesions produced spatial deficits alone in 31.7% of the sample and aphasia in 9.7%.

4. Of the 57 right-handed women, 37% of the left-lesion cases had aphasic signs alone, and 14.8% had only spatial problems. Thirty percent of the right lesion cases had spatial problems, and 6.6% had aphasia alone. No deficits in either function showed in 47.4% of the sample.

5. In the group of 40 left-handed women, left-sided lesions produced aphasia alone in 39.3% of the cases, and only spatial disorders in 3.6%.

Bryden, Hécaen, and DeAgostini concluded that "aphasia is more frequent with posterior lesions in the left hemisphere of right handers, and spatial disability is more frequent with posterior lesions in the left hemisphere of left handers, and in the right hemisphere of right handers" (Bryden, Hécaen, & DeAgostini, 1983). "The majority of individuals will show language and visuospatial functions in opposite hemispheres even though the two are causally independent of one another" (p. 254). Bilaterality occurs only in left-handers for both verbal and spatial functions and in both sexes.

This evidence makes it clear that a simplistic left–right dichotomy of cerebral function in adults is not accurate. Although the *majority* of right-handers fit the right–left pattern fairly closely, the left-handers, especially those with a history of familial left-handedness, show a great deal of variability in cerebral organization.

The left hemisphere in most adults is more proficient in mediating verbal, sequential material, motor skilled performances, the analysis of verbal ideas, and the storage and use of "well-routinized codes" (Goldberg & Costa, 1981). The right hemisphere is better adapted to handle visual–spatial–three-dimensional imagery, holistic or intermodal integrations, and to process new material. Goldberg and Costa (1981) have proposed that the right hemisphere plays an essential role in the initial stages of learning, when the material is new and unfamiliar. The left hemisphere gradually takes over the processing as learning becomes coded in established neural patterns and expressed in familiar mental concepts.

The investigations of hemispheric asymmetry during childhood are relatively new, most studies having appeared since 1960. Researchers divide themselves into two groups on this issue: (1) Those who consider that the two hemispheres are neutral in infancy and permit language to develop bilaterally during the first 2 years. Then, according to this view, language dominance develops gradually until early adolescence when it reaches its mature form. An influential proponent of this view was Lenneberg (1967). (2) Those who hypothesize that cerebral lateralization is potentially established during fetal development, and that structural and behavioral asymmetries are present from birth. Kinsbourne (1975b, 1989) is a strong proponent of this view. More will be said about developmental cerebral organization in the next section and later in the book because knowledge of its functional patterns should help improve understanding of learning during childhood development, and choices of teaching and remedial methods.

Sex Differences in Laterality

Recent evidence from a number of neuropsychological studies strongly suggests that women characteristically are more proficient with their left hemispheres and men with their right. If this is true, it should have significance for special education. McGlone and her associates at the University of Western Ontario have carried out investigations that tend to support a sex difference in hemispheric specialization (McGlone & Davidson, 1973; McGlone & Kertesz, 1973) and other researchers have made similar findings (Buffery,

1976; Hobson, 1947; Kimura, 1969; Lansdell, 1962; Sandström, 1953; Wechsler, 1958; Witkin, 1949).

Because there does seem to be a reliable female verbal superiority and a male spatial superiority, this pattern suggests that "specialization of the right hemisphere for nonverbal functions may be advantageous for space perception, and that males more often than females have this type of neural organization" (McGlone & Kertesz, 1973). Other studies (McGlone & Davidson, 1973) have shown that when a task can be performed by either left- or right-hemisphere mechanisms, males are more likely to use their right hemispheres, whereas females are more likely to use their left. In brief, this means that depending on the sex of an individual, she is more likely to use a verbal strategy to solve a problem, and he a nonverbal strategy, where either is possible.

Buffery (1976) studied boys and girls at each year from age 5 to age 9 and found a preference by both sexes to process easy-to-verbalize problems more by the left hemisphere, although the asymmetry was more pronounced in the girls, especially as they grew older. When he presented problems that were difficult to verbalize, however, both sexes used their right hemispheres predominantly for processing them. He also found that cerebral asymmetry for cross-modal analysis, particularly with spatial material, emerges later in boys (at about 8 years) than in girls (at about 7 years). This evidence suggests several possible practical applications that need experimental investigation. In general we might expect girls up to about age 8 to be more competent than boys in following purely verbal instructions, and boys to be better in understanding spatial diagrams or pictorial material. It may also mean that if an idea is difficult for the child to grasp by verbal explanation alone, he or she should be provided, as much as possible, with accompanying graphic material related to it, because the level of difficulty is a determiner of the child's cognitive strategy and hemispheric emphasis.

In research with normal adults Buffery (1976) found sex differences in those with signs of mixed laterality. His sample included 100 women and 100 men students at Oxford and Cambridge Universities who, we can safely assume, had no serious learning disabilities. Even so, his evidence showed 8%–19% with ipsilateral hemispheric dominance and eyedness and handedness. Buffery concluded that his findings "are contrary to any simplistic hypothesis of crossed laterality being a sufficient condition for learning disorder" as proposed by Delacato (1963). Among the women he found 13% with dominance and handedness on the same side and among the men, 8%. When dominance and eyedness were examined, 14% of the women showed an ipsilateral pattern and

19% of the men. Mixed hand and eye dominance was found in 23% of the women and 28% of the men. Buffery rightly points out that because "a sex difference in cerebral asymmetry of function has been demonstrated in adults which is similar to that found in children, an explanation in terms of a transient lag in male development is not appropriate." It seems that the elementary school's emphasis on acquiring verbal skills may give girls an advantage, which boys later overcome when problem material enables them to exploit their spatial facility.

Townes, Trupin, Martin, and Goldstein (1980) studied the relation between a large number of neuropsychological skills and academic success in 230 kindergarten and 226 grade 2 children. During the 3-year period from age $5\frac{1}{2}$ to $8\frac{1}{2}$, marked improvement was made in most of the neuropsychological variables (motor, perceptual, conceptual, and language skills), and these researchers found the test findings useful in understanding each child's pattern of cognitive strengths, and in planning individual instructional programs. They found the girls superior in verbal reasoning, language skills, and serial–perceptual matching. Boys were superior on tests of spatial memory and motor skills. Because the school program from the earliest grades is heavily loaded with verbal demands, it was suggested that "boys are at a developmental disadvantage with respect to academic achievement during early elementary school years" (Townes, Trupin, Martin, & Goldstein, 1980). Drawing on Witelson's work (1977), these writers suggest that normal-reading boys processed verbal information in the early stages using linguistic strategies, but dyslexic boys preferred a spatial strategy.

Teachers of the early grades are constantly impressed by the greater facility of girls than of boys at reading, and whereas this difference is generally true, the verbal superiority does not include all language skills. In our laboratory, a study of 353 normal boys and girls, ages 6–13, was made to examine their language development on 20 subtests of the Spreen–Benton Aphasia Battery (Gaddes & Crockett, 1975). It was found that girls in this age range were *not* superior to boys in most language skills as measured by the battery. No sex differences were found in 11 of the 20 subtests, and these included visual naming, description of the use of an object, stereognosis in both hands, sentence repetition, repeating digits forward and backward, constructing sentences with a number of supplied words, identification of objects by name, identification of objects by descriptive sentence, and reading names of objects and pointing to them. All these tasks can use a strategy that is maximally verbal or nonverbal, so that in the light of the neuropsychological studies cited above, it seems likely that boys and girls, possibly using different strategies, achieved the same levels of success.

In the nine tests where girls did show superiority it was only a temporary advantage in seven of them. These included copying writing, oral reading, reading descriptive sentences and pointing to objects, visual–graphic naming, writing to dictation, and articulation. By age 9, boys were able to match the girls' performance.

On only two subtests did the girls show any prolonged superiority. These were in word fluency and spelling. Present knowledge suggests that primary age girls *do* possess better abilities in reading and writing, but that boys may match their level of verbal achievement in most basic skills by using a different strategy, which is likely to draw more on spatial or pictorial analysis.

The research of Bakker, Teunissen, and Bosch (1976) showed that in the first three grades, cerebral dominance for language seems to be established sooner in girls than boys. Using a dichotic listening test, they found that in the first two grades, boys and girls tended to use both hemispheres about equally in reading—that is, bilateral reading. By fourth grade, girls tended to use their left hemisphere primarily, but boys did not reach this left-sided unilateral process until fifth or sixth grade. Assuming that the right hemisphere reacts to the visual pattern of a word and the left hemisphere responds more to the linguistic meaning of a word, this finding was in agreement that girls in the early grades tended to be better than boys verbally, and boys tended to be better in spatial-constructional activities. An investigation of reading strategies by these children across grades showed that right-dominant readers are slow but accurate in their reading, whereas left-dominant readers tended to be fast but careless. These findings suggest that girls pass through the successive laterality–reading stages faster than boys, and that boys may get stuck more frequently than girls in the early stages of learning to read. This type of neuropsychological evidence is beginning to provide better understanding of the verbal superiority of girls in the early grades.

These researches draw attention to the assumed development of cerebral dominance. The idea that the small child's brain is probably bilateral for language at first and gradually shows an increasing lateralization was given credibility by Lenneberg with his influential book in 1967. He proposed that in most children there was a progressive increase in the role of the left hemisphere and a gradual decrease in the role of the right hemisphere. The so-called Lenneberg hypothesis described this developmental process as beginning in infancy and becoming complete by puberty. A similar view saw this development occurring more quickly and maturing by age 5 (Krashen, 1973), but some recent research has thrown possible doubt on this popular belief and supports the view that the human cerebral hemispheres are specialized both structurally and functionally in infancy. A persuasive proponent of this view, Marcel Kinsbourne, has even suggested that the concept of progressive lateralization be rejected (Kinsbourne, 1975b). Hiscock (1979) has presented evidence of a right-ear advantage in dichotic listening studies in preschoolers, school-age children, and adults. From this evidence he concluded that if dichotic listening measures a fixed function of the brain, and if this is lateralization for language, then it seems that this function is already established by age 3 and so does not develop. Kinsbourne and Hiscock (1978) made an impressive case against the concept of progressive lateralization, citing evidence from studies of anatomy, neurophysiology, developmental psychology, handedness, and neuropsychology. The case is far from closed, however, because of methodological problems and some conflicting and some unexplained evidence. The school psychologist may want to keep abreast of investigations in this area and the special teacher may want to be aware of the developmental behavioral evidence.

Before we leave the subject of hemispheric specialization, let us look at some common examples of its effect on our social behavior. Printers and poster artists have customarily placed pictorial figures at the top left area of a poster and a standard printed message at the top right corner. Experience shows that, other things being equal, this format usually is more successful in attracting attention. In the theater, play directors will tell you that the most dramatic entrances are made from the theatrical right side of the stage (the viewer's left). At a lecture on the Peking Opera, which has established traditions for about 1000 years, it was explained that entrances were always from the audience's left, and the exits always on the right side of the stage. Presumably the slight superiority of the right hemisphere in processing spatial–pictorial input may have been the underlying neural mechanism that determined these customs. And this common phenomenon seems to have experimental support. Right-handers in some studies prefer pictures with a rightward balance (that is, pictures with their areas of interest to the right of center) and left-handers prefer leftward balance (McLaughlin, Dean, & Stanley, 1983). These researchers concluded that "aesthetic preferences for asymmetric pictures seem determined by the direction of cerebral asymmetry."

Conductors of bands and symphony orchestras nearly always enter from the left side of the stage (the viewer's left), as do also the soloists, and lecterns for lecturers who comment on slide or film shows are nearly always placed at the left side of the screen. These customs, no doubt, have grown out of intuitive feelings of artistic taste, but could these judgments of appropriateness have been defined by the relatively better spatial processing of the right hemisphere in most people?

These observations may mean that it is better to place the teacher's desk at the left front corner of the classroom, and any notices at the right end of the front blackboard. Bakker and Van Rijnsoever (1977) have actually studied the effects of auditory–spatial asymmetries in the classroom. They set up two loudspeakers at the middle of the left and right walls. Pairs of words, some differing in initial consonants, some differing in final consonants, and some identical, were presented from one or the other of the loudspeakers. They found that children seated in the middle of the classroom made fewer errors, that discrimination of different phonemes is better for most children when projected from the right, and of identical phonemes, it is better when they are projected from the left. This is one of the first studies to apply the knowledge of dichotic and monaural listening to classroom management.

Using Knowledge of Hemispheric Specialization in Training the Whole Brain

Teachers have known for years that a number concept can be more easily acquired by using blocks or other concrete objects to count. No doubt this tactic helps the child to use *both* hemispheres in this learning process. In our own work with left-brain damaged adults of normal intelligence we have found that reading is facilitated when objects are left casually on the table, if they are pertinent to the sentence being read. Sometimes the traumatically dyslexic adult is unable to read, "Show me a large yellow square," when the table is bare, but can read it successfully when a large number of colored tokens including yellow, of various shapes and sizes, are spread out. Possibly the spatial stimulation interacts with the impaired verbal skills to assist them.

This tactic appears to be a simple applied use of context effects in perception. This phenomenon has also been studied in reading, where the verbal context is much more complex (Chase & Tallal, 1990). More will be said about this subject in Chapter 8.

The brain's functions are extremely complex, and many or most are not yet understood, but this may be the basic mechanism in learning in an enriched environment. An Armenian friend was born and raised in Egypt, where he learned Armenian at home and

French and Arabic at school and on the street. At age 17, he left Egypt to settle in the United States. Twenty-five years later he and his wife decided to return to Egypt for a visit, but prior to the trip he wondered how he would converse because he had long since lost his Arabic. In fact, he could remember hardly any words, but on landing at the Cairo airport he found a competent working knowledge of the language came back to him with surprising facility. Is it possible that the appropriate environment stimulates the brain more completely and more efficiently?

In summary, the child learns specific cognitive skills with different parts of the left or right hemispheres, but learning may be facilitated by activating *both* hemispheres in the process. Skilled remedial teaching requires an imaginative and experimental approach to arrive at ways of maximizing this bilateral activity.

Clinical Addendum

Measures of Handedness and Lateral Preferences

Probably the best reason for attempting to assess lateral preferences (hand, foot, and eye) in children is to increase our comprehensive knowledge of human development and behavior. Studies have examined the relation of handedness to neuroanatomical asymmetry, to prenatal influences, to genetics, to aphasia and language processes, to differential hemispheric activation, to sex differences in hemispheric specialization, to memory for tonal pitch, to artistic talent, to cognitive abilities and learning disorders, to tactile learning, and to skill in Braille reading (Herron, 1980). The breadth of these investigations suggests the important need for precise assessment techniques to measure handedness and all lateral preferences, behaviors with such a wide spectrum of possible neural and behavioral relationships. A second reason is practical: should researchers reveal proven associations between cognitive functions and handedness, the special educator would be better informed for developing appropriate and effective remedial procedures. But determining a person's handedness is not as simple as it may appear. The procedure "often depends largely on the testing instruments, techniques, and criteria employed, as well as the society from which the individual comes" (Bradshaw & Nettleton, 1983).

At present we have a great variety of techniques for assessing handedness. These include parents' or teachers' ratings, classification by writing hand, performance tests (e.g., watching the subject use scissors, a screwdriver, and so on, or a pegboard test, Annett, 1985), demonstration tests (a subject carries out a unilateral activity, such as looking through a telescope, or stepping on an imaginary bug), observations of specific behavioral activities (e.g., hand movements during speech, Kimura, 1973), and preference inventories (Annett, 1970a; Benton, 1967; Bryden & Steenhuis, 1991; Oldfield, 1971; Spreen & Strauss, 1991). Each of these approaches has its uses and weaknesses and Bryden and Steenhuis (1991, pp. 421–429) provide a useful critical discussion of all of them.

Two Cases of Varying Hemispheric Specialization and Handedness

Jim Lane

Jim was 10 years old when we first saw him because of a developmental language disability and weak arithmetical reasoning. His mother reported nothing remarkable in his medical history; he always appeared bright and mentally quick until he entered school, when he immediately ran into obvious difficulty in learning to read and spell. As a result, Jim had become quiet and socially cautious at school, but there were no serious behavior problems. His family was highly supportive, and his grandmother, a retired teacher, helped him with his reading.

Our tests showed him to have a verbal IQ of 105 and a performance IQ of 115 (WISC), but his grade-point averages on the Wide Range Achievement Tests (WRAT) were: reading (single-word recognition), 3.3; spelling, 2.9; and arithmetic, 3.9. Because Jim, at the time of testing, was 9 years 11 months old, to be academically *average* he should have attained grade-point averages of about 4.5.

His family doctor, who was very interested in the possible neuropsychological variables that might be related to Jim's learning problem, reported that she thought he showed mixed handedness and footedness. Until age 8 he wrote with either hand and his reading and writing were full of reversals.

A family history revealed that Jim's father was ambidextrous but was forced to write with his right hand when he went to school. *Both* of the paternal grandparents and the only paternal uncle were left-handed. This familial pattern of left-handedness seemed to be related to Jim's early manual indecision and led us to anticipate the results of the Dichotic Listening Test with genuine interest. It was impressive, then, to find that the test suggested fairly strongly that Jim was *right*-hemisphere dominant for language (right ear preference, 10 and left ear preference, 34). These findings suggested a cerebral–manual conflict, in that he was right-handed and probably right-hemisphere dominant for language. If our hypothesis were true, Jim had to initiate his language concepts in his right hemisphere, shunt them to the left motor strip, and then convey them to his right hand for writing. This unusual circuitous route is frequently correlated with spelling problems.

To examine this hypothesis further we looked closely at Jim's hand-grip strength (which was weak in *both* hands, although a little stronger in the right), his finger tapping (which was about 10% too slow in *both* hands, although the right hand was better than the left), his finger localization (which was perfect in the left hand and had two errors in the right), and his visual–manual and auditory–manual reaction times (which were slow for *both* hands to a visual stimulus, but which showed a relative *left*-hand superiority to both visual and auditory stimuli). All these indicators together point to the possible hypothesis that Jim was intended to be left-handed by genetic determination, but because of a minimal brain dysfunction in the sensory and motor strips of both hemispheres, his handedness was weak and confused in developing and ended in a conflict pattern.

We were now faced with the problem of whether or not to change his handedness. We decided against it because of his age and the learned establishment of his right hand. Because Jim's tactile and phonetic recognition were strong we recommended a remedial teaching program that stressed these two sense modes. On spatial tasks he was superior (Raven's Matrices, better than 95th percentile) and on a picture vocabulary test he measured an IQ of 118 (approximately 88th percentile).

Although the neurologist's examination turned up no positive findings, the neuropsychological tests revealed minimal but definite signs strongly suggesting brain dysfunction in the sensorimotor strips bilaterally. It is highly likely that these dysfunctions contributed to Jim's indifferent handedness, his brain–hand conflict, his developmental dyslexia, and his spelling apraxia.

Stress on tactile and auditory instruction showed improvement in his reading and spelling after only 6 months.

Sara Fraser: A Case of Reported Mirror Writing

This little girl was referred for neuropsychological assessment because of mirror writing and difficulty in following directions involving written work. At the time of her referral, Sara was 7 years old and in first grade. She was the middle child of five in a supportive and affectionate family. Mrs. Fraser was intelligent and genuinely interested in Sara's progress, and though she realized that Sara was "different" from her other children in learning, she was careful not to communicate this awareness to Sara.

At the end of kindergarten in the previous year, the school psychologist had reported that her large muscle coordination was good (balance, throwing, and catching were normal), but she was unable to copy designs. She had a speech problem (poor articulation) and mixed laterality (she threw and caught a ball with her right hand, but drew and colored with her left). After several demonstrations of skipping, she was unable to imitate it.

In first grade she had learning problems from the beginning, although a Wechsler test (WISC-R) administered in October of that year showed her to have a verbal IQ of 114 (better than about 82% of 6-year-olds). Her speech was unclear until age 4, and during kindergarten and her first-grade years she continued to have speech therapy to improve her articulation problem (dysarthria). She had trouble learning to pronounce her own name correctly until she was 5 years old. Reading was poor and spelling chaotic, and she had difficulty in written arithmetic but not oral counting and number facts. She reversed several digits when writing them. She frequently did not follow oral instructions well although her academic achievement level showed considerable variability from day to day.

Childhood Allergies. Sara's mother reported that the birth was normal, but that Sara was slightly jaundiced. However, it soon became evident that she reacted with stress to a number of stimuli. Her eyes have little tolerance to bright light, and nutritionally she was and is allergic to dairy products, oranges, apples, and tomatoes. Since age 2 Sara has had a skin eczema and scalp irritation, and certain soaps and perfumes aggravate the condition. Three of her siblings are allergic to the same foods, so a family pattern of food allergies is evident.

Handedness

Sara was strongly left-handed for writing and drawing and always had been, although both parents and all four siblings were right-handed. This pattern strongly suggests pathological left-handedness.

I Neuropsychological Assessment (Spring, First Grade)

Verbal Abilities. Her strong verbal IQ of 114 was corroborated by high scores in Sentence Repetition, Word Fluency, following oral instructions (Token test), and tactile naming. Her ability in oral arithmetic was good (WISC-R subtest = 13), but Sara's written arithmetic in school was inferior because of her poor motor abilities. Her oral vocabulary on the WISC-R was superior (subtest score = 14).

Handedness. The lateral dominance examination confirmed her strong left-handedness and left-eyedness. Her footedness was mixed; she kicked a ball with her left foot, but stepped on an imaginary bug with her right. Her hand grip was stronger in her left hand, although both hands were weak. Her finger-tapping speed showed the same pattern: her left hand was faster than the right, but both hands were slower than the 7-year-old average (Spreen & Gaddes, 1969). Sara's visual–manual reaction times were better for her right hand (her nondominant hand) and her auditory–manual reaction times were slow for both hands. Her printing was large and poorly controlled, and her perception of right and left, both on her body and in extrapersonal space, was inferior. These findings indicate that as well as a spatial–perceptual problem, there is a motor disability, and the unsystematic pattern of laterality suggests that the sensorimotor strips on both sides may be involved.

Memory. Sara's ability to draw geometric designs on the Benton Visual Retention Test was poor, but on the Multiple Choice Form she did very well. Her scores on the Embedded Figures test were also superior. This performance suggests that her nonverbal memory per se was above average, but that her motor disability impaired her performance on the drawing version of the Benton VRT.

Test Behavior. Sara was alert and cooperative throughout the test sessions, although at times she appeared to have lapses of attention.

Summary and Recommendations. Sara's problems included difficulty with manual speed and dexterity, an attentional deficit, a visual–motor disability, an inferior directional sense with poor body imagery, and a possible hand–brain conflict (i.e., left-hemisphere language dominance and written left-handedness).

We found that although Sara was referred to us as a mirror writer, in fact she did not write whole phrases or sentences in reverse. She did, however, reverse about half the digits, especially under pressure on a speeded test, and she reversed a number of short words and many single letters. She suffered from a problem of severe spatial confusion. To help her overcome these problems we recommended the following:

1. Body image and large muscle exercises (e.g., "Simon Says").
2. Small muscle activities (e.g., writing spelling words in damp sand with simultaneous multisensorimotor exercises).
3. Color coding (e.g., red sticker on left hand, and green sticker on right hand to learn left and right; Sara should be taught to relate this to navigation lights on boats, ships, and airplanes).
4. Color coding to learn letters in writing (e.g., *d* faces left and is red, *b* faces right and is green, etc.).
5. Tactile reinforcement in learning left and right.

Medical Referral. Because of her allergy condition, her attentional lapses, and her variability in speech and intellectual competence from day to day, we referred Sara to an internal medical specialist in the summer following first grade. All biomedical tests (e.g., urinalysis, PKU screening, etc.) were negative, and genetic studies showed normal chromosome appearance.

The following September Sara entered grade 1 for the second time. The school authorities believed she was not ready for grade 2, so she was placed in a first-grade class with another teacher. We argued that conceptually she was ready in that her verbal intelligence level was better than about 82% of her classmates, but that her learning was disturbed by her spatial and motor problems. Because these were not primary elements of intellectual capacity, but mechanistic processes of its expression, and as such could be improved with skilled remediation, we urged the school to promote her to grade 2 and provide daily remedial training for her learning disabilities. We likened the situation to failing a mentally bright cerebral palsied child because his writing was untidy and his speech unclear. On the basis of performance, not potential, however, Sara was directed to repeat grade 1.

In the following March, during Sara's second year in first grade, Mrs. Fraser was contacted for a progress report. Wondering if Sara would be bored and frustrated in having to endure the same material again, we were pleased to hear that she was enjoying school. The work was well within her grasp and she was acting as the teacher's aide in helping some of the other children who were having problems in learning the academic material. Sara's mother reported that Sara excels in long-distance running and that she could run the 1 kilometer run with the grade 5 students. This repeat year has given Sara a better opportunity to establish herself as an important member of her group. Socially, it has improved her by increasing her self-confidence, but Mrs. Fraser said, "I know that she is not being challenged and I realize that she may not be equipped to meet the stiffer academic demands next year in grade 2."

This case illustrates a common problem: whether or not a potentially bright child in the early grades should be kept back because of a perceptual–motor disability. No one can predict with certainty because of the impossibility of repeating the alternative choice with the same child at the same age. We can, however, study specific cases like Sara's and learn from them.

II Neuropsychological Assessment, July–August, Prior to Entering Grade 2

Sara was still cheerful, but restless during the testing, and she still had difficulty giving prolonged attention to assigned tasks. She frequently made careless errors because of failure to perceive the stimulus accurately. For example, she was inaccurate in counting items and copying designs.

Intelligence. Her Full Scale IQ on the WISC-R was not much changed from a year before (down from a 70th percentile level to a 65th percentile level). The biggest change was a decrease in Verbal IQ (down from 82nd percentile to 70th percentile), and a slight increase in Performance IQ (from 45th percentile up to 60th percentile). Examination of her verbal subtest scores showed that only two tests were down, Arithmetic and Vocabulary. A year earlier her arithmetic score depended largely on counting and providing simple number facts. This year it is beginning to depend more on number concepts, and her poor directional sense may be impairing her achievement.

Memory. Last year on the Token Test she followed oral instructions very well. This year she dropped from a 90th percentile level to a 10th percentile level. This variability appeared to result from Sara's inattention. However, her ability to remember geometric designs and draw them improved from a 20th percentile level to a 50th percentile level.

Perception and Sensorimotor Tests. Sara's auditory perception of language sounds (phonetic discrimination) was weak. It dropped from a 40th percentile level in grade 1 to a 20th percentile level a year later. Her visual recognition of embedded figures (geometric figures against a camouflaged background) also decreased markedly, but this appeared to be due to carelessness. Her right–left orientation for both personal and extrapersonal space was very confused. Her finger localization showed slight improvement in both hands.

Sequencing. Her inability to imitate skipping, in April of her kindergarten year, alerted us to the possibility of a sequencing problem in reading and writing. In both test sessions during her two years in grade 1, Sara was unable to tell which light in a sequence was different from a standard pattern; in fact, even during the second test session when she was 8 years 4 months old, she was unable to understand the instructions, although some 6-year-olds and most 7-year-olds can do this test successfully.

All these findings indicate that Sara still had serious problems in spatial and directional orientation, maintaining attention on a task, and sequential perception and motor response. Her teachers were urged to continue a program of sensorimotor activation in learning to spell, to encourage Sara to use a typewriter or computer to increase her sequential skills and her attention in learning to spell, to have Sara use a tape-recorder to learn the auditory aspects of spelling, and board games such as Parcheesi and computer games to practice sequential perception and more accurate visual attention. Her teachers, of course, drew on their own experience to provide a varied academic remedial program.

Sara's Mother's Report, Summer, Following Sara's Second Year in Grade 1

"Sara has now completed two years in grade 1 and repeating it was not very stimulating. There were no major problems as there had been during the first year, but there were no real challenges, either. She still reverses numbers when under pressure of a speed test. Her speech varies; some days her articulation is good, other days very poor. It will be interesting to see how she deals with the new work in grade 2."

Allergies and Learning Disabilities. Geschwind (1983) reported that childhood allergies such as hay fever, asthma, and eczema tend to occur with abnormal frequency in families of dyslexics. He also found significant interrelationships with food allergies, disorders of the immune system, left-handedness, childhood migraine, and developmental dyslexia. More will be said about these biological associations with left-handedness in Chapter 8.

In spite of the negative findings of the biochemical tests when Sara was 7, an association between Sara's allergies, her left-handedness, and her learning problems will continue to be considered as a tentative possibility for understanding her behavior.

Sara's Mother's Report, in March of Sara's Grade 2 Year

"She is doing well in grade 2. At first she slipped from the top reading group, but in November they began giving her more remedial help and she is back up now. She likes her teacher (a man) very much. Her speech is clear now; the speech therapist 'graduated' her from therapy in October. The reversals have disappeared from her writing, unless she is tired or hurried. Her writing is neat if she takes time; she can write well. She still needs help with her spelling, but the school believes that will be an ongoing process. She is enjoying school, and while not at the top of her class, she is progressing satisfactorily."

When questioned about Sara's allergies: "I keep her on a pretty strict diet. I have found that she can drink milk if I scald it, without developing eczema."

Summary

At this time in Sara's life she is learning to cope successfully with her learning problems. Neuropsychological assessment techniques identified her specific deficits although they did not reveal their cause(s). However, this approach permitted a successful remedial program to be developed. In the future, improved neurological and neurochemical assessment procedures may disclose the etiological mysteries of cases like Sara's.

Clinical Classifications of Handedness

No conclusive evidence points to an exact classification of handedness, but the following may be useful and is strongly supported by current research findings.

1. Pure right-handers. These subjects are consistently right-sided in all their lateral preferences and strongly left-hemisphere dominant for language. On a Dichotic Listening Test they will probably show a strong right-ear preference for verbal stimuli. If they show no neurological signs of brain dysfunction and have at least average intelligence, they should be free of specific learning disabilities. If they are underachieving academically, chances are high that their problem is purely motivational and not organic. According to Annett's theory they make up 64% of the general population.

2. Pathological right-handers. These children are rare and may be missed because they are operating in a right-handed world. They are subjects with some degree of right hemisphere dysfunction who genetically were intended to be left-handed and right-hemisphere dominant for language. Because of the disturbing effects of the cerebral dysfunction, which is maximally in the right hemisphere, they tend to be right-handed (i.e., the right hand is controlled by the healthy left hemisphere), but unfortunately the language dominance may remain in the defective right hemisphere. They may suffer from specific learning problems, depending on the locus of the damage. Because many of these children go undiagnosed, we have no way of knowing their frequency, but it is probably much less than 1% of the population.

3. Mixed right-handers. These children use their right hands for writing and nearly always are left-hemisphere dominant for language. However, because of brain dysfunctions in various loci of the right or both hemispheres, they tend to show mixed laterality for manual skills other than writing and for eyedness and footedness. As beginners in school they manifest a high incidence of letter reversals in writing, and they may show impairment in perceptual and motor skills. In Annett's theory these children would be heterozygotes with brain damage superimposed. Many of them suffer some type of academic learning problem. They may be distinguished from the pathological right-hander by careful neuropsychological diagnostic study.

4. Pure left-handers. These children are assumed to be natural or genetic left-handers. They normally have right-hemisphere dominance for language and are consistently left sided in their lateral preferences. When they are free of brain dysfunctions, they should be as free of specific learning disabilities as the pure right-handers. According to Annett's genetic theory they may make up about 4% of the population.

5. Pathological left-handers. The majority of these children were genetically intended to be right-handed, but because of brain dysfunctions in various loci in either the left or both hemispheres they have used the left hand for writing and some manual skills. However, they are nearly always characterized by mixed laterality for various manual skills and for eyedness and footedness. Their cerebral dominance for language is on the left in about one-half of the cases, and bilateral, to some degree, much more than groups of right-handed subjects (Hécaen & de Ajuriaguerra, 1964; Luria, 1966; Milner, Branch, & Rasmussen, 1966; Satz, 1972, 1973; Shankweiler & Studdert-Kennedy, 1975; Subirana, 1958; Zangwill, 1960). Deficits are common in right–left orientation, body image, visual perception, and visual–motor skills.

Most children with organically based disabilities come from Groups 3 and 5, that is, the mixed right-handers and the pathological left-handers. They seem to make up about 7% of the elementary school population, according to the data of Mykelbust and Boshes (1969).

Continuum of Cerebral Lateralization

We have already drawn attention to the fact that handedness does not manifest itself in discrete groupings. The five classes of handedness above are major constellations of hand–brain organ-ization, but detailed handedness examinations, as we have shown, reveal a continuum from very strong right-sidedness, through degrees of mixed laterality, to marked left-sidedness.

Recent neuropsychological research has supported Hughlings Jackson's early caution (in 1874) that cerebral dominance is not absolute. It is evident that dominance for speech is bilateral in many cases, and that a continuum of lateralization for speech perception exists from complete left-hemisphere dominance, through various degrees of bilaterality, to complete right-hemisphere dominance. Shankweiler and Studdert-Kennedy (1975) assessed this relation-ship on a series of handedness measures and on a dichotic consonant–vowel syllable test.

Numerous researches already mentioned indicate a tendency for earlier left-hemisphere proficiency of young girls, and for earlier right-hemisphere competence of young boys. These abilities fre-quently include better verbal, sequential, or analytical skills attributed to the left hemisphere, and better spatial, imaginative, and holistic ones attributed to the right (Bogen, 1975). These findings suggest that women may use their brains more bilaterally than men when confronted with some types of spatial problems and that they may be lateralized in the left hemisphere earlier for language than men (Buffery & Gray, 1972). It has been suggested that this earlier language lateralization and possible bilateral function accounts for their better recovery from traumatic aphasia in some cases. This whole matter is not clear, however, because Buffery (1976), in studying 100 male and 100 female students at Oxford and Cambridge Universities in England, found greater laterality for handedness and dichotic ear preference in females than males. It seems highly likely that the response of either sex is a function of the task being faced. Van Duyne, Bakker, and De Jong (1977) found that under normal conditions in a dichotic listening experiment girls in the primary grades recalled more words than boys with their right ears (left hemisphere) but under the condition of proactive inhibition boys and girls recalled the same number of words with their right ears (left hemisphere).

Although the whole matter of cerebral bilaterality and sex differences is not yet clear, many studies have shown that girls show a superiority in verbal fluency that seems to be present from infancy, earlier speech than boys, better articulation, fewer grammatical errors, and the production of longer and more complex sentences (Buffery & Gray, 1972). This advanced language ability in girls may result from some subtle cerebral structures and functions not yet identified, and it may be that this earlier language learning provides a stronger defense against cortical disorganization in aphasia. Whereas many women show a better recovery from traumatic aphasia, this is not always the case (Kertesz & McCabe, 1977).

The reader who wishes to pursue this topic further may find pertinent papers in books by Bradshaw and Nettleton (1983); Bryden (1982); Bryden & Steenhuis, 1991; Heilman and Valenstein (1979); Herron (1980); U. Kirk (1983b); Kolb and Whishaw (1990); Maccoby and Jacklin (1974); Miller and Lenneberg (1978); Ounsted and Taylor (1972); Pirozzolo (1979); Rourke, Bakker, Fisk, and Strang (1983); Segalowitz (1983); Segalowitz and Gruber (1977); Spreen et al. (1984); and Wittrock (1980a).

Should Handedness Be Changed?

Many first-grade teachers are faced with the problem of whether a left-handed child should be changed to write with his or her right hand. This subject has been discussed theoretically in the main body of the chapter. Here we describe a simple educational procedure that any teacher can carry out to examine a left-handed child's handedness and writing.

This little examination can be carried out with a left-handed 6-year-old as soon as he can write all the numbers from 1 to 10 and as early as possible in the fall term of first grade. Obviously these two limitations are related.

Ask the child to write the numbers from 1 to 10 as fast as he can. Notice the number reversals (e.g., Σ for 2, $\mathcal{E}$ for 3). Then say, "Now let's try it with the other hand. I know you don't write with that hand, but let's see if you can write the numbers 1 to 10 with that hand." If the child has been writing on a sheet of paper, then turn it over so that he cannot see what has already been written. If the child has written on the blackboard, either rub off what has been written or move to another part of the blackboard so that the child is unable to see his first sample. If the left-handed writing is frequented with reversals and the right-hand writing is free of them, then we should question whether there is a manual–cerebral conflict present. The child should be referred to the school psychologist for detailed study, including a lateral preference examination (Barnsley & Rabinovitch, 1970; Harris, 1958; White & Ashton, 1976) and a Dichotic Listening Test (Kimura, 1961a,b, 1967; Satz, Achenbach, & Fennell, 1967; Zurif & Bryden, 1969). The decision to change should be made only after the neuropsychological evidence strongly suggests the child is left-hemisphere dominant for language and a better speller with the right hand, and after a thorough discussion with the school psychologist, the teacher, the child's parents, and with the child.

Some References on Handedness Examinations and Inventories

Bryden, M.P. Measuring handedness with questionnaires. *Neuropsychologia*, 1977, *15*, 617–624.

Bryden, M.P. & Steenhuis, R. The assessment of handedness in children. In Obrzut J.E. & Hynd G.W. (Eds.), *Neuropsychological foundations of learning disabilities*. San Diego: Academic Press, 1991, 411–436.

Crovitz, H.F. & Zener, K.A. A group test for assessing hand- and eye-dominance. *American Journal of Psychology*, 1962, *75*, 271–276.

Harris, A.J. Harris tests of lateral dominance: Manual of directions for administration and interpretation, 3rd ed. New York: Psychological Corporation, 1958.

Oldfield, R.C. The assessment and analysis of handedness: The Edinburgh Inventory. *Neuropsychologia*, 1971, *9*, 97–113.

Raczkowski, D., Kalat, J.W., & Nebes, R. Reliability and validity of some handedness questionnaire items. *Neuropsychologia*, 1974, *12*, 43–47.

White, K. & Ashton, R. Handedness assessment inventory. *Neuropsychologia*, 1976, *14*, 261–264.

Footedness Laterality

Footedness laterality measures have their own tested methods of measurement. See Vanden-Abeele, J. Comments on the functional asymmetries of the lower extremities. *Cortex*, 1980, *16*, 325–329.

7 Attention Deficit Disorder

Everyone knows what attention is. It is the taking possession by the mind in clear and vivid form one, out of what seems several simultaneously possible objects or trains of thought.
William James (1890)

The reader will remember that in Chapter 4 we discussed the cognitive processes of sensation and perception and their possible alterations with brain damage or dysfunction. In this chapter we examine the cognitive and behavioral aspects of inattention, first looking at the components of attention and the different ways in which these components can be studied. Second, we focus on children with attention deficit disorder and comment on the diagnostic criteria and characteristics of the disorder. Third, we discuss some of the theories about the causes of attention deficit disorder and some of the techniques and procedures for treating the disorder. And fourth, we briefly examine memory processes and how memory is influenced by disturbances in attention.

Nature of Attention

In his first textbook on psychology, William James referred to attention as the "searchlight of consciousness." He meant that attention involves scanning the environment and focusing on selected items (James, 1890). Obviously, as we scan the environment many things can capture our attention at any moment, but it is impossible to attend to them all. Attention, then, is more akin to a "beam of light in which the central brilliant part represents the focus" (Hernández-Peón, 1964).

The two major forms of attention are described as (1) passive and (2) active. Passive attention is involuntary in that it is directed by external events that stand out from their background. A bright flash, a sudden loud noise, or a strong odor might command our attention involuntarily or automatically. In contrast, active attention is voluntary and is guided by alertness, concentration, interest, and needs, including internal states such as hunger and curiosity. Active attention involves effort, but one is often unaware of this effort unless the task is difficult. Posner and Boies (1971) describe active attention as vigilance and sustained attention, divided attention, and selective attention. We look at each of these, for all are important to the child in learning.

Vigilance and Sustained Attention

A child may be considered to have a problem with vigilance (or readiness to respond) if he or she is unable to listen for the next spelling word the teacher presents during a test. The child who is unable to remain "on task" to complete it may be experiencing a problem with sustained attention or persistence (Goldstein & Goldstein, 1990). Vigilance and sustained attention require us to maintain alertness and accurate observation during a long, perhaps boring task. Studies of vigilance began in response to the attentional problems reported by radar operators during World War II. After a time on duty, these operators found that their ability to detect the signals created by incoming planes decreased. In a series of experiments, Mackworth (1950) investigated the problems associated with sustaining attention over prolonged periods. Observers were asked to follow a moving clock hand that occasionally made a double step; they were asked to report detecting this double step by pressing a key each time one occurred. Mackworth found that after thirty minutes of watching, accuracy of detection dropped, and observers began to miss more than one in every four events. Later, Broadbent and Gregory (1964) investigated this performance decrease over time. Their findings suggested that the performance decrement was not the result of fatigue so much as a change in the observer's willingness to say that the signal had been detected. During tasks requiring vigilance, as arousal levels and effort increase, attention becomes narrowly focused. As early as 1908, Yerkes and Dodson described this relationship between arousal and performance as an inverted U, with a midrange of arousal that brings about optimal results. This is referred to as the Yerkes-Dodson Law.

In our laboratory we measure a child's ability to sustain attention on a boring task (usually a minimum of 10 minutes), using a continuous-performance task. The child is asked to monitor a series of letters, usually presented on a screen, and then respond when a specific target is present (e.g., trial one, the letter x; trial two, whenever the letter x is preceded by the letter a). The child must try to suppress any response to nontarget stimuli.

Divided Attention or Alternating Attention

Divided attention refers to the ability to track two sources of information simultaneously, such as reading a book and knitting, or listening to the teacher and taking notes (Goldstein & Goldstein, 1990). Once each of these skills is mastered, it can then be carried out almost automatically. The automaticity of these learned skills enables a subject to divide attention between the two tasks. The ability to alternate one's attention depends upon learning, practice, memory, and the systems that we have developed for storing and retrieving information. In our laboratory, divided attention is measured by having the child complete tasks that involve working with two or more cognitive concepts simultaneously (e.g., alternating between alphabetical and numeric sequences).

Selective Attention

Selective attention can be defined as the ability to maintain attention on a target stimulus when distracters are present. A child who is easily distracted by extraneous events, such as minor noises in the classroom, may be experiencing problems with selective attention. A widely used method for studying selective attention is modeled on a real-life phenomenon called the cocktail-party effect. At a noisy party, one tunes in the voice of the person one is talking to, and the many other voices are somehow filtered out, becoming a background noise. This phenomenon has been studied in scientific, controlled laboratory settings using a method known as shadowing (Cherry, 1953). In these studies, the subject wears a pair of headphones that play a different message to each ear. The subject is then asked to attend only to the message in one ear. To ensure that the subject is completing the task correctly, he or she is asked to repeat or shadow the message as it is heard. These experiments demonstrate what is already known from the cocktail-party example. Under high levels of arousal, attention is restricted and focused on only one train of information at a time. For the interested reader, Coren, Porac, and Ward (1979), provide a comprehensive account of this research.

One way to measure visual selective attention in our laboratory is with a visual search task. For example, we ask the child to find a target letter or shape embedded in a long list of other distracting letters and shapes. Successful completion of such a cancelation task requires selective attention: the child has to pay attention to the main stimulus and ignore the incidental stimulus, scanning the array visually until the target is found.

Brain Mechanisms and Attention

Although some parts of the brain, notably the right hemisphere (Mesulam, 1981; Vallar & Perani, 1986; Hynd et al., 1991a; Matazow & Hynd, 1992) and the right frontal-striatal system, including the prefrontal cortex and caudate nucleus (Heilman et al., 1991; Lou et al., 1989; Hynd et al., 1992), are considered more important in attention than others, there is no "attention center."

Because "attention involves the selection of specific information by the organism . . . it is logical to expect it to be associated with selective facilitatory processes in the brain" (Hernández-Peón & Sterman, 1966). In fact, it seems to be determined by basic neural structures and characteristic functions of which the school psychologist and the special teacher can be aware.

The first of these is the brainstem, reaching upward from the medulla oblongata to the thalamus and the cortex. The sensory nerves connecting into the thalamus branch out, some going directly to their sensory nuclei and thence to the appropriate sensory area of the cortex—visual, auditory, or tactile. The others, several million of them, connect through the thalamus to all parts of the cortex. The function of the main branch is to provide perceptual cues, and the function of the remaining fibers to the nonspecific cortical areas is believed to be an "arousal system" (Hebb, 1972). The reticular activating system appears to have two functions, arousal and selective attention. Although neurophysiological research has confirmed the "arousal" function (Moruzzi & Magoun, 1949) agreement is not complete on how the brain selects objects on which to focus attention while ignoring all others, but this seems to include the inhibition of receptors (Hernández-Peón et al., 1956), the acceptance or inhibition of sensory input (i.e., "gating,") (Milner, 1970) by both the brain stem and the cortex, the amount of experience and knowledge, and the strength of motivation of the person attending.

The upper part of the brain stem mediates arousal and regulates sleep. On the basis of chemical information, it recognizes fatigue level and limits the sensory impulses traveling to upper regions of the brain so that an individual can drift into undisturbed sleep. Groups of cells in the brain stem make chemicals including dopamine, noradrenalins, and serotonin. They then distribute these chemicals through their axons to other parts of the brain. Disruption of these chemical pathways can lead to a number of disorders, such as the disruptions in dopamine pathways that result in Parkinson's disease.

Various parts of the thalamus control the shift of attention from the internal to the external world, and, like the cerebral cortex, the left side of the thalamus is more involved with verbal perceptions and the right thalamus more with visual–spatial input. "The selective attention mechanism seems to be the system turning different brain areas on and off to the external or internal world" (Calvin & Ojemann, 1980, p. 7). These writers propose the interesting speculation that malfunctioning of the selective attention system could lead to weak ability to hold attention on external stimuli (e.g., instructions of a teacher) so that attention could easily be diverted by other external or internal stimuli (i.e., distractibility). This pattern of behavior will be familiar to any experienced teacher as typical of many LD children. Many of them manifest chorea (i.e., minimal involuntary twitching movements of the hands and/or the face) and other neurological signs that might be the result of malfunctioning of the thalamus or striatum (Calvin & Ojemann, 1980).

Ojemann (1983) believes that left thalamic stimulation directs attention to verbal stimuli in the external environment, at the same time blocking retrieval of material from both short-term and long-term verbal memory (i.e., the internal environment). Electrostimulation of the right thalamus provides a similar "gating" function with visual–spatial stimuli and visual–spatial memory. "This thalamic-specific alerting mechanism may well play a major role in learning. . . .When the mechanism is active, the type of material present in the external environment will be more readily available" (Ojemann, 1983). When more is known about this possible interior–exterior–thalamic relationship, it may be an important step toward understanding childhood autism.

While the gross structure of the reticular formation is believed to regulate the incoming neural stream from the receptors to control attention and concentration, single cells function in particular ways to direct it. Some exciting research in the last two decades provide strong evidence suggesting that specific cortical cells respond to specific environmental stimuli. In the visual sphere, Hubel and Wiesel (1959); and Hubel (1963) show that some cortical cells in the cat's striate cortex react to vertical lines of light but not to horizontal or sloping ones. They discovered that some cells are turned "on" by particular forms and contiguous cells are inhibited. The "on" and "off" groupings of cells were found to be mutually antagonistic and to possess not a random distribution and function but an orderly arrangement in the cortex. These were microelectrode or single-cell studies and provided information to support the idea of a one-to-one relationship from retinal pattern to visual cortical coding. Morrell (1961, 1967) found that some cells in the visual cortex, but not all, are subject to stimulation by temporary connections. These cells, which initially reacted to a specific light stimulus, could be primed to respond to a temporally contiguous sound stimulus. This evidence suggests that some cortical cells are unique in their responses and others are more general. Some may be feature-detecting cells (Pribram, 1971) and others may be more connected with arousal functions and with more general tasks of perception and interpretation.

Electrical Changes in the Brain During Attention

In previous paragraphs we said something about the possible specific function of some cortical cells in perception and the evidently more generalized function of other cells. We now examine some research evidence of electrical changes in the brain during attention, perception, and mentation, to increase the clinician's and the teacher's conceptual picture of the LD child's neural functions. Let us look first at experiments with animals, and then at some with human subjects.

E.R. John studied single-cell firing patterns in different parts of the cat's brain. He found that learning and attention activate large numbers of neurons in different parts of the brain in a coordinated way by the spatiotemporal characteristics of the stimuli that happen to be present during a learning experience (John, 1972). John's researches are ingenious, technically complex, and beyond the scope of this present discussion, but his studies of the electrical changes in cat's brains during learning are innovative and informative. He fitted an experimental cat with an instrument with several microelectrode connections to different parts of the brain. When the cat was stimulated visually with a steady flicker, seven parts of its brain showed minimal electrical activity. Electrical activity appeared simultaneously in the occipital and temporal cortex, the brainstem, and the limbic system. The cat was taught that milk could be obtained whenever a lever was pressed, and that on a different flicker frequency he must not press the lever. Microelectrode patterns from the same cerebral loci showed a change in pattern and amplitude following anticipation of the visual stimulus as a cue for food. John's work is important in that it supports a unitary rather than localizationist view of the cat's brain function, and it provides detailed information on the electrical changes in individual cerebral cells following establishment of a newly learned pattern of behavior. Recently, John and a number of other researchers have found marked changes in the EEG tracings of humans when clicks have been sounded (i.e., an auditory evoked potential) and they have been asked to attend to them and then to ignore them by reading a book.

During the 1960s and 1970s considerable research was done with human subjects, leading researchers to revise their view that the neurophysiological changes that control "attention" are not peripheral, but are central, including electrochemical events in the brainstem (the reticular system) and in the cortex itself. With human subjects it has been possible to attain better control of "attention" than in the animal studies.

Näätänen carried out an interesting experiment (Näätänen, 1970) wherein his human subjects were asked to listen to loud and soft clicks. These were alternated and spaced sequentially 1 second apart. His subjects attended to the loud clicks against a background of soft clicks, and vice versa. The attended clicks thus became the "relevant" stimuli and the unattended the "irrelevant." There were 50 clicks of each intensity. Five of the 50 relevant stimuli differed slightly in intensity from the remaining 45, and the subject's task was to detect these "target" clicks. He concluded from his observations that there was somewhat generalized cortical activation preceding the relevant stimuli, which caused enhancement of the evoked potential in the brain resulting from the clicks. This generalized cerebral electrical activation was in agreement with E.R. John's findings, discussed above.

Effects of Injury to the Brain

When the brain suffers an injury to some areas, the normal working of attention breaks down. For example, children with a closed head injury as a result of a motor vehicle accident may exhibit difficulties in the complex processes of attention—that is, in maintaining attention in the face of competing stimuli, in sustaining attention, and in shifting attention, particularly if there has been diffuse damage in the frontal lobes (Johnson & Roethig-Johnson, 1989). A patient with an injury on one side of the brain may ignore events at the opposite side of the body. Patients with such defects in attention (referred to as neglect or agnosia) may exhibit unusual behaviors, such as combing the hair on one side of the head, ignoring food on one side of the plate, or, when writing, crowding the words at one side of the page. Patients with neglect fail to detect stimuli and also have difficulty in focusing and shifting their attention (Rapcsak et al., 1989). Spatial neglect and sensory inattention appear to be more common and more severe with right-hemisphere lesions (Heilman et al., 1991).

A method for marking the cells and their interconnections involved in attention involves using the plant enzyme horseradish peroxidase (HRP). This enzyme is taken up by nerve endings and is transported toward the cell body where the nerve endings originate (Mesulam, 1981, 1985). When HRP is injected into the parietal cortex, the network of nerve cells and their projections is extensive. There are connections with the motor cortex (especially areas involved with eye movements (looking toward the object of attention), as well as extensive connections uniting parts of the limbic lobe (important for generating emotional drive). There are cells extending to the brainstem and reticular system. Mesulam (1981), who carried out the HRP experiments, formulated a hypothesis about how the brain operates in directed attention. First, the reticular structures apply an alerting effect. From here events proceed within a tightly interlocked system involving sensation, movement, and emotion. According to Mesulam, neglect can result from damage anywhere within this network. Attention, then, is a distributed process that involves extensive areas of the brain, and each brain area makes its own special contribution.

Attention Deficit Hyperactivity Disorder

The history of diagnosis and treatment of attention deficit hyperactivity disorder (ADHD) is a long and complex problem. It is the third most common learning problem among children, following reading and other language disorders. It is estimated to affect between 5% and 15% of the population, depending on how the disorder is classified and which review is cited. On average, about one child in every classroom in North America (Goodyear & Hynd, 1992) is affected by this disorder, or 3% to 6% of school-age children (Barkley, 1990; Shaywitz & Shaywitz, 1991). Although excessive activity can be seen in many children, including some with a variety of psychological disorders, the term ADHD is used to describe a specific childhood disorder consisting of inherent weakness in ability to concentrate on relevant tasks and to maintain attention until the task is completed. The cardinal symptoms include inattention, distractibility, and impulsivity, as well as difficulties in delaying gratification, motor restlessness, and hyperactivity.

Little was documented about ADHD until the nineteenth century, and most of what is written on the subject has been published in the past thirty years. The earliest known description of the disorder was published in 1845 in a children's story book, *Der Struwwelpeter* (*Unkempt Peter*), by a German physician, Heinrich Hoffman. Earlier anecdotes from children's stories describe children who today would be identified as hyperactive. They were depicted as always active, always in trouble, and never appearing to learn from their mistakes. A negative value was attached in nursery rhymes and children's stories about "Fidgety Phil," "Harry Hurricane," and "Tommy Tornado." One of the first accounts was provided by an English physician, G.F. Still, who published in *Lancet* in 1902. In his clinical practice, Still described a group of children with poor attention span who were disruptive, hyperactive, and impulsive. They were of nearly normal intelligence, but were aggressive, unresponsive to discipline, and had difficulty controlling their impulses. The behaviors occurred more in boys than girls, and in most cases before age 8 years. Still attributed these behaviors of "wanton mischievousness and destructiveness," to a problem in moral development (Still, 1902). He was quite pessimistic about their future, believing that they could not be helped and should be institutionalized.

Following a 1918 outbreak of influenza encephalitis after World War I, many adult survivors of this acute illness developed Parkinson's syndrome (muscle rigidity, abnormal gait, shaky hands and arms, expressionless face, drooling, and disturbances of attention, memory, and emotion). Some of the children who survived this epidemic showed a constellation of behaviors similar to those of attention deficit hyperactivity disorder (Hohman, 1922). It was believed that this disorder was caused by brain injury as a result of the disease process. The pattern of behavior was later described as post encephalitic disorder (Bender, 1942). During the 1930s, research led to the conclusion that a series of disorders of childhood seemed to involve some type of minimal brain dysfunction. Some of these disorders were a result of brain injury and were associated with mental retardation, and others were linked to toxic reactions to metals such as leaded paint. In other cases, perinatal complications were associated with behavioral problems, hyperactivity, and poor attention. In an effort to combine all these factors under one rubric, Strauss and Lehtinen (1947) introduced the concept of minimal brain dysfunction (MBD), also referred to as the Strauss syndrome.

An important milestone occurred in 1937, when Dr. Charles Bradley, an American psychiatrist, tried to treat this symptom complex with medication. He described a group of emotionally disturbed children who responded to treatment with amphetamine sulphate, a stimulant drug. The children showed dramatic improvement in school-related behaviors, with better work habits and less disruptive conduct. The apparently contradictory response of hyperactive children to stimulant drugs has remained a puzzle until the present. From many studies of head trauma patients during World War II, it was discovered that injury to the brain frequently resulted in a pattern of inattentiveness, restlessness, and overarousal (Goldstein, 1942). This research, together with Strauss and Lehtinen's influential *Psychopathology and Education of the Brain-Injured Child* (1947), contributed to the notion that brain-injured children are hyperactive and distractible. Other potential causes of brain injury such as birth trauma, lead toxicities, infections, and epilepsy in children were also linked to hyperactive children. In fact, the terms organic driveness (Kahn & Cohen, 1934), restless syndrome, Strauss Syndrome, minimal brain damage, minimal brain dysfunction, and hyperkinesis were coined to describe the hyperactive and distractible child. An important observation during this period was the striking similarity between the symptoms of hyperactive children and the behavioral sequelae of frontal lobe lesions in primates (Blau, 1936; Levin, 1938). Frontal lobe ablations were shown to result in restlessness, aimless wandering, poor ability to sustain attention, and excessive appetite. Early investigators suggested that severe restlessness in children was likely to be a result of weaknesses in frontal lobe structures, although gross evidence of such defects was not apparent. Within the last ten years or so, investigators have resurrected this notion, with greater evidence to substantiate it (Mattes, 1980; Chelune et al., 1986; Lou et al., 1984; Lou et al., 1989). During the 1940–1950 period, the milder forms of hyperactivity were attributed to poor child-rearing conditions and delinquent families. This idea was revived in the 1970s (Barkley, 1990).

At the time when the MBD concept was most popular, neurologists began to search for markers that could be useful in helping to make this diagnosis. In 1938, Jasper, Solomon, & Bradley provided evidence to show EEG abnormalities in children with MBD, taking the form of slowing in the EEG. A number of other researchers also reported EEG abnormalities in children with behavioral problems (Knott et al., 1953; Werry et al., 1964). The EEG readings, however, were not specific enough to differentiate between the many subtypes of the disorder (Lubar, 1991).

Definition and Measurement of Attention

The current definition of attention deficit hyperactivity disorder (ADHD) describes it as problematic behaviors reflecting the core symptoms of (1) inattentiveness, (2) impulsivity and motor restlessness, and (3) difficulty with gratification. These symptoms cannot be accounted for by developmental or mental level, thought disorder, affective disorder, or other confounding factors such as high anxiety levels or family dysfunction. Over the past eighty years, this disorder has been referred to by at least thirty descriptive names (Goldstein & Goldstein, 1990).

Research to date suggests that ADHD children have their greatest difficulty in sustaining attention to task (Douglas, 1983). The average 2-year-old can attend without supervision to a constant stimulus such as television for about 7 minutes; 3-year-olds can do it for 9 minutes; 4-year-olds for 13 minutes, and 5-year-olds for 15 minutes (Call, 1985). By the first grade in school, children can be expected to sit and work for up to an hour. The inability of children with ADHD to remain on task often results in "behavioral disinhibition" and the seeking out of more engaging activities (Barkley, 1990). This disinhibition appears as distractibility and impulsivity. As a result, inattention and disinhibition combine to affect their ability to remain on task. Children with ADHD tend to be overactive, easily aroused, and restless. Such children also have difficulty in thinking before they act, and often do not think about the consequences of their behavior. They often appear impetuous, unthinking, and do not learn easily from their experiences. They invariably have difficulty in working toward a long-term goal.

Definitions of ADHD have been shaped mainly by the American Psychiatric Association (APA) and the World Health Organization. Currently, there is definitional confusion about ADHD mostly because of the changes in diagnostic criteria that have taken place in the last twenty-five years. In the second edition of the Diagnostic and Statistical Manual (DSM) (APA, 1968), the disorder was referred to as the Hyperkinetic Reaction of Childhood. This title was modified, elaborated, and renamed in the third edition (DSM III) in 1980, to Attention-Deficit Disorder. Other definitions were developed by the World Health Organization and the International Classification of Diseases (ICD-10), used mainly in Europe. The DSM III (APA, 1980) divided attention deficit disorder into two subtypes: attention deficit disorder with hyperactivity (ADD/H), and attention deficit disorder without hyperactivity (ADD/WO). The authors of the more recent DSM III Revised edition (APA, 1987), collapsed the diagnostic criteria into a single disorder called Attention Deficit Hyperactivity Disorder or ADHD, which does not distinguish between attention deficit disorder with and without hyperactivity. Authors of the DSM IIIR argued that there was little empirical evidence to support the separation of the disorder. The current unidimensional view of ADHD has not met with overwhelming approval, and epidemiological studies have not supported this unified definition (Cantwell & Baker, 1985). Recent research indicates that ADD without hyperactivity may be a distinct behavioral and neurocognitive syndrome (Barkley, 1990; Hynd et al., 1991a). Currently, the APA is compiling DSM IV, and the reader is encouraged to refer to this source for a more recent definition from revised diagnostic criteria.

Presently, ADHD is treated as a unitary disorder but with a variety of features. The onset of the symptoms most typically occurs before age 7 and lasts at least 6 months. The current working definition also implies that ADHD can coexist with severe emotional problems and/or mental retardation if the symptoms of ADHD are excessive. There are fourteen symptoms, and to satisfy the criteria for diagnosis, eight of them must be present (Table 7.1). According to DSM IIIR criteria, a diagnosis of ADHD also includes reference to the environment. Symptoms of ADHD may occur in one situation (e.g., home but not school, or vice versa), or in a number of situations (e.g., both home and school). Hence, ADHD may be situation-specific or pervasive. Because the attentional difficulties of children with situational ADHD are not easily distinguishable from those of other atypical children, Barkley (1990), recommends confining the term ADHD to children who exhibit these difficulties in all situations. In addition to the fourteen criteria outlined by DSM IIIR, the American Psychiatric Association recommends that other diagnostic criteria be used, such as child behavior rating scales and parent self-report scales that the school psychologist can use. The ADHD child should also demonstrate difficulties on objective measures that assess various attention skills. These might include objective and norm-referenced computer-based tests and pencil and paper tasks. One of the difficulties in using the diagnostic criteria from DSM IIIR (e.g., talks excessively or fails to finish chores), is that they have little direct similarity to attention as it is described in attention theories. Barkley writes:

> ADHD consists of developmental deficiencies in the regulation and maintenance of behavior by rules and consequences. These deficiencies give rise to problems with inhibiting, initiating, or sustaining responses to tasks or stimuli, and adhering to rules or instructions, particularly in situations where consequences for such behavior are delayed, weak or nonexistent. The deficiencies are evident in early childhood and are probably chronic in nature. Although they improve with neurological maturation, the deficits persist in comparison to same-age normal children, whose performance in these areas also improves with development. . . . These apparently biological deficiencies in the regulation and maintenance of behavior emanate into the social ecology of the child's social interactions in the family, school, and community, resulting in increased controlling behaviors . . . which over time meet with little success. . . . Left untreated the development of these early antisocial behaviors appears to increase the risk of early and recurrent patterns of delinquent and antisocial behaviors. . . . Managed properly, these social interaction

Table 7.1. Diagnostic Criteria for Attention Deficit Hyperactivity Disorder

---

Note: Consider a criterion met only if the behavior is considerably more frequent than that of most people of the same mental age.

A. A disturbance of at least six months during which at least eight of the following are present:
  1. often fidgets with hands or feet or squirms in seat (in adolescence may be limited to subjective feelings of restlessness).
  2. has difficulty remaining seated when required to do so.
  3. is easily distracted by extraneous stimuli
  4. has difficulty awaiting turn in games or group situations.
  5. often blurts out answers to questions before they have been completed.
  6. has difficulty following through on instructions from others (not due to oppositional behavior or failure of comprehension), e.g., fails to finish chores.
  7. has difficulty in sustaining attention in tasks or play activities.
  8. often shifts from one uncompleted activity to another.
  9. has difficulty playing quietly.
  10. often talks excessively.
  11. often interrupts or intrudes on others, e.g., butts into other children's games.
  12. often does not seem to listen to what is being said to him or her.
  13. often loses things necessary for tasks or activities at school or at home (e.g., toys, pencils, books, assignments).
  14. often engages in physically dangerous activities without considering possible consequences (not for the purpose of thrill seeking), e.g., runs into street without looking.
B. Onset before the age of seven.
C. Does not meet the criteria for a Pervasive Developmental Disorder.

  Note: The items above are listed in descending order of discriminating power based on data from a national field trial of the DSM IIIR criteria for Disruptive Behavior Disorders.

Criteria for Severity of Attention Deficit Hyperactivity Disorder:
Mild: Few, if any, symptoms in excess of those required to make the diagnosis and only minimal or no impairment in school or social functioning.
Moderate: Symptoms or functional impairment intermediate between "mild" and "severe."
Severe: Many symptoms in excess of those required to make the diagnosis and pervasive impairment in functioning at home and school with peers.

American Psychiatric Association: *Diagnostic and Statistical Manual of Mental Disorders, Third Edition, Revised*, Washington D.C., American Psychiatric Association, 1987, pp. 52–53.

conflicts of ADHD children may be maintained at relatively low levels, such that difficulties with school performance may be the primary area of difficulty for ADHD children during adolescence. (Barkley, 1990, p. 71. Reprinted by permission of the Guilford Press.)

Prevalence of ADHD

Problems with attention and arousal are one of the largest sources of referral to child mental health centers (Barkley, 1981). Inattention, overarousal, impulsivity, and difficulty in delaying gratification influence a child's interactions at home and school, as well as academic work and emotional well-being. Recent estimates by Szatmari et al. (1989) indicate that ADHD affects 4% to 6% of the school-age population in North America. Lower estimates, down to 0.1%, have been reported by Rutter et al. (1970) in their Isle of Wight study. British criteria for diagnosing ADHD are more stringent than those in the United States, and require the presence of the problematic behaviors across settings (Pennington, 1991).

The disorder occurs three times more often in males than females, and is more common in the younger child between 6 and 8 years old. The results of a province-wide survey in Ontario, Canada (Szatmari et al., 1989), found the prevalence rates to be 9% in boys and 3.3% in girls. The rates varied by age for boys. In the 4–11 age group, about 10% of boys were identified as ADHD, down to 7.3% in the 12–16 age group. The prevalence for girls was fairly stable across age groups (3.3%–3.4%, respectively). The higher rates of males among clinic samples seems related to expectations and the fact that males are more likely to be aggressive and antisocial and, as such, are more likely to be referred to a mental health center. When males and females are compared to their same-sex normative groups, and controls are added for symptoms of hyperactivity and antisocial behavior, occurrence of ADHD in males and females may be equal (McGee et al., 1987). Females with ADHD may present with problems in mood, affect, and emotion, and with less difficulty with aggression (Kashani et al., 1979). They appear more socially withdrawn and have more internalizing symptoms (depression, anxiety) than boys (Brown et al., 1989). A large majority of ADHD children are referred to mental health clinics because of a cluster of presenting problems, including aggression and poor conduct. In contrast, ADD children without hyperactivity are more frequently shy, socially withdrawn, and moderately unpopular (Lahey et al., 1984).

Developmental Course of ADHD

Retrospective reports by parents indicate that the symptoms of ADHD are often present in infancy. Parents describe their infants as difficult to manage, with high activity levels, irregular sleep, reduced need for sleep, and emotional lability. These difficulties become more apparent between 3 and 4 years and are readily observable in the classroom, where the symptoms become intensified by the attentional demands of school work. Additional symptoms appear, such as short attention span, tantrums, and difficulties in functioning in group settings. Some preschoolers with ADHD develop a combination of symptoms, including impulsivity, noncompliance, fearlessness, boundless energy, and poor judgment (Ross & Ross, 1982). The irregularity of their behavior often leads to family stress. A few cases of ADHD develop after age 7 when the disorder is acquired secondary to a compromising neurological incident such as trauma or hypoxic injury. Findings suggest that it is possible to identify children at risk for developing an early pattern of ADHD symptoms before they enter kindergarten, using a combination of child and parent variables. These include: (1) family history of ADHD; (2) maternal smoking and alcohol consumption during pregnancy; (3) poor infant health and developmental delays; (4) early onset of high activity levels and demanding behaviors in infancy; (5) single parenthood and low educational attainment (Barkley, 1990).

Earlier research (Laufer & Denhoff, 1957) viewed ADHD as a childhood disorder that weakened with age, but follow-up research has shown persistence of the problems of impulsivity, restlessness, poor self-esteem, and poor social skills (Gittelman et al., 1985). As the child with ADHD approaches preadolescence, the presenting problems may change. Activity levels may decrease and other aspects of ADHD may become more important, particularly productivity and completion of assignments. Developing social relationships is often difficult for the child with ADHD, where the roles and perceptual cues that influence activities and relationships are not correctly interpreted by the child. A pattern of academic, familial, and social conflicts becomes established. Between 30% and 50% of ADHD children develop symptoms of conduct disorder and antisocial behavior (Barkley, 1990). About 60% to 80% of children by this time will have tried stimulant medication, and more than 50% will have taken part in individual and family therapy. By the end of grade 6, 30% to 45% will have received formal special educational assistance. Up to 58% will have failed at least one grade in school (Barkley, 1990). Follow-up studies over the last twenty years have clearly dispelled the notion that the ADHD disorder is generally outgrown by adolescence. About 60% of children with ADHD continue to show signs of this disorder into adulthood, and 75% continue to experience problems in inter-personal relations (Gittelman et al., 1985; Weisss & Hechtman, 1986).

Associated Problems

A diagnosis of ADHD is also complex because it often occurs concurrently with other disorders. Apart from the primary prob-lems of inattention, impulsivity, overactivity, and inability to re-gulate their behavior, children with ADHD may have an array of other difficulties. One of the most difficult areas for ADHD children is academic performance. The majority of clinic-referred children do poorly in school and typically underachieve relative to their intellectual level, mainly because of their inattentiveness, restlessness, and impulsivity. Stimulant medication appears to help some of these children improve on their academic productivity and standing (Rapport et al., 1980). Estimates vary depending on which criteria are used to identify learning disabilities, but about 30% to 40% of LD children also meet the ADHD criteria (Lambert & Sandoval, 1980). Because attentional disorders often affect behavior in many settings, including the classroom, some educators consider ADHD and learning disabilities to be com-mon correlates, and ADHD a possible cause for LD. This view is not consistent with that outlined at the National Conference on Learning Disabilities (1988). Learning disabilities and disorders of attention are different entities. The former is characterized by the specificity of dysfunction (e.g., deficits in arithmetic or spelling), whereas ADHD covers a variety of dysfunctional behaviors that may be observed in a wide range of environments. Recent research indicates that primary learning disabilities such as dyslexia, and other factors such as family environment, influence whether dys-lexia leads to symptoms of ADHD (Pennington, 1991).

In an early study, Hagen (1967), was able to demonstrate that some LD children were more deficient in selective attention than non-LD children. Using an incidental learning paradigm, a central stimulus was presented together with an incidental or background stimulus. The non-LD group were able to retain more of the central items, whereas the LD group recalled more of the incidental items. Recent studies comparing LD and ADHD children have supported this finding (Tarnowski et al., 1986; Richards et al.,

1990). Some LD children are deficient in selective attention compared to normal controls, whereas some children with ADHD and no LD are not. In contrast, LD children do not as a group show deficiencies in sustained attention, whereas ADHD children make more errors by responding to nontarget stimuli. Also, ADHD children tend to have problems with rote memory, whereas LD children often do not (Felton & Woods, 1989). These cognitive processing differences between LD and ADHD children are important in both assessing and treating children.

Some ADHD children also have speech and language difficulties related to fluency and organization of speech (i.e., to the higher-order cognitive processes called executive functions, which involve organizing and monitoring one's thoughts and speech). As a group, ADHD children also tend to show poor complex problem-solving strategies and organizational skills (Tant & Douglas, 1982). Their use of strategies is impulsive, poorly organized, and inefficient. Tests that measure complex problem solving, response inhibition, and sustained effort (i.e., primarily tests that are sensitive to frontal lobe functions) reveal some of these difficulties (Chelune et al., 1986).

About 52% of ADHD children have poor motor coordination for tasks such as maze drawings and pegboards (Szatmari et al., 1989). Many of these children also show motor overflow movements indicative of poor motor inhibition, as well as poor handwriting (Denckla & Rudel, 1976). Epidemiological data from the Province of Ontario, Canada (Szatmari et al., 1989), suggest that children with ADHD may have a number of developmental abnormalities. Developmental problems such as slowness to talk and walk, clumsiness, and low birth weight were 1.8 times more common in children with ADHD than those without ADHD. Children with ADHD were 1.9 times more likely to have chronic health problems than children without. The likelihood of family dysfunction was 2.2 times more likely in a family with a child with ADHD.

Estimates vary, but between 21% and 51% of children diagnosed as ADHD also meet the criteria for Conduct Disorder (CD) (Barkley, 1990). Recent evidence indicates that the etiologies of the two disorders ADHD and CD are different. The home backgrounds of children with CD include greater social adversity and more psychiatric disorders among the parents than do ADHD children without significant CD problems (Szatmari et al., 1989). Some children with ADD but not hyperactivity have internalizing symptoms that may lead to greater risk for affective disorders in later adolescence. Goodyear and Hynd (1992) in their comprehensive review of more than thirty behavioral and neuropsychological studies, suggest that ADHD children have more behavior problems, are less popular, tend to be more self-destructive, and are more likely to have a dual diagnosis of ADHD and CD. Children with ADD but not hyperactivity appear to be more socially withdrawn, have a slower cognitive tempo, are more self-conscious, and have a greater incidence of developmental learning disorders.

Causes of Attention Deficit Hyperactive Disorder

Considered a disorder of brain function, ADHD is thought to be a result of biological and/or environmental causes.

Heredity

Children with ADHD often have a positive family history. Hyperactivity has been found in the parents of hyperactive children four times more often than in controls (Cantwell, 1972). Families with a history of ADHD among relatives, particularly parents and siblings, are more likely to have hyperactive children than families without such familial disorders. Some studies show that ADHD is more common in fathers and uncles of children with ADHD than in the relatives of children without ADHD. Having a hyperactive sibling appears to increase the risk of hyperactivity among other siblings. Goodman and Stevenson (1989) estimate the risk to be as high as 17% for female siblings and 30% for male siblings. Twin studies often help to clarify the role of environmental and genetic factors (Goodman & Stevenson, 1989). Monozygotic twins originate from the same fertilized egg and have identical genes. Dizygotic (nonidentical) twins originate from separate eggs fertilized by different sperm. In a study of 93 sets of twin girls, Willerman (1973) found that hyperactivity was common to both members of identical twins, but very few of the genetically dizygotic sets of twins were both hyperactive. Specific genetic disorders which include features of ADHD, are Turner's syndrome in females, and Fragile X syndrome. These findings support a genetic hypothesis on the causes of ADHD.

Allergies and Dietary Sensitivities

Allergy or immunologic sensitivity is an abnormal response to food, chemicals, or inhalants. Food allergens enter the circulation and travel to sites in the body such as lungs, stomach, intestines, and brain. Accounts by some clinicians suggest that foods or chemicals may be a contributing factor in children with learning and behavioral problems. Some of the early studies are anecdotal but present a clinical picture that is marked by restlessness, irritability, bursts of temper, drowsiness, and sullenness (Shannon, 1922; Duke, 1927). These symptoms have been identified in two groups of children: the first was the tired, listless, and sluggish child; the second group the excitable, hyperactive child. It has been suggested that these two groups may represent two stages in the same illness, a tension or "high" stage followed by a fatigue or "low" stage (Mayron, 1979). This pattern of symptoms has been referred to as a tension-fatigue syndrome (Crook, 1963; Speer, 1970).

Other studies suggest that food dyes can produce effects such as hyperactivity. Lockey (1948), was among the first to report such sensitivities. Feingold (1968, 1974), proposed that food additives such as artificial flavors, colors, and salicylate can alter a child's behavior. The types of symptoms attributed to these food additives include restlessness, hyperactivity, asthma, itching, headache, nausea, and lassitude. Feingold (1974), reported that approximately 60% of the children in his clinical practice were cured of their attentional difficulties following a modified Feingold diet. The incidence of food allergies in the general population has been measured as 6% to 7% (Marshall, 1989), yet between 47% and 66% of children with ADHD reporting to clinics were allergic to at least one food substance (Rapp, 1978; Tryphonas & Trites, 1979). It therefore seems possible that food allergies and ADHD may have a common cause, or stress reactions to food allergies may aggravate the symptoms of ADHD in children who are predisposed to develop them (Pennington, 1991).

Arousal Defect

In the 1950s, a proposed model of ADHD suggested that the symptoms of ADHD stemmed from overarousal, and that stimulant drugs acted paradoxically because, although they increased arousal, they led to less activity. The overarousal model has influenced treatment. If arousal is increased by stimulus input, then it will be advantageous to reduce the activity level of children by restricting the level of stimulation. Interestingly, research into this area has found that ADHD children are often indistinguishable from controls in high-stimulation environments and show abnormal levels of activity as the level of stimulation is reduced, not increased. Others interested in the arousal theory have considered that ADHD children suffer from underarousal. Because ADHD children are stimulus seeking, this theory has held some attraction, and it has been proposed that ADHD children may actually have low levels of arousal and seek stimulation to raise the level of arousal (Zentall & Zentall, 1983). Distractibility and stimulus-seeking behaviors may occur because ordinary levels of stimulation are too low. In fact, under minimal-stimulation conditions, the differences between children with and without ADHD is very evident (Kaspar et al., 1971). This relation has been demonstrated objectively using a continued-performance task with infrequently occurring signals. Children with ADHD are able to detect fewer signals than are controls, possibly because the level of stimulation is too low and they seek other sources of stimulation. Children with ADHD learn less efficiently on a paired-associate learning task when the information is presented at slow rates (Conte et al., 1986, 1991).

Support for a low-arousal hypothesis for ADHD has been gathered using measures of electrodermal activity, cortical evoked potentials, and behavioral observations (Satterfield & Dawson, 1971; Satterfield et al., 1973). These authors propose that such children behave as if they were in a state of decreased sensory arousal. Because of their low arousal, these children habituate easily to sensory stimulation and therefore constantly seek stimulation. This hypothesis might explain the disruptive behavior of hyperactive children. The problem of low arousal may be related to the reticular activation system (RAS) and the abnormal production or utilization of adrenergic neurotransmitters within that system. Because the RAS includes the pontine and mesencephalic RAS in the brainstem, and the diffuse thalamic projections that act to inhibit the lower pontine and mesencephalic sections, dysfunction of the RAS could also be reflected in the disinhibition of the frontal lobes. Satterfield's hypothesis helps to explain the positive effects obtained by Bradley with amphetamine sulphate, a stimulant drug.

Neurological Abnormalities

It has long been thought that ADHD was caused by specific brain damage. Earlier, we mentioned the terms minimal brain dysfunction, hyperkinesis, and Strauss syndrome, which were commonly used in the 1950s and 1960s to account for the features of ADHD. Fewer than 5% of children with ADHD have documented brain damage (Rutter, 1977).

In CT-scan studies of ADHD children, no evidence appears of structural differences (Harcherik et al., 1985). More recently, however, Hynd and his colleagues (1990), using MRI scans, failed to find the usual R > L frontal asymmetry in ADHD children that is found in normal controls. A reverse pattern of asymmetry in the head of the caudate nucleus of ADHD children has also been reported (Hynd et al., 1992). In 73% of the normal children, the left caudate is larger than the right, whereas in 63% of children with ADHD, the left caudate was smaller than the right. This asymmetry may be related to asymmetries in the neurotransmitter systems implicated in ADHD. Differences in the morphology of the corpus callosum of ADHD children have also been reported. Using MRI studies, a group of ADHD children were found to have a smaller right frontal region and a smaller corpus callosum, particularly in the regions of the genu, in the anterior area, and splenium, in the posterior areas (Hynd et al., 1991b). Heilman and his associates (Heilman et al., 1991) propose that ADHD children have dysfunction in the right frontal-striatal system (i.e., the area of the prefrontal lobes and the basal ganglia, including the caudate and putamen). The right frontal lobe together with the right striatum appear to be important for inhibiting unwanted actions in response to stimuli. The basal ganglia (which form part of the striatum) function to gate or control sensory input into motor systems. In ADHD children, a dysfunction may appear in this gating system so that volition is not correctly transcoded into action. "This defect leads both to a form of inattention, where the stimuli that should lead to action do not, and to defective response inhibition, where stimuli that should not lead to action do elicit a response" (Heilman et al., 1991, p. 78). This notion of right frontal-striatal involvement is supported by the blood-flow studies of Lou et al. (1989).

Other researchers have attempted to correlate the presence of neurological soft signs or minor physical anomalies with ADHD, but the results have not been conclusive. Minor physical anomalies are slight deviations in physical appearance, such as an index finger longer than the middle finger, a curved fifth finger, or a single transverse palmar crease. There appears to be a weak association between minor physical abnormalities and hyperactivity that is not specific to hyperactivity (Burg et al., 1980).

Other interesting evidence for differences in brain organization in ADHD children comes from studies of brain function rather than brain structure, such as regional blood-flow studies and studies of catecholamine neurotransmitters—dopamine and norepinephrine (i.e., chemicals secreted at the synapses to facilitate transmission of neural energy in the brain). Some evidence supports the model of CNS underarousal in a subgroup of ADHD children. Using regional blood-flow studies, a group of ADHD children were found to have decreased blood flow to the frontal lobes, which was increased following a treatment of methylphenidate (Ritalin). The

treatment with Ritalin also led to decreased blood flow in the
motor cortex and primary sensory cortex, "suggesting an inhibition
of function of these structures seen clinically as less distractible
and decreased motor activity during treatment" (Lou et al., 1984,
p. 829). In a second study by the same investigators, data pointed
specifically to the basal ganglia (a cluster of nuclei near the thalamus, including the caudate and putamen), as the locus of reduced blood flow (Lou et al., 1989). A study involving the parents
of ADHD children who themselves showed residual features of
ADHD, and who had never been treated with stimulant medication, were examined using PET scans. The results indicated
reduced cerebral glucose utilization, especially in the frontal lobes
(Zametkin et al., 1990).

In brain chemistry, increasing research and evidence indicate
that dopamine and norepinephrine are related to ADHD. A group
of researchers has provided an animal model of ADHD related to
dopamine (Shaywitz et al., 1982). In this study, young rats were
given a chemical (6-hydroxydopamine), which selectively destroyed
dopamine nerve endings and caused rapid and permanent loss of
up to 75% of dopamine in the brain. As the rats matured, they
showed increased activity and difficulty in learning. At maturity,
they continued to show difficulty with learning and adjustment to
unfamiliar environments. This form of ADHD, which was produced by reducing dopamine levels in the young rats, was produced not by specific lesions to the brain, but by damage to the
nerve endings that deliver dopamine to other parts of the brain.
Other metabolic studies of children with ADHD (Shaywitz et al.,
1977; Shetty & Chase, 1976), demonstrate a link between ADHD
and altered dopamine synaptic function. Lower levels of a dopamine metabolite (homovanillic acid—HVA) were found in the
cerebral spinal fluid of ADHD children. These studies support the
notion that the clinical syndrome of ADHD is related to dopamine
dysfunction. Other studies have provided evidence of depleted
norepinephrine in the right hemisphere of children with ADHD
(Posner et al., 1988; Shaywitz & Shaywitz, 1988). Norepinephrine
pathways have been identified in maintaining alertness by acting on
the posterior attention systems of the right hemisphere. It seems
likely, however, that the neurochemical mechanisms of ADHD are
more complex, and no one neurotransmitter is exclusively involved
in ADHD (Zametkin & Rappaport, 1987). Here is one plausible
theory of the brain mechanisms underlying ADHD:

> The executive function deficit of ADHD children is caused by func-
> tional hypofrontality, which in turn is caused by either structural
> and/or biochemical changes in the prefrontal lobes and is detectable
> as reduced frontal blood flow. Biochemically, the cause would be

low dopamine levels, which Ritalin treatment reverses, at least in part. . . . One subtype of ADHD children may fall into the group that is related to hypoarousal of the right posterior hemisphere secondary to norepinephrine depletion. While the posterior and anterior systems interact, separate deficits in each system are possible. (Pennington, 1991)

It seems likely that the attention system may coordinate several groups of nerve cells, including dopamine, noradrenaline, and serotonin cells.

> The catecholamine systems of dopamine and norepinephrine are complex and measurements of increases and decrease in these systems are not sufficient to explain but lead us to an important conclusion that the chemical systems that have their nerve-cell bodies in brainstem nuclei are important factors. (Goldstein & Goldstein, 1990, p. 40)

The limbic, right-hemisphere, and frontal cells may also be part of the attention system. The projections from the brain stem center to the basal ganglia and cortex would make possible inhibition of motor activity and restlessness at one time, and releasing it at another. The variable and unpredictable responses that occur with a disorder in attention and motor activity would result from a dysfunction in the mechanism for controlling attention. This model of the attention system

> allows us to understand why the treatment of attention disorders does not help learning disabilities. Learning disabilities can be seen as dysfunctions of cerebral cortical function as opposed to poor function of brain-stem regulatory centers. Chemical agents, such as methylphenidate or amphetamine, which improve the attention system, would not improve the function of cortical neurons. The attention system regulates a child's ability to concentrate on reading, whereas the cerebral cortical centers would determine the child's reading comprehension. Improving the attention center might improve a child's interest in reading or his receptivity to reading, which may secondarily improve his reading skill. The attention system concept explains why ADHD is a separate problem from learning disability and why medications that improve attentional skills may have little direct effect on learning. (Goldstein & Goldstein, 1990, p. 47)

Neuropsychological Studies of ADHD

The earlier focus of interest in the study of ADHD children was activity level. Findings indicated that the quality of activity level differentiated ADHD children from controls rather than the *amount of activity* (Cromwell et al., 1963). Interest then moved to the study of the different aspects of attention, and this led to a major finding that there were no differences between ADHD children, on and off Ritalin, in orienting or reactive attention, but there were differences in selective and focused attention (Porges et al., 1975). Douglas and Peters (1975), demonstrated that ADHD children and controls responded similarly to extraneous stimuli. Of great importance was the finding that ADHD children showed a clear deficit on measures of sustained attention, particularly on long, self-paced tasks (Sykes et al., 1973). More recent work by Douglas (1988), shows that ADHD children may have a generalized self-regulatory deficit that influences the organization of information processing, the role of attention while information is being processed, and the inhibition of inappropriate responding. Some of the cognitive tasks on which ADHD children perform poorly include continuous-performance tasks, perceptual-search tasks, card-sorting tasks, and planning tasks. The extensive work by Keith Conners provides further support for a frontal lobe dysfunction model of ADHD (Conners & Wells, 1986). These authors were able to distinguish six neuropsychological subtypes within a group of ADHD children. The first two groups did not exhibit cognitive disabilities and their overactivity was a result of anxiety. A third group showed LD with symptoms of ADHD as secondary symptoms. The fourth group demonstrated an isolated motor impulsivity that was not responsive to treatment. The fifth group appeared to have visual–spatial deficits similar to those seen in children with a nonverbal learning disability. The sixth group showed frontal lobe dysfunction, as exemplified by their poor performance on the Porteous Mazes. The members of this group were responsive to drug treatment, which helped them control their socially inappropriate responses.

In summary, neuropsychological studies of ADHD children provide some evidence to support a hypothesis of executive-function deficit, but it is inconclusive. An alternative theory of ADHD, or perhaps a subtype of ADHD, with few supporting data, involves a primary deficit in alertness secondary to dysfunction of the posterior right hemisphere.

Treatment of ADHD

The ADHD disorder can be managed but is not cured. It is generally agreed that medication alone is insufficient to treat ADHD successfully, and combined treatments have proven more successful, including educational intervention, medications, psychotherapy for the child, and therapy and education for the parents.

Medication

The most common form of treatment for ADHD is stimulant medication. Ritalin (trade name for methylphenidate) is the most widely used. Stimulants increase autonomic activity such as heart rate, blood pressure, and skin conductance, and potentiate production of the neurotransmitters dopamine and norepinephrine (Cohen et al., 1971; Levy & Hobbes, 1988; Porges et al., 1975). More than 600,000 children annually in the United States, that is, between 1% and 2% of the school-age population, receive medication, primarily Ritalin. In a 1987 study of students in Baltimore County, Maryland, Safer & Krager (1988), reported 6% of public elementary students, 4% of middle school students, and 0.5% of senior high school students were taking medication for hyperactivity and inattention. The highest incidence occurred in grades 2 and 3: 93% of these children used Ritalin.

In general, about 50% to 66% of ADHD children show improvement from stimulants, with improved ability to attend, increased on-task behavior, reduced motor activity, and improvement in learning new material. While on medication, some ADHD children also appear to work more efficiently and accurately on math problems (Pelham, 1986), and respond with more appropriate social behaviors (Douglas, 1980). The behavioral effects of this medication are short-lived and peak and dissipate within 4 to 5 hours. The long-term gains of stimulant medication are less clear. The side effects of Ritalin appear to be minimal. In high dosages, Ritalin may cause poor appetite and insomnia, and in a small percentage of cases, children may develop symptoms of Tourette's syndrome (recurrent, involuntary, repetitive, purposeless motor movements). The response of ADHD children to stimulant medication is not unique. Some normal children exhibit a favorable response to stimulant medication, with increased attention to tasks and less activity (Rapport et al., 1980).

Behavior-Modification Techniques

Behavior modification is a form of treatment based on the classical behaviorism of Skinner. Using this approach, rewards may be given (such as verbal praise) for on-task behavior, or punishments (such as removal of tokens), may follow less desirable behavior. Barkley views this treatment approach as a way of establishing the regulation of behavior by its consequences. Although it is possible to increase the levels of appropriate behavior using this method, there are a number of shortcomings. Not all children respond to behavior-modification techniques and some who do fail to continue beyond a one-year follow-up (Pelham and Murphy, 1986). In one study, 50% of parents of ADHD children discontinued the treatment (Firestone et al., 1981). The combined effects of psychostimulant medication such as Ritalin and behavior modification techniques are the two most common, effective, and safe interventions for ADHD (Barkley, 1989, 1990). This approach has more appeal because the benefits obtained from stimulant medication make it possible for children to gain greater benefit from behavior modification.

Cognitive Behavior Modification

Cognitive behavior modification uses a set of procedures to train behaviors such as self-regulation, planning skills, and problem-solving skills. The rationale for these procedures comes from the work of Luria and Vygotsky, two eminent Russian psychologists who stressed the role of verbal mediation in the control of behavior. Using this approach, ADHD children are taught to use self-talk or "to think aloud" to direct their behavior. Another procedure involves teaching how to use strategies to solve problems. Children with ADHD are taught to define the problem, generate a solution, monitor the solution, and provide self-reinforcement when the problem is solved. Meichenbaum (1977), and Kendall & Braswell (1984), have provided manuals and workshops to train professionals and parents in these procedures. To date, few encouraging data have been gathered to demonstrate the effects of this type of treatment over time (Conte, 1991). Children with ADHD appeared to use these strategies in the training situation, but failed to generalize from them when they were returned to their treatment situation months later.

Parent Training

Because the transfer of training over time and to other situations using behavior-modification techniques has been poor among ADHD children, interest has been increasing in training parents to deal with problematic behaviors (DuPaul et al., 1991). Programs have been developed, studied, and adapted for use with parents and preschoolers with ADHD (Forehand & McMahon, 1981; Pisterman et al., 1989). The techniques involve teaching how to enhance the value of parent attention, giving positive attention, using a token economy of rewards and punishment, and using time out for noncompliance. One study using a parent-training program over a twelve-week period found that the program was effective in improving the child's compliance and improving the parents' management techniques. Changes in the child's behavior were maintained up to the twelve-week follow-up. One significant finding was that the training did not generalize to nontrained behaviors or carry over to the school environment when the children started school.

EEG Biofeedback Techniques

Electroencephalogram biofeedback, or neurofeedback, is a treatment for ADHD in which brain-wave activity is used as the parameter for feedback to the subject. Since 1976, several clinicians have used neurofeedback to produce clinical improvements in ADHD children (Hodes, 1989). Lubar (1991) reports that more than 90% of the approximately 250 children treated have made significant improvement. Other clinicians report similar success rates (Carter, 1985; Tansey, 1985). The use of neurofeedback for treating children with ADHD incorporates:

1. Satterfield's theory (1971), on the relationship between low arousal and poor attention. As the reader will recall from the section on causes of ADHD, Satterfield proposed that children with ADHD have a low arousal threshold and are easily habituated to sensory stimulation and therefore constantly seek it. This condition is likely to be caused by an abnormality in adrenergic neurotransmitters in the RAS including the thalamic projections.

2. The early EEG studies (Berger et al., 1938), which demonstrated that when one is resting, the dominant EEG activity is in the alpha and theta range (4–8 Hz). As one becomes excited, EEG activity begins to shift toward the beta region above 14 Hz. Lubar (1991) suggested that children with ADHD might be less able to produce beta activity above 14 Hz and would experience excessive slow activity, primarily in the theta region of 4–8 Hz. Also, children with ADHD often have problems with alpha blocking; that is, they tend to produce excessive alpha activity (8–12 Hz) while on task.

3. The management and reduction of seizures through EEG biofeedback and sensorimotor rhythm training (Sterman & Friar, 1972; Seifert & Lubar, 1975). The first clinical application of neurofeedback was for treating epileptic patients who were resistant to drug therapy. This application developed out of research in the late 1960s by Dr. Barry Sterman, a neuropsychologist at the National Institute for Mental Health. Sterman found that cats trained to produce more sensorimotor rhythm activity (SMR) in the lower range of beta (13–16 Hz) were resistant to chemically induced seizures. In the early 1970s Sterman began to treat a few epileptic patients, whom he trained to produce more SMR activity while inhibiting theta activity (4–8 Hz).

Lubar's recent work shows (Lubar, 1991) that the brain-wave patterns of children with attention disorders vary from those of other children. Children with ADHD have trouble shifting their brains into faster brain-wave patterns needed for effective attention and concentration. When confronted with tasks requiring concentration, they remain stuck in slower brain-wave patterns more characteristic of daydreaming and lack of focused thought. In neurofeedback, specialized computer equipment provides the subject with information about his or her brain-wave patterns. Changes in the graphic display on the computer screen indicate when faster brain-wave patterns are being produced. With this information, children learn to decrease the slow waves and to increase the faster brain waves needed for concentration and attention. Lubar reports that about 80% of the children treated show improvement as measured in grade scores, standardized academic tests, I.Q. scores, and parent and teacher ratings. Most of these findings need to be replicated in well-controlled studies because it is not yet clear what factors contribute to the success. Is it the attention the child receives in completing the treatment, or brain maturation, or brain-wave feedback?

Dietary Changes

Reviewing the studies of dietary intervention in children with ADHD raises several important points. First, food allergies are more common in ADHD children than in normal children. This finding does not necessarily imply that food allergies cause ADHD; they may have a common cause. Second, a weakness in the literature on the effects of dietary intervention is the method for selecting subjects. Some studies have chosen subjects from the population of ADHD children, whereas others have picked ADHD children with allergic responses. The former group of studies (Conners et al., 1976; Harley et al., 1978), did not produce consistent findings, whereas others such as Rapp (1978), using a modified Feingold diet that is free of dyes, preservatives, and salicylate for children with allergic symptoms, found improvement in almost 50% of the children monitored. Favorable results were obtained also by modifying the diet of children who had ADHD as well as allergies (Trites et al., 1980). In a study of ADHD children with skin rashes and rhinitis (i.e., head cold), improvements in behavior were obtained when food substances such as artificial flavors and colors, chocolate, monosodium glutamate, preservatives, and caffeine were eliminated from the diet (Kaplan et al., 1989). In this study 42% of the children showed a 50% improvement in behavior.

Third, the age of children who are treated by dietary changes is also an important factor. In one major study (Harley et al., 1978), it was found that fewer school-age children responded to changes in diet than did preschool children. As with other forms of treatment for ADHD children, diet may improve the behavior, but it does not normalize it, and ADHD children continue to have problems with their behavior (Conte, 1991).

Summary

In this section we have looked at many issues related to the topic of attention. The distinction between the concept of attention in attention theory and ADHD was discussed. Attention refers to processes of vigilance, selection, and sustained effort that can be measured with a number of attention tasks. In discussing ADHD we saw that conclusions about attention disorders are based on observing a child's behavior as outlined in the diagnostic criteria in DSM IIIR and reported by parents, teachers, and others who interact with these children. One of the difficulties in using the DSM III criteria is that they have little similarity to attention as described in attention theories. The topic of ADHD and its behavioral effects has received increasing attention in the past few years because it is one of the major sources of child referrals to mental health clinics. Because the diagnostic criteria for ADHD have changed and are still changing, our conclusions about ADHD should be interpreted cautiously. In fact, "generalizations about ADHD must be tempered by the definitional confusion that still besets this area of study" (Conte, 1991).

No one factor that contributes to attention disorders has been found to account for its onset. As a consequence, "it may be prudent to view ADHD as the final common pathway of a number of possible etiological events, much as mental retardation or other developmental disabilities are conceptualized" (Barkley, 1988). Findings in twin studies and epidemiological studies support the idea that there are biological reasons for this disorder. As a group, children with ADHD have a high incidence of developmental problems (such as delayed motor milestones and low birth weight). There also appears to be a high incidence of ADHD in families. Psychosocial factors such as low socioeconomic status or family dysfunction alone are not significant in ADHD.

Specific neurological and neuropsychological models of ADHD also are presented, including discussion of research on the influence of brain damage, neurotransmitter deficiencies, and deficiencies in the arousal system. Current research suggests that ADHD children may suffer from chronic low arousal (involving the frontal-striatal system and/or the right posterior regions of the brain), which may help to explain why these children are characterized as attention seeking and why stimulant medication is effective.

Because of the variety, pervasiveness, and chronicity of behavior problems associated with ADHD, varied treatment techniques across settings are necessary. There is no cure for ADHD, and it appears that, "even the most effective treatments are short term in nature and symptomatic in focus" (DuPaul et al., 1991, p. 121). In reviewing the treatment techniques used to manage ADHD, the use of stimulant medication is reported to provide the most consistent results. Most treatment centers, however, use a combination of treatment approaches, including parent education, behavior modification, cognitive behavior modification, and medication. A group of ADHD children with allergic symptoms show some improvement in behavior when their diet has been modified. The evidence so far suggests that behavior-management techniques provide short-term alterations in a child's behavior, with minimal generalization of skills beyond the treatment time. The most encouraging results have been obtained when a combination of treatment techniques have been applied, which professional staff can support, particularly when the child moves from the preschool or home environment to the school.

Memory

Attention and memory are different but related processes fundamental to learning. Attention to a stimulus allows it to be more fully and permanently entered into memory, whereas unattended input is flecting and may be lost. Memory enables the past to be recorded and accessed so that it may affect the present. The act of remembering involves a number of cognitive processes related to the acquisition, retention, and retrieval of information. To remember, one must first have learned or acquired the information. Next, the information is filed away or retained for later use. The final stage is retrieval, the point of trying to remember. Many failures to remember are failures of retrieval and not of storage. Previously acquired information can be obtained in two ways: by recall or by recognition. Not all the components of memory develop at the same rate. Some appear to function more or less in the same way in five-year-olds and adults, and other processes continue to develop throughout childhood, adolescence, and adulthood (Kail

& Hagen, 1982). The study of these complex memory processes has generated a great deal of information, some of which is summarized here and will be useful to teachers and school psychologists in understanding children with learning difficulties.

The logic for relating attention and memory was established by William James. In his chapter on attention (James, 1890), he wrote that the immediate effects of attention are to make us perceive, conceive, distinguish, and remember better than we could otherwise. Aristotle, usually considered the first psychologist (R.I. Watson, 1963), appears to be the first to write systematically on memory. In his essay "On Memory and Reminiscence," he clarifies mental processes relative to time. He points out that "to remember the future is not possible, but this is an object of opinion or expectation . . . nor is there memory of the present, but only sense-perception . . . but memory relates to the past." Aristotle recognized that perception and attention must precede memory. Hebb, 2000 years later, commented on "the commonly held opinion that no learning is possible without intention to learn, no memory of a sensory event is possible unless it was attended to at the time of its occurrence" (Hebb, 1949, p. 151), but he warns that this statement, though mainly true, needs qualification. Sometimes events peripheral to the focus of attention are remembered, but usually attention enhances learning and memory, which appears to be true in most of academic learning.

Memory can be conceptualized as an information-processing model in which information is transformed, reduced, elaborated, stored, retrieved, and used (Atkinson & Shiffrin, 1968; Newell, 1980). The general components in this "computer" system include: (1) a structural component similar to the hardware of a computer; the structural component includes the sensory storage, short-term memory, working memory, and long-term memory; (2) a strategy (or control) component, comparable to the software of a computer; (3) an executive process during which strategies are overseen and monitored (Boyd, 1988; Swanson & Cooney, 1991).

Structural Components of Memory

The Sensory Register

Sensory memory refers to the first representation of information that is available for processing for a limited time—about 3 to 5 seconds. At this stage the information in the initial store is believed to be a copy of the original physical stimulus. Sensory registers probably exist for all the senses, but the ones studied intensively thus far are vision and audition. In the visual modality, the image is referred to as the icon (Sperling, 1960). In the auditory modality it is referred to as the mental echo (Darwin et al., 1972). The icon and mental echo last for only a brief period. They represent un-analyzed sensory information that is a copy of what the receptors provide.

Transfer from Sensory Register to Short-Term Memory

The transfer of information from the sensory register to short-term memory is believed to be controlled by the processes of pattern recognition and attention. These are referred to as control processes because they control the flow of information between the memory storage systems. Pattern recognition is the process of recognizing that information in the sensory register is familiar or meaningful. As the information is recognized, it is transferred into short-term memory. The sensory register can hold a large amount of information for a limited time, but short-term memory has limited capacity. The control process of attention governs which information will pass from the sensory register to short-term memory. This procedure can be demonstrated by the cocktail-party phenomenon described earlier in this chapter, which involves being able to attend to only one channel of information at a time. Even though the sensory register takes in a large amount of information, control processes such as attention will help determine what portion of this information will be transferred into short-term memory. The information in the sensory register is encoded in a replica of the physical stimulus. By the time the information arrives in short-term memory it may be encoded in a different way. Most verbal information in short-term memory is encoded acoustically through sound, even when it is presented visually (Salame & Baddeley, 1982). Abstract visual images that cannot be described are encoded visually (Brooks, 1968).

Short-Term Memory

Information is transferred from the sensory register into short-term memory, which is a temporary storage system with capacity to store a limited amount of information for a limited time. It processes information for about 3 to 7 seconds and primarily deals with storage and not retrieval. Of the several short-term memory systems, the most intensively studied are verbal short-term memory, visual-verbal short-term memory, and visual-spatial short-term memory. Selective disorders of these systems correlate with localized brain regions (McCarthy & Warrington, 1990).

Most people can remember 7 (±2) random digits, but only 4 or 5 random words. This restriction in the "span of apprehension" was first investigated by Jacobs in 1887. He asked subjects to write down, from memory, sequences of numbers that he had read aloud to them. He found that the maximum span was 7 to 8 digits. He also reported an increase in the number of digits recalled between ages 8 and 19, and suggested that this increase was linked to the growth of intellectual abilities. Binet and Simon (1908), incorporated the digit span task in their measures of intelligence, a tradition carried on in more recent intellectual tests. In the experimental literature of short-term memory, it has become conventional to differentiate between limitations in *capacity* and the amount of information that can be retained and reproduced, and limitations in *duration* of short-term memory and the rate at which material is forgotten. The capacity of short-term memory is about 7 items, ±2 (Miller, 1956). For normal subjects the capacity is also determined by the subject's ability to chunk or recode information into higher order units (McCarthy & Warrington, 1990). A chunk is any piece of information that is represented as a single meaningful item. Grouping information allows more to be stored in short-term memory. Meaningful information is more easily stored than nonmeaningful information. For example, subjects can repeat sentences that are longer than the span of apprehension for digits.

Short-term memory is limited by the amount of information that can be stored and also by its duration. For example, when we take down an unfamiliar telephone number, we need to rehearse the number mentally so that we will retain it long enough to write it down or dial it. Ebbinghaus (1885) was among the first to study the effects of rehearsal on duration of information. He memorized lists of nonsense syllables to a strict rhythm. He found a mathematical relation between the number of times he recited the list on one day and how fast he could perform the task the next day. He concluded, as did Aristotle, that repetition increased the likelihood of subsequent recall. In more recent times, the investigation of forgetting in short-term memory has been enhanced by a technique developed for studying storage and decay of information: the Brown-Petersen task (Brown, 1958; Petersen & Petersen, 1959). To prevent the subject from attending to and rehearsing information in short-term memory, the subject is asked to perform a distracting task continuously for a set time. Using this technique, Petersen & Petersen were able to demonstrate that normal subjects forget a large proportion of "meaningless" information in less than 1 minute. If subjects were not allowed to rehearse, some information was lost after 3 seconds and almost all after 18 seconds.

Visual span for meaningful stimuli can be assessed by having subjects briefly view arrays of visual stimuli (100–200 milliseconds) and then recognize the stimuli from a multiple-choice selection. The brief exposure prevents the subjects from recoding the stimuli into spoken form. Using these conditions it has been found that normal subjects can report between 4 and 5 items. Information stored in short-term memory depends upon control processes that enable the subject to choose which information to scan and which to rehearse. An important control process is rehearsal (i.e., consciously and meaningfully repeating information). Other processes involve ways of organizing information (such as ordering or classifying) and mediation processes (such as comparing new information with that already in memory). Organization strategies include chunking (or grouping), clustering (or categorizing), mnemonics (abbreviated associations) and imagery. Mediation is promoted by employing preexisting associations or by giving direct and explicit instructions to the child, or by cueing (Swanson & Cooney, 1991).

Information is retrieved from short-term memory by a scanning process. Research shows that subjects scan short-term memory one chunk at a time using a strategy called serial search pattern, during which each item is searched for separately (Sternberg, 1966).

Working Memory

Working memory is dynamic and active because it focuses on active interpretation of newly presented information as well as on integration of previously stored information (Baddeley, 1986). The working memory model is conceptualized as having three major components: the articulatory loop, the visual-spatial sketch pad, and the central executive. Working memory allows for temporary storage of information in the articulatory loop or in the visual-spatial sketch pad, which is overseen by a central executive function. The ability to hold material verbatim in working memory is important in problem solving. For example, performance on an auditory-verbal span task requires the operation of the articulatory loop under the direction of the central executive system (McCarthy & Warrington, 1990). The central executive system monitors and coordinates the functioning of the memory systems and decides the order in which processes will be performed (Neisser, 1967).

Long-Term Memory

Long-term memory is storage of information, permanent as long as the brain is free of pathology. The information that is stored is primarily semantic. As in the transfer of information from the sensory register to short-term memory, transfer from short-term to long-term memory is governed by a control process, referred to as elaborative rehearsal. Maintenance rehearsal is the simple repetition of information that can be used to keep information in short-term memory. To transfer information into long-term storage, elaborative rehearsal is thought to take place. The meaning of new information is analyzed and related to information that is already in long-term memory (Craik & Tulving, 1975). The more elaborate the rehearsal, the more analysis takes place, the better the recall of information. Transferring information into long-term memory also requires effort, but some information can be transferred quite effortlessly by automatic processing (Hasher & Zachs, 1979). For example, one does not actively rehearse the events that have happened during the day. These can be recalled effortlessly. Most information in long-term memory is stored by semantic coding—that is, by remembering the general meaning of a word or sentence. A second way to encode meaning is by imagery (i.e., creating a mental image of an object or scene).

Information stored in long-term memory can be broken down into two major categories: procedural and declarative memory. Procedural memory is the memory of skills, knowledge about how to do things, such as riding a bicycle or driving a car. These are memories of actions and motor skills that have been gained by observing others and by practice. Procedural memory is older in human evolution than declarative memory and is less susceptible to insult. The exact brain structures that mediate procedural memory are not clearly understood, but the cerebellum has been implicated as a possible source as well as the basal ganglia, hippocampus, and amygdala.

Declarative memory (or memory of facts) is memory for specific information such as dates of birth. Declarative memory can be subdivided into two types: episodic memory and semantic memory (Tulving, 1973). Episodic memory is autobiographical and is responsible for storing the events of our lives. It is linked to place and time. Semantic memory is more general and includes information such as rules, concepts, and facts. The transfer of declarative memory into long-term memory is mediated by the hippocampus, amygdala, and other closely associated structures. The storage sites for long-term memory, however, are in cortical networks that are distributed throughout the cortex, probably in networks that initially processed the information (Squire, 1987) . . . "so storage is hard to disrupt (hence Lashley's failure to find the engram), but the mechanism of transfer into long-term memory is quite localized and vulnerable to insult" (Pennington,

1991, p. 19). The brain structures that mediate short - and long-term memory are different and short- and long-term memory disorders for verbal and visual material are mediated by different structures, as we shall see in the discussion that follows.

Information can be retrieved from long-term memory according to the principles of organization and use of retrieval cues. Long-term memory can be compared to a library of information, a highly organized collection of material with related material stored in the same general location. Retrieval cues help locate the information. Thus it is possible to facilitate retrieval by storing information in an organized manner. By carefully organizing information when it is stored, it can be more easily retrieved, provided a cue or place to start is identified (Tulving & Pearlstone, 1966).

Physiological Correlates of Memory

The pioneering work on memory and the brain was begun in 1915 with Karl Lashley's work on the neural locations of learned habits. Lashley spent a great deal of his time studying which parts of the brain in rats were involved in memory. In his experiments he cut fiber pathways or removed portions of the neocortex in the rat brain and observed the effects of these lesions on the rat's memory for a maze. Even after hundreds of such experiments, Lashley was not able to disrupt specific memories or identify a single area of the rat's brain that was critical to memory. He concluded that it was not possible to isolate memory traces anywhere in the rat's nervous system, and that although some regions of the brain were involved in retention of an activity, the engram was represented throughout the region (Lashley, 1950). Therefore, lesions to a number of brain regions may interfere with memory, but these regions do not store memories. It seems likely that "groups of neurons in different parts of the brain, especially in the cerebral hemispheres, are more or less important for the remembering of different types of information [e.g., verbal, pictorial], but even this specialization is relative rather than absolute" (Kolb & Whishaw, 1990, p. 526). Not long after Lashley's work, the neurosurgeon William Scoville and a neuropsychologist, Brenda Milner, made an important discovery about localization of memory in the human brain (Scoville & Milner, 1957). Their research involved a young man (H.M.) who had been suffering from epileptic seizures. Because medication had not helped the young man, it was suggested that a neurosurgical operation be performed to remove the anterior portion of the temporal lobes. Previously the operation had been restricted to one temporal lobe. During the surgery, Scoville removed two-thirds of H.M.'s temporal lobe and the hippocampus in the right and left hemispheres. Within a few hours following the operation, the seizures had stopped, but H.M. could not find his room or recognize members of the hospital staff. The surgery had produced severe anterograde amnesia (i.e., inability to store new memories). When anyone was introduced to him, he forgot the person's name and face within minutes. The most striking disturbance was H.M.'s inability to encode new memory traces such as who cared for him, or what he had eaten at his last meal. When given something new to remember, he could do it perfectly as long as there was no delay between hearing the information and repeating it. In other words, H.M. was unable to recall events following the operation. The case of H.M. provided an important contribution to the understanding of memory: the realization that memory is not one system stored in a particular region of the brain, but consists of many processes and systems. It is significant that apart from H.M.'s memory disorder, his other intellectual functions were normal. His I.Q. remained unchanged and his speech was normal (Milner, 1966).

In contrast to the patient H.M., a man unable to form new memories, Luria, in his *Mind of the Mnemonist* (Luria, 1968) describes his patient S., a man of unlimited long-term memory, but without a short-term memory. In testing patient S. Luria was unable to reach the limit of S's memory. S. was able to look briefly at a table of numbers and repeat them verbatim. When he was tested several years later, he was able to recall the table without error. Similarly, he was able to recall lengthy transcripts verbatim, without error.

A number of areas of the brain are associated with memory loss. Most information about the relation of memory and temporal lobe function has come from four research methods: (1) autopsy studies of patients who, in their final months or years, have developed serious memory deficits; (2) observations of memory loss after surgical removal of various parts of the cerebral cortex; (3) electrical stimulation of the human cortex in conscious patients during brain surgery; and (4) use of the Wada amytal technique to produce temporary amnesia in conscious patients. Milner draws attention to Bekhterev, the famous Russian physiologist and contemporary of Pavlov, who was the first to suggest (in 1899) "that the mesial parts of the temporal lobes might play a critical role in human memory processes" (B. Milner, 1966). He examined the brain following autopsy of a patient whose most striking behavioral abnormality had been a severe memory impairment. The brain cutting revealed a bilateral softening or deterioration of cerebral tissue in the region of the uncus, the hippocampus, and the adjacent mesial structure of the temporal lobes. Milner, in the same publication, lists a number of clinical studies in which hippocampal damage and memory disorder appear to be related. Most of these studies, however, have included some form of infection (encephalitis) and the resulting tissue damage has been diffuse and poorly defined. Though such studies are valuable in providing gross neuropsychological relationships, they lack the exactness that results from studies of more homogeneous experimental samples.

Evidence from studies of patients after surgical removal of parts of the cerebral cortex is more definitive. Some of the work of W.B. Scoville, the neurosurgeon, has already been mentioned. Frontal lobotomies had shown some undesirable behavioral effects and it was important to discover whether fractional lobotomies would be successful in alleviating psychosis. For example, it had been found that undercutting the orbital surfaces of both frontal lobes (i.e., the area above and behind the eyes) actually did have a favorable therapeutic effect in psychosis without any new signs of personality deficit. Because the orbital frontal surfaces and the mesial temporal cortices are closely related, it was hoped that surgery in the mesial temporal area might have the same salutary effect. Scoville and Milner (1957) have reported that when the mesial or inside surfaces of both temporal lobes are undercut in the hippocampal area, severe impairment of recent memory results. When only the uncus and amygdala were removed bilaterally, no memory impairment occurred, although the relation of these structures to memory is not clear. Their studies led them to conclude that the anterior hippocampus and hippocampal gyrus were critically related to recent memory, but their removal, with the lateral temporal cortices left intact, did not impair early memories or habitual memory, technical skills, general intelligence, or perceptual abilities. Such cases also showed no deterioration in personality such as is seen in more nearly complete bilateral temporal lobectomy. Their studies suggested that the lateral temporal cortices are needed for long-term memory, but that the mesial temporal areas, particularly the hippocampus and hippocampal gyrus, at least on one side, are crucial to short-term memory.

However, if a memory test includes a series of line drawings of common objects that are chosen so that they can be categorized as to physical shape or lexical category, normal subjects will organize them either way. But subjects with unilateral right temporal lobectomy grouped the pictured objects according to lexical category, and those with left temporal lesions grouped the objects by their shape (Moscovitch, 1979). This type of evidence reminds us that verbal memory draws on both hemispheres, and may make more or less use of the right hemisphere, depending on the degree of semantic or visual imagery involved in the memory performance (Paivio & Linde, 1982).

The third research technique is electrostimulation of the cerebral cortex. Wilder Penfield's studies at the Montreal Neurological Institute during the 1930s and 1940s, reported in the 1950s, provided considerable new knowledge using this technique. The details of how this research was done are described by Penfield and Roberts (1959). With a local anesthetic to reduce discomfort from the incision, the patient remains conscious during the early part of the operation so that he or she can report any sensations or experiences as they occur following cortical electrostimulation. Penfield found that in one patient, stimulation of the posterior cortex with a weak current could produce a false sense of familiarity regarding her present experience. In many patients suffering from temporal lobe epilepsy the phenomenon of déjà vu was not uncommon. When different points on the temporal cortex were stimulated, previous experiences, such as the patient's place of work, a scene from a play, her small son's voice, in fact any experience stored in memory, were revived. These experiences were more vivid than normal remembering, however, and Penfield reports (Penfield & Roberts, 1959), "The patients have never looked upon an experiential response as a remembering. Instead of that it is a hearing-again and seeing-again—a living-through moments of past time." Penfield's findings also have been repeated and extended by other researchers (Mahl et al., 1964; Ojemann & Whitaker, 1978; Ojemann, 1979). This evidence suggests that the electrical activation of memories in the brain may be somewhat similar to the action of a tape recorder. A story, a song, or some pattern of meaningful material may be permanently stored on the tape in a magnetized pattern. When this pattern is appropriately stimulated the original material may be retrieved as many times as it is wanted. This concept of the brain depicts it as an electrochemical repository of experiences neurally stored for future reference. It is interesting that only the temporal lobes produced these "flashback" experiences when stimulated; no such responses resulted from stimulating any of the other lobes.[1]

The Wada technique, the fourth method for studying the relationship between brain function and memory, has been described. Although it was originally developed to establish hemispheric dominance for speech prior to therapeutic surgery for severe epilepsy, it has been useful in demonstrating transient memory disorders

[1] The reader is referred to an excellent, inexpensive paperback on cortical electrostimulation: W.H. Calvin and G.A. Ojemann, *Inside the Brain* (New York: Mentor Books, 1980).

produced by this method of single-hemispheric anesthetization. Wada's original technique (Wada & Rasmussen, 1960) was to have the patient lie on a bed with forearms up in the air and fingers either moving constantly or gripping the examiner's hand. The knees were drawn up with the feet near the buttocks, and the patient was asked to begin counting as the injection was made into the carotid artery in the neck. If made on the left side, the left hemisphere soon became anesthetized or maximally affected, and the arm and leg on the opposite side (contralateral) would slump to the bed. This flaccidity of the contralateral limbs and cessation of counting would usually occur by the time the injection was completed. The ipsilateral arm and leg (i.e., those on the left) would remain in the air and could be moved voluntarily to command, although the patient was unable either to speak or move his right arm or leg. The aphasia (inability to speak) and the right hemiplegia (paralysis of the right limbs) usually was complete for from 1 to 3 minutes, after which time normal speech and voluntary limb movement gradually returned as fresh blood replaced the drug in the left hemisphere. When the injection was on the language nondominant side (i.e., the right side in most people), the patient was able to speak, read, and write, but unable to remember and interpret pictorial material accurately (B. Milner, 1958) during the period of the left hemiplegia. Although this technique has great value for studying cerebral dominance, for providing preoperative information to the brain surgeon, and for shedding light on phenomena associated with amnesia, it is helpful here in providing evidence for the importance of the temporal lobes in memory functions.

The role of the temporal lobes in memory was identified around 100 years ago. Specifically, four major sites within the temporal lobes have been identified as contributing to memory functions, including the anterior temporal cortex, the amygdala, the hippocampus, and the entorhinal cortex (the cortex located on the medial surface of the temporal lobe), which sends out and receives input from the hippocampus. Patients with Alzheimer's disease show deterioration of the entorhinal cortex. The hippocampal formation is made up of two major structures: (1) the hippocampus or Ammon's Horn, which has an outline in cross-section of a ram's horn, and (2) the dentate gyrus, a tooth-shaped fold of cortical tissue. Parts of Ammon's Horn are especially susceptible to damage and are associated with memory disturbances. Recently, neuropsychologist Larry Squire hypothesized that the hippocampus is very important in declarative memory (remembering facts), but other brain structures are involved in procedural memory (Squire, 1987). The amygdala also is involved in memory functions. It lies in front of the hippocampus and is vulnerable to damage following stroke, infection, or removal of the anterior temporal lobe for management of intractable epilepsy (Kolb & Whishaw, 1990).

Unilateral temporal lesions of the left hemisphere may result in difficulties of verbal recall and understanding and retention of verbally expressed ideas (receptive aphasia). In dichotic listening experiments with normal subjects, it is usual for more words to be recognized by the right ear (contralateral) than by the left (ipsilateral), because most people are left-hemisphere dominant for language (Kimura, 1961a,b). This normal pattern is disrupted, however, in cases of unilateral temporal lobe damage; in these cases better dichotic perception for speech stimuli may occur in the ipsilateral ear (Berlin, Lowe-Bell, Cullen, Thompson, & Stafford, 1972) when both ears are stimulated at normal and similar intensities. When the ipsilateral ear is stimulated below threshold, then the contralateral ear may approach normal function (Berlin, Lowe-Bell, Jannetta, & Kline, 1972).

Right temporal lesions are usually accompanied by impaired spatial perception and imagery and comprehension of pictorial material. Children with temporal lobe seizures tend to be more impaired than normals in stereoscopic vision (Webb & Berman, 1973). Whereas unilateral temporal lesions result in relatively mild or moderate memory deficits, bilateral damage to the hippocampal areas produces severe and generalized loss of recent memory.

Although the temporal lobes (including the amygdala and hippocampus) are important in memory, they are not the only structures involved. Dysfunction in parts of the thalamus and mamillary bodies are associated with memory problems such as Korsokoff's syndrome (a metabolic disorder associated with chronic alcoholism). The area of the basal forebrain lying in front of the optic chiasm served by a major artery called the anterior communication artery, is also involved with memory functions. Patients with severe interruption of blood flow in this area may experience memory dysfunction. Some patients with damage to the prefrontal cortex exhibit disturbances in memory (Schacter, 1987). Such patients seem to have difficulty in recalling information in serial order, are susceptible to interference, and have difficulty with short-term memory, particularly spatial information (Kolb & Whishaw, 1990).

Long-term memory difficulties such as color amnesia or face amnesia can occur as a result of damage to focal cortical areas. Structures that mediate short-term and long-term memory are different. For example, adults with amnesia who have profound long-term memory deficits may perform normally on immediate memory-span tasks such as the Wechsler Digit Span (Shallice, 1988). It seems likely that deficits in short-term recall occur as a result of dysfunction in one or more of a number of sites. ". . . Since there are multiple systems for processing sensory input and because the input must be held for processing, there are likely to be multiple places to demonstrate short-term memory deficits. The most likely places are the polymodal areas of the posterior parietal cortex, posterior temporal cortex and frontal lobe" (Kolb & Whishaw, 1990, p. 550). A detailed and comprehensive account of the anatomical correlates of memory can be found in Kolb and Whishaw's book (1990).

Another important avenue of research on memory studies the chemical events in the brain that occur when new information is stored in memory. One theory states that when new memories are stored, a change makes the synapse (the gap between two adjacent neurons) more proficient. The neurotransmitter acetylcholine seems to be related to memory disorders that accompany Alzheimer's disease. Recent research suggests that patients with Alzheimer's have a decrease in brain acetylcholine (Coyle et al., 1983). The chemical basis of memory, however, is very complex, and presumably many neurotransmitters are involved.

Learning Disabilities and Memory

Research with LD children on the initial stages of memory (i.e., the sensory register) suggests that in most cases the sensory register functions adequately. Learning-disabled and NLD children perform equally at the encoding stage of word recognition (Lehman & Brady, 1982; Elbert, 1984), but LD children need more time to carry out a memory search. Although some researchers suggest that LD children "may have poor recognition for quickly presented information . . . or a slower rate of information pick-up from the iconic sensory store" (Swanson & Cooney, 1991, p. 107), there appear to be minimal differences between LD and NLD children in attention to visual and auditory stimuli. In general, current research findings suggest that in a large majority of LD children, the attentional processes are adequate for performance on many learning and memory tasks (Swanson, 1983a, 1987).

Problems of immediate and short-term memory are common among children with learning disorders (Pennington, 1991). Swanson and Cooney (1991), conclude that short-term memory problems in LD children are associated with the way in which information is strategically processed (e.g., using rehearsal, organization, and elaborative processing) and in the way in which information is mentally represented (e.g., using effective phonological coding). Researchers have studied the lip movements of children during a memory task and recorded the extent of lip movements as an indication of rehearsal (Torgensen & Goldman, 1977). Some data suggest a rehearsal deficiency in LD children. Other researchers suggest that LD children rehearse material in a qualitatively different way (Koorland & Wolking, 1982). Other LD children have been found to experience difficulties in employing organizational strategies when they rehearse information, and they appear to be deficient in elaborative processing (Swanson, 1983). Short-term memory processing in some LD children is also influenced by errors in phonological coding and poor access to phonological codes, as in recalling similar and dissimilar-sounding names (Shankweiler et al., 1984; Siegel & Linder, 1984). The results of a study by Swanson et al. (1989), indicate that working memory in LD readers is inferior to that of NLD readers.

The prevalence of defects in long-term memory in children is unknown and research is limited. Unlike other adult neuropsychological syndromes, there is not a recognized developmental equivalent of the amnesic syndrome. Pennington (1991) suggests two plausible explanations. First, failure of declarative memory or episodic memory would undermine cognitive development in a pervasive manner and lead to mental retardation, with or without autism. Alternatively, the structures subserving declarative memory may be more resilient to developmental insult because some of them (i.e., the hippocampus), develop quite late. In contrast, children who acquire neural insults through closed head injury or anoxic episodes often develop an amnesic disorder.

Research on long-term memory problems in LD children suggests that these children experience difficulties in both storage and retrieval. A fairly consistent finding is that LD children are less proficient in using rehearsal strategies. Bauer (1979) analyzed the ability of LD children to learn a list of words over a series of trials and found little evidence of a primary effect (i.e., improved recall of items at the beginning of the list). The primacy effect is thought to be a good indicator of more rehearsal of those items at the beginning of the list and less interference (Swanson & Cooney, 1991). Other researchers have found that although LD children choose less efficient strategies to store information, they also seem less rigorous in using retrieval cues (Wong, 1982). Long-term memory for tasks that require semantic processing seems especially difficult for some LD children (Swanson, 1986).

Improving Memory Abilities in Children

The research findings above suggest important implications for improving the LD child's ability to learn. "A number of memory researchers have converged on the notion the LD student's ability to access information remains inert, unless they are explicitly prompted to use certain strategies. . . . When LD children are encouraged to use strategies their performance improves and thus the discrepancy between their general intellectual ability and contextually related memory deficits is lessened" (Swanson & Cooney, 1991, p. 115). Moely et al. (1986) provide practical concepts and principles to help LD children improve their memory skills and become more efficient learners. Swanson & Cooney elaborate on these in their review (Swanson & Cooney, 1991). Table 7.2 provides some examples of these strategies.

Summary

Attention and memory are distinct but associated cognitive processes. Attention facilitates the processing or encoding of information, prior to its being recorded in memory and later accessed or retrieved. The information-processing model of memory outlined here views memory as a "computer system" with its unique hardware or structural components (including the sensory register, short-term memory, long-term memory, and working memory), and software or control processes (e.g., selective attention and pattern recognition are processes involved at the stages of the sensory register, and rehearsal, ordering, and classification are processes involved at the short-term memory stage). The physiological correlates of memory have been intensively studied and research shows that brain structures mediating short-term and long-term memories in various modalities are different. Short-term memory deficits may result from disturbances in the posterior parietal, temporal, and frontal cortices. The storage sites for long-term memory also are distributed in cortical networks throughout the cortex. The lateral temporal cortices are important in long-term memory, whereas the mesial temporal areas are important in short-term memory. The mechanism of transfer from short-term memory into long-term memory may be localized in the hippocampus, amygdala, and closely related structures, and is vulnerable to insult. Unilateral lesions of the mesial temporal lobes produce less severe memory problems than bilateral lesions. Current findings on LD

Table 7.2. Classification of Memory Strategies

1. Rehearsal
   Students are told to rehearse stimuli verbally or to write, look at, go over, study, or repeat the stimuli in some other way. The children may be instructed to rehearse items just once, a finite number of times, or an unlimited number of times.
2. Elaboration
   Students are instructed to use elements of the stimulus material and assign meaning by, for instance, making up a phrase or sentence, making an analogy, or drawing a relationship based on specific characteristics found in the stimulus material.
3. Orienting (attention)
   These strategies direct students' attention to a task. For example, teachers may instruct children to "follow along" or "listen carefully" during lessons.
4. Specific Attentional Aids
   This strategy is similar to the attention strategy, but students are instructed to use objects, language, or a part of their body in a specific way to maintain orientation to a task.
5. Transformation
   Transformation is a strategy suggested by teachers for converting unfamiliar or difficult problems into similar or simpler ones that can then be remembered more easily. Transformations are possible because of logical, rule-governed relationships between stimulus elements.
6. Categorical Information
   Teachers might direct students to use taxonomic information (e.g., pictures accompanying a category) or to analyze the item into smaller units (e.g., looking for interitem associations).
7. Imagery
   This strategy usually consists of nonspecific instructions to remember by taking a mental picture of something or to maintain or manipulate them in the mind.
8. Specific Aids for Problem-Solving and Memorizing
   This strategy involves the use of specific aids in problem-solving or memorizing. For example, teachers may tell children to use blocks or other counters to represent addition or subtraction operations in a concrete way
9. General Aids
   In contrast to specific aids, teachers recommend the same general aid for a variety of different problems. These aids are designed and used to serve a general reference purpose. Examples include the use of dictionaries or other reference works.
10. Metamemory
    Teachers instructing this strategy tell students that certain procedures will be more helpful for studying and remembering than others. The strategy frequently includes giving hints about the limits of memory, asking students about the task factors that will influence ease of remembering, or helping them understand the reasons for their own performance. Teachers can also tell students that they can devise procedures that will aid their memory or indicate the value of using a specific strategy.

Source: Swanson, H.L., and Cooney, J.B. 1991. Learning Disabilities and Memory. In B.Y.L. Wong (ed.) *Learning about learning disabilities*. New York: Academic Press, p. 117. Adapted from Moely, B.E., Hart, S.S., Santulli, K., Leal, L., Johnson, T., and Rao, N. 1986. How do teachers teach memory skills? *Educational Psychologist*, 22, pp. 55–57. With permission of the authors and publishers.

children and memory suggest that the attentional processes of many LD children are adequate. In contrast, problems of short-term memory are fairly common among LD children, partly as a result of inefficient strategies for rehearsing and organizing information. Poor phonological processing also contributes to problems with short-term memory. Learning disabled children experience difficulties in both storage and retrieval in long-term memory. Some research shows that when LD children are assisted in using strategies, their performance improves.

Clinical Addendum

A Case of ADHD with Food Allergy Problems

Kelly Carter, an adopted child seen in our clinic, was selected for discussion because he was hyperactive, impulsive, had an attention deficit problem, suffered from a number of food allergies that were related to his explosive and destructive behavior, and his social behavior was a constant problem both at school and at home.

The Carters, childless for a few years following their marriage, adopted Kelly when he was two years old. They were told by the adoption agency that the natural parents were unable to manage Kelly and as a result "the boy had never had any discipline." Both Mr. and Mrs. Carter were university graduates, were eager for a child, and in their youthful enthusiasm they were sure that when Kelly had his own room and a loving and stable family his undisciplined behavior would disappear. From the first day that the Carters had him, Kelly was hyperactive, highly distractible, impulsive, and destructive. When he started school, the first-grade teacher asked if he was on some form of medication to control his behavior and when told that he was not, she advised the Carters to consult a doctor. This led to a prescription of Ritalin, which became a permanent part of his behavior management.

In addition to his behavior problems, Kelly suffered from many food allergies that required his mother to prepare a separate diet for him. The allergies were discovered by Mrs. Carter in a discussion with other parents in a parents' self-help group. Mrs. Carter described Kelly's destructive behavior and another mother replied that it sounded like her own son's behavior, which resulted from severe food allergies. She advised Mrs. Carter to get a copy of Feingold's book, *Why Your Child Is Hyperactive*, to study the lists of foods that might be causing the problem, and to use these to monitor her observations. Mrs. Carter kept a strict account of the limited number of foods that she fed Kelly so that she would be better able to identify those which might be disturbing his behavior, and within a few days he had improved so much that he could now sit and look at a book. If his diet was not strictly observed and maintained, Kelly could explode, in a few minutes, into sudden violent and destructive behavior. Because no pediatric allergist practiced in the small town where the Carters lived, Mrs. Carter on her own put Kelly on a modified Feingold diet which excluded sugar, corn, wheat, and any foods based on or including those. By careful observation, she developed a long list of foods that were taboo. They included apples, avocados, all berries, butter and margarine if they included corn oil, chocolate, dates, figs, oranges, peas, pears, peanuts, salmon, tomatoes, and many more. She found that he could eat rice in any form, potatoes, any meat except processed (e.g., wieners), most vegetables (but not corn, peas, tomatoes, or carrots), eggs, cottage cheese, small amounts of milk, yogurt, home-made bread, pasta, pineapple, kiwi fruit, and a few other foods. This meant that Kelly was deprived of many of the foods that most children are able to enjoy spontaneously, although by adolescence he had developed a tolerance to some foods that had been previously banned.

In the late spring in grade 1, Kelly was referred for psychological assessment because of his disruptive behavior in the classroom. On the WISC-R he measured a verbal IQ (VIQ) at the 79th percentile and a performance IQ (PIQ) at the 70th percentile, which suggested a 6-year-old of average to above-average intellectual abilities, but with marked problems in visual–motor skills. His drawings and printing were substandard scrawls.

By grade 3, Kelly's classroom behavior had become so disruptive that his mother was called to the school numerous times to take him home. This, of course, was only an immediate and temporary solution to a behavior problem that was so serious as to be almost beyond the normal management capabilities of the school system. Kelly had also become unpopular with most of his classmates, and this frustrated his needs for acceptance.

On the positive side, Kelly was affectionate and responded positively to attention from his parents, both of whom were striving strenuously to help him learn the normal social skills that would gain him acceptance by his peers and result in a happy family

Table 7.3. Kelly's Results on a Continuous-Attention Test[a]

	Test 1 (Ritalin)	Test 2 (No med.)	Test 3 (Mellaril)	Test 4 (Placebo)
1. Simple task	90	65	87	82
2. More difficult	90	0	83	84
3. Combined 1 and 2	180	65	170	166

[a] Possible score = 90.

life at home. By the time he was 8, Kelly enjoyed trips to the public library with his mother, and he selected and read books regularly. He was reasonably normal in his behavior on outings with his grandparents, but not if one of his siblings was also included.

A second assessment, when he was in grade 3, indicated a VIQ at the 77th percentile and a PIQ at the 66th percentile, almost identical with the measures two years before. But by this time Kelly had been transferred several times to different special programs in different schools because of his disruptive behavior.

At age 11, when he was in grade 6, Kelly was referred by a child psychiatrist for a complete medical-psychological assessment at a short-term (8 weeks) residential treatment center for older children. Included in the six-hour battery of neuropsychological tests was a computerized continuous-attention task designed to assess his ability to sustain attention, reduce his impulsivity, and regulate the speed of responding. Four trials of this test were done at different times, one with Ritalin, one with no medication, one with Mellaril, and one with a placebo. His results are listed in Table 7.3.

The test results indicate the negative effects of hyperactivity on sustained attention, and the value of an appropriate and monitored medication program for Kelly. Both Ritalin and Mellaril controlled his hyperactivity so that his attention was not interrupted, and his scores were perfect (on Ritalin) or nearly perfect (on Mellaril). Without medication he was unable to control his impetuous and angry behavior and as a result his responses were so erratic as to be unscorable, except on the simple task. The placebo situation, in which Kelly *thought* he was on a calming drug, enabled him to do almost as well as on Mellaril. This result implies that psychological intent, if it can be established, can be a powerful force in helping to control hyperactivity, although it is likely that some of Kelly's success on Test 4 resulted from the practice effect. Nevertheless, such findings are encouraging for those therapists attempting to use motivational procedures (see previous discussion in this chapter).

During his stay at the treatment center, Kelly received daily behavioral training sessions in a small-classroom setting, on field trips, in social situations with other children in the center, and in individual therapy sessions. His behavior responded to the individual treatment, but in the group situations (e.g., field trips), where he was free to show some degree of self-control, he still found himself in trouble and needing extra attention from his counselor. On the assessment test battery he now measured a VIQ and a PIQ at the 55th percentile level, a noticeable drop from his previous measures 3 and 5 years before.

On the haptic-perceptual tests (replacing blocks in a form board while blindfolded), Kelly showed an unusual result. The test requires the child first to replace the blocks with the dominant hand, then with the nondominant hand, and finally with both hands together. Scores on the test are calculated for accuracy and speed. Most children get better scores as the trials proceed because of the learning and practice effect, and the final test with both hands is usually completed quickest. Kelly's scores were in the *reverse* order. On his first trial (dominant hand) he got his best score, 84%. His next trial (nondominant hand), even though he was replacing the same blocks, gave him a lower score of 79%. His last trial (with both hands) produced his worst score, of only 8%. This performance suggests a serious incoordination between his hands, a pattern similar to that of split-brain patients. Though it might mean a deficit in function of the corpus callosum, such a diagnosis cannot be made on this type of evidence alone. Behaviorally, however, it does suggest a problem with bimanual tasks that can interfere rather seriously in any type of learning that draws on bimanual functions. His mother reported that whenever he received a balsa-wood model to build, Kelly always ended up smashing it in a fit of anger and frustration.

The clinical neuropsychologist concluded that Kelly had (1) an inability to monitor and regulate his behavior and thinking efficiently (i.e., ADHD); (2) poor fine-motor coordination; (3) problems in visual–motor integration in copying written material; (4) a weak visual short-term memory especially for stimuli presented in a temporal sequence; (5) a specific LD in math; and (6) mild perseverative tendencies in his thinking.

When last seen, Kelly was 14 years old and he was transferred twice during the year to special school programs attempting to deal with his aggressive and socially destructive behavior.

The causes of Kelly's abnormal behavior and inability to learn from parents, both of whom spend much time attempting to train him and to meet his needs, may never be known for sure. But it was known that both natural parents drank alcohol to excess, and both smoked, and this continued during Kelly's mother's pregnancy. The father also was a confirmed heroine addict, and the mother, an epileptic, was on anticonvulsive medication during the pregnancy. Although Kelly does not fit the pattern of fetal alcohol syndrome (FAS) he does fit the pattern of fetal alcohol effect (FAE). To complicate the picture, his mother's use of dilantin during the pregnancy may have had an added negative effect on his behavior (see Chapter 1).

Many of these children never learn to develop normal adult behavior, and this provides a poor prognosis for children like Kelly. How the FAE is related physiologically to the food allergy problems is not clear, but because both are biochemical it seems likely that they interact in their influence on Kelly's behavior. When more is known about the behavioral effects of prenatally consumed alcohol and postnatally consumed specific diets, and when more exact physiological and psychological methods of intervention are developed to meet them, children like Kelly, and their families, may have a brighter future.

Suggested Readings

Barkley, R.A. *Hyperactive Children: A handbook for diagnosis and treatment*. New York: Guilford Press, 1990.

Barkley, R.A. *Attention-deficit hyperactivity disorder: A clinical workbook*. New York: Guilford Press, 1990.

Goldstein, S. & Goldstein, M. *Managing attention deficit disorders in children. A guide for practitioners*. New York: J. Wiley & Sons, 1990.

Kendall, P.C. *Stop and think workbook*. PA: Marion Station, 1988.

Kendall, P.C. & Braswell, L. *Cognitive-behavioral therapy for impulsive children*. New York: Guilford Press, 1985.

Moghadam, H. *Attention deficit disorder: Hyperactivity revisited*. Calgary: Detselig Enterprises Ltd., 1988.

Quinn, P.O. & Stern, J.M. *Putting on the brakes. Young peoples guide to understanding attention deficit hyperactivity disorder (ADHD)*. New York: Magination Press, 1991.

Ross, D.M. & Ross, S.A. *Hyperactivity: current issues, research & theory*. 2nd edition. New York: J. Wiley & Sons, 1982.

Swift, M.S. & Spivack, G. *Alternative strategies: Helping behaviorally troubled children achieve*. Champaign, Illinois: Research Press, 1975.

Weiss, G. & Hechtman, L. *Hyperactive children grown up*. New York: Guilford Press, 1986.

8 Language Development, Aphasia, and Dyslexia

It is known that the study of the function of separate parts of the brain began with observation of cases of speech pathology.
A.R. Luria (1964)

. . . there are major and fundamental differences between rules of language and rules of games. The former are biologically determined; the latter are arbitrary.
Eric H. Lenneberg (1967)

The concept (of aphasia) always has entailed both physiological and behavioral facets; this is one reason for its being difficult.
Helmer R. Myklebust (1971b)

Probably the most compelling argument in favor of professional educators' including neuropsychological knowledge in the understanding and treatment of children with learning problems is the close relationship between brain structure and function and the development of language. As Lenneberg (1967) has shown, the rules of language are biologically determined, because "all behavior, in general, is an integral part of an animal's constitution." It is related to structure and function, one being the expression of the other. Psychologists for many years have been interested in this dynamic interaction. "If a behavior sequence matures through regular stages irrespective of intervening practice, the behavior is said to develop through maturation and not through learning" (Hilgard, 1948). Put more simply, some forms of behavior result just because the animal grows older. Maturation must always precede learning, for all learning, and particularly for this discussion, verbal learning, is biologically dependent. By adopting the view that language is an aspect of a human's biological development, "we may regard the language capacity virtually as we would a physical organ of the body, and can investigate the principles of its organization, functioning, and development in the individual and the species" (Chomsky, 1978).

A simple example of this principle is the emergence of speech in the human infant. Not only does language first appear at about 9 months, but the same phonetic sounds begin to appear in different children regardless of their geographical or cultural location. This means that until the speech centers in the cortex and the necessary sensory and motor tracts in the central and peripheral nervous systems have matured, the child is unable to produce words. No matter how potentially bright a 6-month-old child is, and no matter how skilled the teaching, it is impossible to teach him or her to talk. Six months later, when the brain is older, the child now can produce two or three words. Not only that, but there is a system to the appearance of the sounds that appear, because "the onset of speech is regulated by maturational development of certain physiological and perceptual capacities" (Lenneberg, 1966). This development is complete in most children between the ages of 5 and 7 years, so that by this age the phonetic repertoire is complete; of course, the child will continue to learn new words beyond this age, but no new phonemes in English. To acquire language normally the child must learn to hear and discriminate different phonetic sounds and to recognize the subtle auditory speech cues that occur in a temporal sequence. He or she must also master the motor skills of articulation and motor–speech expression and, finally, must build up "the store of linguistic knowledge that eventually forms the basis for both the production and reception of speech" (Fry, 1966).

English has more than 40 phonetic units for the child to master, some relatively simple to produce because of the earlier cortical and neuromuscular maturational changes, and some much more difficult, presumably because of the later developmental changes in the human brain and central nervous system. Lenneberg (1966) has told us that "man's brain-maturation history is unique among primates" and determines the onset and development of language.

A child's first utterances will include those phonetic sounds easiest to produce, and these usually include p, b, m, n, d, t, and the vowel a (as in sofa), although he or she may use only three of these at first. For example, one child may say "mama" and "dada," thus using only three phonemes in his or her first recognized words that emerge from the babbling stage, a period usually lasting 4 or 5 months prior to the first word. Another child may first use p, m, and a, and say "papa" and "mama." These variations may occur because of different environmental demands, but all children, regardless of culture, will tend to produce the same earliest phonetic sounds. For this reason, the names for the parents are composed of sounds from the early list. North American children usually call their parents "mama" and "dada," which later become "mum" or "mom" and "dad." German children say "papa" and "mama," and "Vati" and "Mutti" before they articulate the final form of "Vater" and "Mutter." Their grandparents are called "Opa" and "Oma," later to become "Grossvater" and "Grossmutter." French children say "papa" and "maman." Russian children say "mama" and "papa," and "baba" for the grandmother. Chinese children use "pa" and "ma," although the more formal Mandarin forms are "foo" and "mo."

A little later, the child learns to master k, g, f, w, and s, and much later, sometimes 4 or 5 years later, the more difficult sounds, such as j, l, r, h, th (as in thin), th (as in this), sh (as in she), n (as in sing), and finally, probably the most difficult blend in English, thr (as in thrift). The 2- and 3-year-old who has not yet learned to master these difficult phonetic sounds will adapt his or her speech to the use of the simpler sounds. The 18-month-old child may call his or her older sister Janet, "Dan'dan," and her older brother Stephen, "Dee-dee." Rachel may call herself "Ay-oh" at first, and Neill refers to himself as "Neeno." The 3-year-old, when asked his age, will almost certainly say, "I'm free." Because cortical development in all children, regardless of color or race, seems to be similar, their first words are likely to be similarly based phonetically. This is an example of what Lenneberg (1967) called "behavioral specificity." Whereas some behaviors are similar across species because they are structurally determined, others are unique to some individuals because they are specifically trained. Specificity results in a common repertoire of basic speech sounds for all humans, and plasticity in the different languages of different cultures. Both processes coexist.

Studies of the phonetic speech perception of human infants during the first 8 months of life (i.e., before the first words appear) show that "when given a choice among sounds young infants prefer to listen to 'Motherese,' a highly melodic speech signal that adults use when addressing infants" (Kuhl, 1991). The higher pitch, slower tempo, and exaggerated intonation of Motherese appears to be universal across languages (Grieser & Kuhl, 1988), and it is this acoustic quality rather than its syntax (grammatical structure) or its semantics (word meaning) that appeals to infants.

Infants as young as 6 months have been shown to perceive a word produced by different speakers as the same (i.e., "peep" spoken by a man, a woman, and a child), although computers have difficulty classifying words when they are produced by various speakers (Kuhl, 1991). This finding seems to indicate that the infant brain by the age of 6 months is better able to detect changes in timbre (i.e., different patterns of overtones) than a computerized auditory receiver. Also, as early as six months, the beginnings of specific phonetic speech perception have been recorded. Infants in America and in Sweden were tested with both native and foreign-language vowel sounds (American /i/ or "ee" sound and Swedish /y/) and results showed, in each group, a more accurate response for their native language speech sound (Kuhl et al., 1992).

Lenneberg has shown a remarkable regularity in the emergence of language. Single words begin about the eighth or ninth month and show the same developmental pattern of increase whether the child is raised in Austria, Great Britain, or the United States. The emergence of two-word phrases among British children showed a pattern similar to those in the other two languages and about 10 months later than the first single words in all three.

Normal Language Development

How language develops is not fully understood but it depends on the maturing of cortical cells (Lenneberg, 1967), social reinforcement (B.F. Skinner, 1957), and social learning (Piaget, 1965). A large number of theorists have described the development of language, and most recognize the importance of perceptual reception, understanding, adaptation, imitation, and expression. The infant, in order to learn language, must have normal hearing for a wide variety of speech sounds and normally obtains visual cues by watching the gestures and facial expression of the speaker or those in the immediate social environment. The blind child has to rely mainly on the auditory sounds of spoken speech and the tactile perceptions of environmental objects to acquire verbal concepts and linguistic understanding of the social and physical world. All these processes involve decoding and understanding. The child then imitates the sounds of words he has heard and learns to formulate them to express the ideas and feelings he wants to communicate.

Myklebust's (1964) developmental hierarchy of the human language system includes the above three linguistic processes in a practical and useful model. It conceives of the development and acquisition of language proceeding from meaningful auditory experience to motor–expressive behavior. In detail, the behavioral stages are as follows:

1. Birth to 9 months. The child hears language and gradually begins to understand it, developing an "inner language" or a conceptual understanding that is largely nonverbal.

2. Up to 12 months: auditory receptive language. The infant learns to comprehend much of what is said and, by 9 months, is beginning to imitate specific words, usually "Muhmuh, buhbuh, dada," and similar easily produced sounds, which later may become enunciated as "momma," "baby," and "daddy."

3. From 12 months to about age 7 years: auditory expressive language. This stage includes the auditory perception of words and the motor–speech imitation of them. This is the period for developing oral speech and a passive vocabulary of about 3000 words.

4. Age 6 years and up: visual receptive language (reading). On entrance to school the child must learn to acquire an auditory-graphic match between what he knows auditorially and the printed or written representation of speech. This demands a crossmodal integration.

5. Age 6 years and up: visual expressive language (spelling and writing). Where reading is a receptive process, in which the child recognizes letters and words and attaches auditory meaning to them, writing is a reversed process. To write, the child must convert the verbal idea into an oral word, analyze it phonetically, and translate the word into a motor–manual–linguistic pattern that is socially understood.

This scheme is useful for the teacher because it recognizes the order in which language is learned, but it is important to remember that this whole perceptive, motor, integrative process is reinforced by the *meaning* that language conveys. Lenneberg (1964) has reminded us that "understanding is more significant for language development than the capacity for making speech sounds."

Because the acquisition of language involves visual and auditory perception, verbal abstraction, understanding, imitation, and motor–speech expression in a correct sequence, all of the brain parts subserving these various behavior processes must be functioning normally for the child to learn to listen, to talk, to read, and to write. In the next section we describe the speech centers in

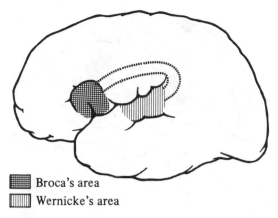

Broca's area
Wernicke's area

Figure 8.1. Receptive auditory speech cortex (Wernicke's area) and motor-expressive speech cortex (Broca's area or contiguous tissue) showing the subcortical connections (arcuate fasciculus) between the two speech areas. (© 1984 William D. West)

the brain and consider how their dysfunctions may lead to a verbal learning disorder.

Language and the Functional Anatomy of the Human Brain

Some of the major language cortical circuits have been known for a little more than 100 years. In 1861 Broca, a French neurologist, identified the area in front of the left[1] motor strip that controls the muscles of the face, jaw, tongue, and speech muscles. This area is known as Broca's area (Fig. 8.1) and it is the cortical center largely involved in the articulation and expression of spoken speech. In 1874, Carl Wernicke, a young German neurologist, published his first paper, identifying the superior lateral surface of the left temporal lobe as the cortical area for decoding oral speech. It was Wernicke who made the assumption that the two areas, Broca's and Wernicke's, were connected. We now know this to be true, the two areas being connected by a subcortical bundle of fibers known as the arcuate fasciculus (see Fig. 8.1). Geschwind (1965, 1972) has proposed the very logical theory that a person who is asked to repeat a word, hears it and decodes it in Wernicke's area

[1] Because about 90% to 95% of the population are left-hemisphere dominant for language, our discussion of brain processes includes only left-hemisphere function.

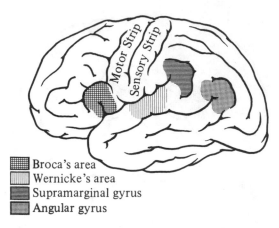

Figure 8.2. The primary speech centers in the left cerebral cortex. (© 1984 William D. West)

and relays the auditory pattern, by way of the arcuate fasciculus, to Broca's area, where the necessary cortical changes take place for the word to be pronounced. Geschwind (1972) pointed out that "this model may appear to be rather simple, but it has shown itself to be remarkably fruitful," and it has been supported by numerous clinical and autopsy studies.

The classical model of language representation in the human cortex of the left hemisphere has been developed since the conceptual establishment of Broca's area in the 1860s and Wernicke's area in the 1870s. By 1890, William James described in some detail the classical cortical areas involved in aphasia. These included the auditory linguistic receptive cortex (Wernicke's area) in the posterior portion of the superior temporal gyrus (usually the left); the motor speech area (Broca's area) in the inferior frontal gyrus; the arcuate fasciculus joining the Wernicke and Broca areas; the motor and sensory strips in the pre- and post-Rolandic gyri; the supramarginal gyrus located around the posterior extremity of the Sylvian fissure; and the angular gyrus in the parieto-temporal region. This model (Figs. 8.1 and 8.2) has survived for a century, although it soon became evident that some cases with known lesions did not respond as predicted by this theory. Two possible reasons for these discrepancies are: (1) Most brain lesions are not highly localized, so that although the focus of the brain dysfunction might be known, the extent of its "distance effects," named *diaschisis* by von Monakow in 1911 (A. Smith, 1975), were frequently unrecognized. (2) The theory, originally based exclusively on studies of brain lesions, assumed that all human brains were structurally and functionally identical.

We know now that there is great variability among subjects. Most of this new knowledge has come from cortical electrostimulation and brain-scan studies. These procedures, which are relatively recent, provide more accurate indicators of brain function than the earlier methods of inferring brain dysfunctions from the atypical behavioral signs that usually follow traumatic brain injury.

Cortical electrostimulation of conscious patients undergoing brain surgery was first done in 1909 by Harvey Cushing, the eminent American neurosurgeon (Ojemann & Whitaker, 1978), and was well established by Wilder Penfield and his associates in the 1930s and 1940s (Penfield & Roberts, 1959). In fact their discoveries led to the identity of a new language cortical area, the supplementary motor area, not previously detected from behavioral studies of brain-injured patients. Later studies (Fedio & Van Buren, 1974) led to the conclusions that "much anatomic variability seems likely in the language association cortex" and "the detailed functional anatomy of our brains may be as individualized as is the detailed anatomy of our faces" (Ojemann & Whitaker, 1978).

For example, three patients studied by Ojemann during craniotomy showed great variability (Fig. 8.3). Patient A produced naming errors when the normal function of Broca's area was interrupted with electrostimulation (filled circle in Fig. 8.3) but no naming errors when Wernicke's area was electrically interrupted (open circles in Fig. 8.3). This is the result we would predict using the classical model of cortical language representation. But patient B does not show as clearly localized a picture. Stimulation of this patient's Broca's area produced naming errors, as we would expect, but so too did one spot in the temporal lobe. Patient C was even more atypical: stimulation of Broca's area produced naming errors, but so too did Wernicke's area, and spots in the parietal and frontal lobes. Cortical electrostimulation of large numbers of patients shows expressive language deficits when Broca's area is stimulated, but among some patients, areas remote from Broca's area may also produce the same language disturbances (Fedio & Van Buren, 1974; Ojemann & Whitaker, 1978).

This same variability is shown quite clearly when a composite picture is made from brain scans of a number of patients with expressive aphasia. When 14 patients with Broca's aphasia had their CT scans superimposed (Kertesz, Lesk, & McCabe, 1977), they showed a wide area of variability (Fig. 8.4). Although the focus of dysfunction centered on Broca's area, some of the patients showed additional pathology in areas quite remote from it.

In summary, this means that the localizationist model of language representation in the human brain, established in the last

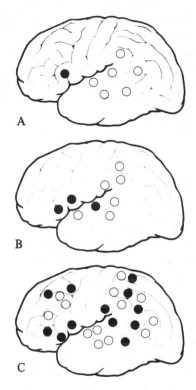

Figure 8.3. Mapping of language centers with electrostimulation in three patients. Filled circles are sites where stimulation produced naming errors; open circles are sites with no errors. (Adapted from W.H. Calvin and G.A. Ojemann, *Inside the Brain* Mentor Books, 1980, p. 28. With permission of the authors and the publisher.)

quarter of the nineteenth century, is no longer tenable. Despite a strong tendency for expressive language to involve cortex contiguous to Broca's area, and for receptive language to include Wernicke's area in most people, in some subjects additional functional cortical areas may be involved.

Subcortical Connections

Although the cortical language areas are essential to normal linguistic function, so too are certain vital centers in the brainstem. In Chapter 2, the cortical connections with the thalamus were described (Fig. 8.5), and it has been found, by subcortical surgical procedures and with brain-scanning techniques, that when localized lesions occur in the left thalamus, frequently deficits in language and short-term verbal memory may result (Ojemann, 1975). When

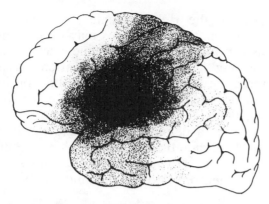

Figure 8.4. A composite diagram of the brain scans of 14 patients with Broca's aphasia superimposed. Notice the concentration of pathology in the region of Broca's area, but also the diversity of some of the cases. (From Kertesz, Lesk, & McCabe, *Archives of Neurology* 1977, *34*, 594. With permission of the authors and the publisher.)

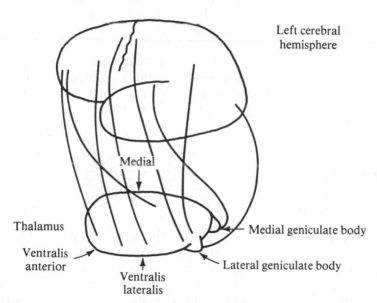

Figure 8.5. A diagrammatic representation of some of the many connections from the left half of the thalamus to the cortex of the left cerebral hemisphere. The thalamus is drawn proportionately larger than life (actually it is made up of two ovoid masses about 4 cm or $1\frac{1}{2}$ inches in length). Many more fibers connect the thalamus to the cortex than are shown in this simplified drawing, and many more connect the cortex to the thalamus. This is a good reminder of the important involvement of the subcortical structures in cognition and learning and the complexity of the neural circuitry.

isolated lesions occur in the right thalamus, deficits in visuo–
spatial memory and arithmetic calculations may occur (Ojemann,
1974). Ojemann has hypothesized that thalamic electrostimulation
acts as a "specific alerting" circuit "that directs attention to verbal
material in the external environment, while simultaneously blocking retrieval of . . . material from either short-term or long-term
memory" (Ojemann, 1983).

For the student wishing a detailed neurophysiological explanation of the thalamocortical radiations, a fine graphic presentation is
made by Netter (1972, Plate 47, p. 72), and discussions are available in any good text in neurophysiology (Schmidt, 1978a, p. 58 ff.;
Schmidt, 1978b, p. 252 ff.).

Also to be recognized in the subcortical functions are the more
recently discovered contributions of the cerebellum to cognitive
and language skills (Leiner, Leiner, & Dow, 1991).

When the brain mechanisms that subserve language functions
are normal and healthy, the child, if motivated to do so, can learn
to read, write, and spell with little difficulty. However, if these
brain centers are damaged, diseased, structurally malformed, or
functioning at a less than optimal level, the child will have difficulty
in acquiring language skills, the degree of difficulty correlating
directly with the severity of dysfunction and the locus of the
damage. When the dysfunction is in the language centers and is
mild, the child is said to have a specific learning disability involving
reading and the language arts; when it is severe, the child is said to
have aphasia.

Aphasia

Why Include Aphasia?

It may seem irrelevant to introduce the study of aphasia in a book
designed for educators, but we do so for three reasons. This book
is intended for clinical psychologists, school psychologists, and
special educators, and these professionals need all the information
they can get to help them hypothesize about the possible causes of
the subtle learning problems of their students. Because most
learning disabilities include language deficits, it is highly probable
that a mild form of childhood aphasia may be involved. Because it
is easier to understand a borderline form of pathology by studying
its full-blown form, this is the first reason for including a study of
aphasia in this chapter. The second reason is to assist rehabilitation
therapists who are faced with teaching severely brain-injured
children and adults. Traumatically brain-injured adults frequently

have been neglected by society once they have been discharged from the hospital, with the conclusion that they have recovered from the medically treatable sequelae of their injuries. More recently, long-term treatments and occupational training centers have been established to meet the needs of the traumatically brain-injured adult. The teaching personnel in these centers may profit from an understanding of aphasia.

Our third reason is probably the best. A great deal is known conclusively about aphasia and, by tying a theory of dyslexia to a theory of aphasia, we are on tested ground. School psychologists who are knowledgeable about the theories and clinical manifestations of aphasia are more thoroughly equipped to provide better diagnoses and predictions than are those with no systematic knowledge of language development or impairment.

Definition of Aphasia

What is aphasia? It is the loss or impairment of the use and/or understanding of language resulting from some type of brain injury or dysfunction. When it affects spoken language it is medically described as aphasia; when it affects reading it is called alexia or dyslexia; and when it affects writing it is called agraphia or dysgraphia. Educators may prefer other terms for deficits in reading and writing, but the medical terms imply accompanying brain dysfunctions.

The classifications of aphasia are almost as numerous as the researchers attempting to make them. For readers who want a quick review of the field, Benson has provided a comprehensive discussion of aphasia with most of the major classifications since 1885 (Benson, 1979). During the past 100 years, the three "classical" groupings of aphasia have been recognized: Broca's aphasia (motor or expressive); Wernicke's aphasia (receptive); and conduction aphasia (the inability to repeat orally presented material). These brain lesion−language-deficit relationships grew out of clinical investigations by Broca and Wernicke in the nineteenth century.

During the past few years, however, research aphasiologists have begun to question the theoretical inadequacy of the classical groupings (Caramazza, 1984; Poeck, 1983; Schwartz, 1984). They soon discovered that Broca's aphasia was not a "pure" or reliable classification because different patients so diagnosed usually had varying degrees of impairment in comprehension in addition to their expressive problems. Because human brains vary structurally and functionally, the classical categories are "polytypic," or have several symptoms (Schwartz, 1984), so that symptoms overlap category boundaries (Poeck, 1983). Because any language deficit may occur in more than one category, Poeck (1983) has proposed that language disturbances can be classified on at least three levels: (1) clinical (observing the various symptoms displayed in a patient's spontaneous speech); (2) psycholinguistic (observing the semantic and syntactical confusion in the patient's spontaneous speech); and (3) anatomical (observing the nature and location of the neuroanatomical damage or dysfunction). The latter may include a cerebral hemorrhage or "stroke" (the cause of most cases of traumatic aphasia) and a collection of causes not due to a CVA (e.g., brain tumor, abscess, trauma, or diffuse inflammatory or degenerative brain disease). Poeck has pointed out that each of "these different levels do not have a hierarchical relation, and each of them serves a different purpose" (p. 80).

Because the validity of aphasiological theories is beyond the scope of this book, we shall stress the linguistic behavioral symptoms in aphasia so as to help the teacher, the school psychologist, and the parent to recognize subtle deviations in the language of a LD child or adult that they might otherwise overlook.

Receptive Aphasia

The most severe aphasic disorder includes an inability to carry on inner language functioning, and hence a difficulty in perceiving oneself with any clarity. Johnson and Myklebust (1965) described the development of inner language as the first linguistic step in the hierarchical development of language; it occurs during the first few months of life in the preverbal stage of cognitive development. The infant has meaningful, pictorial experiences (e.g., he reacts with enthusiasm to the sight of the bottle at feeding time), but has not yet learned to associate verbal symbols or words with these experiences. Gradually the infant learns to integrate experiences in all the sense modes and to attach nonverbal symbolic meaning to them. A dog or cat remains at this stage of development of *inner language*. Once this stage of cognitive understanding is reached in the human infant, however, he or she is ready to develop receptive and expressive language as described above. "Because of this developmental hierarchy, no child speaks until he has learned the meaning of words. . . . Input precedes output" (Johnson & Myklebust, 1965).

This description indicates the basic priority of *inner* and *receptive language*. Inability to interpret one's own subjective experiences is called *central aphasia*, and because of its severity it is difficult to diagnose. No doubt it is sometimes confused with childhood autism or psychosis.

From reports of Annie Sullivan's first struggles with Helen Keller, it seems that Helen as a child was subject to explosive temper outbursts and socially meaningless behavior similar to that of an autistic child. Once she learned to interpret her world and herself by tactile language symbols, her potentially superior mind developed and her disorganized behavior disappeared. It seems possible that she may have moved out of a condition similar to *central aphasia*, in which she could not communicate with herself, to one in which, through verbal symbols, her mind took on order and clarity.

Receptive aphasic children may be able to understand their own mental lives but have difficulty understanding what is said to them or remembering specific words they wish to use. In one form of receptive aphasia, *amnesic aphasia*, the adult patient cannot remember the name of an object he can describe (anomia). For example, when shown a key, the patient may say, "I know what it is but I can't tell you. You do that with it (makes a twisting motion with his hand) in a door to open it. It's a lock, no, but that's close." When the therapist supplies the word, the patient will say, "Yes, a key." We have all had this experience when tired; we cannot find the word for the idea we wish to express.

An adult with a classic receptive aphasia will have a left temporal lesion (in Wernicke's area) and a number of behavioral symptoms, including a word-finding difficulty (anomia), impoverished verbal content, and frequent paraphasias. Paraphasias are of two types: (1) verbal substitutions, and (2) nonsense words (neologisms) or mixtures of two words. Examples of substitutions are "chair" for "table" or 6 when one conceptually intends 8. We have all had such verbal slips when we are fatigued; these types of errors suggest that the cortical mechanisms have triggered the wrong ready-made cortical circuit. Abnormal mixtures of words are limitless, and when they dominate the person's speech it may be referred to as "jargon aphasia." Such a patient, when asked to describe a key, might say, "Kay (pause), that's what I want, it's dorent—I'm in the floor, door. It's all away." Whereas the receptive aphasic's speech is usually fluent and generally manifests normal grammar and articulation, it sounds like "doubletalk." Very little is communicated and much of it is confused. The condition appears to stem from the person's inability to mobilize the words he or she needs in the correct order, and to attach the appropriate conceptual meanings to them. Ojemann has produced most of these types of speech errors by electrostimulating the left thalamus (Ojemann, 1975).

Military personnel subjected to decompression-chamber experiments will have had these same difficulties when the oxygen content of the air was severely depleted. Potential air-crew members during World War II were frequently tested for their ability to do simple arithmetic calculations as the air pressure was systematically reduced to simulate flying conditions in a nonpressurized cabin. Most people began to find difficulties in concentrating above 10,000 feet (simulated), and as the air became more rarefied it became increasingly difficult to remember the conceptual meanings of numbers. This type of mental impairment in fact was an artificially imposed and temporary receptive aphasia. As soon as the air pressure was returned to normal, the testees' word-finding and conceptual associations returned to their intact functional level.

Motor Aphasia

The so-called motor aphasic might answer, when asked to name a key, "Bay—no! Day—no! Cow—no, no! Kay—no!" He may hit on the right word or may never get it until the therapist supplies it. In any case, motor aphasia includes the understanding of words but the inability to produce them fluently and accurately. The motor aphasic's failure to say the word is not caused by an inability to say it, for he may be able to produce it when prompted, or on other occasions. In any case there is no impairment in function of the tongue, teeth, lips, or vocal cords in most cases. When there is a problem of peripheral articulation this is known as *dysarthria*. Such a patient may or may not be completely free of aphasia. A bright person with poor articulation because of a harelip is an example; he or she is dysarthric (has poor articulation) but is not aphasic.

The motor aphasic has difficulty producing, in his own imagination, the exact sensorimotor pattern prior to pronouncing the word. Many normal students mispronounce the word "statistics" because they have never taken the care to analyze it and therefore cannot imagine its correct muscular form. Consequently, they may hurry over "stastistics" knowing it is not quite correct, but not knowing how to correct it. The motor aphasic patient may have enough damage or dysfunction in the left hemisphere to be unable to produce the desired word, although understanding and intent are quite clear. These patients understand language reasonably well, but their speech may be elliptical and telegraphic. Their language may be devoid of connectives, articles, and small parts of speech, like that of a 2-year-old learning to talk.

Conduction Aphasia

People with conduction aphasia may speak fluently and have complete understanding of what is said to them, but they will be unable to repeat a word or phrase when asked to do so. If asked in 1993 to say the word "president," a patient might answer, "I know who that is, Bill Clinton," but still be unable to repeat the requested word. This curious inability in verbal repetition, a simple task for normal small children, was explained by Wernicke in 1874 (Geschwind, 1965) as the result of a lesion in the bundle of fibers (the arcuate fasciculus, Figs. 8.1 and 8.6) that joins the Wernicke and Broca areas. However, he later withdrew this neuroanatomical explanation for lack of autopsy evidence, although the theory, at least in part, still has credibility for some. Regardless of its etiology, the syndrome of conduction aphasia has been recognized clinically for more than 100 years.

Although it is unlikely that a child so impaired would be found in the public school system, many children are unable to repeat sentences accurately. Understanding the possible neural mechanisms underlying conduction aphasia and the awareness that some school children may have minimal neural dysfunctions in the language areas of their brains, should lead teachers to greater tolerance for a poor performance on a sentence repetition test. All well-developed aphasia batteries include such tests, which can easily be administered by a school psychologist to measure a child's competence in this skill. If a consistent weakness appears in the child's ability on the sentence repetition test relative to the other tests in the aphasia battery or to the norms for that particular age, this inability could strongly suggest an organic basis. Such a hypothesis would contraindicate such diagnoses as "lazy, isn't trying, needs to settle down," which are all too frequent in such cases. Normative data are available for children aged 6–13 on a 26-sentence form of the Spreen–Benton battery (Spreen & Gaddes, 1969) and a 22-sentence form (Gaddes & Crockett, 1975; Spreen & Strauss, 1991, 177–183).

Isolation of the Speech Area (Mixed Transcortical Aphasia)

A particularly rare form of aphasia can occur when the speech area is isolated from the rest of the cortex (Fig. 8.6), and the lesson to be learned from this type of case has significance for understanding normal brain function. Benson (1979) has called this condition "mixed transcortical aphasia." Geschwind, Quadfasel, and Segarra (1968) reported the case of a young woman brain damaged by carbon monoxide poisoning and studied for 9 years prior to her death. Postmortem examination revealed a remarkable lesion that isolated the speech area from the rest of the cortex. "A detailed study of serial whole brain sections showed intactness of auditory pathways up to and including Heschl's gyrus, of Wernicke's area

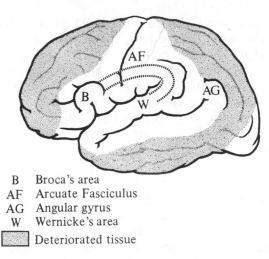

B   Broca's area
AF   Arcuate Fasciculus
AG   Angular gyrus
W   Wernicke's area
▨   Deteriorated tissue

Figure 8.6.   A pattern of cortical deterioration that results in cortical isolation of the healthy speech areas of the left hemisphere. Geschwind, Quadfasel, and Segarra reported such a case. (© 1984 William D. West)

and Broca's area and of the arcuate fasciculus connecting these two cortical regions, of the lower Rolandic cortex and of corresponding portions of the pyramidal tract." Also, both the limbic system and the reticular structure of the brainstem were intact. However, extensive cortical deterioration was present in the prefrontal, upper and posterior parietal, and inferior temporal cortices, thus sparing the essential cerebral mechanisms for the production of speech but isolating them from a total healthy cortex.

Behaviorally, she never spoke spontaneously and she appeared to have no understanding of oral speech. She could, however, repeat, parrotlike, what was said to her, and she could complete certain phrases and familiar and rhyming statements begun by the examiner. She could also learn to sing a song by imitation. Because the brain damage was outside the speech and auditory areas, she could recite speech mechanically, but with no understanding. Thinking requires the whole cortex to feed into the cortical speech production areas. By themselves these areas have no more understanding of their speech production than a tape recorder, record player, or talking mynah bird.

This type of clinical evidence seems to point to a widespread cortical stimulation in order to develop language skills. No doubt this explanation shows why a multisensorimotor approach is remedially successful with most children.

Developmental Aphasia

All of the discussions above have related to traumatic aphasia in adults. In these cases the adults had already acquired normal or superior language use prior to their brain damage. That is, they lost something that they had already acquired.

In developmental aphasia the pattern is different. Here, because of maldevelopment or injury to the language centers of the central nervous system prenatally, perinatally, or postnatally during the first year of life, the child is unable to develop or has difficulty in developing a normal understanding and use of language. However, because of the plasticity of the young brain, this child may adapt to the inherited neuropathological condition either by becoming right-hemisphere dominant for language or by developing a bilateral shared dominance. For this reason the loci of cortical lesions in children may show a pattern different from that of the adult. In this case Broca's area, Wernicke's area, the arcuate fasciculus, and the acoustic area (Heschl's gyrus) of the left temporal lobe are usually impaired in whole or in part and in differing degrees.

So different is childhood aphasia from adult aphasia, both behaviorally and cerebrally, that Bender (in West, 1962) suggested that knowledge of adult aphasia may at first blind us to a clear understanding of the syndrome in children. The plasticity of the child's brain appears to enable him to overcome to some degree both the number and the severity of language impairments, which in an adult with the same cerebral pathology would probably be more serious.

Children with normal hearing and intelligence who fail to acquire oral speech were recognized at least as early as 1825, when Gall published a treatise on the function of the brain and each of its parts (Wilson, 1965). Myklebust (1971b), in his scholarly review of childhood aphasia, records a continuing interest in the subject since Gall's early publication and the use of the term "congenital aphasia" by Broadbent in 1872. Myklebust draws attention to Binet's early work in 1908, in which Binet identified the four basic operations in language development: understanding, speaking, reading, and writing. Binet wrote; "and each of these operations may be suppressed separately by a cerebral accident" (quoted by Myklebust, 1971b).

Although a few special schools have been interested in treating aphasic children since the first such department was established at Central Institute for the Deaf in St. Louis, there was no wide interest in their diagnosis and teaching until Myklebust's important book in 1954 (Wilson, 1965).

During the 1950s, progress was made by a number of investigators in refining the terminology and classification system. These contributions led to a recognition of these children as being mentally normal, having normal hearing and no evidence of cerebral palsy or obvious disease, but showing marked delay in the development of speech.

Because the normal acquisition of speech is through auditory sensation and perception, imagery, symbolization, and conceptualization (Myklebust, 1954), it is not surprising that the most impressive gains in understanding and treating aphasic children were made in special schools for the deaf. In fact, developmental aphasia in some cases may reveal a mixed picture of brain damage and partially defective hearing. In small children, because of their inability to introspect and to follow complex instructions, it is frequently difficult or impossible to be sure whether the child suffers only from auditory imperception or weak auditory sensation, or both.

Teachers of special classes and psychologists and therapists in rehabilitation centers will certainly have to teach some children with aphasic symptoms. Awareness of the common symptoms may help the teacher recognize the problem and the school psychologist make a differential diagnosis.

Traumatic or Acquired Aphasia in Childhood

In the above discussion of developmental aphasia, we included, in one of the etiological classifications, traumatic brain damage prior to the age of 1 year. After that age the child begins to acquire language, and any left-hemisphere damage between age 2 and puberty, normally referred to as acquired or traumatic childhood aphasia, will interfere with language habits already learned. During growth and development the brain-injured child experiences language learning (from the social environment) and language interference (from his brain injury). Earlier researchers reported fairly rapid recovery from traumatic aphasia for preschoolers (Lenneberg, 1967) but slower recovery for children between 4 and 10 years of age. This finding was also supported in a study of 50 unilaterally brain-damaged children whose trauma occurred between infancy and adolescence (Woods & Teuber, 1978). These investigators found that children suffering brain lesions before the age of 8 years recovered what appeared to be normal nonaphasic speech, but those with lesions after that age suffered permanent aphasic disturbances in their speech. Subsequent studies of these same children on a large battery of language tests, however, indicated that although the children with early trauma were clinically nonaphasic, their language skills showed subtle deficits compared to a normal matched group (Woods & Carey, 1979). Such subtle language symptoms are common among many LD children and adults.

Denckla (1979) has reported that, in her clinical experience, there seem to be very few cases of acquired aphasia in young children; during 7 years as director in a large neurological institute, she saw only seven such cases under the age of 10 years. Still, there may be some children with early left-hemisphere damage who can be described as "aphasoid," and who are somewhat inept in most types of verbal learning and linguistic expression.

It should be made clear at the outset that aphasic children with definite evidence of early brain damage or cerebral agenesis are not numerous, but children with congenital language disorders are. The latter group, whether their language deficits are acquired or developmental, makes up a major group of all LD children, and because their diagnostic features are similar to aphasia, understanding its symptoms is essential to the special educator and the school psychologist.

Severe left-hemisphere damage in preadolescence frequently is followed by recovery of spoken language in a year or two, but much slower recovery of reading and writing skills. Adolescents and adults tend to recover the latter more quickly, presumably because of the greater degree of practice and overlearning. The case of Robbie Yates (discussed later in this chapter) is a good example. He was injured at age 3 years 9 months, and by age 6 his oral speech appeared normal to a casual observer. However, his reading and writing skills were chronically inferior even with skilled remedial teaching.

A reluctance to speak is common among most aphasic and some aphasoid children. Denckla (1979) has proposed that this condition may result from the child's relative inexperience and lack of practice in learning "the articulatory rules and social habits of speech" as compared to the adult aphasic. As a consequence, the lack of language knowledge (which draws heavily on the posterior left hemisphere) is not enough to produce a normal volume or quality of spoken language even though the mechanisms of motor speech (in the left frontal lobe) are intact. The case of Sam (in Chapter 4, pp. 169–172) illustrates such repressed verbal expression.

Readers who wish a more thorough examination of traumatic or acquired childhood aphasia may find useful discussions in Denckla (1979), Lenneberg (1967, pp. 145–150), Myklebust (1971b), and Satz & Bullard-Bates (1981).

Common Symptoms of Developmental Aphasia

Language Retardation. Although language retardation is the primary symptom, it is essential to remember that not all impaired speech is aphasic. The most common causes of inferior speech development in children, other than aphasia, are peripheral hearing loss, mental retardation, emotional disturbance, social deprivation, and/or a peripheral articulation problem. By the time the child reaches school age it is usually possible to make a differential diagnosis of developmental aphasia versus some other nonaphasic syndrome, but sometimes the aphasic child may be mistakenly labeled mentally retarded or emotionally disturbed, when in fact the child may be potentially mentally bright or superior.

Receptive Signs. Receptive signs include poor auditory perception. The child can hear sounds but cannot decode them meaningfully. This condition frequently results from cortical damage to Wernicke's area (Luria, 1973) and may include the auditory projection pathways connecting from the medial geniculate nuclei (Benton, 1963a) and possibly the parieto-occipital areas (Landau, Goldstein, & Kleffner, 1960). Benton (1963a) feels that "the most extreme degree of disability is shown by children who show 'auditory imperception.'"

Central Processing Defect. If damage or dysfunction occurs in the left inferior parietal or parieto-temporal–occipital area, adults may have difficulty in associating individual words or ideas into a meaningful whole. They have difficulty understanding sentences, and for this reason this condition has sometimes been called "semantic aphasia" (Luria, 1973). Because it may also include poor memory and defective association of abstract concepts and symbolic thinking, it has also been called "central aphasia." Considerable clinical evidence exists to localize brain lesions in aphasic adults, but few cases of children with developmental aphasia have come to postmortem study. Three who have are described below, and whereas the language areas are generally similar in location to those in adults, the impaired behavioral responses are less intense and may show a greater degree of recovery.

Expressive Signs of Childhood Aphasia

1. Little or no expressive speech with near-normal understanding.
2. Telegraphic speech. There is an absence of connectives (articles, prepositions, conjunctions) and a presence of what

Benton (1963a) has called "syntactical poverty." This lack may also show in the child's writing.

3. Articulation may be normal or nearly normal on repetition but poor in spontaneous speech.

Personality Disturbance. Because the development of language enables one to control oneself and one's environment, any retardation in language in a child with average intelligence may serve only as a frustration and source of anxiety. It is common to find the aphasic child subject to temper tantrums, mood swings, hostility, destructiveness, apathy, and/or a desire to be left alone. It seems highly likely that some children who are diagnosed as "autistic" are in fact aphasic, because their social behavior improves as their language is developed.

The Neurology of Developmental Aphasia

Because it is generally accepted, even by the most enthusiastic behaviorists (B.F. Skinner, 1938), that aphasia is a direct result of brain damage or dysfunction in the speech centers of the dominant hemisphere (Luria 1966, 1973), it seems essential for the school psychologist and useful for the special teacher to know something about the possible neurological deficits of the aphasic child. A major literature is available on the aphasic adult (Bay, 1964; Brain, 1961; Geschwind, 1965; Lhermitte & Gautier, 1969; Weisenburg & McBride, 1935/1964) and these findings indicate a strong reliability in locus of lesion and behavioral sequelae in normal adults who have suffered injury to the speech centers (Luria, 1966, 1973).

For children, however, the clinical literature is not as rich and the behavioral deficits are more varied. Because much can be learned from in-depth studies of individual cases, these appear throughout this book.

Probably the most thorough clinical early report made on a child with developmental learning disabilities was that by Drake (1968), in which he reported in detail the medical history, the physical and neurological examination, the psychiatric findings, the educational record, the psychological test results, and the neuropathological report of a boy who died suddenly at the age of 12 and whose brain came to postmortem study. Billy was a likable boy of average intelligence who was subject to marked mood swings, some "dizzy spells and blackouts," and trouble with most academic learning. He was retarded in reading and had difficulty remembering what he read; he had some problems with arithmetic, spelling, and writing; he was slow in learning to tell time (he learned after he was 11 years old); and he showed extreme slowness in completing homework assignments. In the sixth grade he read at a fourth-grade level, and his word analysis and spelling were at the fifth-grade level. Arithmetic was about 1 year retarded.

A postmortem examination of his brain showed abnormal growth of the parietal cortices *bilaterally* and poor development of various parts of the corpus callosum. There was also an unusual and abnormal pattern of cortical gyri or convolutions. Subcortically there were abnormal structures of the blood vessels and displacement of some of the subcortical cerebral cells. In view of this major disorganization of Billy's brain, it is remarkable that he learned to read at all or to show any academic progress. Lenneberg (1968) has described such a process by concluding, "the child with a perinatal cerebral injury only gradually 'grows into his symptoms,' and that both lesions and symptoms have their own ramified consequences." More simply, it might be inferred that the congenitally brain-damaged child learns to make the optimal compromise between structure and function. Because his brain is young he can shift to the healthier parts with greater freedom than can the traumatically brain-damaged adult.

The first autopsy study of a child with developmental aphasia (Benton, 1963a) was reported by Landau, Goldstein, and Kleffner (1960). This 6-year-old boy seemed mentally bright but had almost no understanding of spoken language. His speech was a chaotic mass of jargon and he resorted to gestures in order to communicate. After 3 years of special speech training he developed a moderate vocabulary and learned to say simple sentences. He also learned to read and write simple material and arithmetic at about the first-grade level. During those 3 years his nonverbal IQ rose from 78 to 97, which suggested average nonverbal intelligence. Audiometric testing showed normal hearing in the right ear with a possible high-frequency loss in the left. These findings eliminated the possibility of a hearing loss to account for his language retardation and suggested localized cerebral damage and dysfunction.

This hypothesis was supported with the postmortem findings following the boy's sudden death at age 10. Autopsy study showed considerable evidence of inadequate growth of the cortical layers in *both* temporal lobes. Because this growth anomaly was *bilateral*, it was difficult for the boy's brain to shift his defective Wernicke's area to the other side, assuming that healthy tissue adapts more easily. The posterior portions of the parietal, temporal, and occipital lobes were reduced in size on both sides, and the medial geniculate nuclei, connecting the auditory nerves to the Heschl's gyri on both sides, were severely degenerated. It seems highly likely that the registration of language sound patterns in his brain was so distorted that learning to understand oral speech was impossible for him except to a limited degree, and only with specialized language training.

In commenting on this very interesting case, Benton (1963a) draws attention to the fact that comparable lesions in adult patients would have produced central deafness. Again, however, it seems that this boy responded to the special speech training by using whatever healthy cerebral tissue he possessed. This type of evidence supports the belief in skilled remedial teaching as early as possible, to exploit to its fullest the plasticity of the child's brain.

Roberts (1962) reported a very interesting case of a girl whom he followed from age 6 years until her death in early adolescence. Her development was normal until the age of 15 months, when she incurred a high fever associated with convulsions and the development of a right hemiparesis. The seizures continued and could not be controlled by medication.

Examination at age 6 showed a smallness of the left side of her cranium and the right side of her body. She had a mild right hemiparesis, which indicated pathology in her left cerebral hemisphere. Her oral speech was so garbled that only her mother could understand her, and her attempts to vocalize normal phonetic sounds were quite abnormal in most cases. She developed idiosyncratic speech with a consistent meaning for herself.

An EEG showed spike discharges over the left side of her brain mainly in the parietal area. Brain surgery revealed diffuse atrophy of the left hemisphere especially in the parietal lobe, which was surgically removed.

Treatment of Aphasic Children

Two of the early major contributors in the treatment of developmental aphasia are Helmer R. Myklebust, who worked extensively with deaf and aphasic children for many years, and Mildred A. McGinnis, a gifted teacher who worked for more than 40 years at the Central Institute for the Deaf in St. Louis, and latterly at the Pathway School in Norristown, Pennsylvania.

Mykelbust (1971b) has stressed the importance of a competent identification and diagnosis of the aphasic child. It is important, as already stated, to differentiate the aphasic from the mentally retarded, hard of hearing, or emotionally disturbed. A deficit in auditory (oral) language may be recognized during the preschool years, whereas aphasia may not be suspected until after completion of first grade, or not recognized as a chronic problem until third or fourth grade. The diagnosis will provide information on auditory perception, comprehension, integration, and expression, thus indicating the pattern of deficits and relative strengths the child may have. The diagnostic procedure lies in showing a significantly inferior ability in auditory language relative to his or her nonverbal intelligence level, hearing, emotional adjustment, and motor ability. The study of the child with language retardation must include both a detailed audiometric examination by a qualified language pathologist and a comprehensive battery of psychological tests (Myklebust, 1954), and we would add neuropsychological tests. Myklebust (1971b) recommended an exhaustive evaluation of the child's perceptual processes, which include the ability to give attention; the rate, intensity, and duration of response to both verbal and nonverbal, meaningful and nonmeaningful, and rhythmical and nonrhythmical auditory stimuli; sound recognition and phonetic discrimination; ability for auditory figure–ground recognition, perception and manual production of rhythm, and intersensory perception. For many years, Myklebust has recognized the importance of intraperceptual and interperceptual functioning. In his own research he has used cross-modal tasks as one of the most sensitive behavioral tests for the presence of brain damage, or particular cortical dysfunctions.

Along with perceptual processes, verbal functions must be carefully evaluated. These include auditory verbal memory, comprehension and integration of language, verbal memory using both methods of recognition and recall, and motor expressive functions. How all of this evaluation is done clinically is discussed by Myklebust in summary but detailed form (1971b) and in full detail (1954). The school psychologist not thoroughly familiar with clinical evaluation of childhood aphasia is well advised to study these and other sources.

Remediation is highly individualized, being determined by the child's particular strengths and weaknesses in perception, auditory memory, comprehension, integration, recall, and expression. Myklebust for a long time has emphasized the importance of including both verbal and nonverbal skills in evaluating any child with a learning problem, and he has given these two functions equal weight psychometrically in his formula for the learning quotient (Myklebust, 1967a). For the evaluation of the potential abilities of the aphasic child this balance is particularly important.

Although there is great variability among aphasic children, Myklebust stressed certain basic homogeneities. The first of these is that input precedes output. The child's understanding of a word should be ensured before one attempts to teach him to say it. Similarly he should be able to read a word before being taught to write it. A second basic assumption is: Do not use the multisensorimotor approach indiscriminately. It is necessary first to find out the child's perceptual strengths and weaknesses and any possible motor deficits. An unsystematic use of multistimulation may interfere with learning in some cases. "Overloading may be deleterious to attention, orientation, motivation, and in rare instances may cause severe fatigue, if not seizures" (Myklebust, 1971b).

Myklebust's approach is practical and is based on a sound knowledge of learning principles, neurology, neuropsychology, and classroom teaching of children with special needs.

Mildred McGinnis's approach, which she called the association method, has many differences. She reported (1963) that "the opinions, suggestions, and judgments contained in this book are based upon the author's accumulated first-hand experience of daily contact over a period of forty years with the problem of assessing and teaching children with deficiencies in the ability to communicate orally." Miss McGinnis was a gifted and very successful teacher and she concerned herself only with the behavioral aspects of oral communication, and not the organic deficits underlying the child's aphasia.

From her experience with hundreds of children with communication disorders she developed a clear clinical judgment that enabled her to differentiate the aphasic child from the deaf, mentally retarded, autistic, emotionally disturbed, or the child with delayed speech. Her book illustrates each type of differential diagnostic problem with many detailed clinical case studies.

The association method is systematically adhered to, and if "one step is by-passed a gap in learning becomes apparent, and the steps must be retraced" (McGinnis, 1963). The aphasic child is first trained to develop attention to directions, and then to say and read 50 common nouns. This exercise begins with single sounds; sounds are then combined to form the whole word, and finally, activities are used to associate meaning with the word. This is primarily a phonetic and articulatory attack, leading to reading and then writing. Once the 50 nouns are mastered, the next stage provides for developing an increased memory span by teaching simple sentences using the familiar nouns. From here the training increases the knowledge of concrete nouns and moves on to abstract ideas and more complex grammatical forms of language.

By contrast, McGinnis stresses a teaching method, whereas Myklebust stresses a thorough neuropsychological analysis of the child's ability that will indicate a particular teaching program for that child. McGinnis's book is a rich compendium of opinions, suggestions, and judgments drawn from her own experience, but there are no references to research. Myklebust was a vigorous researcher himself and his writings are thoroughly documented with numerous references to current research studies in neurology, psychology, and special education. The writings of both writers have their special value for the new worker in the field of childhood aphasia. One comprises the insights and practical recommendations of one of the major living scholars in this field, and the other the detailed first-hand account of a particularly gifted teacher.

Psycholinguistic Analysis of Reading

Before examining reading disabilities and their possible causes and treatments, we will look briefly at some of the current views of the *psychology of reading*. The literature in psycholinguistics is immense, and no brief account can do it justice. But for the reader with little or no background in this field, this abbreviated discussion may be useful.

Linguistics, or the study of language, was, until the late 1950s, primarily objective and impersonal. It was mainly the study of the *structure of language*, with a greater emphasis on grammatical structure than on psychological meaning. But in 1957, Noam Chomsky's book *Syntactic Structures* revolutionized traditional linguistics (Kess, 1976), not only by including an understanding of linguistic structure, but also its psychological function. With this change in emphasis, linguistics became more directed toward the study of the cognitive process of how a person extracts *meaning* from language (Downing & Leong, 1982; Leong, 1987) both spoken and written. Chomsky's new direction made the study of language a branch of cognitive psychology (Chomsky, N., 1968).

In the study of the psychology of language there are two broad classes of data, the *behavioral* (e.g., measuring language acquisition in children), and the *intuitional* (e.g., one's personal judgment about the accuracy or appropriateness of a statement) (Catlin, 1978). Our "intuition" or "common sense" enables us to recognize the sentence, "John believes in honesty," as a rational statement that is acceptable in the real world. But "Honesty believes in John" makes no sense, unless we know that Honesty is a person. The pragmatic use of language refers to the construction of reality by the speaker/listener through his or her knowledge of the social and physical environment and the particulars surrounding the present utterance.

Under normal conditions all children learn to understand and speak their native tongue. How this learning occurs is not yet fully understood, but in the last thirty years psycholinguistic research has produced theories to try to account for it. Initially the small child learns to understand words and their meanings by *hearing* them—that is, by attending to their *phonological content*, and gradually, with much repetition and observing the social situations in which the word is used, its meaning (or its semantic value) slowly becomes evident. When two words sound the same or have the same pronunciation, their phonological pattern is recognized as the same though their semantic value may be different (e.g., sew and so). The child "with command of a language has in some way internalized the system of rules that determine both the phonetic shape of the sentence and its intrinsic semantic content" (Chomsky, 1972). And as indicated at the beginning of this chapter, these changes are a product of the person's biology and experience.

In summary, the acquisition of one's native language includes (1) its semantic structure (word meaning), (2) its syntactic structure (grammatical rules and how words are related), and (3) its phonological structure (Downing & Leong, 1982).

Chomsky conceptualizes the awareness of language as involving two levels of mental function, a "deep structure," whose contents are beyond the level of consciousness of the speaker-hearer, and a "surface structure" that includes the words, phrases, and sentences that are written, printed, or spoken. The so-called deep structure might be compared broadly to the contents of the "unconscious mind" of the Freudian's, although it has no theoretical relation to Freudianism. Chomsky's surface structure might be seen as somewhat similar to the observable behavior of the Behaviorists, although it has no theoretical relation to Behaviorism. "Deep structure provides the grammatical relations of predication, modification, and so on, that enter into the determination of meaning. On the other hand, it appears that matters of focus and presupposition, topic and comment, the scope of logical elements, and pronominal reference are determined, in part at least, by surface structure" (Chomsky, 1972). By "focus" he meant "that part of the sentence which presents new information," and by "presupposition," those "propositions not asserted directly, which the sentences presuppose to be true" (Downing & Leong, 1982). If we attempt to relate this proposed theory to brain function, the various cerebral areas involved in long-term verbal memory (Chomsky's deep structure), could include at least the left temporal lobe, some brainstem structures, and various areas of the cortex (Ingvar, 1983, 1991; Petersen et al., 1988). From this unconscious repository of learned words, word phrases, sentences, and grammatical rules, the appropriate words from the person's neurally stored vocabulary, and the needed verbal phrases and sentences are mobilized and transformed into grammatically acceptable forms before appearing on the surface, where they are expressed in spoken speech or writing.

This hypothetical source of words has been named the *internal lexicon* by some psycholinguists. It is conceived as an internal mental dictionary containing not only all the words that a person has learned, but all the information (e.g., meaning, pronunciation, spelling) necessary for the correct use of each word in both spoken and written language (Downing & Leong, 1982). In conversation we must access and retrieve from the *lexicon* each word that is needed in its correct serial order. Word-finding problems may follow brain damage, especially when in the left hemisphere, as we have seen in the discussion of traumatic aphasia. It may also occur when we are tired, and it is common among elderly people. This evidence suggests that learned words are neurally stored in the brain and coded in complex patterns of neural excitation and inhibition (Pribram, 1971). The difficulty of accessing and retrieving specific words when we are fatigued or hungry suggests possible temporary electrochemical inadequacies at the synapses (Hebb, 1972). Difficulty of lexical access following traumatic brain damage indicates that certain functionally healthy brain structures are essential to normal language function.

All children learn to speak before they learn to read. Many 2- and 3-year-olds with a high verbal aptitude and a strong curiosity to discover how to break the code in printed language will learn to read many words and numbers by asking their names and "what they say" (i.e., their phonological coding). Many of these children are reading independently when they enter grade 1, but most children will have to wait for formal training in school. The possible process by which they do this is examined in the following discussion.

The various cognitive processes involved in fluent and successful reading are several. The order in which these functions occur is not agreed by all linguists (Stuart & Coltheart, 1988), but there is general agreement that they are present. They include (1) visual processes, (2) phonological processes, (3) word retrieval, (4) the ability to use contextual information to facilitate word recognition, (5) short-term memory, and (6) comprehension common to reading and listening (Stanovich, 1985). Until the research findings of recent years, it was thought that deficits in early visual information-processing operations were an important cause of reading difficulty. However, "it appears that deficits in visual processing account for an extremely small proportion of the variance in reading ability, and that verbal–linguistic rather than visual factors are implicated" (Stanovich, 1985). In this same vein, Vellution (1987) in discussing dyslexia concluded that "Far from being a visual problem, dyslexia appears to be the consequence of limited facility in using language to code other types of information."

Benton (1984), in examining spatial thinking, concluded that "there appears to be no substantial evidence that impairment in spatial thinking plays an important role in the genesis of developmental dyslexia." For the reader who is confused by these conclusions, it should be remembered that the basic processes in reading are carried out *in the brain* and that the eye carries the visual impulses to the brain but does not process them. A visually impaired person who has mastered visual reading of printed matter can read it if the printed page is held close to the eyes. It is possible, however, that in some cases of cortical brain damage the images of print or writing are distorted and could lead to difficulty in reading (see case of Mrs. Stanley on pp. 350–351).

During the past decade the research evidence supporting the relationship of phonological processes to successful reading and spelling has shown it to have major importance (Shankweiler & Liberman, 1976). It has been estimated that there are about two or three dozen separate vocal sounds[2] in human utterance and, "What a phonology does for us is to provide a basis for constructing a large and expandable set of words—all the words that ever were, are, and will be" (Liberman & Shankweiler, 1985). In learning to speak one's native language the process of hearing the phonetic sound of each word (the phonological process) and acquiring its meaning (the semantic process) and of learning the grammatical structure in which it occurs (the syntactic process) is automatic and unconscious. But to learn a foreign language in school the learner has to acquire all of these processes consciously and with effort. Studies have shown that young children having difficulty in segmenting words (i.e., identifying the phonemes and syllables) and blending their phonemes have difficulty learning to read and spell (Liberman & Shankweiler, 1985; Wagner & Torgesen, 1987). A study in Sweden indicated that the ability to segment words into phonemes was the most powerful predictor of future reading and spelling skills in a group of children tested at the end of their kindergarten year (Lundberg, Olofsson, & Wall, 1980). However, there is speculation by some "whether the ability to perform phonemic segmentation is a necessary precursor to, or is the result of, reading in an alphabetic script" (Stuart & Coltheart, 1988). Regardless of the variation in theoretical opinions, most researchers and educators agree that phonological or auditory

---

[2] Readers with no background in the analysis of speech sounds and their function in phonological processing will find a useful and brief discussion in Wagner, R.K. and Torgesen, J.K., The nature of phonological processing and its causal role in the acquisition of reading skills, *Psychological Bulletin*, 1987, 101, 2, page 194. See also Downing, J. and Leong, C.K., *Psychology of Reading*, New York: Macmillan, 1982, ch. 5.

processing is an essential part of understanding and using language, both spoken and written.

Several research studies suggest a strong relation between speed of name retrieval and reading. Disabled readers were found to be slower in naming various stimulus types such as colors, letters, numbers, and objects (Denckla & Rudel, 1976). Spreen (1988), using a word fluency test in which the subject is given 1 minute to say as many words as possible beginning with a given letter, found groups of LD adults with confirmed identifiable neurological signs significantly inferior to normal controls in this skill.

A reader may use contextual information to facilitate word recognition during reading, and also to aid comprehension. F. Smith (1971) has argued that because sentences provide the reader with two sets of cues (semantic and syntactic), this "contextual redundancy" facilitates word recognition by providing a variety of hypotheses about words, thus assisting the reader in predicting the correct meanings of words as they are being encountered in the reading process. This enriched information was believed to enable the reader to identify individual words using only some of their visual features. This is an interesting theory, but Stanovich (1982b) believes there is little evidence to support it, and much that contradicts it. His research leads him to believe that "the rapid word recognition ability of the better readers appears to be a direct cause of their reading skill" (i.e., competent word analysis). Speed and automaticity of decoding are essential to successful reading comprehension (Samuels, 1976). Poor readers do make use of context effects on word recognition *when they understand the context* (Stanovich, 1985). It is not unusual to see a student in a cooking, automotive, or other applied course read the instructional manuals competently though his previous reading scores in academic courses had been inferior.

Many writers agree "that the comprehension of both written and spoken language depends on some form of working memory" (Baddeley, 1986). As we saw in Chapter 7, in the past 25 years, many theories of short-term and working memory have been proposed, and working memory has provided a fruitful concept in the better understanding of the psychology of reading. In reading, the printed image of the word is retained until it is identified (usually about 500 ms) and then the reader moves on to the next letter, letter cluster, whole word, phrase, or sentence, depending on his or her competence. "A primary function of phonetic representation is to yield an adequate span in working memory to permit linguistic interpretations of the temporally arrayed segments of the message" (Shankweiler & Liberman, 1976).

Two possible explanations account for poor readers' memory deficits: (1) the deficient formation and maintenance of phonological codes in short-term memory, and (2) the failure to employ verbal rehearsal and other memory strategies. But because these two processes are not mutually exclusive, Stanovich (1985) has concluded that "poor readers may display inferior short-term memory performance due to deficits in *both* phonological processing and strategic planning," and with instruction in the use of memory strategies it is possible to improve the performance of poor readers (Stanovich, 1982b).

Because a child learns to speak before learning to read, learning by listening precedes learning to read, and in fact, may actually form a basis for acquiring skills basic to reading (Sticht, 1972). "One view of the reading–auding relationship is that there is one holistic ability to comprehend language by ear and by eye. The further corollary is that one should be able to comprehend equally well by listening or by reading, if one has learned auding and reading equally well" (Downing & Leong, 1982), but learning to do this may take as long as 7 school years (Sticht, 1978). In a study of fifth-grade good and poor readers (matched for sex, chronological age, and IQ), who were asked to report what they remembered from selections which they listened to on a tape and which they read from typescript, the researcher concluded that "reading and listening comprehension are closely related. Teaching the disabled reader is not only a matter of developing decoding skills and sight word vocabularies." Although these skills are essential, skilled reading also "requires an understanding of the structure of language, an ability to abstract the essential elements of a verbal message, and knowledge of which key words or letters signal an action, an object of that action, and which words convey critical meaning in a sentence" (Berger, 1978).

This brief discussion of the psychology of normal reading is meant to prepare us for the neurolinguistic examinations of disordered reading.

Dyslexia

Up to this point we have considered auditory receptive and expressive speech, and the psychology of normal reading. Let us now examine the defective form of reading, or dyslexia. Money (1962) has written, "the reading defect may represent loss of competency following brain injury or degeneration; or it may represent a developmental failure to profit from reading instruction."

Definition of Dyslexia

Because dyslexia is not yet fully understood, it is difficult to define, and as a result all early attempts were descriptions of dyslexic people rather than analyses of the process itself. Three examples follow. In 1968 the World Federation of Neurology proposed the following two definitions of dyslexia (Critchley, 1970):

1. Specific Developmental Dyslexia: "A disorder manifested by difficulty in learning to read despite conventional instruction, adequate intelligence, and socio-cultural opportunity. It is dependent upon fundamental cognitive disabilities which are frequently of constitutional origin."
2. Dyslexia: "A disorder in children who, despite conventional classroom experience, fail to attain the language skills of reading, writing and spelling commensurate with their intellectual abilities."
3. Arthur Benton produced a definition of developmental dyslexia, recognizing the transitory nature of the problem by writing, in part, "it refers to (as of today) inexplicable failure to learn to read by a child whose intelligence level, oral language development, and sensory capacities appear to be fully adequate to permit the development of reading skills. . . ." (Benton, 1975).

Harris and Hodges (1981) have produced an operational definition that includes three conditions: (1) failure to read despite normal sensory processes, intelligence, and opportunity; (2) the reading disability must be severe; and (3) it must be due to CNS dysfunction. Hynd and Hynd (1984) have expressed a preference for this definition because it avoids exclusionary conditions and includes aspects that are useful in recognizing and assessing dyslexic subjects. It has been estimated that the number of children defined in this way exceeds the combined number of children suffering cerebral palsy, epilepsy, and severe mental retardation (Duane, 1979). "This translates into an expected frequency of between 15 and 30 dyslexics per 500 children" (Hynd & Hynd, 1984), or 3% to 6% of the general population.

These descriptive definitions raise two points: (1) The reading disability may stem from congenital deficits, that is, it may be "developmental," or (2) it may result from postnatal traumatic brain damage after the child or adult has acquired the skill of reading. These types of reading deficits (i.e., developmental and acquired) we classify as "primary reading retardation." Cases in which potential ability to learn to read is normal but insufficiently utilized we classify as "secondary reading retardation." These "secondary" cases may result from environmental (e.g., hostile family pattern, or other social and/or educational deprivation) or intrapersonal causes (e.g., negative attitude). Calling reading problems "primary" when they result from organic dysfunctions does not imply greater importance than the "secondary" emotional ones, but they are more refractory to conventional teaching methods because of central processing dysfunctions. The "secondary" group retains an intact capacity to read (Quadfasel & Goodglass, 1968), which can function normally when the emotional conflicts are resolved. For this reason, the remedial teacher will want to know at the outset whether he or she is dealing with an "organic" or "purely motivational" type of reading problem. This knowledge will indicate a basically different remedial approach depending on the causal pattern of the reading deficit.

Descriptive definitions can be useful to the practitioner, but the scientist needs a more precise interpretation. The early idea that dyslexia is a homogeneous disorder with a single cause has been abandoned by most researchers and "attempts to specify subtypes of reading disability have followed three courses: clinical observations (e.g., observation reveals that all readers normally rely on a semantic code, a phonological code, and a visual code [Coltheart, 1981]); single case studies (e.g., in-depth study of single cases can provide knowledge of the coexistence of neurological, psychological and educational variables, not possible in any other way [see the many cases cited throughout this book]); and large multivariate studies" (Newman et al., 1989). Each method has its advantages and its limitations. The single case study has great clinical value but one is unable to generalize to the general population from this detailed and specific knowledge. Large group studies employing statistical analytic methods are useful but they frequently are inconclusive because it is difficult or impossible to include and control all of the pertinent variables. Their obvious value, when they are successful, is in providing knowledge with which to generalize and add to the understanding of a specific problem or area of scientific knowledge.

Because of its neurological, perceptual, and intellectual complexity, reading impairment cannot be defined in a simple statement. In the past, neurologists have defined it in neurological terms (Déjerine, 1892) and cerebral dominance (Orton, 1937), and psychologists have used models stressing perceptual-motor (Kephart, 1960), language (Vellutino, 1987), multisensory (Fernald, 1943), or auditory perception (Gillingham, 1965). All have merit but none is complete.

All of these descriptive definitions appear to reinforce the popular notion that dyslexia is a discrete diagnostic entity quite different from ordinary poor reading. Because of its recognizable status it can and should be defined. The idea of distinctness was given scientific respectability by the impressive Isle of Wight study (Rutter et al.; 1970), in which poor or backward readers had a mean IQ of 80, and the retarded readers (i.e., the specific reading retardates or dyslexics) had a mean IQ of 102.5 (Yule & Rutter, 1976). Rutter and his colleagues, in studying a large sample of 2300 9- and 10-year-olds, found a "hump" or excess of cases at the lower end of the normal curve of distribution of these readers, and they interpreted this collection of retarded readers to be a distinct collection superimposed on the normal distribution of readers. After more than 20 years this bimodal distribution and its interpretation is still commonly accepted.

Recently, Shaywitz and her colleagues at Yale have challenged the bimodal model on the grounds that no one else has been able to replicate it (Shaywitz et al., 1992). They contend that "dyslexia occurs along a continuum and is best conceptualized as the tail of a normal distribution of reading ability." Although accepting the model of distinctness or continuity will make no difference to the choice of a successful remedial program in a particular case, it will affect the direction of future research and the delivery of services to children (Rennie, 1992). Discrepancy scores between IQ and reading achievement are used to identify dyslexics but in the United States, because the cut-off score for identification is not universal, a child could receive special help in one state and be denied it in the one next door. "The quilt of conflicting standards that covers the U.S. is a by-product of the difficulty that educators, policymakers and researchers have faced in defining dyslexia" (Rennie, 1992).

More than 30 years ago, Money (1962) pointed out that "medicine and pedagogy have been slow to come together" in the study of dyslexia. This professional parallelism has given way to a greater blending of these two disciplines in the last few years mainly because of dramatic advances in neurological research (e.g., CT, PET, BEAM, and MRI scanners), the investigation of possible organic correlates of dyslexia by histological examination (e.g., Galaburda & Kemper, 1979; Galaburda & Eidelberg, 1982), the advances in assessing functional cerebral asymmetires, the marked increase in neuropsychological and neurolinguistic studies of dyslexia and other learning problems, and the greater availability of these findings in psychological and educational journals. Until the mid-1970s, most educators and school psychologists attributed reading failure exclusively to psychogenic causes; neurological factors were seldom considered.

By the beginning of the 1980s the significance of the brain in learning was at least recognized, if only superficially understood, by large numbers of educators and school psychologists. They were gradually becoming aware of convincing evidence in some cases and, in others, of knowledge with peripheral usefulness in the better understanding of linguistic impairments.

Let us look at some of this evidence. The first neurological evidence correlated with the inability to read came from adults suffering cerebral strokes. The various categories of reading retardation that we shall use in this discussion follow:

A. Primary reading retardation (alexia or dyslexia)
   1. Adults
      a. Traumatic dyslexia
      b. Developmental dyslexia
   2. Children
      a. Traumatic dyslexia, after 1 year of age
      b. Developmental dyslexia, when trauma was prenatal, occurred at birth, or occurred postnatally before 1 year of age
B. Secondary reading retardation (weak motivation because of poor environmental influences).

Terminology

The terms "alexia" and "dyslexia" receive different definitions from different writers. *Webster's New Twentieth Century Dictionary* (2nd ed., 1968) defines "alexia" as the "inability to read, caused by lesions of the brain; word blindness," and "dyslexia" as "the loss of power to grasp the meaning of that which is read." The implication here, though not specifically stated, is that the reading disability in alexia is caused by brain damage but in dyslexia is unknown. Benson and Geschwind, both neurologists, accepted this classification with greater definitive specificity. For them, "alexia refers only to *acquired* defects in contrast to dyslexia, a term designating an *innate* or constitutional inability to learn to read" (Benson & Geschwind, 1969).

It is notable that some current dictionaries have produced definitions of these two words that have lost any basic difference. They include brain injury or dysfunction in both definitions (The Random House College Dictionary, 1988; Webster's New World Dictionary, 3rd Edition, 1988). It is possible that the rapid development of neuropsychology during the past 25 years and the increased general awareness of brain behavior relationships may be related to this definitional change.

Many educators use the term "alexia" to indicate a complete or very severe inability to read, and "dyslexia" to mean a mild dysfunction or moderate retardation in reading, but this use of the words to indicate a degree of severity of the same condition has been rejected by some neurologists (Quadfasel & Goodglass, 1968). Obviously this confusing situation in naming a phenomenon they are all studying has resulted from a lack of communication between educators and neurologists. Neurologists in the past have made a greater effort to share their knowledge with educators (Binet & Simon, 1908; Montessori, 1965; Orton, 1937; Critchley, 1970) than educators with neurologists. There are a few notable exceptions, such as Myklebust, but many psychologists and educators, impressed with the value of neuropsychological data, have been told by many in the Educational Establishment that it is irrelevant to the educational process. That contribution is a poor return for the wealth of knowledge neurology has to offer education.

Let us look at the evidence.

Primary Reading Retardation in Adults

Traumatic Dyslexia

In Chapter 3, we described the Wada Amytal Test. It will be remembered that following injection to affect the left hemisphere, the patient for several minutes is unable to speak, to understand what is said, to read, or to write. The patient's understanding of nonverbal tasks is normal or nearly normal, but he or she is temporarily aphasic, *dyslexic*, and agraphic. In our study of dyslexia, we are primarily concerned with this patient's temporary inability to read because of the chemical effects on the left-hemispheric cortical centers essential to reading. As fresh blood replaces the drugged supply, the patient's normal ability to read returns after a few minutes. Thousands of amytal tests have been carried out in most parts of the world since 1948, when this technique was first developed by Dr. Juhn Wada in Japan. The response to this procedure is highly reliable for predicting the side of speech dominance. It is evident that when the cortical "reading centers" are rendered powerless by controlled chemical means, reading is temporarily impossible, although visual recognition of nonverbal stimuli is usually normal and intact. However, although this clinical experiment tells us that there is a reliable causal relationship between the normal functioning of the language-dominant hemisphere and the ability to read, it does not tell us *what parts* of the hemisphere are vital.

Prior to the introduction of the present brain scanners, to search for the vital reading centers in the cerebrum, researchers had to go to another type of clinical study, the study of localized lesions. One of the best of these is the impressive report of Russell and Espir (1961) in England in which they examined the medical reports of almost 1200 men suffering brain wounds during World War II. Most of these men were injured during the invasion of Normandy in 1944, and they reached the hospital in Oxford a few days after being wounded. The brain wounds were mostly caused by small fragments of metal from shrapnel or high-explosive shells so that they usually produced highly localized lesions. Russell and Espir developed a system for recording the site of the lesion or wounds. A tracing was made of the lateral view of the skull, and X-ray information was transferred to this outline drawing. They then composed a cumulative tracing of all those men suffering aphasia and those free of it. The two tracings were basically complementary to each other, the one being the negative of the other. The aphasics suffered injuries to Broca's area, the inferior part of the left motor strip, the related parts of the sensory strip (controlling the speech muscles and right hand), the left angular gyrus, and Wernicke's area. Left-hemisphere wounds not causing aphasia were outside the speech areas, in the prefrontal cortex, lining the longitudinal fissure, and in various scattered loci. Of the aphasic subjects—and these made up about one-third of the total sample—we are particularly interested in those in whom reading ability was impaired. In their Chapter XIII on alexia, Russell and Espir report seven cases with graphic information regarding the brain damage on the lateral brain tracing outline. Six of these showed lesions in the left parietal cortex near to or involving the angular gyrus and one with left anterior parietal damage. It is interesting that this last case, several years after his injury, regained his ability to speak and he could read accurately, although slowly. From the tracing of this man it appeared the angular gyrus was spared.

Another source of evidence comes from the work of Norman Geschwind in Boston. He has written at some length on the anatomical basis of language, pointing out that the angular gyrus and the supramarginal gyrus do not appear in subprimate species. They appear only in rudimentary form in the higher apes (Geschwind, 1965). In neural development these areas are among the last to myelinate, and some evidence shows that this region matures structurally very late, often in late childhood. Geschwind believed, from this neurological knowledge, that the angular gyrus is in evolutionary terms a new association area interconnecting other cortical regions. Put more simply, it seems to function as a "junction box" interconnecting the visual, auditory, motor, and sensory

cortices. As explained in Chapter 2, this transcortical interconnecting center appears only in humans and provides an integrating
neurological basis for language. "Early language experience, at
least, most likely depends heavily on the forming of somesthetic-
auditory and visual-auditory associations, as well as auditory-
auditory associations" (Geschwind, 1965). Thus, the acquisition of
speech requires an ability to form cross-modal associations, and
because only humans possess these transcortical connections, inner
language develops in subhuman forms, but not speaking, reading,
or writing as in humans.

   A.R. Luria, the famous Russian neuropsychologist, has made a
monumental contribution to the study of language development
using neuropsychological knowledge. His first major work to be
translated into English, *Higher Cortical Functions in Man*, was
published in 1966, and since that time several of his translated
books have appeared. In Chapter 2, we presented his ideas on the
functional organization of the human brain, but here we shall
concentrate on his conception of dyslexia.

   In reading Luria's writings one is immediately impressed with
the depth and breadth of his thinking. He gives an integrated
concept of reading, writing, and language and he objects to the
classical neurologists who discussed these matters as entirely
separate processes. For Luria, reading and writing are special
aspects of speech activity, although their "psychological structure
and functional characteristic . . . are considerably different from
those of oral speech" (Luria, 1970). When there is a disturbance in
language functions (i.e., aphasia) there are also disturbances of
reading and writing, and Luria considers these the most common
symptoms of traumatic aphasia.

   In analyzing speech and reading, Luria points out that in
oral speech a person usually speaks spontaneously and unself-
consciously, whereas in reading, he must be able to carry out a
conscious auditory analysis of syllables from the written or printed
page. In reading, the letters representing the sounds of words
are supplied directly to the reader, who must translate them into
a correct acoustic pattern or verbal concept. The reader then
recognizes the sound of the word and associates its meaning. This
is what Luria (1970) calls "acoustic analysis and synthesis," and
this process is disturbed and impaired with lesions in the left
temporal lobe or Wernicke's area (Luria, 1970, 1973).

   Phonetic analysis and synthesis of words may be the first stages
in reading. The first-grader may sound out "c—a—t" and then
synthesize or blend the three sounds into the monosyllable "cat,"
but as these processes become automatized, the child soon learns
to recognize whole words as visual ideograms. The experienced

reader recognizes words from the general contour of the word or from its major letters. The context of meaning in the sentence may also facilitate the recognition of the word. Only when readers encounter a new or difficult word do they need to revert to phonetic analysis and synthesis, otherwise familiar words are read by direct recognition.

Luria's examination of the dyslexic patient is based on this systematic analysis of the psychological structure and function of the reading process (1970, p. 349):

1. Recognition of individual letters. The subject is asked (a) to choose identical letters in a list and (b) to read letters aloud from both written and printed pages. Failure on task (a) indicates a disturbance of the visual perception of single letters (i.e., literal alexia), but the person may have no trouble recognizing common objects, only letters. This inability to perceive written or printed symbols results from lesions in the parieto-occipital zones of the dominant left hemisphere (Luria, 1973). Failure on task (b) may result from either impaired visual recognition of the letter as in task (a) and/or an auditory imperception leading to impaired ability to associate the appropriate phonetic sound.

2. Reading simple and complex syllables. The patient is asked to read syllables varying in phonetic complexity, e.g., "ba, mo," and "bat, mit," and "bake, mote." This test shows whether the subject can pronounce the syllable as a whole or has to spell it out letter by letter.

3. Reading simple and complex words. Three simple tests are used with single words: (a) recognition of familiar words, such as the subject's own name; (b) silent reading of less familiar words, some of which will require phonetic analysis; (c) reading aloud words requiring phonetic analysis. Failure on (a) may indicate a failure to recognize words regardless of their familiarity (verbal alexia). This may result from disturbed visual form recognition or, if the recognition of letters is intact, the subject may be unable to remember their meaning (literal amnesia).

4. Reading sentences. Sentences are provided with various structures, some deliberately designed to provide a set or context to assist the interpretation of the word. Other sentences lack such a facilitating set, enabling an understanding of the various strategies the reader employs.

Lesions of the primary and secondary visual cortices result in visual alexia, both literal and verbal. Such lesions may also result in a reduction of the "reading field" (Luria, 1970); that is, the patient may be unable to perceive more than two or three letters at a time. This condition seems to be a lack of simultaneous organization of visual material, and to overcome this defect the patient may recite the letters one by one, then recognize their auditory pattern and identify the word. In other words, he carries out the process of word synthesis not in the visual mode but in the auditory mode. It will be noted that although Mrs. Stanley, described in the following section, Alexia without Agraphia, suffered an almost complete loss of single-letter recognition, she could recognize the same words instantly if they were spelled orally to her. Although her visual word recognition and synthesis were almost completely lacking, her auditory word synthesis was intact. This is the characteristic pattern of the "Déjerine syndrome," as will be explained in the later section. Visual–perceptual disturbances in reading, or optic alexia, always result from lesions of the occipital and occipito–parietal cortices, which Luria calls "the visuo-gnostic systems" (Luria, 1970).

Different types of reading problems result from disturbances of the speech processes, especially the auditory analysis and synthesis of words. Traumatic temporal lobe lesions in young children may be more devastating than in adults because children have not had as much time to automatize the reading process. When there is a disruption of the acoustico-gnostic systems, the patient is not able to resort to phonetic analysis to interpret the word. The adult who has had more time to perfect the process of direct visual recognition has a greater repertoire of sight words and hence is less disturbed by traumatic temporal lobe damage. Thus the child with a dysfunctional left temporal lobe will have to learn to read by a visual–motor method. This technique bypasses the acoustic features of the word, and though this approach is ultimately slower than a phonetic method, it provides some immediate success for the child.

Auditory analysis, as well as helping in the identification of letters, syllables, and words, also provides an ability of *inner articulation* (Luria, 1970). If one is asked to pronounce the word "sister" covertly—that is, with the mouth closed and no lip movement—the awareness of each letter and phoneme is introspectively muscularly clear. This process occurs in normal hearing subjects during silent reading. However, a person with *afferent motor aphasia* (i.e., lacking normal sensations of muscle activity) who has lost the inner articulatory ability, will have difficulty with both reading and writing. Such a person will misread and confuse letters because he or she has lost their phonetic meanings. This person will resort to a lot of guessing in order to recognize some letters or parts of most words by visual recognition, but will not have the advantage of phonetic analysis to establish their correct identities. Luria believes that afferent motor aphasia results from a lesion in the left sensory strip, affecting the kinesthetic sensations in the face, lips, and tongue (Luria, 1973) and that sensory aphasia or acoustic agnosia (phonetic auditory imperception) results from lesions of the secondary areas of the left temporal lobe, i.e., Wernicke's area.

Efferent or *kinetic motor aphasia* has a different psychological and neurological structure and function from afferent motor aphasia. It has two types, both of which result from lesions in the left (dominant) motor strip or pre-Rolandic area. The first involves lesions in the inferior zones of the premotor strip (i.e., the cortical motor centers for the face and speech muscles). In contrast to afferent (kinesthetic) aphasia, patients with lower motor strip lesions have no trouble with inner articulation of single letters, and they can pronounce individual sounds but cannot blend sounds smoothly into words. Consequently their speech is blocked and grotesque. Although this type of aphasia interferes mainly with expressive language, both oral speech and writing, it may also impair reading.

Premotor lesions also interfere with smooth, integrated sequential motor responses and, if deep at the subcortical level, may result in an inability to inhibit sequential motor actions, such as tapping. The latter phenomenon is known as elementary motor perseveration (Luria, 1973).

In summary, Luria's concept of dyslexia makes a detailed psychological analysis of the structure of language and the integration of visual, auditory, tactile, and motor sensations involved in the complex process of reading. He relates systematically the various loci of lesions producing the numerous defects that contribute to an inability to read normally. All of his evidence is drawn from careful clinical studies of traumatically brain-damaged adults.

Electrostimulation mapping of the human cortex during craniotomies under local anesthesia has led Ojemann to conclude that cortical organization for some language functions (e.g., naming or word-finding) has a mosaic pattern. He has found that "when a response has been reliably evoked, the transition from the site where that response occurs to one where it does not occur is often quite abrupt, appearing over a distance of a few millimeters" (Ojemann, 1983, p. 136). Naming, short-term verbal memory, and reading usually have separate stimulation sites outside of Broca's area "where all speech output and all types of facial mimicry are altered" (p. 139). Outside of the motor speech area, he found syntactical errors in reading resulted from stimulation of the peri-

Sylvian region and certain spots on the lateral surface of the left temporal lobe. These findings have corroborated the involvement of the classical language areas of the brain but have added more definitive information. Electrical stimulation mapping has provided evidence suggesting that language is mediated in the dominant hemisphere of both the cortex and the thalamus. The peri-Sylvian region appears to be a control center for speech and reading, short-term verbal memory, phonetic discrimination, and sequential motor responses. All of these processes are essential to successful reading, and we can assume that dysfunctions at any of the sites mentioned can produce dyslexic symptoms.

The introduction of the various brain-scanning methods introduced in the 1970s has improved the imaging of the brain, and has provided more detailed knowledge of the structure and function of the human brain and its role in reading. The CT and MRI can provide pictures of brain structure that are useful in identifying morphological abnormalities and growth anomalies (Hynd & Semrud-Clikeman, 1989; Semrud-Clikeman et al., 1991) and in correlating them with cognitive reading tasks (Semrud-Clikeman et al., 1991), but they tell us very little about brain function during mental activity. The PET scan (Frith et al., 1991; Gross-Glenn et al., 1991; Ingvar, 1991; Kushner et al., 1988; Parks et al., 1988; Petersen et al., 1988) and studies of cerebral blood flow (Flowers et al., 1991; Hynd et al., 1987) can provide us with serial measures of regional changes *as they occur* during reading, spelling, and mental association. BEAM, a method of enhancing the amount of information available on a standard EEG (Duffy, 1982; Duffy et al., 1979) has been combined with PET to provide more accuracy in purely medical diagnoses (e.g., studying brain tumors, Restak, 1984) and has also shown promise in examining the neurophysiological differences between normal and disabled readers (Lyon et al., 1991), but there are some constraints with its technical and statistical procedures (Duane, 1986). As well, because it has been developed by Duffy and his colleagues at the Harvard Medical School, in spite of its usefulness it may not be as widely available nor as well known as the CT, MRI, and PET.

Microscopic analyses at autopsy of the brain tissues of known dyslexics have shown a variety of growth anomalies (Rosen et al., 1986), and neuroimaging techniques, including CT and MRI, have also revealed abnormal neural structures in the brains of diagnosed dyslexics, but in the latter, certain methodological problems exist that imply caution in their interpretation (Hynd & Semrud-Clikeman, 1989; Hynd et al., 1991c).

Benson and Geschwind (1969) have described a number of highly specific and severe reading disorders that, because they are rare, are usually seen clinically by a neurologist. These are the cases of hemialexia, alexia without agraphia, alexia with agraphia, and aphasic alexia. Because the neurological dysfunctions are well understood in most of these syndromes they provide a sound basis for the educator and the school psychologist to broaden their knowledge of dyslexia and its possible neurological etiology.

Hemialexia. Although hemialexia is a somewhat rare type of reading disability, we include it because it is a powerful reminder of the close causal relationship between specific types of brain function and successful reading ability. Geschwind (1965) has written very clearly and convincingly on this syndrome. To understand it clearly one must be reminded that the primary visual tracts connect to the language decoding areas of the left hemisphere. The two eyes connect to the two occipital lobes, and the neural impulses stimulated by printing or writing are then shunted to the left angular gyrus and then to the left temporal lobe (Wernicke's area) for verbal interpretation (Fig. 8.7). The right occipital lobe, which registers visual sensations from the left visual field, is connected to the left angular gyrus by a band of fibers that passes through the posterior part of the corpus callosum. This posterior part of the corpus callosum is called the splenium.

The first reported case of the cutting of the splenium during brain surgery was made by Trescher and Ford in 1937 (Benson & Geschwind, 1969), and it was discovered that the patient postoperatively suffered from a permanent unilateral reading disturbance. He was unable to read anything placed in his left visual field, but reading was normal for printed material placed to the right of his midline. However, it was particularly interesting to note that vision for nonverbal stimuli was normal in *both* full visual fields. The authors concluded that the right occipital lobe was isolated from the left angular gyrus by their cutting of the splenium, thus obstructing the verbal–visual input from that visual cortex. Because the connection of the left occipital lobe to the left angular gyrus was intact, all printed stimuli reaching it from the right visual field were decoded normally. A large number of similar cases in which the splenium has been cut or destroyed by a pathological condition (Maspes, 1948; Gazzaniga, Bogen, & Sperry, 1965) have since been reported, and they provide evidence to support the left visual field reading problem in hemialexia.

Although destruction of the splenium in an adult patient will produce hemialexia, failure of the corpus callosum to develop from birth does not. Several patients with congenital callosal agenesis have been studied and found to react differently from comissurotomized adult patients. Two siblings (ages 9 and 18) with

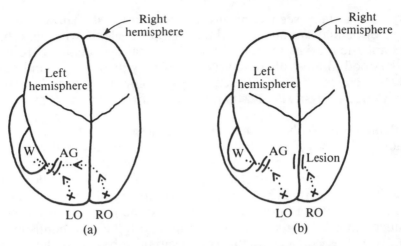

Figure 8.7. Two views of the human brain showing slightly more of the left hemisphere, including the left temporal lobe and Wernicke's area (W). (a) Normal cerebral function during reading. The visual stimulus (written or printed letter X) in the right visual field is registered in the left occipital lobe (LO), and the X from the left visual field, in the right occipital lobe (RO). Both occipital areas feed into the left temporal lobe through the area of the angular gyrus (AG) for phonetic analysis. (b) A lesion in the splenium (posterior part of the corpus callosum) that blocks passage of neural input from the right occipital lobe (RO). Only input from LO (hence stimuli from the right visual field) is processed. This is the phenomenon of hemialexia, or the ability to read material only when it is shown in the right visual field.

total agenesis of the corpus callosum were studied (Sauerwein & Lassonde, 1983) and found to be able to recognize both letters and geometric designs tachistoscopically and to compare them when presented simultaneously in one visual half-field and in both. This type of presentation required the subjects to process both verbal and nonverbal material intrahemispherically and interhemispherically. Sauerwein and Lassonde found that their acallosal subjects did not differ substantially from normal-IQ and IQ-matched controls, although they tended to respond more slowly. The ability of the subjects to react to bilaterally presented stimuli demonstrated their ability to cross-integrate visual information. To account for this the researchers proposed residual secondary commissures located lower in the brain stem, and/or cerebral reorganization in terms of abnormal hemispheric specialization. Regardless of the exact cause, this does demonstrate the marked difference in the results of traumatic damage in normal adulthood and fetal damage or agenesis. As is well known, early brain injury is less damaging than later because of the plasticity and adaptability of the developing human brain.

Alexia Without Agraphia: The Subject Cannot Read But Can Still Write. One of the most interesting cases of acquired reading disability in an adult is the "Déjerine syndrome," known by neurologists since 1892 but generally unknown to most teachers and psychologists. Geschwind (1962) presented a detailed explanation and discussion of Déjerine's famous case along with a number of very interesting line drawings reproduced from the original report. This is the classic case of *pure word blindness without agraphia*, and all school psychologists not familiar with the syndrome could profit from reading Geschwind's account. To see one of these patients is very compelling and quickly lays to rest the delusion that all reading problems are psychogenically produced.

Very briefly, Déjerine's case described an intelligent man of 68 years who suddenly discovered he could not read a single letter. He was sent for ophthalmological examination but his eyesight was within the normal range. He spoke fluently and understood all spoken speech normally. He could name objects perfectly (i.e., there was no word-finding difficulty) and he could identify his morning newspaper but he could not read anything in it, even its name.

His writing was perfect, both to copy and to dictation, but once he had written, he was unable to read what he had just written. Whereas he could not decode writing or print visually, he could identify and recognize letters both tactually and auditorially. If his fingers felt the letters of a tactile alphabet, or if a word was spelled orally to him, the patient had no difficulty in decoding the words presented. Although he could not read letters visually, he had no problem with Arabic numerals or complex written calculations. He could not read musical notation but could write musical notes on command. His ability to sing and play instruments was normal. From the time of the cerebrovascular accident that had caused his sudden dyslexia, he suffered from a right hemianopia. This, of course, implied a left hemisphere dysfunction, which was to be expected because a language function was impaired.

About 4 years later he suffered a second cerebrovascular accident (stroke), which left him with paraphasic speech and a sudden loss of his ability to write. He died 10 days later and Déjerine performed an autopsy within 24 hours of his death.

Two major lesions were found in the brain, the 4-year-old lesion and the recent one. It was possible to discriminate these by their different discolorations and the presence of atrophied tissue in the older lesion. Examination of the brain enabled Déjerine to

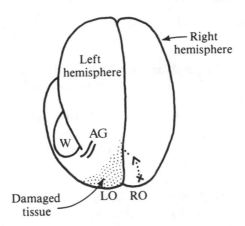

Figure 8.8. The human brain from above, showing the area of damage resulting from a hemorrhage of the left posterior cerebral artery. The primary visual cortex of the left occipital lobe and the splenium are damaged, thus destroying visual input from the left occiput (LO) and blocking input from the right side (RO). This is the basic neurological pattern of the Déjerine syndrome, in which a person is unable to read but can still write and interpret spelling words through auditory and tactual presentation.

conclude that the presence of alexia with the ability to write was caused by localized damage of the left occipital lobe and the splenium, with sparing of the left angular gyrus (Fig. 8.8). This meant that no visual–verbal input could reach the angular gyrus because the left occipital lobe was destroyed and the right occipital lobe, although normal and healthy, was isolated from it (Geschwind, 1962, 1965; Benson & Geschwind, 1969). At the same time, the left temporal acoustic analyzer (Wernicke's area) was still normally connected to the sensory and motor strips, and so the man had no difficulty interpreting words by the tactile and auditory modes, or in expressing them in speech and writing. In other words, the oral speech and writing cortical circuits were still intact.

The second hemorrhage 10 days prior to his death damaged the angular gyrus, thus disconnecting Wernicke's area from the sensory and motor strips. This appeared to cause the aphasic speech and his inability to write.

Mrs. Stanley, aged 66, seen in our laboratory, exhibited the classic signs of the Déjerine syndrome. On a visit from her home in London, England, she suddenly suffered a cerebral hemorrhage, presumably of the left posterior artery. Although a highly intelligent woman, she suddenly discovered she could not read, but she could write normally. In fact, she wrote long letters to her friends in England that were perfectly spelled, but she was unable to proofread or reread them. She could recognize letters moderately well if her hand traced them in the air or on the page, and she was quick and accurate at identifying all words spelled orally to her.

To test the possibility of her regaining her ability to read, she was seen twice a week for 2 hours each for remedial teaching, for a 4-month period. She was highly motivated and she tried very hard but she still could not read any words. Toward the end of the 4-month period she learned to read five or six letters sometimes, but her performance was erratic and unreliable.

When asked to write "London," she printed in a large, firm style. She could point to each letter and identify it if she spelled the word orally, but if started on the second letter without her noticing, she identified the letters quite wrongly and was surprised to find she ran out of letters one from the end. In other words, her oral spelling, both receptive and expressive, was quite intact because, presumably, the left angular gyrus was spared, but her optic dyslexia was permanent. It is possible to speculate on the cause of this and similar cases because of the large number that have come to autopsy examination since 1892.

Alexia with Agraphia: The Subject Cannot Read or Write. Although the preceding syndrome, alexia *without* agraphia, is not common, alexia *with* agraphia is frequent in left-hemisphere stroke cases. Structurally the difference in the two syndromes stems from the sparing of the angular gyrus in the first instance and the destruction of it in the second. Déjerine discovered this in 1892 at the autopsy study of his famous case. The hemorrhage that occurred 10 days before the man's death destroyed his angular gyrus and as a result the writing circuit was erased. In other words, the Wernicke's area was disconnected from the manual writing area in the left motor strip.

This deficit has been observed numerous times since Déjerine's report, and all cases that have come to postmortem have shown damage or destruction of the angular gyrus, with accompanying alexia and agraphia. There is frequently a mild receptive aphasia, because damage to the angular gyrus can sometimes affect Wernicke's area, which is nearby. Mrs. Stanley had mild word-finding problems that she found frustrating, and even picture identification and naming was slow.

Aphasic Alexia. Patients suffering from severe receptive (Wernicke's) aphasia will have great difficulty understanding the conceptual words spoken by others. Similarly they will have difficulty bringing meaning to the printed word. Motor (or Broca's) aphasia may interfere with the ability to produce inner articulation. Even though the perceptual and cognitive aspects of reading may not be impaired, the expressive functions in normal reading are lacking or distorted.

Just as the aphasic patient produces paraphasias in his speech (i.e., substituting the wrong word for the desired word, e.g., "table" for "chair"; or a neologism or fabricated nonsense word in place of the desired word), some dyslexics when reading aloud may misread a word and substitute a different one for it (paralexic error). The important point to note in both paraphasias and paralexias is that they possess a *semantic relationship* with the desired word (e.g., "chair" for "table," or 6 for 8), or they have a rhyming and semantic association. The aphasic patient who recognized a key but could not name it, said, "Kay . . . it's dorent [probably a contraction of "door" and "not"]. I'm in the floor [floor rhymes with door, which semantically is related to the desired word, key]. It's all away" (the subject knows all the words are wrong).

Paralexias have been known since 1928 (Marshall & Newcombe, 1980), but a systematic study of them has existed only since the mid-1960s, and a name for this syndrome, *deep dyslexia*, was originated in the early 1970s. The patient with deep dyslexia is an adult who, after acquiring reading skills, suffers traumatic damage to the language-dominant hemisphere, and manifests semantic errors while reading aloud (e.g., "act" may be read as "play"), derivational errors (e.g., birth → born), visual errors (e.g., saucer → sausage), misreading functional words (i.e., articles, prepositions, conjunctions; e.g., his → she, or for → and), and inability to read nonwords (e.g., wep → wet). Deep dyslexics read concrete and high-imagery nouns best, then adjectives, then verbs, and function words the poorest. They often complain that "the small words are the worst" (Marshall & Newcombe, 1980; Newcombe & Marshall, 1981; Coltheart, 1981).

Attempts to provide a neuropsychological theory for deep dyslexia have included drawing on our knowledge of right-hemisphere reading. Coltheart, Patterson, and Marshall (1980) have proposed a model that includes integrated hemispheric specialization. They summarize it thus: "When the deep dyslexic is asked to read a word aloud, then his problem . . . is this: orthographic input to a right hemisphere linguistic system is possible, but speech output is not; speech output from a left hemisphere linguistic system is possible but orthographic input is not. If so, the task of reading aloud will require (a) orthographic input to a right-hemisphere reading system, followed by (b) transfer from the right hemisphere to the left of information which can be used (c) to select from amongst the phonological forms of words stored in the left hemisphere that form which corresponds to the word being looked at" (p. 352).

This theoretical proposal has much to recommend it. Some split-brain experiments have shown that the separated right hemisphere is superior to the left in reading calligraphy and numbers (E. Zaidel, 1973) and it is unable to speak. Bliss Symbolics, a form of picture writing, can frequently help a severely cerebral palsied child, with maximal damage in the left hemisphere, to learn to read and write using the Bliss symbols. Presumably this technique makes use of the better right hemisphere and avoids the damaged left one.

Deep dyslexia is the only form of acquired dyslexia in which the person makes *semantic errors* while reading single words out of context (Coltheart, 1981, p. 276ff.), possibly because of semantic confusion in accessing words with some similarities in meaning from the internal lexicon, hypothesized to be in the unconscious and hence "deeper" recesses of the mind. By contrast, *surface dyslexia* is characterized by more difficulty in reading irregularly spelled words than matched regularly spelled words, and misreadings of irregular words often take the form of "regularizations" (e.g., none—acquainted with, known). If the surface dyslexic reads a word aloud, it may be misinterpreted by what is said (e.g., enigma, an image or picture) but spelling is determined by what is seen (Coltheart, 1981, p. 270ff.). The reader will recognize these cues as perceptually evident or "surface" features of language. In reading individual words a surface dyslexic will have the least difficulty in reading nouns, more problems with adjectives and verbs, and more success in reading concrete rather than abstract nouns. Visual confusions (e.g., spy: shy) and partial failures of grapheme–phoneme conversion (e.g., incense: increase) are common (Marshall & Newcombe, 1973). It is significant that surface dyslexia occurs not only as an acquired but also as a developmental dyslexia. "Exactly the same pattern of reading errors . . . occurs in some children who have failed to acquire competence in reading despite apparent neurological normality, as well as in some adults who had learned to read competently but then suffered a brain injury which left their reading impaired" (Coltheart, 1981).

Word-form dyslexia is characterized by patient's having to name each letter of a word and, after hearing the letters, recognizing the whole word (Coltheart, 1981, p. 263ff.). This condition is similar to a modified Déjerine syndrome, in which the patient can still read individual letters but cannot read words visually without first converting them into their auditory or phonological form. Some Déjerine cases can do that, but in "pure" cases, such as Mrs. Stanley, this ability is impossible because they are unable to read even single letters.

Patients with *phonological dyslexia* can usually read single-morpheme content words, but they are impaired in the ability to read nonwords aloud (e.g., cruft). Visual errors are made in reading nonwords (e.g., bef read as beef), derivational errors in reading aloud (e.g., running read as run), function-word substitutions (e.g., yet read as that), but all the symptoms of this form are not yet certain. The first case was reported in 1979, and only a few cases have been seen to date. It is described in more detail by Coltheart (1981, 265–269).

Before leaving this discussion of different types of paralexias we must recognize that all of these cases of acquired dyslexia had visual deficits that interfered with their reading (Coltheart, 1981; Coltheart, Patterson, & Marshall, 1980; Luria, 1973; Marshall & Newcombe, 1973; Russell & Espir, 1961). This may seem contradictory to the preceding discussion of the psychology of normal reading, in which visual processes were discounted as major determinants of successful reading (Stanovich, 1985; Vellutino, 1987), and linguistic competence was recognized as important. This view appears to be valid for readers with healthy, normally functioning brains, and possibly with those with minimal cerebral dysfunctions, but with cases of severe brain damage in which normal visual images are frequently distorted, visual deficits can cause disturbances in perception of individual letters (i.e., literal alexia, Luria, 1973), or can result in a complete inability to recognize any letters even in the presence of normal object recognition (see the case of Mrs. Stanley, pp. 350–351). In brief, the discussions of the acquired dyslexias included cases of severe brain damage, but the discussions of developmental dyslexia included, for the most part, children in the school system, whose cerebral dysfunctions, if they had them, were minimal and subtle, but just disturbing enough to make normal reading difficult.

Developmental Dyslexia in Adults

An unknown segment of the adult population is unable to read, or they read so minimally that they hide it as a sign of inadequacy. These people are of average or superior intelligence level, so that their disability is even more mystifying and humiliating to them. Some of them have successful careers in business, athletics, or construction work; and they are on constant guard to keep their secret, because reading is so common in modern Western society that they feel many people would consider them stupid if their disability were known.

The evidence on acquired dyslexia from traumatically brain-damaged adults that began in the early 1890s with Déjerine's autopsy studies, though interesting and definitive, cannot be used to explain the disability of all congenital nonreaders. When the first such case was reported by Morgan in England in 1896, however, he used Déjerine's evidence to hypothesize that a 14-year-old boy who was academically bright but had great difficulty in learning to read and write probably suffered from an underdeveloped angular gyrus. This was a logical association, to reason from a known cause of reading disability to an unknown, and it is still a temptation for the neurologist or neuropsychologist who has worked with any one of the types of traumatic dyslexics in the preceding discussion. But most cases of developmental dyslexia subjected to a standard neurological examination show no signs of neurological pathology, and many of these subjects possess unusual talents in other areas. These are the children who may be gifted artists, superior mathematicians, or charismatic social leaders. As adults many of them have become successful business people, artists, or scientists. The fact that Albert Einstein was said to be dyslexic is well known. According to "the family legend, when Hermann Einstein asked his son's headmaster what profession his son should adopt, the answer was simply: 'It doesn't matter; he'll never make a success of anything'" (Clark, 1971).

It soon became evident in the early part of this century that among the population of dyslexics there were too many with superior intellects and special talents, and many more with normal levels of intelligence, to accept an etiology of brain damage or cerebral atrophy for all of them. This realization led to a search for some type of brain dysfunction without identifiable brain damage that might interfere with the complex neuropsychological processes demanded by reading.

The first influential proposal was that of Orton (1925, 1926, 1937), who suggested that incomplete cerebral dominance may be the major cause of developmental reading retardation. Since Orton's proposal, many researchers have also described dyslexia as having a single cause, though the causes varied from cerebral dominance (Orton, 1937), to maturational lag (Bender, 1958; Delacato, 1959), to perceptual–motor deficiencies (Cruickshank, 1968, 1978; Frostig & Maslow, 1973; Kephart, 1960), to genetic traits (Hermann, 1959), to language deficits (Vellutino, 1979), to parietal dysfunctions (Jorm, 1979).

By the 1960s, dualistic theories began to appear (e.g., visual and auditory dyslexia, Johnson & Myklebust, 1967; visual–spatial and auditory–linguistic dyslexia, Bakker, 1979; Pirozzolo, 1979). By the late 1960s and early 1970s, multicausal theories were produced as more experimental discoveries about dyslexia appeared. Three subtypes of dyslexia (e.g., Bateman, 1968; Boder, 1973), four subtypes (e.g., Mattis, 1978), and five subtypes (e.g., Denckla, 1977) have been proposed by various medical, neuropsychological, neurophysiological, linguistic, and educational researchers and practitioners. The many theories reflect the present incomplete knowledge of dyslexia, but their diversity is encouraging as a sign of increasing understanding and promising possibly greater remedial competence.

Since the late 1970s, much new knowledge relating reading to brain function and dysfunction has come from experiments in cerebral blood flow, brain scanning, cortical electrostimulation, histological studies, and correlational studies in biopsychology. The first three techniques have already received brief explanations; their findings suggest that dysfunctions in any part of the cerebral cortex (particularly on the left), and anywhere in the brainstem (particularly in the thalamus and cerebellum) may result in impaired reading.

Autopsy studies of the brains of dyslexics are relatively recent (Drake, 1968; Galaburda & Kemper, 1979; Galaburda, 1983; Rosen et al., 1986). These histological examinations have revealed abnormal neural tissue growth. Drake (1968) reported excessive numbers of neurons in the subcortical white matter, which is abnormal. Galaburda and Kemper (1979) studied the brain of a 20-year-old left-handed male dyslexic and found an abnormal amount of white matter in the whole left hemisphere and evidence of disordered neuronal migration in the left peri-Sylvian area.

The brain of a 14-year-old dyslexic (Galaburda, 1983) also showed abnormal growth. Collections of neurons were found in layer one of the cortex, and in the subcortical white matter of the left hemisphere, a condition not seen in normal brains. By contrast, the right hemisphere appeared architectonically normal and mature. Galaburda's findings suggest that the brains of developmental dyslexics may have acquired anomalous lateralization, and that their left hemispheres may contain structural distortions.

Geschwind (1983) has reported an interesting association of food allergies, immune disorders, left-handedness, and childhood migraine among developmental dyslexic children (mostly males) and their families. The biological aspects he related to brain development by proposing the following hypothesis: It is known from fetal studies that the right hemisphere tends to grow faster than the left, but in dyslexics there appears to be a slowed migration of neural cells to the language areas of the left hemisphere.

This slowing of the left may produce compensatory growth of the right hemisphere, thus resulting in left-handedness and superior spatial and artistic skills.

During intrauterine life the male fetus produces huge quantities of testosterone, a male sex hormone, and Geschwind suggests that this over-production may retard the growth of the left hemisphere in males. He points out that his hypothesis possesses some empirical support in animal studies, in which testosterone injected into rats and birds has shown resulting brain changes. Excessive testosterone may also result in impaired migration of cerebral nerve cells, and in disturbances of the immune system. Although this theory is far from complete it does point to a possible relation among biochemical processes, neural brain growth, and developmental dyslexia.

A more recent proposal by Livingstone and her colleagues (1991) suggests that the brains of dyslexics may process visual information more slowly than normal subjects because of an atypical development of the two major neural pathways connecting the retinae to the two lateral geniculate nuclei (LGN) and from there to the two primary visual cortices (see Fig. 2.7 on p. 69; or Netter, 1972, p. 63). The human LGN and optic nerve have six clearly segregated layers of cells; the four more dorsal layers are composed of small cells, named the parvocellular layers. The two more ventral layers, composed of larger neurons, are called magnocellular layers (Shapley, 1990). It has been known for a long time that a larger neural fiber conducts impulses at a faster rate than a small one (Gardner, 1968, p. 102), and as may be expected the magnocellular layer conducts faster than the parvocellular layer. Visually the two layers also show differences in color selectivity, contrast sensitivity, temporal resolution, and acuity, and with this knowledge, Livingstone et al. hypothesize that due to a magnocellular defect in dyslexic subjects their visual systems are deficient in processing visual stimuli which are fast and transient and which have high contrast sensitivity and low spatial selectivity. The latter processes are required in normal reading.

Because the flicker fusion rate of perception of dyslexic children is abnormally slow (Martin & Lovegrove, 1987), and because both dyslexic children and adults are abnormally slow in perceiving sequentially presented light patterns and single letters (Gaddes, 1982), the proposal of Livingstone et al. that developmental dyslexia may result from a magnocellular defect is particularly appealing. Their proposed theory, for which they have supplied both physiological and anatomical supporting evidence, is a possible explanation that does not stress brain damage or resulting dysfunction, and instead conceives of two major visual processing pathways that, because of variations in neural cellular growth, function at relative speeds that interfere with normal reading. Presumably these developmental variations could be within the normal distribution of individual differences, and could be the physiological basis for some specific aptitudes, in this case the aptitude for verbal processing and reading.

Context Effects

In Chapter 6, a brief mention was made of the clinical use of context effects in reading single sentences by dyslexics and aphasics, and the discussion of the psycholinguistics of normal reading, earlier in this chapter, described how contextual information facilitates word recognition and comprehension. Chase and Tallal (1990) have studied this effect in reading letters and words among normal adults, dyslexic children, and children matched for reading age and children matched for chronological age. Because adults can more accurately identify letters in a word than when they are alone, or in other random displays (i.e., the word superiority effect or WSE), Chase and Tallal examined the abilities of the three groups of children to respond to the WSE. They found that young normal readers demonstrated the WSE, but their pseudoword advantage was less than that of adults. The dyslexic children showed no WSE at all, presumably because their linguistic knowledge (semantic, syntactic, and pragmatic meanings) was relatively much weaker.

Mr. Darwin. Mr. Darwin was referred to our laboratory at the age of 32. He had an engaging manner and was successful in managing his own logging business. The only word he could read and write was his own name, because he needed to sign checks in managing his business, and he could recognize and name about 12 individual letters.

He had attended a small rural school during the 1940s and because he could not read he was left to look at picture books while the other children completed their academic exercises. He could read arabic numbers and was able to do arithmetic calculations at about the grade 5 level, which had enabled him to manage a small logging business, hire skilled help, do his own bookkeeping, solicit business, and direct the whole operation. When we first saw him, his business management was so successful that he earned half again as much that year as the local high school teachers at the top of the salary scale (i.e., with an M.A. degree and at least 10 years' experience). This achievement was particularly impressive because he could not read "cat."

Being a gregarious fellow, he mixed socially a good deal, and this necessitated the development of a number of social coverup strategies. When he was in a restaurant with a number of people he would pick up a menu and pretend to read it for a few moments and then pass it to one of the others. When the waitress came to take their orders he would listen to what the others requested and either pick the most appealing order from what he heard or order a standard dish that was certain to be available. Because he could read numbers he was able to read price lists, which was of some help.

The neurologist who referred Mr. Darwin originally reported that although he complained of frequent headaches, his neurological examination and EEG were both normal, as was his skull x-ray. His neuropsychological test findings were also unremarkable. He measured a verbal IQ of 88 and a performance IQ of 106 on the Wechsler Adult Intelligence Scale. His general information was inferior and his vocabulary below average because of his dyslexia, but his diagnostic understanding of common problems (Comprehension) was nearly superior. His visual, auditory, tactile, and motor scores were all in the normal range, and so his pattern suggested a man of above-average intelligence with a specific reading disability. Because the neurological and neuropsychological examinations revealed no deficits, his reading failure may have been genetically determined or the result of a minimal and atypical cortical function too minute to show on a standard neurological examination. That his two sons were also poor readers, but his daughter was not, reinforced the possibility of a familial pattern in the male members.

Because the neurological and neuropsychological tests were negative we felt confident in recommending a multisensorimotor remediation program. This proved successful, because when he returned a year later he could read 200 words correctly and had learned good methods of phonetic attack, although he still occasionally confused the sound of "i" and "e." On the Gates–McKillop reading test he could read at the early grade 3 level and his perception of visual and auditory sequential stimuli had improved markedly.

On his third visit to our laboratory, $2\frac{1}{2}$ years after we had first seen him, Mr. Darwin could read about 500 words and was reading the newspaper headlines and brief bits of news reports. Tachistoscopically he could read single letters at half a second and most common words from the Dolch lists (Dolch, 1945) at 1 second (e.g., dish, sister, brother, wife, pen). Within another year he was able to read at a fifth-grade level and to write well enough to fill out a job application.

It seems almost certain that Mr. Darwin's reading problem resulted from some undetermined constitutional source (possibly a subtle neurological deficit, a genetic defect, or a magnocellular defect?) because he was so refractory to normal teaching methods as a child and had suffered educational neglect in the school system.

Reginald Simmons. Reginald Simmons was referred to us because of an inferior ability to read. This case is an interesting comparison with that of Mr. Darwin; whereas no abnormalities showed in either Mr. Darwin's neurological or his neuropsychological examinations, Mr. Simmons's neurological exam was negative but very specific left-hemisphere signs showed on the neuropsychological exam. Both men were 32 years of age when first referred and both were competent athletes. In fact, Mr. Simmons was a professional hockey player.

On the neuropsychological test battery Mr. Simmons showed himself to be of average intelligence level but left-handed and most likely left-hemisphere dominant for language (right-ear preference, 26; left-ear preference, 5). Figure 8.9 shows the significant findings in brief summary. His tactile form recognition (stereognosis), finger localization, and tapping speed were all poor with his right hand, though normal with his left. His right–left orientation and sequencing abilities were also poor. All of these signs point to possible minimal dysfunction in the medial part of the left hemisphere (particularly the left sensory and motor strips). Because nothing showed on the neurological tests, this lesion, if it exists, must be minimal and subtle but potent enough to make him use his left hand. The dichotic findings suggest that normally he should have been right-handed.

Because his auditory perception was good, a modification of the Gillingham method was used in conjunction with a color-coding system. At the beginning of a remedial program (6 hours a week) he read at a grade-point level of 4.2 on the Gates–McKillop test, and so he was not severely alexic to begin with, as Mr. Darwin had been. After 3 months of special tutoring his reading measured at the grade 7.0 level. The presumed lesion would seem to have retarded his sequential skills with visual and auditory tasks and visual–motor abilities.

Summary. These two cases of developmental dyslexia in adults provide some interesting clues to guide us. First, whereas the traumatically damaged adults had highly specific reading deficits that showed a close relation to the locus of damage and a reliability of prediction, the adults with developmental dyslexia as a group

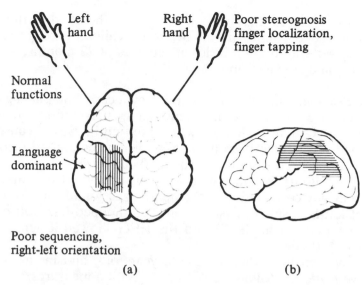

Figure 8.9. Case of Mr. Simmons, showing neuropsychological signs of possible minimal left-hemisphere dysfunction: (a) top view of his brain with arms outstretched; (b) the left hemisphere with the inferred lesion shaded. (© 1984 William D. West)

were highly variable both neurologically and behaviorally. This would seem to result, in the traumatic cases, from a normal nervous system being damaged after the cortical language centers had been locked in, whereas in the developmental cases, the child during his or her development was using the functional areas of the brain and making the optimal compromise. Consequently, the child or adult with developmental dyslexia will need to be studied in great detail both neurologically and behaviorally, and a remedial program constructed making maximum use of this knowledge. This procedure is in basic agreement with Myklebust's (1971b) recommendation for the treatment of children with developmental aphasia.

Primary Reading Retardation in Children

Traumatic Dyslexia

Quadfasel and Goodglass (1968) have made the point that brain damage incurred between birth and about the age of 2 years (i.e., prior to the acquisition of established speech) and damage incurred after 2 years may have some unique differences. One would expect the first type to be similar to developmental dyslexia, and the second to be increasingly specific, the older the child at the time of injury. To examine this point, three children are presented here who suffered brain injuries at the ages of 22 months, 3 years 9 months, and 6 years 9 months.

Max Pearson. This boy had been hit by a car while playing on a residential street in front of his home. He was 22 months old at the time of the accident. When he was picked up he was unconscious and blood was issuing from his left ear. He made a good recovery and was discharged from the hospital 10 days later.

His head injury left him with a squint in his left eye that was later medically corrected, and the neurologist found some minimal signs of left-hemisphere dysfunction ("He hopped less well on his right foot than on his left") and the EEG showed a generalized grade iii dysrhythmia.

We saw him first when he was 6 years old, and in the next 3 years we made the following Wechsler (WISC) measures:

Age (years)	Verbal IQ	Performance IQ
6–1	86	99
8–4	80	108
8–5	82	104 (Tested in another clinic)
8–11	72	96
Average	80	101.75

By themselves these findings were congruent with inferior left-hemisphere function. This conclusion was reinforced by a relatively inferior performance with the right hand on hand-grip strength, finger-tapping speed, and stereognosis. In addition, his ability on sequential tasks (largely a left-hemisphere function) was also poor.

At age 6 his handedness was mixed even for writing, but by our last testing (age 8–11) he was writing consistently with his right hand and the dichotic test suggested that he was markedly left-hemisphere dominant for language but not strongly so (right-ear preference, 18; left-ear, 8). By this time he was in grade 3, although he was beginning his fourth year of school. Though mildly aphasic (he could not follow oral instructions except in small bits), he learned to read at a level that his teacher considered "average" for the class. His arithmetic was very weak because his abilities for abstraction were so poor. Socially, Max was well adjusted, he spoke well to adults, and he gave an impression of normal alertness, which would tend to obscure his "invisible disabilities." However, studies of his development suggest that as an adult he will most likely be employable, because of his cheery personality, in some type of unskilled work.

Considering the seriousness of Max's head injury, his brain had made a remarkable adjustment. He is minimally aphasic to oral instructions, has learned the mechanics of reading, but has weak comprehension. The early brain damage has impaired his competence in arithmetic much more. Although he can write numbers neatly, his very weak conceptual ability has impaired him seriously. Had an adult of average intelligence received this pattern of brain damage, he would likely have become aphasic and alexic but retained most or all of his ability in simple arithmetic facts. Max's pattern is in the reverse direction, possibly because of the bilateral functional reorganization following his brain injury.

Robbie Yates. This boy was struck by a car at the age of 3 years 9 months and sustained bilateral, diffuse brain damage, with greater injury in the left hemisphere. Because oral language is becoming pretty well established by this age, the average child having an active vocabulary of about 1400 words (M.E. Smith, 1926, adapted by Thompson, 1962), we can logically expect his language development to be impaired.

The neurological and neuropsychological evidence indicated bilateral damage resulting from a violent closed head injury. This type of injury reduces the possibilities of compensation by preventing the child from using healthy tissue, as is possible by a localized injury. At age 4 years 10 months his Stanford–Binet IQ measured 63, mainly because the tester had so much difficulty communicating with Robbie. He was quiet and extremely noncommunicative.

At age 7 years 11 months, when we first saw him, he was unable to read anything. The school put him on a multisensorimotor remedial program, purposely not stressing phonics, but including them, because his phonetic discrimination was not strong. By the time he was 11 years 5 months, he could read slowly and he was able to sound out and blend three- and four-letter words competently. Because of a mild receptive aphasia, it was necessary for the teacher to speak slowly, at a tempo Robbie could decode. Wechsler (WISC) measures at age 11 years 4 months showed a verbal IQ (VIQ) of 72 and a performance IQ (PIQ) of 94. Two months later he was tested again for medical–legal reasons and his WISC measures were VIQ, 75 and PIQ, 90. The permanent lesion in his left hemisphere, which by this time had existed for almost 8 years, was showing itself in a pattern of chronic verbal inferiority and relatively better, but not strong, spatial–constructional skills. His teachers, in a special school for brain-damaged and aphasic children, understood this condition and developed a remedial program and set of expectations Robbie could manage successfully. As a result, he made slow but steady academic progress and a healthy and normal social adjustment.

Vera Brown. This girl was normally healthy and happy until she suddenly suffered a spontaneous cerebral hemorrhage at 6 years 9 months. This incident occurred the day before she was to enter grade 1, so that fortuitously this case provides a pattern of normal preschool health with all formal academic learning being impaired by the effects of left-hemisphere brain damage.

Vera was playing with some other children on the day of the subarachnoid hemorrhage, when she felt ill, was nauseated, and became unconscious. She was rushed to the hospital, and a large hematoma was evacuated and the bleeding stopped. The bleeding originated in the inferior left parietal–occipital area, and until it was stopped it caused some permanent damage in the left temporal–parietal–occipital region.

One of the obvious sequelae of this damage was a right visual field defect, which, when Vera was learning to read, caused her to have to move her head a great deal, because her restricted visual field extended from the vertical midline to the normal left extremity. To make it easier for her in school we advised her teachers to seat her at the right side of the classroom.

Vera spent 6 weeks in a hospital recovering from the brain surgery and 2 weeks at home, and she was ready to enter first grade by early November. Although the other first-graders had a 2-month start on Vera, she caught up enough to pass into grade 2 the following June. Her mother, a primary school teacher, was unusually skillful and supportive in helping her learn. Even so, she had great difficulty in learning to read, and an analysis of her weaknesses showed that they included a below-average vocabulary (a mild anomia) and poor phonetic discrimination, although an audiometric test showed her hearing to be normal. She also had difficulties in visual sequencing, spatial imagery, visual–motor speed, and rhythmic sequential tapping.

Vera's mother reported that she was one of the most promising students at the end of kindergarten in the previous year, but at the end of grade 1 she slipped to an average level (Table 8.1).

Ten months after her brain injury we tested Vera for the first time and found a Wechsler (WISC) verbal IQ of 105, a performance IQ of 101, and difficulties in reading, writing, and all the language arts. Her mother's persistent and skilled help no doubt had a great deal to do with Vera's steady progress during the next few years.

Table 8.1. Kindergarten and First-Grade Achievement: Vera Brown

Name	Kindergarten (Pretraumatic)	Name	Grade 1 (Posttraumatic)
Vera	*High*	Richard	High
Richard	High	Susan	High average
Susan	High average	*Vera*	*Average*
Louise	Low average	Louise	Low
Gordon	Low average	Gordon	Low

The next year, about 22 months after her cerebrovascular accident, we found a WISC verbal IQ of 103 and performance IQ of 96. The drop in the performance IQ resulted mainly from an inferior score on the Picture Completion Subtest. Her hemianopia was making it difficult for her to scan pictures thoroughly and notice some small details. Reading was still a problem, but Vera was doing well enough that she was almost keeping up to the average of the class. With all her remedial help at home she rated "low average," which was a passing grade.

About 3 years later we saw her again. By this time she was beginning grade 6, and her mother reported that during the previous summer she began to read spontaneously for her own pleasure. The intensive remedial work in the language arts during the past 5 years was beginning to pay off, because her vocabulary was now above average and her teacher reported that she wrote interesting stories with a competent choice of words. She did well in arithmetic and very well in art. In fact, she took private lessons in drawing because she showed a special artistic talent.

Vera's musical ability remained defective. Her mother reported that "she cannot carry a tune and her sense of rhythm never has returned."

Academically, Vera did moderately well in grade 7, but in high school she had many difficulties because many of the high school teachers *did not believe she had a learning problem.* In grade 10 she was able to keep up in the English course with tremendous effort, which usually meant 3 hours of homework each night.

At the end of grade 10, Vera's mother wrote:

Looking back, I feel sure, as a teacher, that we should not have put Vera into grade one immediately after recovering from her brain hemorrhage. Speaking as a primary teacher, we find children who have had a great deal of hospitalization before six years of age are really not ready for grade one. Also, we must remember how disoriented children with sudden brain damage are. They need time to adjust to their old world before embarking on a new venture.

How many adults who have had a stroke would one recommend to start a new job one month later—especially one that requires a new set of values, and a lot of new language skills?

Very has managed "to keep up to her grade level," whatever that means, but I feel she has done this at the loss of her social development. She feels she is dumb and has few close friends, but she has never been one of the crowd, any crowd.

I would suggest to parents of children who have sudden brain damage to be very careful of the school placement of their children when they return home from hospital. Doctors and most other professionals encourage you to think that these children are normal, but they are not, in the sense that they cannot cope immediately with their new life. They need help in the transition from their memory of their former life and the acceptance of their new impaired one. I don't mean that they should be treated as invalids, but only helped to recover from the shock, in the same way we allow adults.

Also, I want to suggest that some sort of help be available to the parents, perhaps through the Association of Children with Learning Disabilities. Everyone forgets what a shock it is for them. I think so much stress is placed on the medical aspects of the case the psychological ones are overlooked. Once the child is free of the hospital, everyone writes "finis" to the case. There is much emotional adjustment to be made by both parents and child, and some counseling would be welcome.

The frustrations of the brain-damaged child and his or her parents are usually obscured to society and are just as "invisible" as the child's disabilities. As a result, some teachers deny the existence of the so-called learning disability and frequently blame the parent for trying to manipulate the school. More will be said about the roles of the child, the parent, and the teacher in Chapter 10.

Developmental Dyslexia in Children

In the past, the child with a congenital reading problem was usually referred for an ophthalmological examination. Because reading obviously requires visual functions it was believed that dyslexics must have some deficit in the structure or functions of their visual systems. In almost all cases the dyslexic is normal or superior in reading an eye chart. The ophthalmologist or optometrist with this evidence will report that the child's vision is normal, and this seeming contradiction has only added to the etiological mystery of dyslexia. As more became known about brain structure and function, however, a preference for a *central* or brain dysfunction to account for reading problems became established, and *peripheral* or visual deficits have come to be recognized as rarely associated with retarded reading.

One exception to this view has been expressed by Pavlidis (1979, 1983). His research indicated "that dyslexics' erratic eye movements are present not only during reading but also in other non-reading tasks such as trying to follow moving lights." Similar results were found in research with the Dynamic Visual Retention Test (DVRT) (see Appendix for description of the DVRT) by one of us (Gaddes 1982, 100–102) in which both dyslexic school-age boys and adults were found to be inferior to matched normals in visual tracking and remembering moving sequential patterns of lights, and this skill deficit increased with greater speed of presentation. Certainly visual processing is related to success in reading. Certain capital letters (A, E, L, P, T, W, X, Z) have been found to be the least confused perceptually (Kinney et al., 1966), and visual crowding of musical notation, contrast sensitivity, visual accommodation, and convergence have all been found to be possible causes of the inferior sight reading of music by dyslexics (Atkinson, 1992). However, whether eye movements and other visual skills are a primary cause of dyslexia, or a secondary interference in the reading process, is still not clear. Pavlidis (1986) has made the important point that defective visual skills might "be seen as the results of the same or parallel but independent brain malfunctions" and "the dyslexics' erratic eye movements can be further perceived as being complementary to their language problems, rather than being causally related."

Frequently, a child with a severe reading problem reveals no deficits on a neurological examination. If he or she possesses normal intelligence, is free of any sensory deficits and is well motivated, a possible remaining cause appears to be a genetic one. Drew (1956), Hallgren (1950), Hermann (1959), and Sladen (1970) all have provided support for a genetic theory of dyslexia. A more recent report by a team of behavioral geneticists provides evidence that might link specific reading disability to chromosome 15 (S.D. Smith, Kimberling, Pennington, & Lubs, 1983). They found a lod score of 3.241 where a score of 3.0 is traditionally accepted as significant. A lod score is a measure of linkage between a specific behavior and a particular locus on a designated chromosome.

When no deficits show on a neurological or neuropsychological test, this does not necessarily mean the person is free of some slight but crucially located dysfunction, as was described in the case of Mr. Simmons. Prior to the neuropsychological findings, nothing had ever been found that might account for Mr. Simmons's dyslexia, and so he was left to think he was stupid. Counseling, based on interpreting these findings, was basic in improving his self-image.

Children brain injured prenatally, at birth, or up to about the age of 2 years or less constitute a subgroup of developmental dyslexics. Numerous studies have appeared for the past 70 years relating perinatal events as precursors of learning and reading disabilities. Balow, Rubin, and Rosen (1975–1976) have reviewed more than 30 of these studies and conclude that "it is most probable that some neurologic function or functions mediate between perinatal factors and later reading ability." They point out wisely that abnormal perinatal conditions are likely to have only a long-term impairing effect to the extent that they have permanently damaged neurological functioning. This effect can explain why many premature babies or infants suffering anoxia at birth have no learning problems; presumably their perinatal discomfort was temporary enough not to result in a neurological insult.

When the injuries are severe and bilateral, as they were in the cases of Max and Robbie, the reading retardation is permanent and only partially responsive to therapeutic teaching. Probably many children with chronically severe reading difficulties have had early brain injury or some obscure genetic anomaly (Lubs et al., 1991) that interferes with normal reading. At present, the best diagnostic and remedial approach to the treatment of these children is to discover as much as one can about the child's perceptual, intellectual, motor, cross-modal, sequential, and sensorimotor skills. Ideally the school psychologist should be equipped to do this and to supply this detailed information to the teacher, who, in collaboration with the psychologist, develops a tentative remedial program. Such a program is always tentative, contingent on regular and ongoing evaluations of its effectiveness.

Secondary Reading Retardation

This category includes children of average or superior intelligence level; normal sensory, motor, and cognitive abilities; a normal and healthy central nervous system; and no genetic defects, but who are underachieving in reading and academic learning. When tests have removed the possibility of any seriously impeding organic causes, then the logical origin would seem to be psychological and environmental determinants. What are the family pattern, sibling relationships, parental attitudes, the subcultural view of reading (lazy, effeminate, second or third rate), and television viewing habits? The etiology of this type of reading retardation is primarily psychological and social, and skilled methods of behavior management coupled with proven methods of teaching reading usually are all that are needed to correct the problem.

Behavior-modification techniques, of course, can also be successful with the child with brain damage and/or a specific reading disability, but a careful neuropsychological analysis is needed first to help in devising a prescription for teaching. This analysis can help to provide a more effective learning climate for the child and reduce the chances of frustration by trying to reinforce a type of behavior that may be impossible or difficult for the child.

Mrs. Semmes was referred to our laboratory because she was unable to read. At 31, she was happily married with two young children but constantly frustrated by her problem. A neurological examination was completely normal, and neuropsychological study revealed average intelligence with no defects in perception, motor, sensorimotor integration, sequencing, or oral language.

The story of her childhood read like something out of Dickens. She was orphaned at the age of 5 years and placed in a residential school operated by a religious order of women. Finding her a bright and active child, they soon had her working all day, washing floors or windows or doing whatever had to be done. She was a strong girl and evidently considered more useful on the housecleaning staff than in school; and because she had no family to defend her rights she was never sent to class. This treatment continued until she was 16 years old, when she ran away and married, to escape her unhappy life. This first marriage did not survive long, but by the time she was 22 she married Mr. Semmes, who provided a stable and happy marriage.

At the age of 31 she heard of the experimental program in our laboratory and sought help. She was put on a remedial program that employed visual, auditory, tactile, and motor association and reinforcement. Within a month she was able to read a large number of words on the Dolch lists and was excited because she could now read street and traffic signs. By the end of 3 months she could read at a grade 5 level and could spell about 200 words with a fairly strong level of assurance.

This case is the classic Cinderella story, and her dyslexia was purely the result of educational neglect. Our own studies, although covering short training periods so far, have shown that many non–brain-damaged adults, when strongly motivated, can be taught to read at a rate of 1 year's progress for each month of training. How permanent the results are will not be known without further training and evaluation.

Individual Studies of Dyslexia: What Do They Teach Us?

So far in this chapter we have examined individual cases of children and adults who have suffered unusual reading problems. The reader may find some of these cases interesting as case histories but still feel no closer to a confident diagnostic and remedial approach. To clarify a neuropsychological model of dyslexia, the following summary of neuropsychological signs is proposed.

A Neuropsychological Analysis of Dyslexia

The reading circuits in the brain are extremely complex, including specific centers usually in the left-hemispheric cortex with thalamic connections to other subcortical areas. There are probably as many types of dyslexia as there are loci of cerebral lesions in this circuit and its contiguous brain tissue. Figure 8.10 is a simplified diagram showing the cortical areas of the left hemisphere that are strongly involved in mediating reading, spelling, and writing. Following are the various processes involved in reading, with their cerebral functional correlates.

Visual Letter and Word Recognition. Lesions in the left occipital–parietal cortices and the splenium may produce a visual agnosia that results in literal dyslexia or an inability to recognize individual letters and to associate their linguistic meanings (Benson and Geschwind, 1969; Geschwind, 1962; Luria, 1970, 1973). The term used for verbal dyslexia has been "word blindness" since before the turn of this century, but Orton (1937) correctly pointed out that the term "is somewhat misleading since the (alexic) individual . . . can still see the word but the grasp at sight of the meaning of the word is gone."

Visual Searching and Scanning. Visual searching and scanning, so essential to normal reading, can be impaired by lesions in the right parieto–occipital region (Karpov, Luria, & Yarbuss, 1968) and in the dorsolateral areas of the frontal lobes (Calvin & Ojemann, 1980; Luria, 1973).

Figure–Ground Perception. Necessary for letter and word re-cognition, figure–ground perception may be disrupted by cortical lesions anywhere in the cortex (Teuber & Weinstein, 1956) or in the frontal lobes, in particular (Luria, 1973). Although figure–ground perception of pictorial material has long been known to be inferior in brain-damaged children and adults (Cruickshank, Bice, Wallen, & Lynch, 1957; Strauss & Lehtinen, 1947; Werner &

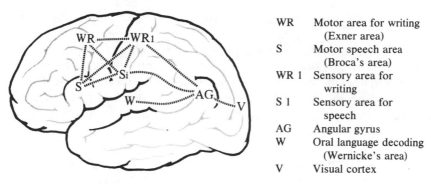

WR	Motor area for writing (Exner area)
S	Motor speech area (Broca's area)
WR 1	Sensory area for writing
S 1	Sensory area for speech
AG	Angular gyrus
W	Oral language decoding (Wernicke's area)
V	Visual cortex

Figure 8.10. Cortical reading, spelling, and writing circuits of the left hemisphere (simplified). (© 1984 William D. West) This is the classical view of the language centers in the cerebral cortex; it does not recognize the variability among human subjects (see discussion on pp. 310–313). Therefore it cannot be accepted as valid for every case.

Strauss, 1941), visual agnosia for letters while other vision remains normal attracted little attention until Orton (1937), Geschwind (1962), Johnson and Myklebust (1967), Myklebust (1967a, 1971a, 1975a), Luria (1970, 1973), and many others began to report significant research studies in this field. Because letters and words must be perceived against a background of writing or print, the same perceptual function seems to be involved, although the cognition of pictures and of letters stresses opposite hemispheres.

Visual Sequential Perception. Essential to the reading process visual sequential perception (Gaddes, 1982; Gaddes & Spellacy, 1977; Leong, 1975; Pavlidis, 1986) is interrupted with lesions to the left frontal lobe or the left motor strip (Luria, 1973).

Phonetic Auditory Discrimination. A child with auditory imperception may be suffering from some degree of peripheral deafness (a lesion or dysfunction located somewhere between the eardrum and the medial geniculate body), or some degree of central deafness (a lesion or dysfunction in the dominant Heschl's gyrus or Wernicke's area). Frequently, a child may have normal perception of pure tones on an audiometric test (Heschl's gyri are functioning normally) but he cannot discriminate "deer" and "dare" when presented auditorially on a tape recorder (possible evidence of a lesion or dysfunction in Wernicke's area). Luria has described this phenomenon clearly: "in local lesions of the secondary zones of the left temporal lobe in man [i.e., the Wernicke area] the ability to distinguish clearly between the sounds of speech is lost" (Luria,

1973). The reader will recognize this as a basic causal factor in sensory or receptive aphasia.

Most reading involves some degree of recoding from the visual to the auditory modality. Any receptive aphasic impairment in comprehension at the individual word level is likely to result in a corresponding difficulty in reading. Indeed, Wernicke (receptive) aphasic patients usually show similar difficulties in reading as in auditory comprehension.

Auditory Memory. As has already been discussed, standardized sentence-repetition tests can be used to detect a defect in a child's short-term memory. Left temporal lesions can produce it (Luria, 1973). Short-term verbal memory can be disturbed by electrical stimulation at various sites in fronto–parieto–temporal cortex of the left hemisphere (Ojemann, 1983).

To avoid confusion, it should be noted that a sentence-repetition test, as well as being sensitive to conduction aphasia (see pp. 318– 319) is also a test of memory. In fact, Spreen and Benton call their Sentence Repetition Test the Sentence Memory Test, and they have found that it shows a significant correlation with the memory quotient (MQ) of the Wechsler Memory Scale of .377 (Spreen & Strauss, 1991, 177–183).

Auditory–Verbal Understanding. Luria (1973) has described clearly the process of auditory perception of a sentence, followed by a simultaneous survey of the words, ordering them into a logical scheme, and extracting the meaning. As sentences proceed from simple subject–verb forms to complex logical–grammatical relationships, the demand on this ability increases. Following oral instructions that become more and more complex is an example of this ability, which is impaired by generalized dysfunctions in the left temporal, parietal, and occipital areas. The Token Test designed by DeRenzi and Vignolo (1962), is a useful clinical test for measuring this ability in aphasically impaired adults (Spellacy & Spreen, 1969; Spreen & Benton, 1969/1977), in normal children up to the age of 10 years (Gaddes & Crockett, 1975), and in language-impaired children of any age.

Understanding oral speech depends on a number of prerequisite skills. Some children and adults of normal or above-average intelligence are unable to process rapidly presented nonverbal tones (Lowe & Campbell, 1965; Tallal & Piercy, 1973a). They also have difficulty in decoding certain subtle phonological cues (Tallal & Stark, 1983) and organizing rapidly incoming linguistic concepts systematically. Certain LD children may be able to cope with classroom demands if the teacher will slow the tempo of oral delivery when giving instructions. See the case of Derrick White in the addendum at the end of this chapter.

In narrative comprehension the listener constructs a mental model of the situation being described, which will include descriptions of the people involved and a mental map of the spatial setting in which the action occurs (Bower & Morrow, 1990). Although LD students are less able than their average-achieving classmates in detecting inconsistencies and other subtle features in a written story, their comprehension can be improved if cued to look for these inconsistencies prior to beginning reading (Bos & Van Reusen, 1991). Experienced teachers and lecturers know that the same practices assist the student in listening to an oral explanation or lecture. The speaker must help the listener with cues to what is being said.

Auditory Sequential Skills. It is artificial but analytically useful to extricate the sequencing abilities, because they are an essential part of auditory–verbal understanding. Examining auditory receptive and auditory expressive processes in children suggests that the auditory sequencing skills, subordinate to the visual sequencing skills in grades 1 and 2, increase in importance so that by grade 5, visual and auditory expressive skills seem to dominate the reading processes in both sense modes (Gaddes, 1982; Gaddes & Spellacy, 1977).

Repetitive Speech. Because oral reading requires a repetition of verbal concepts originating from an extrapersonal source, the simple ability to repeat words may be a very small aspect of the complex reading process. A child with a minimal conduction aphasia may be impeded in learning to read. A standardized articulation test can measure this ability, although it is useful to watch for competent imitation on the the test coupled with inferior articulation during spontaneous speech. It is possible this ambivalent association is a sign of a mild expressive aphasia. The Spreen–Benton Articulation Test is useful for measuring 6-, 7-, and 8-year-olds (Gaddes & Crockett, 1975). Difficulty in articulation so that literal paraphasias are produced may result from lesions in the left inferior sensory strip (Luria, 1973). Any good sentence-repetition test is useful here; the Spreen–Benton Test has the advantage of normative data for children (Gaddes & Crockett, 1975) and for adults (Spreen & Benton, 1969/1977).

Mattis, French, and Rapin (1975), in a study of 82 carefully selected dyslexic children, found that almost half of the developmental dyslexics in the study (i.e., 48%) suffered from problems of articulation and poor visual–motor skills. This was their major deficit; language problems affected 28% of this group and visual–spatial deficits only 14%. Because the mean age of these children was between 11 and 12 years, the findings of Mattis and his colleagues support the evidence of the increased importance of *expressive*-motor processes after 5 years of school over receptive-perceptual ones in reading.

Word Fluency. The ability to recite the letters of the alphabet (Satz, Taylor, Friel, & Fletcher, 1978) and to produce words fluently usually correlate positively with reading ability. Tests of word fluency and sentence construction can be useful in evaluating this skill (Gaddes & Crockett, 1973).

Right–Left Orientation. A number of researchers have reported a conclusive relationship between directional confusion and reading retardation (Benton, 1958, 1959) and the Benton Right–Left Discrimination Test has been found to discriminate good and poor readers (Hundleby, 1969). The lambchop test of direction sense is also useful for investigating this condition (Bannatyne, 1971, p. 626; Silver & Hagin, 1975; Wechsler & Hagin, 1964). Bilateral parietal lesions will usually produce a directional deficit (see the case of Donald, Chapter 6).

Tactile Sensitivity. There is considerable evidence that the sensory and motor areas of the cortex are among the first to be myelinated, and in that sense they are neurologically older than most of the rest of the brain. It seems highly likely that this is a major contributing factor to the fact that the infant's first learning is sensorimotor (Piaget & Inhelder, 1956; Phillips, 1975). Many educators consider tactile learning "primitive" and hence particularly potent in reinforcing cross-modal skills. For this reason it is useful to know whether the input mechanisms for sensorimotor activity are functioning normally, and to find this out, a test of tactile sensitivity can be useful: to do this an esthesiometer may be used. This instrument is a series of plastic rods, each equipped with a nylon hair of decreasing diameter. The nylon hairs are applied to the subject's fingers or palm in order of size, using a method of ascending and descending stimulation. In this way the threshold of tactile sensitivity may be measured for each hand. Norms for children are available (Spreen & Gaddes, 1969) and a deficit in one hand can indicate possible dysfunction in the contralateral sensory strip, the parietal lobe, or the sensorimotor area. A deficit in the right hand frequently is associated with poor reading because both draw on the left parietal cortex (see the case of Mr. Simmons, p. 360).

Tactile Form Recognition (Stereognosis). Clinical tests of stereognosis are believed to draw strongly on the sensory and motor strips mainly on the side contralateral to the exploring hand (Reitan, 1959). Because sensory and motor processes are reciprocal and interacting, "they are expressed in the single word *sensorimotor* and cannot be considered separately in analyzing the problems of the learning disabled child" (Ayres, 1975). Numerous educators stress the importance of sensorimotor development in their remedial prescriptions (Ayres, 1975; Bannatyne, 1971; Barsch, 1967; Beery, 1967; Cratty & Martin, 1969; Frostig & Maslow, 1970; Kephart, 1966) and experimental investigation has indicated markedly improved scores on word recognition and oral reading by those LD children receiving remedial activity designed to enhance specific types of sensory integration (Ayres, 1972b). These activities have included proprioceptive, vestibular, tactile, thermal, somatosensory stimulation, and motor activity. The Benton Stereognosis Test is a useful and inexpensive test for exploring visual–motor integration in children, and normative data are available for children aged 8–15 years (Spreen & Gaddes, 1969).

Finger Localization. Awareness of which finger has been touched, both when the subject can see the finger being touched and when a screen obscures the view, is mediated by the sensorimotor strips and the contiguous parietal cortices on the contralateral side. Studies of finger localization in mentally defective, in brain-injured, and in normal children have shown the first two groups to be inferior to normals (Benton, 1959). However, a subject's impairment in this perceptual skill appears to be related to the locus of the cerebral damage. Some mental defectives may achieve perfect scores on a finger-localization test (Strauss & Werner, 1938) and we have seen dozens of cases of localized brain-damaged children with no deficit in this area. This result seems to imply that in these cases the sensorimotor and parietal areas essential to this skill have been spared.

In our own clinical analysis of LD children and adults we have found a frequent correlation between retarded reading and defective finger localization in both hands or, particularly, the right hand (Mr. Simmons is an example, p. 360). Because reading and finger localization of the right hand draw primarily on left parietal function, a dysfunction in this area can affect both behavioral skills. It is highly significant that in a 6-year longitudinal study of 442 children from kindergarten to grade 5, Satz and his colleagues found the finger-localization test to have the best predictive value for competence in reading of any test in a large battery (Satz, Taylor, Friel, & Fletcher, 1978). More is said about this important study later in this chapter.

Visual–Manual Reaction Time. When a subject is asked to watch a signal light and to press a telegrapher's key as fast as possible following the appearance of the light, it seems certain, from knowledge of clinical neurology, that a large circuit is involved in the brain. The right-handed person sees the light, and the neural impulses travel along the optic nerves and tracts and through the thalamic level of the brainstem to the occipital cortices. The situation is recognized and responded to by presumably large cortical areas, the "decision" is concentrated on the manual area of the left motor strip, and the right hand is stimulated to press the key. A test that activates so many areas of the brain is likely to be more sensitive to random cerebral dysfunction. For this reason, a visual–manual reaction-time test has been used for many years to examine both brain-damaged and mentally retarded subjects. Brain-injured subjects have been found to be significantly slower than normal controls for both simple and choice reaction time tasks (Benton & Blackburn, 1957). When brain-injured subjects with unilateral lesions were studied, their reaction times for *both* hands were slower than normal, but the hand contralateral to the lesion was the more impaired.

Because of the complexity of neural involvement and the certain activity of the posterior cortices, the chances are increased that the child with slow visual–manual reaction times is also suffering from brain damage or dysfunctions in parts other than the immediate visual–manual circuit described above. If that is so, and the left parietal lobe is involved, the child may be suffering from some of the Gerstmann signs, which could be part of a larger syndrome that could include receptive aphasia or dyslexia (Benton, 1977).

Normative data for visual–manual reaction times are available for children aged 6–12 years (Spreen & Gaddes, 1969), and they are useful for providing evidence that indicates chronic brain dysfunctions producing a continuing impairment to normal reading.

Auditory–Manual Reaction Time. One may use an apparatus with earphones in which an auditory signal is given to each ear singly. It is then possible to ask the subject to press the telegrapher's key with his right hand or left hand in response to a tone in the right or left ear. This produces reaction times from six different sensorimotor combinations: (1) right ear–right hand, (2) right ear–left hand, (3) left ear–right hand, (4) left ear–left hand, (5) both ears–right hand, and (6) both ears–left hand. It is interesting that the average reaction times for normal adults on this test are about 75 milliseconds faster than for the visual–manual reaction time test. No doubt this is because of the much shorter cerebral circuit. The auditory stimulus is picked up in the ear drum and has to travel to the temporal lobes. By comparison with the visual circuit described above, the auditory–manual circuit is about half the length or less.

There are no data relating reading retardation with poor performance on this test, but diagnostic knowledge from it can help to understand the cerebral functioning of a child or adult. For example, a right-handed subject with left-hemisphere dominance for language and normal hearing would be expected to have the fastest reaction time to the right ear–right hand combination, or to the both ears–right hand pattern. The subject who does not may be suffering from a left-hemisphere lesion or dysfunction that may be related to the retarded reading.

Hand-Grip Strength. Normative hand-grip strength data for children aged 6–12 years are available (Spreen & Gaddes, 1969) and are useful for indicating the presence of nonlocalized brain damage or dysfunction. Clinical experience has shown that large numbers of traumatically brain-damaged adults, especially when the brainstem is injured, do poorly on this test regardless of their muscular development.

Lateral Preferences. In Chapter 6 the problems of cerebral dominance and handedness were discussed at some length. At this point, it is sufficient to observe that when there is a conflict between manifest handedness and cerebral dominance there is usually, but not always, a reading problem. There are more reading problems among left-handers, but when they are competent readers it may be that they are "pure" left-handers (i.e., genetically intended to be left-handed and right-hemisphere dominant for language), or that they are partially bilateral for language, or that they compensate with a superior intellect, or that the lesion producing the left-handedness is outside the language areas. The school psychologist needs to know the dominance–handedness pattern, and with detailed neuropsychological data he or she can describe the unique cerebral pattern and prescribe a remedial program in collaboration with the special teacher. Each case is different and needs to be understood on the basis of its own evidence.

Sequencing. We have already referred to visual and auditory sequencing and their relation to reading and assisting in localizing a brain lesion. However, sequencing in its relation to reading is much more comprehensive. Bakker (1972), a neuropsychologist in Amsterdam, carried out an exhaustive developmental study on more than 400 Dutch children aged 6–8. He recognized four types of serial-order behavior: (1) verbally imitating (i.e., receptive or perceptual), (2) nonverbally imitating, (3) verbally expressive, and (4) nonverbally expressive. He examined temporal sequences in these four categories and three sensory modes—visual, auditory, and haptic. He found that temporal-order ability was clearly related to age and that girls at ages 6 and 7 were superior to boys. Between 7 and 8 years, girls were almost equally good in sequential recall tasks in all three sense modes; by 8 and until 11 their haptic sequencing fell off and they emphasized visual and auditory sequencing. Girls showed a superiority in recalling temporal sequences when all three sense modalities were grouped, but from age 9 to 11, boys matched their performance exactly. Bakker concluded that "the temporal perception of verbal and of verbal codifiable stimuli is mediated by the language hemisphere" (i.e., the left hemisphere in most people).

As explained earlier in this chapter, the faster the speed of presentation of tests of both verbal and nonverbal stimuli, the more sensitive they are to impaired sequential processing. This has been discussed in some detail elsewhere (Gaddes, 1982).

Cross-Modal Integration. In Chapter 2 we presented Luria's classical model of lobular brain function. The reader will remember that these functional areas include (1) the primary or projection areas of the cortex, which contain neurons that are highly specific and react to visual, auditory, and tactile stimuli; (2) the secondary or association areas, which are contiguous to the primary areas, and provide a synthetic function leading to an understanding of the perceived stimulus in a particular sense mode; and (3) the tertiary zones, or "the zones of overlapping of the cortical ends of the various analysers," as Luria (1973) called them.

As an illustration, the sounds of oral speech are recorded in Heschl's gyrus of the left temporal lobe (primary area); these sounds are decoded in the auditory speech analyzer, called Wernicke's area (secondary area), and it is related to visual input in the occipital lobes by way of the angular gyrus (tertiary area).

Geschwind has clarified the importance of the interconnections in the human brain among the three basic perceptual and motor areas and credits this cortical association with our ability to acquire speech. In subhuman animals each sensory area is largely connected to the subcortical limbic system; the visual, auditory, and tactile cortices have few transcortical interconnections. In humans, however, the left parietal cortex is a vigorous and flexible association center, connecting the primary, secondary, and motor areas. "In man, with the introduction of the angular gyrus region, intermodal associations become powerful" (Geschwind, 1965). Because animals other than man have no arcuate fasciculus they have very limited oral communication, and because their intermodal associations are weak by comparison with humans, their conceptual language is limited and their reading ability almost nonexistent. "The ability to acquire speech has as a prerequisite the ability to form cross-modal associations" (Geschwind, 1965).

The probable function of the angular gyrus in reading has already been explained (Geschwind, 1962, 1965; Orton, 1937). Neural associative dysfunctions always impair learning. For this reason, a LD child may score normally on individual tests of visual, auditory, and tactile perception, but if he or she cannot switch quickly from one to another of these, this may be the key to the disability and the index to its remediation. The importance of intersensory perceptual functioning in the learning of children has been recognized for a long time (Ayres, 1972a; Birch, 1964; Johnson & Myklebust, 1967; Myklebust, 1971a; Myklebust & Brutten, 1953) and its malfunctioning as a sensitive indicator of cerebral cortical damage and/or dysfunction (Myklebust, 1963).

Neuropsychological knowledge can direct us to the various possible causes of dyslexia. As already indicated, there are probably as many types of reading impairment as there are loci of brain lesions, but most studies suggest that behaviorally they may include abnormal language development and competence, impaired perceptual skills (in all three sense modes), poor motor-expressive abilities, disturbed sensorimotor integration, faulty sequencing, and mixed cerebral dominance and lateral preferences.

A neurological approach by itself is not enough, however, the educational neuropsychologist is only one member of a diagnostic team that may include the child's teacher, a neurologist, and, where appropriate, a neurosurgeon, a pediatrician, a social worker, and a speech therapist. It is unlikely that these people will always find it convenient to meet as a group, but detailed reports from all of them should be provided for the child's file, and a social history will be supplied by the parents. Because remediation is a psychoeducational process, all relevant information should be directed toward that goal.

Developmental Aspects of Reading

One of the major longitudinal studies of reading was done by Satz and his colleagues (Satz, Taylor, Friel, & Fletcher, 1978). They followed 442 boys from kindergarten through grade 5. Of many tests administered early in the kindergarten year, five showed themselves to be powerful predictors of reading problems for the next 6 years. These were (1) finger localization, (2) visual recognition–discrimination, (3) Beery Visual–Motor Integration Test, (4) alphabet recitation, and (5) the Peabody Picture Vocabulary Test. Initially the children were divided into four criterion reading groups using a discriminant function analysis computed on classroom reading level. This analysis provided the following groupings: (1) severely retarded, (2) mildly retarded, (3) average, and (4) superior. By combining the first two groups, it was evident that 120 children, or 26% of the kindergarten children, were retarded in reading readiness. By the end of grade 2, reading achievement tests showed agreement with the initial measures at the beginning of kindergarten of 89% of the severely retarded group and 94% of the superior group. This evidence indicates that in Satz's large sample, most of the superior readers were still in the top category and most of the severely retarded readers had not improved. In fact, there were now 144 children or 34% falling in the reading disability group. A few children from both extreme groups moved toward the center, but most did not. By the end of grade 5, of the 49 severely retarded readers in grade 2, 3 improved to the average group and 6 improved to the mildly retarded group, but 30% of the average readers were now retarded. Of the 62 mildly impaired readers in grade 2, 3 improved to superior readers by the end of grade 5, 8 improved to average, and 24 deteriorated to the severely retarded group. This assessment showed almost no improvement in the problem readers (severe and mild) between grades 2 and 5, and a 30% chance that average readers in grade 2 would decline to become problem readers by grade 5. The initial tests predicted the superior readers accurately, in that 97% of them continued to be reading at grade level or above at the end of grade 5.

Satz, Taylor, Friel, and Fletcher concluded, "these findings, while generally discouraging for children having reading problems in early grades, are compatible with four recent longitudinal follow-up studies using generally smaller samples" (Muehl & Forell, 1973; Rourke & Orr, 1977; Trites & Fiedorowicz, 1976; Yule & Rutter, 1976). These data showed a steady increase in the incidence of both the severe and mild groups from the beginning of kindergarten to the end of grade 5. The increases were most marked during the first year (kindergarten) and the last (grade 5).

Another longitudinal study covering the 6-year period from kindergarten to grade 5 was carried out by Spreen (1978). It differs from Satz's study in that it included more children ($n = 1282$) but fewer predictor tests ($n = 4$). The four tests included the Peabody Picture Vocabulary Test (Dunn, 1965), the Revised Visual Retention Test (Benton, 1963b), the Coloured Progressive Matrices (Raven, 1965), and the teacher's five-point rating scale to predict the future reading ability of each child. Achievement tests in reading, writing, arithmetic, science, and social studies made up the criterion variables. Spreen found the best predictors were the PPVT and the Benton VRT; he reported an accuracy of prediction rate ranging from 63% to 86%.

In a later study, Fletcher, Satz & Scholes (1981), found some additional evidence for developmental changes in linguistic performance correlates of reading achievement. They took measures of morphological knowledge (word segmentation), semantic encoding (retrieving a word from the semantic memory system and bringing meaning to it), and syntactic comprehension (recognizing whether the meaning of a sentence is the same or different when its grammatical structure is altered) of reading disabled (RD) and matched controls (C) at ages 5.5, 8.5, and 11 years. They found performance differences were age dependent on some of the language measures but not all. Word fluency was about the same for the two groups (C and RD) at age 5.5 and increased with age for both groups at 8.5 and 11, but the difference between groups was not significant until age 11. The morphological measures showed significant differences across ages and between groups, but there was no interaction between age and group. The syntactic comprehension measures showed increased scores with age for both groups, but the two reading groups differed significantly only at age 11, although not all disabled readers in this older group had difficulty with the syntactic problems.

More recently (1988), Spreen reported on a 15-year follow-up study of 191 young adults (median age almost 25 years). These young people had been assessed in our laboratory originally at the age of about 10 years. Spreen has reported a large body of data on neurological status, neuropsychological assessment, educational achievement, and personal and occupational adjustment. All measures were compared by categories 1, 2, 3, and 4 (see Table 1.1, p. 11). Spreen found that retarded readers at age 10 tended to be retarded readers at age 25. On the Peabody Individual Achievement Test (PIAT) Reading Comprehension, he found that the subjects in Category 1 (brain damaged; $n = 55$) were reading at a grade 8.0 level; Category 2 (MBD; $n = 59$) at grade 9.2; Category 3 (LD with no neurological signs; $n = 26$) at grade 9.8; and controls ($n = 51$) at grade 12.5.

Frauenheim and Heckerl (1983) followed 11 severe developmental dyslexics for about 17 years. At age 11 their mean verbal IQ was 84, and at mean age 27 (range 25–30) their mean VIQ was 85. Their mean performance IQs at these two ages were 105 and 104. Their reading-achievement scores showed a similar reliability. Their childhood grade level for reading at age 11 was 1.9; by mean age 27 it had increased to only 2.6. As adults, these dyslexic subjects still had severe deficits in associating sounds with symbols, they read at a painfully slow speed, and they still reversed some short words. The authors concluded: "Patterns of skill weaknesses and cognitive abilities, as measured by academic and psychological tests, have remained remarkably consistent over a period of approximately seventeen years" (p. 345).

These findings can be explained by a neurological model: the chronicity of both neural dysfunction and reading achievement, despite remedial teaching, are causally related. The increase in the incidence of reading retardation probably results from the inability of the dysfunctional brain to handle material that makes increasing demands in complexity and flexibility.

Although such evidence is discouraging in showing retarded readers likely to remain below average in reading skill, it in no way implies that remedial teaching is useless. That short-sighted view produced the adult dyslexia in the cases of Mrs. Semmes and Mr. Darwin and in numerous other adult dyslexics. Had their teachers understood that, as children, they needed the best remedial teaching, they would have been slow but competent readers now, and both would have avoided the personal frustrations and unhappy experiences that haunt the nonreader in our society.

Pragmatics

Pragmatics is the study of how language is used rather than, as in linguistics, how it is structured. Though it emphasizes the social use of language, it still covers the aspects of language structure that depend on the immediate social context (Prutting & Kirchner, 1987). A simple example may clarify this. A 10-year-old boy may use a different vocabulary and mental attitude and manner when he is talking to the school principal than when he is with his peer group. Pragmatics has developed as a product of both philosophy and linguistics, and its theories can be highly erudite and abstract. For our purposes we will look briefly at how it might be used in comparative analysis of the language of LD and non-LD (NLD) children.

A clinical discourse analysis (Damico, 1980; cited in McCord & Haynes, 1988) may be used to measure the various aspects of speech. These include, in condensed form: (1) Quantity of information—Did the speaker provide enough specific information for the listener to understand fully? (2) Relation of information—Is the subject of the discourse well organized, or does the speaker skip from point to point without adequate transitional cues? (3) Manner of information—Is speech production fluent or nonfluent? Does speaker answer questions well and quickly? Does speaker include others in the conversation? Using Damico's guidelines, McCord and Haynes (1988) found no significant differences between the LD and the NLD groups, but their findings suggest that some of both groups showed mild pragmatic deficits.

Some investigators have found that the conversational abilities of LD children provide less information, use shorter utterances, make more requests for information, and are less assertive and persuasive than NLD children (McCord & Haynes, 1988), but because there are limitations to free sampling of conversations in naturalistic settings, conclusions are mixed and tentative. In a review of 19 studies of pragmatic skills of LD children, Dudley-Marling (1985) concluded that "the evidence presented here, although sparse, does at least suggest that the communications of LD students are less likely to be as effective as their NLD peers."

Summary

It has been established for more than 100 years that traumatic damage to specific cortical and subcortical areas of the human cerebrum will result in alexia, or the inability to read (Déjerine, 1892). But the causes of developmental dyslexia are far from clear and possibly more complex. Most CT and MRI studies of developmental dyslexics have shown no detectable brain injury (Hynd et al., 1991b), and this suggests a possible genetic, developmental, or physiological dysfunction.

The past decade has seen considerable activity in producing psycholinguistic theories of reading and developing ingenious techniques for observing and studying the structure and function of the human brain. A number of comprehensive survey books on child neuropsychology have appeared (Obrzut & Hynd, 1986a,b, 1991; Reynolds & Fletcher-Janzen, 1989), which have covered the psychological processes in academic learning and the physiology of the brain. This trend is encouraging because such books include many of the best researchers in both fields, but in many of their chapters the authors discuss these topics quite separately. Where attempts have been made to relate them, many of the discussions are speculative, as they are in this book, and this bespeaks the difficulty of the whole study of human neuropsychology.

Although the new scanning techniques are encouraging, some limitations lie in their technology. If irregularities at a cellular level occur enough to disrupt reading, a CT scan may not reveal any structural irregularity because of the limitations of its resolution (Hynd & Semrud-Clikeman, 1989). In spite of such limitations the CT, MRI, PET, regional cerebral blood flow (rCBF), and topographic brain electrical activity mapping (BEAM) at present have the greatest promise in revealing the neuropsychological nature of both normal and disordered reading.

Clinical Addendum

Derrick White: A Case of Mild Receptive Aphasia

Derrick was 9 years 7 months old when first seen by a psychologist in private practice. A large battery of tests was administered and the psychologist reported that Derrick scored in the average to superior range on the sensorimotor tests and that he had difficulty with most of the verbal tests. On the Wechsler (WISC-R) he measured a verbal IQ of 96, a performance IQ of 90, and a full-scale IQ of 92.

Derrick was a healthy, pleasant boy, popular with his peers, and a better-than-average athlete. However, he had had difficulties with academic work from the beginning of grade 1. The teachers told his mother that Derrick had a learning disability, and for that reason she had sent him to the psychologist. However, the psychologist told her very little that she did not know already, and he provided no suggestions on what to do about Derrick's frustrations at school.

His mother then sent Derrick to see a pediatric neurologist, who found Derrick had normal hearing and no abnormalities on the formal neurological examination. He reported, "The general physical examination likewise was within normal limits." He referred Derrick to our laboratory for an assessment of his learning problems and a recommendation for remedial follow-up.

Education History

In kindergarten Derrick first showed signs of being upset. His parents were surprised and mildly alarmed because until then he had always been a happy and sunny little boy. The parents attributed it to their having moved in the middle of the kindergarten year and Derrick had to enter a new class in a different school at midyear.

In grade 1, however, he continued to be frustrated and unhappy, and his teacher reported that "his semantic skills are poor." In grade 2, Derrick was placed in a "learning assistance" class because his language skills, both reading and writing, were so poor. By the end of grade 2 he was much behind his peers and was being teased by them. In grade 3 he was the top scorer on his class's soccer team and was popular with his classmates on the playground, but with typical 9-year-old behavior they teased him unmercifully for being in the "dumb class." He begged his parents to get him out of the learning assistance class, so they hired a tutor who met Derrick twice a week for remedial help.

At the beginning of grade 4 the school agreed to put Derrick back into a regular class full time, but by late November he was falling behind and he was returned to the learning assistance class, which he hated. At the same time he was captain of the soccer team and was the best sprinter in his class. Physical education and art were his only successes in school. It was in this year that the parents sent him to the psychologist.

By the fall of his grade 5 year, Derrick was approaching a crisis. At home there were increasing episodes of frustration, bouts of tears, and begging to be freed from the special class. His mother in turn, was requesting additional homework so that between the extra time with his tutor, Derrick had almost no time to himself, and he was developing a strong hatred for school.

At this time the parents took Derrick to the pediatric neurologist. He recognized the presence of the learning disability and wisely analyzed the situation in which the boy found himself—a school setting that was unhappy for Derrick but in which the teachers casually minimized the seriousness of Derrick's learning problems, and his home, which was supportive but where his parents were obviously distressed by his learning problems and his poor achievement. The ambivalence of his peers added to Derrick's misery and resulted in model behavior at school and violent outbursts at home. The neurologist remarked in his report: "I think that this cannot go on much longer before there will be a breakdown." It was at this point that Derrick was referred to our laboratory.

Analysis of Derrick's Problem

In the spring of his grade 5 year we first saw Derrick, who by now was 11 years old. He was a well-spoken, personable boy, who was sociable and pleasant. The school had placed him every year for 5 years in a learning assistance class for part of the year. Obviously this was not working because Derrick was still having trouble with arithmetic, reading, spelling, and writing.

Because the neurological examination was clear it was evident that we were dealing with a Category 3 case (i.e., LD with no evidence of neurological deficit). We then subjected Derrick to a detailed battery of neuropsychological tests, academic achievement tests, and the full Spreen–Benton Aphasia Battery. The latter, along with some of the verbal memory tests, gave us the clue to the mystery of Derrick's learning and resulting behavior problems.

Test Results

On the sensorimotor tests (e.g., finger-tapping speed, reaction time, tactile sensitivity, hand-grip strength) Derrick's scores were all above average. This result was expected because of his good athletic abilities.

The Wechsler Test (WISC-R) gave him a verbal IQ of 101 and a performance IQ of 96, so we knew that he was at least mentally average. Two of his low scores (Digit Span and Picture Arrangement) are particularly vulnerable to anxiety, so it seemed very likely that his real mental potential under optimal conditions was above average.

The Peabody Individual Achievement Test (PIAT) showed Derrick not to be below grade level in reading. Because he was tested in March of his grade 5 year, any score at or above 5.6 was not below average. Derrick measured 5.6 on Word Recognition and 6.8 on Reading Comprehension. Other measures were below average: Mathematics, 4.9; Spelling, 4.1; and General Information, 4.7.

The memory tests and aphasia battery revealed the basis of Derrick's problems. He had difficulty following oral instructions, but when he understood clearly what was wanted, he frequently had a perfect score on most subtests. He was unable to process *auditory sequential language* at a fast speed. However, if we slowed our tempo of speech, he usually had no trouble.

Because of his strong desire to succeed, Derrick would give an answer based on what he *thought* was said. For example, when asked to construct a sentence with the words "drive—street—car", he misperceived the words and said, "There was a drive-in at McDonald's and there was an accident in the street." Note the paraphasia, "drive-in" for "drive," and the omission of "car." When he was advised to listen again to the three words and they were delivered at a slower pace, he produced a correct sentence.

On the memory tests he did well on Sentence Repetition, better than average in drawing geometric figures from memory, and very well remembering paired-associated nouns. These findings contraindicate a primary memory deficit and suggest that his problem is one of semantic and syntactic comprehension. When he was asked to listen to short stories and then report what he could remember, he produced gross distortions and paraphasic associations that rendered his scores inferior. After listening to a story of a ship that struck a mine, he described "a man who struck it rich" and an accurate fragment about people in lifeboats who were rescued. He made no attempt to relate the paraphasic phrase and the correct episode; he simply reported them.

Derrick's teacher early in grade 5 soon recognized that he would ask for her oral instructions to be repeated immediately after she had given them. Understandably, she found this irritating, and, crediting it to inattention, she refused to repeat her instructions. Had Derrick been too careless to give concentrated attention, the teacher's strategy might have encouraged him to learn to attend more accurately. But because he suffered from a minimal receptive aphasia, it simply had a devastating effect on his learning and his self-confidence, and he kept getting further behind.

In the tactile naming test he also produced some paraphasias, namely, an "egg-beater" for a "can opener." When he was asked what it was used for, he continued the distorted association by saying "to open cans." On the Boston Naming Test, he named pictures of common objects at a normal level for his age, but when we tried a few items above his age level and provided him with a phonetic cue, he produced a nonsense word (e.g., target word, "muzzle"; oral cue, "mŭ"; Derrick's response, "mout." (It is interesting to note that "mout" and "mouth" are phonologically close, and "muzzle" and "mouth" possess a semantic association.) It seems likely that Derrick produces many paralexias during his unsupervised reading (see the discussion of deep dyslexia earlier in this chapter).

Analysis of the Problem

Why, after 5 years in school, was Derrick's academic record so poor? Basically it was because no in-depth diagnostic examination had been done until the spring term of his grade 5 year. The school each year for 5 years had assigned him to a learning assistance class and this remedial program had been determined by *administrative decision* rather than on a diagnositc understanding of Derrick's cognitive structure and his learning strategies. This is not to dismiss administrative decisions completely. In most cases they need to be the *first* decision, but *no child should be left for 5 years in a program that is not working*. If it is not working within a very short time the child should be studied in depth and experimental teaching programs should be developed, based on the collected diagnostic knowledge. The results of the teaching procedures should be continually monitored and assessed and readjusted in terms of their success or failure.

Evidence from Derrick's Social Behavior

When Derrick's problem with processing oral instructions was explained, his father looked relieved. "That explains his confusion at lacrosse," he said. He explained that because Derrick was so successful in soccer, he had taken him this year with one of his friends to a lacrosse coach. At the first practice the coach explained the rules to the two boys and Derrick's father could see that Derrick looked more and more confused, but his friend followed the instructions with no difficulty. During play Derrick made several errors because he did not understand the rules. By the second practice a week later, the errors had diminished, and by the third practice Derrick had a complete understanding and was a valuable member of the team. When we saw him 6 months later he was the established top scorer and a valuable player.

Remedial Program

Derrick's basic learning problem is a slowness in processing large quantities of sequential material, especially oral material. Instructions should be presented (1) at a slower tempo, and (2) in bits or single ideas.

His tutor, with this knowledge, organized a detailed program of remedial measures in arithmetic, reading, and spelling, drawing on multisensorimotor exercises and multiple activities to improve his language development.

A follow-up one year later in April of his grade 6 year showed steady improvement for Derrick. His grade 6 teacher was keen and interested, and was aware of Derrick's learning problem. The mild aphasic tendency to confuse oral messages is a constant handicap, but Derrick compensates by doing well in written work that he can prepare in advance. It is possible that he may have to tape some lessons when he enters junior high school. This technique will give

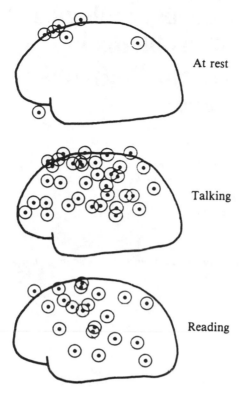

At rest

Talking

Reading

Figure 8.11. Language functions and regional cerebral blood flow were first studied in 1974 by Ingvar and Schwartz in Sweden, using the intraarterial rCBF 133 Xenon clearance method (pp. 75 & 346). Their findings during rest, talking, and reading are shown. Only peaks more than 25% above the mean hemisphere flow are indicated. (After Ingvar & Schwartz, 1974. With permission of the authors and Oxford University Press.)

Derrick the opportunity to replay and repeat some lessons as they become conceptually more complex. He now understands that he is not stupid and his attitude toward himself has improved markedly in the past year (see Fig. 8.11).

9 The Neuropsychological Basis of Problems in Writing, Spelling, and Arithmetic

Man's language systems, the auditory and the written, develop sequentially according to a pattern determined phylogenetically and ontogenetically, neurologically and psychologically.

Helmer R. Myklebust (1965)

The indispensable instrument of the writer is not so much the pen as the left cerebral hemisphere.

Oliver L. Zangwill (1976)

In this chapter we discuss the processes of writing and spelling as the logical sequence to the discussion in Chapter 8 of reading and reading problems, because a child who "has difficulty in the comprehension and use of spoken or read language . . . will probably have difficulty learning to use written language" (Chalfant & Scheffelin, 1969). The reader will remember that according to Myklebust's developmental hierarchy of language skills, written language is the last to be acquired and is only learned normally if all of the preceding stages have been successfully established. Not only is writing the last language function to be acquired, but it is practiced and used least, even by highly educated people. This may account for its being the first language skill to suffer following any type of diffuse brain damage or deterioration. It is a common observation that many elderly people lose their ability to write letters while still retaining the competence for normal simple conversation.

Arithmetic, though primarily concerned with quantitative concepts and their interrelations, also depends on verbal understanding and communication, although on a comprehensive battery of neuropsychological tests, the skills necessary for success in arithmetic and in language show significantly different patterns (Rourke & Finlayson, 1978). But let us look first at writing and spelling.

D.W. Reed (1970) has pointed out that whereas speech in some form is probably more than a half-million years old, writing is only about 5000 years old. Although all present human societies have oral languages, many still have no system of writing, and in our own society all normal adults are able to speak, but only a very few can write with the same level of competence.

Although oral speech is normally acquired spontaneously and without conscious effort, the ability to communicate by writing not only comes later but as the result of conscious effort and intensive study. "From the very beginning written speech is a voluntary, organized activity with the conscious analysis of its constituent sounds" (Luria, 1966).

The Process of Writing

Learning to read and to write differ because they depend on different psychological and neurological processes. Whereas reading is a perceptual–cognitive process that begins with visual stimuli in the *outside* environment and ends with a meaningful interpretation of those stimuli within the cerebral cortex, by contrast, writing begins with an idea and an intent to communicate that originates *within* the brain and ends with a psychomotor act (writing) that leaves a tangible record (the written message) in the outside environment. In a simplistic sense, reading and writing are reverse neuropsychological processes.

Learning to write involves integrating both sensorimotor and cognitive–linguistic functions, and different forms of agraphia may occur, "each resulting from breakdown at a different level within one of the several neuropsychological systems upon which symbolic expressions depend" (Marcie & Hécaen, 1979). These systems include the perceptual (visual, auditory, and tactile–kinesthetic), motor, and cognitive–linguistic. These same writers have categorized the agraphias in the following clinical subgroups: (1) those associated with aphasias; (2) those associated with severe reading disability; (3) "pure" agraphia with no other language impairment, which may be a result of impaired phonemic hearing (Luria, 1973) or a widespread acute cerebral disorder such as acute confusional states (Chedru & Geschwind, 1972); (4) apraxic agraphia, where a disturbance of normal neuromuscular patterns interferes with the writing process (actual cases of agraphia resulting from traumatic brain damage appear later in this chapter); and (5) spatial disorders in writing (inability to align letters and orient the lines properly). An analysis of these groupings shows that they tend to fall into two broad types: (1) the apraxic agraphias with little or no linguistic disorder, and (2) the agraphias with a marked degree of language disturbance.

Neurological Determinants of Writing. The neuromuscular patterns in normal writing originate in visual, auditory, tactile–kinesthetic, and linguistic images in the human cortex that stimulate the motor area where manual–motor images are aroused. These are conveyed to the writing hand in a delicate blending of visual–, auditory–, tactile–, and kinesthetic–linguistic processes. Dysfunction at any point or points in this neuropsychological structure may result in impaired writing ability. Such disruption in the involved neural pathways may result in (1) motor impairment (e.g., tremor, letters clumsily drawn, letters overlapped or not linked, absence of loops, reduplication of strokes, micrographia, etc.); (2) spatial disorders (poor alignment of letters, crowding of words, omitting a margin, orienting the lines upward or downward, etc.); (3) syntactical disorders (agrammatic written answers, following instructions to write answers in *full* sentences, in the presence of grammatically normal oral expression); and (4) reluctance to write (Chedru & Geschwind, 1972).

Let us look at a case of this type, seen in our laboratory, in which writing was altered but not severely impaired by traumatic brain damage, and with no signs of aphasia. Following a head injury from a traffic accident, Mrs. Galloway was seen for neuropsychological assessment. She was 34 years old at the time of testing, which was 2 years after the accident. Her brain injuries affected the left frontal part of her brain and her cerebellum, so that she was very unsteady on her feet and her speech was slurred. Her articulation was so impaired that naive observers were likely to interpret her as mentally retarded. In fact her verbal intelligence measured better than about 77% of other adults, so that Mrs. Galloway found this most frustrating.

Her spoken speech was severely dysarthric (inarticulate) but her verbal organization was normal. Her pretraumatic writing was small and neat (Fig. 9.1) but the brain injury had resulted in her writing being larger (Fig. 9.2) and she now needed lined paper to guide her, although her writing was still neat and its contents well organized.

Summary. Agraphia in traumatically brain-damaged adults may result from lesions or dysfunctions in (1) Wernicke's area or contiguous parts of the left temporal lobe, (2) the occipital lobes or the left parieto–occipital area, (3) the motor strip or premotor

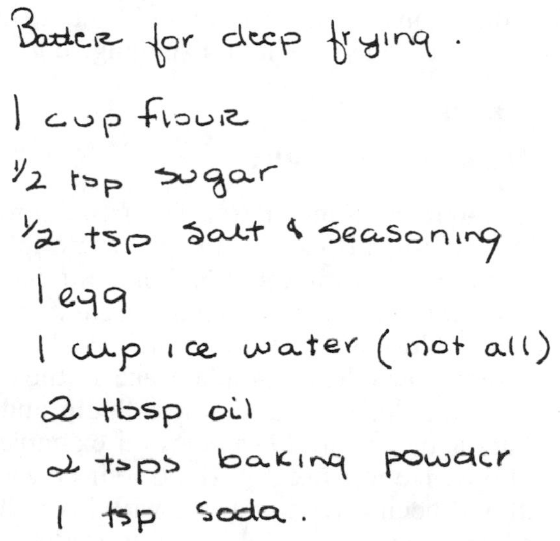

Batter for deep frying.

1 cup flour

½ tsp sugar

½ tsp salt & seasoning

1 egg

1 cup ice water (not all)

2 tbsp oil

2 tsps baking powder

1 tsp soda.

Figure 9.1. Sample of Mrs. Galloway's writing prior to her head injury.

area, or (4) the left sensory strip or the left parietal lobe. No one
has written in as much clinical detail as Luria on the neuropsychology
of agraphia, and his clinical studies have led him to believe that:
(1) Lesions in the left temporal lobe impede subjects in writing to
dictation, although they can still write overlearned motor stereotypes
such as their own signatures (Luria, 1973); (2) lesions in the two
occipital lobes or in the left parieto–occipital lobes result in an
inability to write either to copy or to dictation, since there is an
inability to imagine or remember the visual form of letters (Luria,
1970, 1973); (3) lesions in the left sensory strip may produce mirror
writing (Luria, 1970); and (4) lesions in the left motor strip or
premotor area can produce motor perseveration that may cause

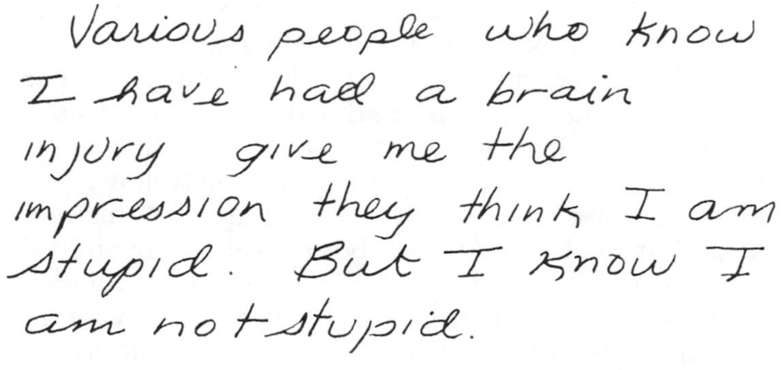

Various people who know
I have had a brain
injury give me the
impression they think I am
stupid. But I know I
am not stupid.

Figure 9.2. Sample of Mrs. Galloway's posttraumatic spontaneous
writing.

repetitions and omissions of single letters (Luria, 1973). This last syndrome leads to problems of chaotic spelling, e.g., "Abbr" for "Abner."

Psychomotor Disorders in Children

Paralysis of the Dominant Hand. Paralysis of the dominant hand, because of either left-hemisphere damage or peripheral injury, forces the child to write with the nondominant hand. Because control must now travel from the language-dominant hemisphere through the corpus callosum to the motor strip of the nondominant hemisphere and then down the pyramidal tracts to the nondominant hand, writing with this hand usually is less fluent and more awkward. Many years ago, Orton (1937) showed examples of writing of a 15-year-old boy. He was not paralyzed, but he was genetically left-handed and had been forced to write with his right hand, and his right-handed writing at age 15, although a product of 8 years of training, was more cramped and less legible than his spontaneous writing with his left hand, which nature had intended (Fig. 9.3). Such evidence suggests that children forced to write with the nondominant hand for any reason, including paralysis, are likely to be dysgraphic. Those who continue to write with the affected hand, because the paralysis is mild, are likely to be dysgraphic because of the minimal motor interference.

Cerebellar Ataxia. Cerebellar ataxia is a condition of neuromuscular coordination that may affect any motor activity, including walking and manipulating. When it affects the hands, the legibility of writing may be impaired, although the spelling and sentence structure may be normal or nearly normal. Myklebust has provided an excellent case of this with a sample of the subject's writing (1965, p. 17). From our own files, Chuck Becker is a good example. When he was 10 years old, Chuck received a severe head injury in an automobile accident, including, among other things, a severe blow to the back of his head. He was riding in the back seat of the family station wagon, and on impact, a heavy metal box packed on the rear deck of the car was hurled forward, hitting Chuck in the base of his skull. So severe were his injuries that he remained unconscious for a period of 3 months, and following that his recovery was slow and partial. Because of injury to his cerebellum his gait and manual control were both severely impaired. In fact, he fell down so much in the early stages of his rehabilitation that he was required to wear a protective helmet. Along with the injury to the back of his brain he also sustained a contrecoup effect, which centered in the left frontal cerebral area. This injury showed

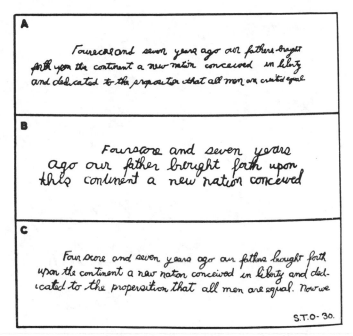

Figure 9.3. Samples of writing of a 15-year-old boy who was originally left-handed but who was forced to write with his right hand. (A) An example of his right-handed writing when first examined. (B) His left-handed writing at the same time. It was more legible but much slower (half as fast). (C) The effect of 2 months' training of the left hand for writing. In this time it had acquired the same speed as the right hand. (After Orton, 1937. Reproduced with permission of The Orton Society.)

itself in an articulation problem (dysarthria) and a manual difficulty in his right hand, which was both sensory (reduced manual sensitivity) and motor (partial paralysis). For more than 2 years after his injury he was unable to recognize forms of blocks with his right hand (astereognosis) and to write. On our fourth testing session with Chuck, which was $2\frac{1}{2}$ years after his injury, he was able to attempt the Coding subtest on the Wechsler (WISC) for the first time, but symbols were poorly drawn and one square was omitted. At age 13 he could spell words orally at an above-average level for his age as measured by the Wide Range Achievement Test, but he could not write them. The psychometrician wrote the words to Chuck's dictation. He learned to write again later that year, at the age of $13\frac{1}{2}$ years. He wrote: "I wish to announce something. I can now write" (Fig. 9.4). His first writing, though grammatically correct, was briefer in content and larger in size than it had been pretraumatically, 4 years before (Fig. 9.5).

Dear Daddy and Mommy,
& I wish
to arrounce something, I can
now write

yours lovingey
your Son
Chuck

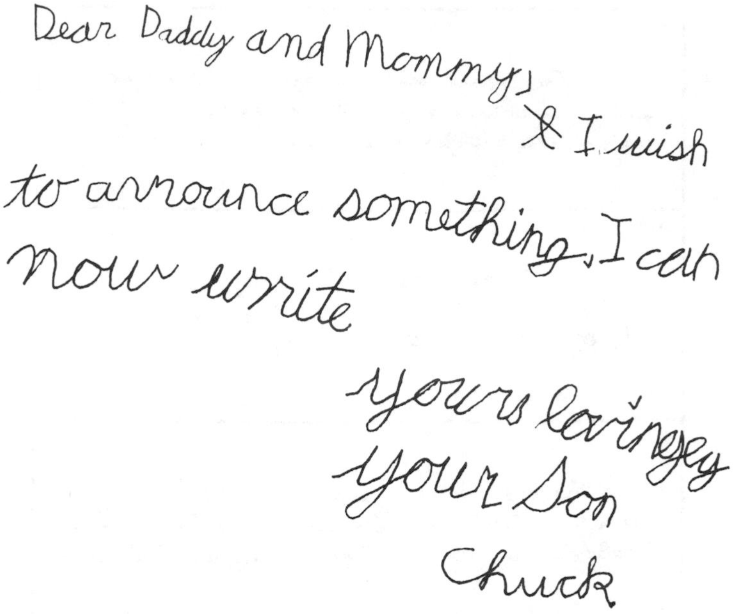

Figure 9.4. Example of Chuck Becker's first writing $3\frac{1}{2}$ years posttraumatically (age $13\frac{1}{2}$ years).

By the age of 16, $6\frac{1}{2}$ years posttraumatically, Chuck could write the symbols more firmly in the Digit Symbol subtest of the Wechsler (WAIS) but he was so slow that he obtained a very poor score (scaled score, 6). It was his poorest score. His best score was on Arithmetic (scaled score, 12). He attended a remedial school for about 7 years, during which time his writing showed slow improvement (Figs. 9.4, 9.6, 9.7, and 9.8).

An examination of his writing from his first attempts at age $13\frac{1}{2}$ to the last sample at age $21\frac{1}{2}$ shows a steady improvement in his ability to compose verbal ideas and to increase their variety and level of social insight. Because of his permanent cerebellar damage he will always be apraxic, and this is reflected in a cramped and jerky style in his penmanship. In spite of his rather extensive brain damage, Chuck has shown persistent determination to gain independence like any normal young adult (Figs. 9.7 and 9.8).

EEG Dysrhythmia in the Dominant Motor Strip. The case of Mark, described in detail at the end of Chapter 5, illustrates a case of agraphia that was caused purely by a motor disability (apraxia). The EEG dysrhythmia was highly localized in the upper left motor strip (Exner's area, Fig. 8.10) so that motor speech was normal, but fine movements of the right hand were abnormally slow. It

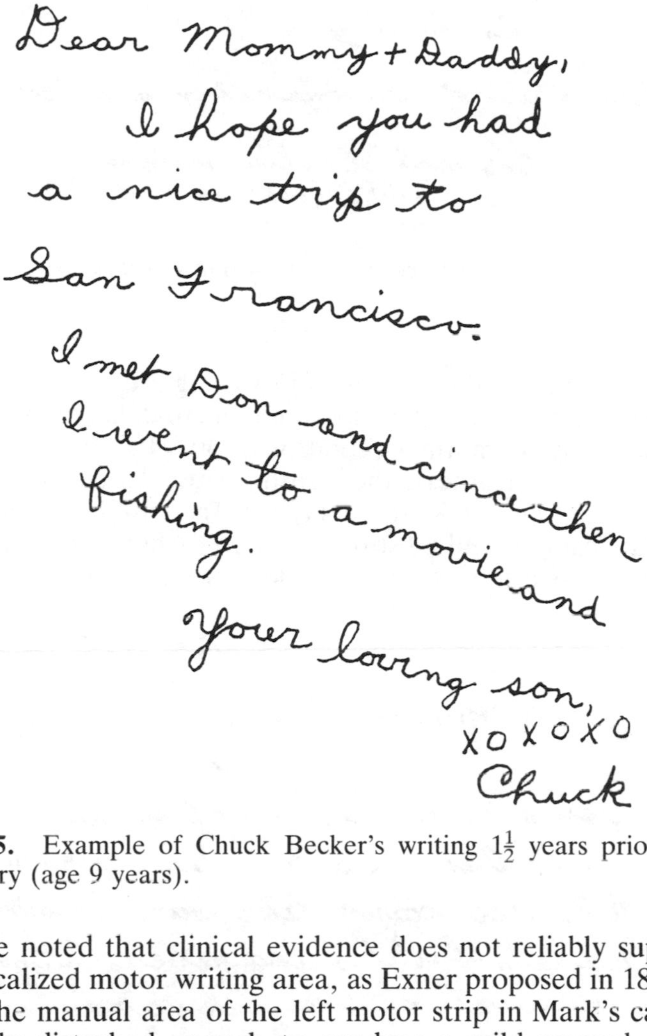

Dear Mommy + Daddy,
I hope you had
a nice trip to
San Francisco.
I met Don and since then
I went to a movie and
fishing.

Your loving son,
XOXOXO
Chuck

Figure 9.5. Example of Chuck Becker's writing $1\frac{1}{2}$ years prior to his brain injury (age 9 years).

should be noted that clinical evidence does not reliably support a highly localized motor writing area, as Exner proposed in 1881, but at least the manual area of the left motor strip in Mark's case was electrically disturbed enough to produce a mild manual apraxia resulting in slow but accurate writing.

Delayed Visual Feedback. Delayed visual feedback can produce a transient dysgraphia by introducing an abnormal delay between the act of writing and the appearance of the script. Van Bergeijk and David (1959) carried out an ingenious experiment to investigate the visual–motor processes in writing, using a technique similar in design to delayed auditory feedback. Because it is well known that delaying a speaker's auditory awareness of his own speech will interfere with normal fluent speech, Van Bergeijk and David asked subjects to write words on a *telewriter*, a device that can reproduce a person's writing on a separate viewing screen. Normally, the

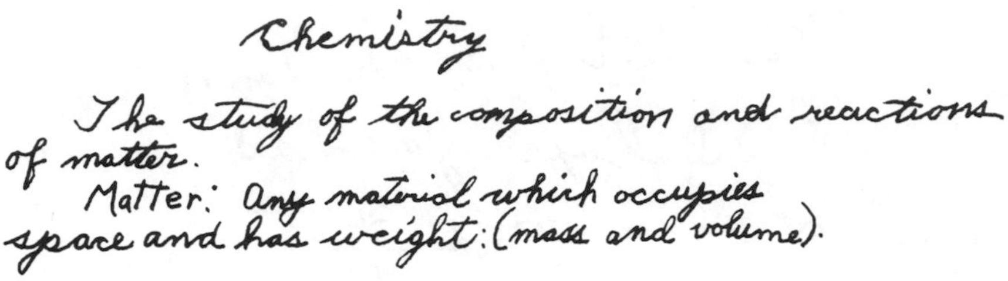

Chemistry

The study of the composition and reactions of matter.
  Matter: Any material which occupies space and has weight: (mass and volume).

Figure 9.6. Sample of Chuck Becker's writing $4\frac{3}{4}$ years posttraumatically (age 15 years).

kinesthetic and visual experiences in writing are simultaneous, but the telewriter permitted the experimenters to delay the visual input by 0 (no delay, or normal conditions), 40, 80, 150, 270, and 520 milliseconds. In neatness, the writing deteriorated monotonically with increased delay. As the delay was increased, errors of omissions, duplications, and substitutions (i.e., spelling errors) appeared. Frequently extra letters or wrong letters were inserted when the

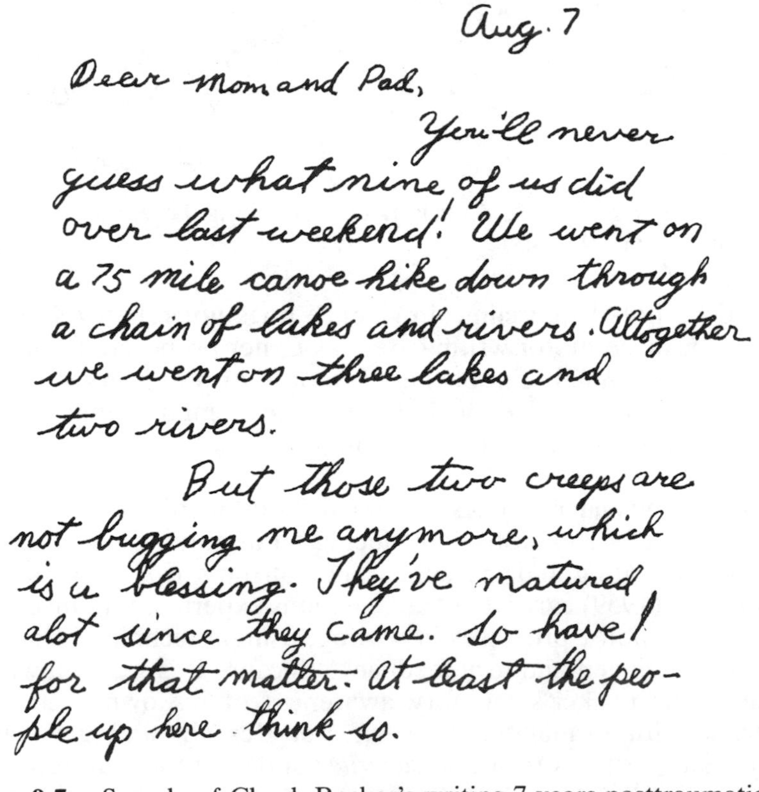

Aug. 7

Dear mom and Pad,
        You'll never guess what nine of us did over last weekend! We went on a 75 mile canoe hike down through a chain of lakes and rivers. Altogether we went on three lakes and two rivers.
        But those two creeps are not bugging me anymore, which is a blessing. They've matured, alot since they came. So have I for that matter. At least the people up here think so.

Figure 9.7. Sample of Chuck Becker's writing 7 years posttraumatically (age $17\frac{1}{2}$ years).

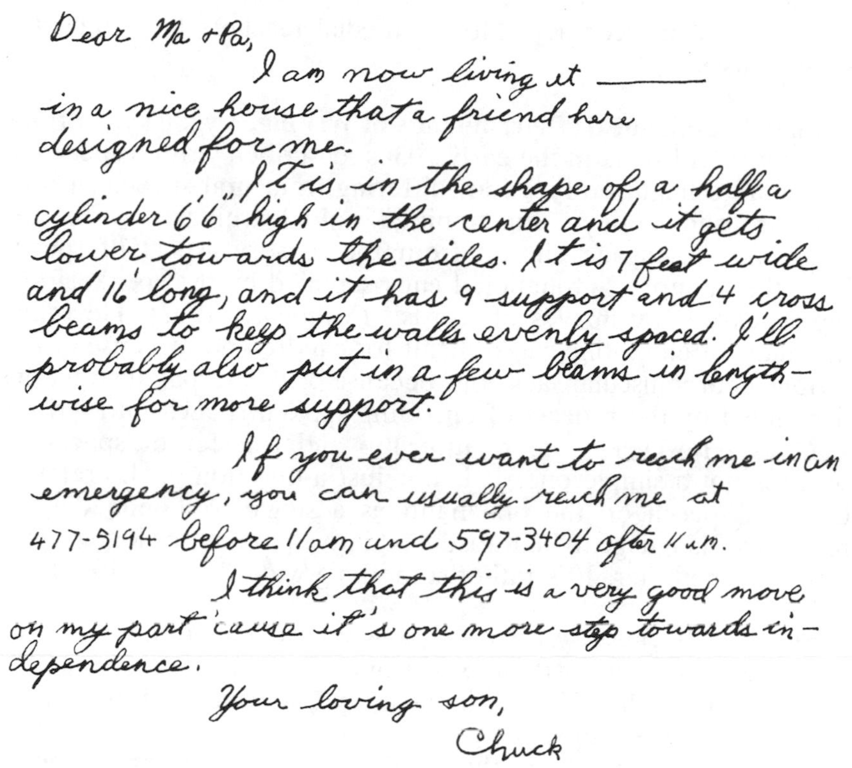

Dear Ma & Pa,

I am now living at ———
in a nice house that a friend here
designed for me.

It is in the shape of a half a
cylinder 6'6" high in the center and it gets
lower towards the sides. It is 7 feet wide
and 16' long, and it has 9 support and 4 cross
beams to keep the walls evenly spaced. I'll
probably also put in a few beams in length-
wise for more support.

If you ever want to reach me in an
emergency, you can usually reach me at
477-3194 before 11am and 597-3404 after 11 a.m.

I think that this is a very good move
on my part 'cause it's one more step towards independence.

Your loving son,
Chuck

Figure 9.8. Example of Chuck Becker's writing 11 years posttraumatically (age $21\frac{1}{2}$ years).

subjects were instructed they were to be scored on speed and neatness.

This experiment is an interesting reminder of the importance of the cerebral motor patterns in writing. They are integrated with visual input, visual imagery, visual and auditory memory, cerebral sequencing, language structure, and a number of other psychological and brain processes. Whenever one of these systems is disturbed, the behavioral product (writing) may also be impaired.

Occasionally, a brain lesion may disrupt the visual–motor integration of a dysgraphic child's ability to copy written material; such children may write better when they cannot see what they are writing. For example, in the above experiment of Van Bergeijk and David, the subjects could easily have escaped from the effects of the telewriter by writing with their eyes closed. In our laboratory some years ago, we saw a 10-year-old boy who was unable to copy correctly from either the blackboard or a page near at hand. It was discovered that when his hand was shielded so that his writing was screened from view, his writing improved markedly both in neatness and in accuracy. Most remedial teachers have reported similar cases.

Cognitive-Linguistic Determinants of Writing. Vygotsky, working with Luria in Russia in the early 1930s, described written speech as "a separate linguistic function, differing from oral speech in both structure and mode of functioning. . . . In learning to write, the child must disengage himself from the sensory aspect of speech [i.e., the auditory, intonational cues supplied by the speaker] and replace words by images of words" (Vygotsky, 1962). He found that most often writing was difficult for children not because of any serious neuromuscular lack, but because of the verbal abstractions demanded by the process of encoding spoken speech into written symbols. However, "the relationship and transfer of speech to script is not a simple one. It is not just a question of the relation between speech on the one hand as a single well-defined basic medium of language to be transduced into alphabetic or logographic script on the other. It is rather something wider" (Lotz, 1972).

Spelling. Because writing single words to dictation is less demanding for the writer than expository or narrative writing, and in that sense it is relatively the simplest type, we shall look first at the cognitive processes in spelling.

To learn to spell a word the writer must be able to pronounce it correctly and to remember its spoken form. One must either (1) remember the auditory sequence of its phonetic sounds or syllables, and transcribe (encode) this auditory pattern into the correct series of letters (i.e., the word's orthographic pattern), or (2) retain the visual sequence of its letters in one's visual memory and copy the visual–motor pattern of the word from that memory. First-graders with good phonetic analysis skills may write words from their oral lexicon that have "phonetically correct" errors (e.g., Qcomeber for cucumber). Small children who are weak in these skills (i.e., dysphonetic; Boder, 1971) must depend mainly on their visual memory of words already learned, and hence they lack the diagnostic skills to spell new words. From neurolinguistic research it seems highly likely that the phonological accessing of words is a left-hemisphere function and that direct accessing of graphemes from the mental lexicon is largely a right-hemisphere function (Friederici et al., 1981). In normal subjects it is possible that both systems are used both alternately and together, and in some left-hemisphere-damaged subjects there may be a tendency for the two systems to act independently. In any event, the ability to segment words into phonemes is essential to successful spelling, as it is for reading (Liberman & Shankweiler, 1985).

Dysgraphia and Aphasia

Localized lesions of the "speech area" of the left hemisphere typically produce an aphasic disturbance of both oral and written language. Penetrating brain injuries, closed head injuries, tumors, abscesses, intracerebral hematomas, and vascular accidents are common causes. Left-hemisphere "strokes" may result in transitory or permanent disability in writing. Such a disability is a frequent symptom of traumatic aphasia and led Luria to observe (1970) that "writing disorders accompany almost every form of aphasia."

We will begin by examining some cases of traumatically brain-damaged adults, and then look at some cases of dysgraphic children.

Adults with Dysgraphia and a Spelling Deficit

Left Anterior Temporal Lobe Excision and Damage in Broca's Area

John Hall. John Hall was a bright young man who on completing high school entered the Air Force and was assigned to the Military Police branch. He was friendly and pleasant and he got along well in the security force.

At the age of 29 he developed severe headaches and a number of signs of a neurological problem. Neurosurgical examination revealed the presence of a cyst embedded in the anterior part of the left temporal lobe, and because of an abnormal arteriovenous malformation, a large piece of the frontal part of the left temporal lobe was removed. Because this surgery did not destroy Wernicke's area, John's understanding of oral speech was normal, but because the frontal and inferior temporal area was affected by the surgery, his speech was postoperatively plagued by a serious word-finding problem and an unreliability of oral expression. He usually knew what he wanted to say but another word would come out. In oral arithmetic he frequently would conceptualize one number and say another, although he was aware of his aphasic problem.

Enough brain damage had resulted to affect both his reading and writing. We saw him for assessment 6 years postoperatively when he was 35 years old. At that time he measured a grade-point average (GPA) in reading (single-word recognition) of only 2.2, and in spelling of only 4.0. He was well above average in spatial tasks (mainly right-hemisphere function), and this seemed to help his written arithmetic, which measured a GPA of 6.1.

His ability to name simple objects and to write their names was impaired (Fig. 9.9). When shown a toy pistol he wrote "gun" correctly. For a plate he wrote "pain" (paraphasia). For a lightbulb

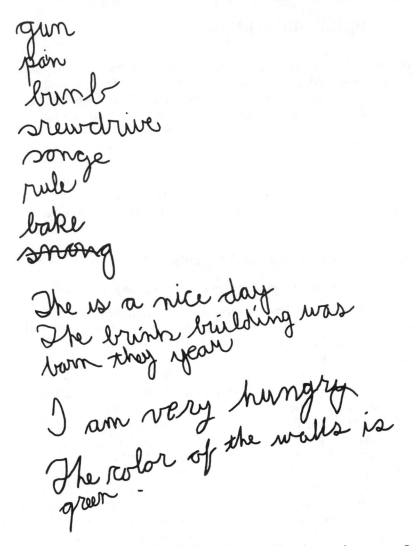

Figure 9.9. Samples of John Hall's writing to dictation and to copy. See text for the discussion of these samples.

he wrote "bunb," (another paraphasia, both of which indicated he was having difficulty in the sequential production of the correct letters). "Screwdriver" was correct except for the missing last letter. "Sponge" and "ruler" were both misspelled, although he recognized them and named them correctly in oral speech. For "eggbeater" he said "mixer" and wrote "bake," another spontaneous substitution. For "spring" he wrote "snoug" (paraphasia), which he recognized as incorrect and stroked it out.

Following the list of names, he tried to write two sentences to dictation. These were: "This is a very nice day" and "This brick building was built last year." His attempts had omissions of words, substitutions, and misspellings (see Fig. 9.9).

The next two sentences, "I am very hungry" and "The color of the walls is green," were both copied correctly. His visual–spatial skills were good and it seems likely he was drawing on his right hemisphere to copy these sentences as spatial patterns rather than samples of sequential language.

His handwriting postoperatively was large but well-enough formed and was different in style from his writing prior to the brain damage.

John Hall's dysgraphia is a good example of a language deficit resulting from aphasia and it includes some paralexias, with semantic associations, of the type described in Chapter 8 in the discussion of deep dyslexia.

The case of John Hall, because it provides us with neurosurgical data to correlate with his language and spelling problems, is particularly valuable in investigating the neuropsychological variables in an aphasia-related spelling deficit. However, such cases are relatively rare in the experience of special-education teachers, clinical neuropsychologists, and occupational counselors. Most cases with which they deal include children or adults with a developmental spelling problem. Francis Martin is such a case.

Francis Martin was referred to our laboratory early in his freshman year because of a serious spelling and writing problem. His verbal IQ on the Wechsler (WAIS) was 121, and so it was no surprise that he liked to read and he enjoyed school. Neuropsychological testing, however, revealed a persistent weakness in all the sequencing tests, including auditory sequencing. He enjoyed lively conversation on a topic with verbal ideas because his understanding was superior, but he was unable to write essays because his spelling deficit impaired his level of language expression. His reading on a standardized test was only average and his spelling, atrocious.

Samples of his writing to copy (Fig. 9.10a) and his writing to dictation (Fig. 9.10b) prior to remedial teaching, and a spelling list of 20 words reveals numerous errors (Fig. 9.11). His performance 6 months later (Fig. 9.12) showed marked improvement.

Because Francis's sequential skills were weak, his tutor gave him practice in serial-order exercises in all three sense modes. Because Francis possessed stronger auditory imagery than visual, the tutor stressed an auditory–tactile match in learning to write the spelling words, and he drew partially on Boder's teaching method for dyseidetic spellers (Boder, 1971). The tutor soon discovered that in spite of Francis's breezy, friendly manner, his spelling deficit was a

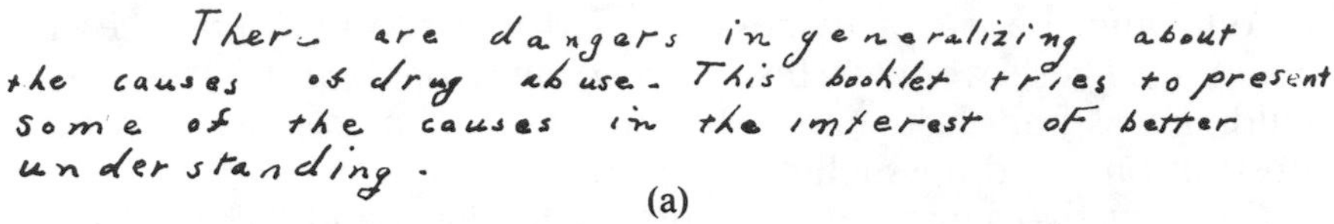

There are dangers in generalizing about the causes of drug abuse. This booklet tries to present some of the causes in the interest of better understanding.

(a)

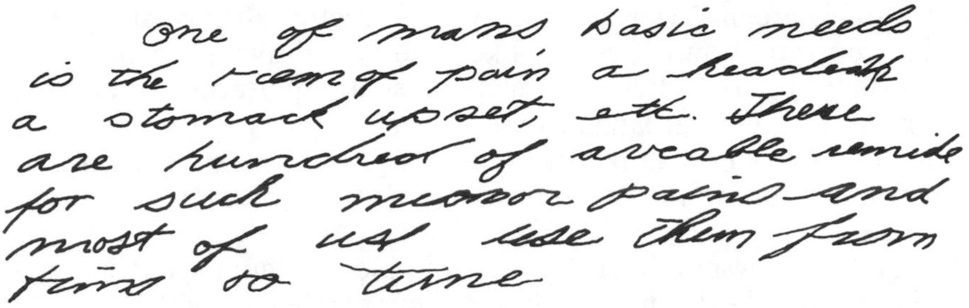

One of mans basic needs is the r-em of pain a headash a stomack upset, etc. There are hundred of avcable remide for such meoor pains and most of us use them from time to time

(b)

One of man's basic needs is the relief of pain—a headache or a stomach upset. There are hundreds of available remedies for such minor pains and most of us use them from time to time.

(c)

Figure 9.10. Samples of Francis Martin's writing prior to remedial teaching program. (a) Writing to copy; (b) writing to dictation; (c) text & dictated paragraph.

constant worry to him and a threat to his self-confidence. With this insight the tutor worked on Francis's self-image, and the total remedial effort paid off in a brief 6 months. Francis went on and completed a B.A. degree in history.

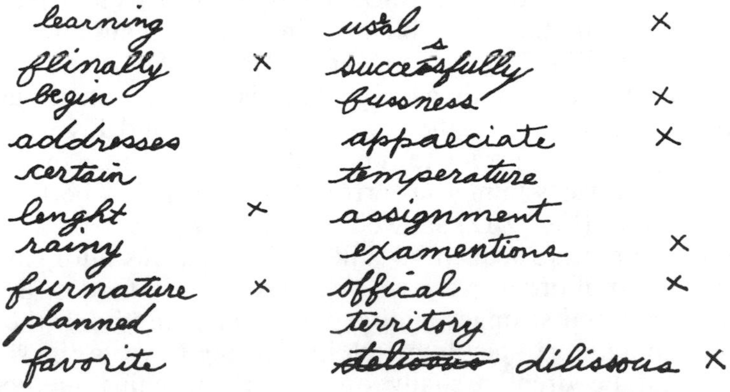

learning		*usal*	×
flinally	×	*succesfully*	
begin		*busness*	×
addresses		*appaeciate*	×
certain		*temperature*	
lenght	×	*assignment*	
rainy		*examentions*	×
furnature	×	*offical*	×
planned		*territory*	
favorite		~~*delicous*~~ *dilissous*	×

Figure 9.11. Sample of Francis Martin's written spelling prior to the remedial teaching program.

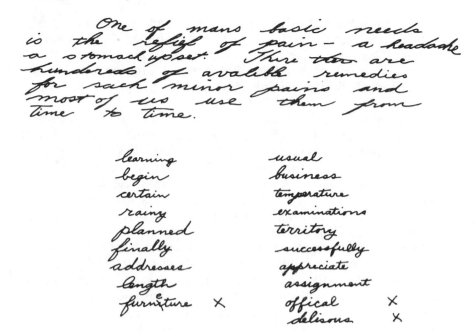

Figure 9.12. Samples of the same dictated paragraph and spelling list after 6 months of remedial teaching.

Agraphic and Dysgraphic Children

Having examined two types of agraphia in two adults, one traumatic and one developmental, let us turn to the same problems in children.

Visual Processes in Writing and Spelling

We have already been introduced to the visual–motor processes in the above discussion. Here we will recall that visual copying of letter forms is a primary function in the initial learning to write, but as the motor engrams become established they gradually become less strongly associated with the visual–perceptual aspects of writing and more strongly related to the visual and auditory imagery of the child, and to developing a knowledge of language.

Luria (1970) has pointed out that we investigate a person's writing by examining his ability (1) to copy written or printed material and (2) to write spontaneously. The first tests the level of visual–motor competence in writing, and the second taps all the concomitant psychological, linguistic and neurological processes necessary to successful adult writing.

If the agraphic child can copy sentences accurately and neatly, then we know that the visual–motor integration necessary in writing is intact. This knowledge will then direct us to look at his auditory phonetic discrimination, oral verbal memory, auditory sequencing, abilities for syllabication and/or phonetic blending, or the possibility of an aphasia.

If the child's visual–motor integration is defective so as to produce visual–spatial disturbances in writing, there is a possibility of a bilateral brain lesion in his parietal–occipital lobes, or unilaterally in the same area of the language-dominant hemisphere (Luria, 1973). The writing of Donald, shown in Fig. 5.5, illustrates his poor visual memory for the letter forms and his chaotic visual scanning. Figure 5.7 shows his marked improvement after 8 months of skilled remedial teaching.

Poor visual memory can lead to poor visual learning, defective writing, and chaotic spelling. So many deficits suggest the possibility of widespread or diffuse brain dysfunction, typical of the chaotic speller of normal intelligence. Every teacher has had these students; they sometimes appear even at the university level, although the less bright have usually dropped out before this to seek a less frustrating line of activity.

In Chapter 6, we observed that it is easier to draw a line from left to right with one's right hand, and from right to left with one's left hand. This motor act is even more pronounced if one attempts a series of loops in continuous form like cursive writing. How then do Israelis write from right to left, because most of them are right-handed? The answer seems to be that Hebrew does not include a cursive style of writing; each letter or grapheme is spatially independent so that it is as easy to write in either direction. It is interesting to note that adult patients with progressive neurological deteriorating diseases frequently abandon cursive writing for printing in the last stages of their illness (Ferguson & Boller, 1977) because isolated letters are easier to produce. These observations can provide greater insights into the writing of children who tend to produce many reversals, to mirror-write, and to produce other left–right writing disorders. The educational diagnostician will need to look at handedness, cerebral dominance, and the relative frequency of errors in cursive and printed writing.

Carl. Carl was 7 years old when we first saw him and 11 years old when he wrote his mother from camp (Fig. 9.13). His birth had been a difficult one and he was cyanosed at 6 weeks (a "blue baby" because of lack of adequate oxygen in the blood). At the age of 1 year, seizures first appeared, which seemed to be clear evidence of a brain lesion or lesions in the medial parts of the brain, near enough to affect the motor strips.

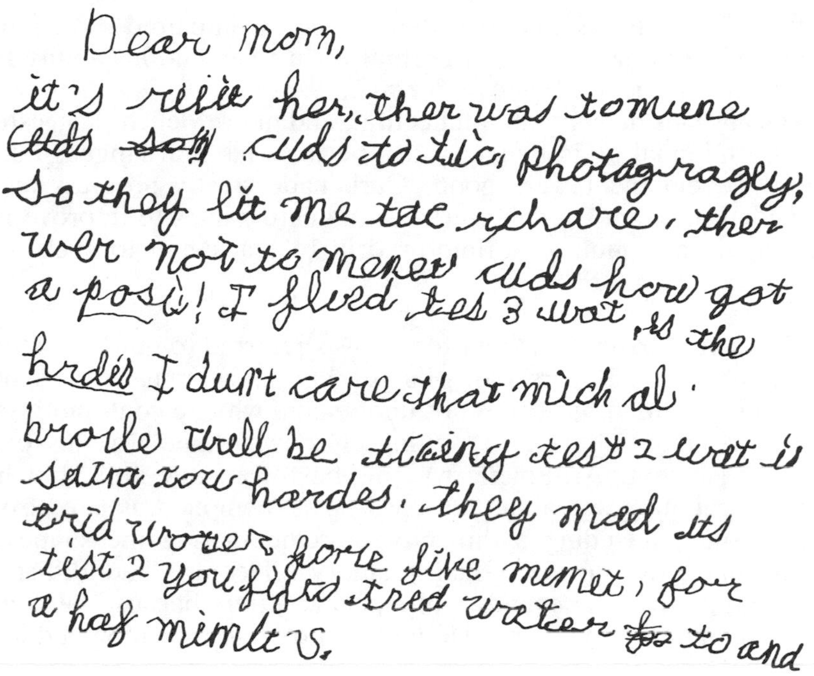

(Mother's Translation)

Dear Mom,

It's raining here. There were too many clouds to take photography so they let me take archery. There were not too many clouds, have got a picture. I failed test 3, what is the hardest. I don't care that much although I will probably be taking test 2 that is second to hardest. They made us tread water for five minutes for test two. You first tread water two and a half minutes.

Figure 9.13. Sample of writing of Carl Morris, age 11 years.

By the age of 7 the seizures were well controlled with anti-convulsive medication, and although he had numerous learning problems in first grade, Carl was a likable and socially bright boy. His Wechsler (WISC) showed a verbal IQ of 91 and a performance IQ of 89. He did well on the Block Design test (spatial imagery of nonverbal figures) but badly on all the other visual–perceptual tests. His memory for words (sentence repetition) and numbers (digit span) was weak. His auditory recognition of nonverbal sounds (e.g., a church bell, people clapping), normally an easy test for average 7-year-olds, was done poorly. His right–left orientation was so poor as to be in the defective range. Obviously, then, Carl had numerous deficits: poor visual memory, poor auditory memory, a defective visual–sequential ability, and an impaired directional sense. His oral language was normal for his age and his ability for productive ideas much above average.

Because his perceptual, intellectual, and motor deficits suggested diffuse minimal brain damage, and because his oral language and social development were good, Carl made steady progress on a remedial program stressing puzzles and card games to improve his arithmetic and multisensorimotor drill to teach him to spell and write.

Pearson Morsby. Pearson Morsby was referred to our laboratory when he was 11 years old. His teacher knew that he was not mentally retarded but could not understand why he could not read above a grade 1 level. In writing, his own name was his only accomplishment. Arithmetic was his best academic area, but his sight vocabulary was about 45 words. His memory was poor from day to day, including a difficulty in remembering the shape of individual letters (poor visual memory). He also had difficulty associating phonetic sounds with specific letters because he could not remember their shapes. He had no problem repeating auditory stimuli.

Detailed neuropsychological testing revealed a developmental aphasia with an aphasic dyslexia. At a special remedial school they began by trying to teach Pearson the letters of the alphabet, but after 4 months he was still able to write only some of the letters and his recall for most of the rest was erratic. Because he was musical, the teacher decided to try singing. When it was put to the tune of "Baa-baa black sheep," Pearson learned the alphabet perfectly in 3 days.

Neuropsychologically this learning may be understood in terms of laterality. Because his brain dysfunction almost certainly was in the left hemisphere, or bilaterally in the occipito–parietal areas, when his language learning was shifted through singing to the right hemisphere he was able to learn the alphabet quickly. His teacher also encouraged him to sing the letters while writing and this improved his writing markedly.

Pearson was left-handed although left-hemisphere dominant for language, and his sensorimotor skills were poor in his right hand. This is the picture of a "pathological left-hander" (Soper & Satz, 1984) with probable dysfunction in the left temporal–parietal area.

Examples of Pearson's writing on his arrival at the special school are shown in Fig. 9.14. His marked improvement resulted from a detailed knowledge of his strengths and weaknesses and a skilled remedial use of his abilities. After 4 years of remedial teaching, Pearson was able to return to a special program in a public high

Dictated words	Writing of Pearson
go	
cat	c a t
in	i n
boy	b o y
and	a n d
will	
make	h
him	h
say	s a h
cut	c ' t
cook	c
light	n

Figure 9.14. Pearson Morsby's attempts to write to dictation, age $11\frac{1}{2}$.

school, where he can read and write accurately, but slowly, at a seventh-grade level.

Auditory Processes in Writing and Spelling

A Case of Temporary Deafness. Janet was a child of above-average intelligence with no particular academic learning problems. In grade 3 she developed an infection in both ears, which resulted in moderate peripheral deafness. Following recovery from the infection she returned to school, but a residual deafness persisted. She missed much of what was said in school and she was unable to gain much from phonics instruction. Gradually her hearing returned to normal, and by grade 7 she measured normally on a phonetic discrimination test, but her spelling continued to suffer from her hard-of-hearing period, so that as an adult she still produces original spellings of many infrequent words. Obviously this type of case can be remedied with skilled teaching with a basic phonetic approach, because her hearing is now normal.

Diagnosis and Remediation of Spelling Disability

To a person who has learned to spell with no difficulty, it seems incredible that any bright person might be unable to do what seems so common-place. However, once an analysis of the whole complex process involved in written language has been done, it begins to become more believable.

There are probably as many causes for a spelling deficit as there are loci of brain lesions in the language circuits. Very simply, however, the cause will stress (1) a language deficit (aphasia); (2) a visual–perceptual dysfunction; (3) an auditory–perceptual problem; (4) a motor–expressive sequential impairment, or (5) a combination of two or more of these.

Although it is useful for diagnostic purposes to isolate language, visual, auditory, and motor processes, in reality that is a misrepresentation because all of these are integrated functions of *one process*—human behavior.

Much attention has already been given to visual and auditory perceptual processes in reading, and so only a brief comment is needed here. In writing, the tactile–somesthetic functions take on more importance because a person can read without writing skills and can write without direct visual cues. Nevertheless, phonetic analysis is still needed to direct the manual–motor activity of writing legibly and spelling correctly. The recent interest in left-hemisphere trauma and profound reading difficulties (deep dyslexia) has been extended to writing and spelling. A patient, aged 57 years, who suffered a left cerebrovascular accident at age 47 and who was diagnosed as a deep dyslexic, also exhibited the same linguistic errors in written and oral naming and writing to dictation (Nolan & Caramazza, 1983). These researchers have proposed that any linguistic performance requiring lexical mediation (e.g., reading, writing spontaneously and to dictation, and oral and written naming) may exhibit the typical symptoms of deep dyslexia. This same patient could copy and repeat single words correctly because, as Nolan and Caramazza hypothesized, an intact phonological processing system can bypass lexical mediation and be accessed directly by auditory input. One can repeat or echo a word without semantic understanding.

The remediation of any form of impaired or undeveloped behavioral skill requires the exercise of neuromuscular *movement*. This is important to improve perception, understanding, and expressive response, whether that response is oral or written. All behavior is a holistic system of input, integration, and output, and the best type of remediation will activate all areas of this system. In diagnosing a spelling problem, the diagnostician needs to survey the behavioral skills and decide on the areas of dysfunction and the correlative behavioral deficits. Because the writing process requires a phonetic analysis of the flow of speech, examining the child's auditory skills is a good place to start.

Auditory Processes and Aphasic Signs in Oral Speech

1. Is hearing normal on an audiometric test? Has there ever been a history of ear infections and periods of partial deafness?
2. If hearing is normal, can the child perform normally on a phonetic discrimination test?
3. Can he recite all the letters of the alphabet?
4. Can he associate all the phonetic sounds of all the letters?
5. Is his auditory memory normal on a digit-span test and a sentence-repetition test?
6. Can he follow detailed oral instructions? (e.g., Token test)
7. Can he name common objects without hesitation?
8. Can he describe the use of common objects?
9. Word fluency: How many nouns can the child produce in one minute?
10. Can he construct a meaningful sentence if given three words?
11. Can he read new words using phonetic analysis?
12. Can he blend syllables into words?
13. Does he have any obvious articulation problems? Did he when he was growing up?
14. Can he write single letters to dictation? Can he write one-syllable words to dictation?
15. Can he analyze a word phonetically aloud? Can he explain how he does this?
16. If you spell a word aloud can he tell you what it is?
17. Is his auditory sequencing normal?

Once the diagnostician has identified the auditory skills that are giving trouble, then remedial drills can be selected to strengthen them.

A patient with a phonemic hearing disturbance may be able to write familiar words (e.g., his or her own name, country, city, and street address, etc.) because such words remain in the cortex as "optical ideograms" and do not require phonemic analysis (Luria, 1973).

Visual Processes

1. Can the child look at pictures of common objects and match them with a similar picture? (The 1916 Stanford–Binet test used this procedure with a number of animal pictures.)
2. Can he name each picture? (e.g., any picture vocabulary test)
3. Can he match geometric figures?
4. Can he name geometric figures?
5. Can he read all the letters of the alphabet?

6. Can he write all the letters of the alphabet?
7. Can he read words and sentences at the expected level?
8. Can he copy sentences accurately from the blackboard or a book?
9. Is his figure–ground visual perception normal?
10. Can he remember figures on a visual retention test? (e.g., Benton VRT)
11. Is his visual sequencing normal?
12. Can he identify right and left on a person facing him or on a picture of a person?
13. Is his visual–motor performance normal: (e.g., Frostig tests)

Tactile Processes

1. Can the child write while blindfolded or with his hand obscured?
2. Can he "read" letters and numbers "written" on his palm or back with a stylus?
3. Can he trace letters and then write them correctly?
4. Can he recognize and name, by touch alone, common objects placed in his hand? If he can name an object by sight but is unable to name it by touch he is said to be suffering from "tactile aphasia." This may occur when the somesthetic areas of the parietal lobes are isolated from Wernicke's area and the occipital lobes. It may also occur in a lateralized way with a lesion of the corpus callosum that isolates the two somesthetic areas (Geschwind, 1965, I, pp. 287–290).
5. If an object that is similar to one of a group of objects scattered on the table is placed in the child's hand, can he match the two objects, i.e., the one he feels with the one he sees? This is cross-modal matching. If he can do this but cannot name the objects, the somesthetic and occipital cortical areas may be normally connected, but the speech areas may be isolated from both of these areas.
6. Is his tactile recognition much better in one hand than the other? Is it normal? (Spreen & Gaddes, 1969).

Motor–Expressive Processes

In spelling, the motor–expressive acts that are most important are manual (writing) and articulatory (oral speech). The diagnostician will want to know:

1. What is the child's finger-tapping speed for each hand? Are they both normal? If not, which one is not? What is their relative pattern?

2. What is the child's hand-grip strength for each hand? Is there a difference between hands? What is the pattern?
3. Is his motor sequencing normal? Can he imitate tapping patterns?
4. Is his spontaneous speech clear and free from articulation problems?
5. Can he imitate words on an articulation test?
6. Is his oral reading smooth and accurate?

Intersensorimotor Integration

It is obvious that spelling requires a subtle and smoothly running integration of many neurological and psychological functions. Knowing the locus of a brain lesion or an area of cerebral dysfunction may help the diagnostician, the school psychologist, or the special teacher to understand an uneven or isolated behavior in a child with a writing or spelling problem. For example, Geschwind's explanation of tactile anomia resulting from a disconnection of the sensory strip and the speech areas is logical and should direct the diagnostician to stress a visual–auditory–motor prescription. It is difficult to teach spelling to a child with this type of defect, but if a skilled remedial program is begun early it can be taught by stressing the child's strengths.

Numerous multisensorimotor methods for teaching spelling have been used for many years (Fernald, 1943). Writing letters on the child's back (Blau, 1968) and having him or her sound them phonetically is an attempt to link the somesthetic and auditory centers of the brain. Asking the child to write spelling words in damp sand with the index finger while sounding the word simultaneously reinforces the tactile (granular feel and temperature differential), auditory, and visual sense modes with the manual–motor activity. This exercise attempts to build engrams linking the occipital, temporal, parietal, and motor strip areas that are crucial to correct writing.

If the diagnostician can provide the special teacher with a clear inventory of the child's strengths and weaknesses, and a prescription for remedial procedures that he or she believes on an a priori basis should be successful, then the teacher may select from his or her own repertoire of remedial techniques. Once a clearly defined diagnostic understanding of the child's strengths and weaknesses is made available to the special teacher, a suitable battery of remedial techniques can be selected. Any experienced teacher already has an armamentarium of teaching skills to draw from.

Before we leave the topic of spelling, it is useful to note that the phonetic inaccuracy of a person's spelling is a reliable measure that discriminates LD from normal groups and it correlates with other measures of language (O'Donnell, 1991).

Expressive, Expository, and Narrative Writing. Cognitive psychologists in recent years have investigated children's abilities to comprehend and to compose stories and other forms of written expression. Original compositions might be classified as (1) expressive writing (writing to satisfy the interests of the writer with little or no concern for the reader, e.g., a diary); (2) poetic writing, designed to have some artistic value in its form or emotional impact; and (3) transactional writing designed to affect the reader, such as a letter, an informative report, or a story (Britton, 1970; Nodine et al., 1985). A mature novel may possess characteristics from all three of these categories, but in this discussion we will confine ourselves to the writing of school-age children.

Narrative comprehension involves "recognition of words, decoding them into meanings, segmenting word sequences into grammatical constituents, combining meanings into statements, inferring connections among statements, holding in short-term memory earlier concepts while processing later discourse, inferring the writer's or speaker's intentions, schematization of the gist of a passage, and memory retrieval in answering questions about the passage" (Bower & Morrow, 1990). Although this list details the processes of the reader or listener of a story, the writer, after deciding on the subject matter and the plan for the intended composition, is also required to master all of these skills and more. Young writers of expository prose, which is typical of school essay or project assignments, face at least three types of difficulties: (1) a lack of knowledge about text structures, major and minor ideas, and logical order and plan; (2) holding in short-term memory two or more major ideas in the composition, to avoid redundancies, irrelevant comments, omissions, and/or early termination of the discussion; and (3) the need to learn the various text structures (e.g., comparison and contrast, description, sequence, and enumeration; Thomas et al., 1987).

In brief, writing disorders are due to (1) deficits in underlying processes required for writing (e.g., oral receptive and expressive language, reading ability, selective attention, verbal concept formation, reasoning, problem solving, verbal categorizing, learning strategies, and the ability to create a nonverbal reality (Litowitz, 1981).

The interesting effect of writing for an audience or for oneself is mentioned briefly above. Vygotsky, writing in the early 1930s, realized the importance of an audience as a motivation for the writer. "Writing is also speech without an interlocutor, addressed to an absent or imaginary person or to no one in particular—a situation new and strange to a child" (Vygotsky, 1962). He explained that in conversation every sentence is prompted by a desire or need to question, or request, or answer, and the direction of the conversation is guided by the responses of the person to whom one is speaking (i.e., the interlocutor). Syntax has been found to be more complex in compositions written by grade 10 students for a teacher than for a best friend, but these differences did not show for grade 6 students (Crowhurst & Piche, 1979).

Developmental Agraphia

Within the neuropsychological model, a congenital deficit in writing is a form of developmental expressive aphasia. Typically, there is an impaired ability to express oneself in writing with no disorder of the peripheral speech mechanisms or the writing hand and arm (Orton, 1937). Children suffering from a developmental agraphia are retarded in learning to write "because the necessary areas of the brain do not develop in the normal manner, or at the usual rate" (Myklebust, 1965).

If born with a dysfunction, even very minimal, in the left motor or premotor area of the brain, the child is likely to have problems with awkward or slow handwriting and/or sequential problems in spelling. Minimal dysfunctions in the posterior parts of the child's brain may result in poor letter and word recognition. Temporal lobe dysfunction in the language-dominant hemisphere may result in poor phonetic discrimination and any number of aphasic symptoms. Diffuse and minimal brain dysfunctions are likely to impair the cross-modal integration relating these different cortical areas. Behaviorally this condition may result in poor handwriting, defective spelling, and/or inferior linguistic expression. The child whose penmanship is untidy but who can spell and write written language normally for his or her age is no real problem. The "nonspeller" and the child who cannot generate verbally expressed ideas and commit them to paper are definitely educational responsibilities.

Arithmetic

"On the one hand, a great deal is known about mathematics, far more than any learning disabled child or professional working with the child will ever have to know. On the other hand, very little is known about disabilities in mathematics, less about effective measurement and diagnosis, even less about effective intervention,

and still less about children who manifest problems in mathematics"
(Cawley, 1981). Keller and Sutton have echoed this view (1991).
Most educators agree that there is a relative lack of adequate
research into, understanding of, and development of validated
remedial programs for children and adults with particular difficulty
with arithmetic. Like any scientific study, new knowledge will
come from various relevant sources. In this section we will examine
briefly some findings from clinical physiology and neuropsychology
that promise to enrich what the educator already knows. We will
look at (1) the neuropsychological–cognitive aspects of the learner,
and their relation to some basic arithmetical functions, and (2)
the educational environment and the learner's emotional–social
perception of and response to it.

The following discussion includes an examination of (1) an acquired disorder of calculating ability in adults as a result of traumatic
brain damage (this is known medically as acalculia), and (2) developmental arithmetical retardation in children. While teachers
are concerned almost exclusively with the second of these, an
examination of the first may aid an understanding of both.

Arithmetical Functions

In any clinical–psychological study of a learning disorder, it is
necessary to make a task analysis of the particular learning behavior
and relate the findings to a neuropsychological examination of
the learner. First, then, we will investigate some basic processes
involved in mathematical calculation and then look at evidence
of impairment resulting from known brain lesions or cerebral
dysfunction.

Number Concept

The normal adult, when told the number "seven," can produce a
mental concept that has meaning for him in terms of quantity.
Seven can be represented concretely with seven environmental
objects, but the normal adult also associates with the word "seven"
an abstract concept that can be manipulated as realistically, and
much more easily and quickly, than the concrete objects. In periods
of malnutrition, extreme fatigue, or illness, or following brain
damage or dysfunction, a person may be unable to produce, or
have great difficulty in producing, the necessary symbolic operation
to give meaning to a perceived number.

Soldiers subjected to decompression-chamber experiments were
rendered temporarily aphasic when the oxygen content of the air
was reduced below certain critical levels (see Chapter 8). If asked

to write "seven" they could usually do it because of the overlearned motor stereotype involved, but they might have great difficulty in trying to remember what the quantity "seven" meant.

This type of evidence tells us that there is a relation between acalculia and aphasia, that the perception and writing of numbers is more resistant to the debilitating effects of aphasia than their abstract conceptual aspects, and that competent abstraction depends on healthy metabolism in the brain.

Relative Value

Although number concept demands an association of a meaningful mental image, numbers are rarely if ever, used in isolation. Social behavior makes constant demands to decide, for example, How far am I from that? Is this bigger or smaller than that? Is its increase linear or erratic? How do I walk through this room full of furniture? As Cohn (1971) has pointed out, "Interacting organisms must be aware of inhomogeneities in their environment in order to make necessary physical adaptations." Put in simpler words, a person must be able to count, to judge relative size, and to estimate immediate distances in order to move about and carry on a normal social life, because mobility implies a three-dimensional spatial perception of the world. In fact, Luria (1966, pp. 158–162) gave great emphasis to the close relationship between arithmetical operations and spatial imagery and spatial concepts.

Number Imagery

Some years ago one of the present authors (W.H.G.) was interested in exploring the relation between the vividness of number imagery, which was spatial, and competence in arithmetic. This investigation was initiated by a sophomore student who had unusually vivid number imagery. He thought of the digits as on the circumference of a circle, with one at 6 o'clock and the numbers from 1 to 9 and zero arranged clockwise and in correct numerical order. As well, each number was in a different color: 1 was always white, 2 blue, 3 yellow, and so on. If he thought of any number it always had the same color, and this was consistent even with multidigit numbers. He was surprised when told that everyone had his or her own system for imagining numbers; until then he had assumed that everyone conceptualized numbers in color on a circle as he did. It seems reasonable to think that anyone who could visualize numbers so vividly would have an advantage in learning arithmetic, but as it happened this student had had great difficulty getting through the freshman course in mathematics.

To investigate the problem, the arithmetic scores from the college admissions test of 147 freshmen were correlated with their responses on a questionnaire designed to investigate their number imagery. These responses were dichotomized as "vivid" or "unclear." Most respondents who used number imagery saw numbers from left to right in a straight line, a few saw them in circles, and very few associated color with them. Many were unable to describe any kind of visual or spatial number imagery, or it was so vague as to be relegated to the "unclear" category. A biserial correlation between the 147 arithmetic scores and the two classes of number imagery showed a correlation close to zero. In other words, as many students with vivid as with vague imagery did well, and those with poor scores also came equally from the two groups. Those with vivid number imagery claimed it helped them to calculate, but those with no definitive imagery who were skilled mathematicians could see no real meaning in the question. Sir Francis Galton, himself a brilliant mathematician, possessed no visual number imagery. In a fascinating discussion of "Number Forms," he wrote, "I see no 'Form' myself" (Galton, 1907).

Although vivid visual number imagery appears to be unrelated to success in arithmetic, basic spatial skills are related. Luria (1966) found that lesions of the parieto–occipital areas of the brain result in impaired spatial imagery and in acalculia, and Hécaen (1962) included the "spatial type" of dyscalculia as one of the three major categories of the disorder.

Electrostimulation of the left and right thalamus has been found to impair arithmetic ability differentially (Ojemann, 1974). Left thalamic stimulation tended to accelerate the rate of counting backwards and to increase calculation errors. Right thalamic stimulation tended to slow the counting rate and to increase calculation errors. Ojemann believes that the right thalamus is related to somesthetic and spatial functions, and it may have a role in number reading. This relation seems quite likely because the right thalamus and the cortex of the right hemisphere are structurally interconnected and the disconnected right hemisphere has been found better than the left in reading calligraphy and numbers (E. Zaidel, 1973). This could explain why most dyslexic subjects, who cannot read words, can usually read numbers (see the case of Mr. Darwin, p. 358 ff.). Bradshaw and Nettleton have provided a brief but detailed summary of a number of studies investigating arithmetic and the right hemisphere (Bradshaw & Nettleton, 1983, p. 155).

It is obvious that written arithmetic contains many spatial demands. Multidigit numbers must be written horizontally from left to right and spaced evenly. Addition sums usually are written in vertical columns, and the answer is measured from the decimal to the left, the units, tens, hundreds, and thousands having their value indicated by their spatial position. Multiplication and long division demand not only horizontal and vertical spacing but oblique spacing to the left in multiplication and to the right in long division.

To help a child to develop a number concept the teacher may place objects spatially on the table or mark "tallies" on a sheet. The spatial ability appears to be related to the concepts of larger than, smaller than, farther, closer, and all relative measures. Cuisinaire rods and other concrete number-teaching aids are designed to assist the learner to improve spatial imagination, relative value, and number concept.

Accurate Reading and Writing of Numbers

Because Luria was working with traumatically brain-damaged patients, and because he wanted to discover the relationships between brain function and the various cognitive processes demanded by mathematics, he developed a very detailed clinical examination of his subjects' mathematical knowledge, extending from the simplest arithmetical skill to the more complex demands of problem solving. He would ask his subject first to count aloud to check memory of numbers in the correct sequence, to recognize quantities, to read and write single digits, to read and write multidigit numbers, to show an understanding of the decimal system, to recognize relative values, to show competence in the basic arithmetical skills, and to attempt more complex calculations (Luria, 1970, p. 358). His researches, and those of others (Hécaen, 1962) identified three areas of acalculia: (1) associated with alexia and agraphia for numbers; (2) associated with spatial disorders; and (3) the inability for calculation in a subject free of the first two disabilities. Benton's clinical examination covers the same cognitive processes and is described by Levin (1979, p. 137).

Luria's studies of traumatically brain-damaged adults led him to conclude that damage to the language-dominant parieto–occipital areas may result in alexia for numbers or confusion of one number with another. This is a somewhat rare occurrence, because the dyslexic individual usually is able to read numbers. A lesion in the left temporal lobe may result in a difficulty in attaching conceptual meaning to spoken numbers, and this type of patient can usually read numbers normally but has difficulty writing long numbers because of a deficit in inner speech.

Clinical vigilance usually shows a combination of poor number reading and writing and calculation and arithmetical reasoning, no doubt because they all draw markedly on the left hemisphere (Hécaen, 1962). Spatial dyscalculia results largely from right-hemisphere lesions, and acalculia involving all of these impairments implies bilateral dysfunctions.

Spatial Acalculia. We have already referred to the important presence of spatial processes in arithmetical calculations in our discussion of number imagery. Because spatial perception and imagery are mostly mediated by the right hemisphere in most people, it is understandable that spatial acalculia usually involves lesions in the right hemisphere (Hécaen, 1962), and that patients with this disorder usually suffer accompanying "right-hemisphere symptoms" among others, such as visuoconstructive impairment, directional confusion, and visual–motor disturbances (Levin, 1979). It is not uncommon for a severe dyslexic, although unable to read letters and words, to be able to read arabic numbers (Coltheart et al., 1980; the case of Mr. Darwin in Chapter 8). This may be explained by the fact that the right hemisphere can mediate the perception of nonverbal forms and ideographic writing, but it cannot process alphabetic letter and word forms that need to be phonologically coded. The latter process is normally a function of the left hemisphere.

A related "right-hemisphere symptom" has been reported by Bogen (1979) in commissurotomy [split-brain] patients. Because disconnecting the two hemispheres can cause a right-hand disability for drawing spatial forms, Bogen has reported such patients having difficulty solving written arithmetic problems, although some of them were able to do the same problems if presented orally. Warrington (McCarthy & Warrington, 1990, p. 264) has reported a case with reversed symptoms. Because of this possibility, in our laboratory we always compare the scores in written and oral arithmetic of each testee. A marked difference can provide useful information in the diagnosis, and possible clues to improve the remedial program.

Retrieval of Numbers. Some aphasic patients may have difficulty saying the name of the number that they have in mind (i.e., verbal paraphasia). They may conceptualize one number but say another one involuntarily in its place (see case of John Hall earlier in this chapter). Benson and Denckla (1969) have reported such a patient who could not say the correct answer but could point to it in a multiple-choice situation. When given the written problem "4 + 5" the patient said "eight," wrote "5," but chose "9."

Calculation. The ultimate aim in mathematics is to calculate or to make a computation to arrive at a quantitative solution based on the provided numerical data, and using the various cognitive skills described above. It is a complex and multiprocess behavior that draws on an understanding of the meaning of numbers and their rules of relative position, which has been termed the syntax of reading numbers—the accurate reading, speaking, and writing of number names (McCarthy & Warrington, 1990). With all these skills is needed a successful mix of judgement, creative imagination, and self-confidence.

Although it is invalid to translate findings of acalculia in traumatically brain-damaged adults to children with developmental number retardation, it should be useful to use neuropsychological clinical diagnostic procedures to examine the cognitive deficits in their disability.

Developmental Number Retardation

The neuropsychological model of the basic causes of disturbances in arithmetical operations (i.e., spatial, visual–gnostic, and auditory–gnostic) is useful in helping us understand how normal number skills develop and how to diagnose a developmental number retardation. Although we are concentrating on neuropsychological deficits in this discussion, it is obvious that there are other psychological and environmental reasons for poor arithmetical achievement, such as anxiety, cultural attitudes, or poor teaching. Because of its uncompromising structure and function, arithmetic seems to stimulate anxiety in students more than reading, writing, and artistic endeavors. In arithmetic, reality is imposed rigidly on the child, and one who cannot meet its demands, has failed. In creative drama, the child creates his or her own reality, and so in that sense, cannot fail. However, assuming that the child is reasonably happy and secure in the classroom setting, is motivated to learn, and is taught imaginatively, and still is unable to learn arithmetic as well as might normally be expected, a developmental disability may be suspected. The teacher or diagnostician will then proceed to carry out a task analysis to determine the areas of trouble.

The precise origin of developmental dyscalculia is not known, because, like developmental aphasia, it is less clearly defined than in the acquired or traumatic type in older children or adults. However, the few cases that have come to postmortem suggest very strongly, that it is related to the abnormal or underdevelopment of the parietal, temporal, and occipital cortices on both sides and the intracerebral mechanisms with hearing and language.

In Billy's case (Drake, 1968), described in Chapter 8, he was reported to have "some trouble with arithmetic" and a table of his achievement from grade 1 through grade 6 showed him to be near or slightly below average each year. However, his spoken language was normal, as was his spatial imagery (WISC Block Design score

9 at age 10, and 10 at age 12). His visual perception for small details as measured by the WISC Picture Completion subtest was 11 at age 10, and 9 at age 12. In oral arithmetic, as measured by the WISC Arithmetic subtest, he measured only 6 at age 10 (which is poor), and 9 at age 12 (which is low average). The evidence from this case suggests that with normal auditory language, and average visual–cognitive and spatial skills, Billy, in spite of his biparietal and callosal underdevelopment, was able to manage classroom arithmetic for his age nearly at an average level. Put another way, he was not aphasic, and his spatial and visuocognitive skills were nearly normal.

The second case (Landau, Goldstein, & Kleffner, 1960), also discussed in Chapter 8, concerned a boy who seemed mentally bright enough but had no speech. At age 6 he measured a performance IQ of 78, and 2 years later, after specialized teaching in a class for aphasic children, his performance IQ measured 97. At this time, at age 8, he could count to 5 (something that is common to many preschoolers) and his number concepts were poor. By the age of 9 he could add and subtract numbers up to 10, an achievement normally reached before the end of first grade. At age 10 he measured an educational quotient of 76, but no information was provided regarding his arithmetical skill. By comparison, this boy showed progress much inferior to Billy's, and probably the major contributing factor was his aphasia. We are provided with no detailed information about either his spatial imagery or his visual–perceptual competence, as we were in the case of Billy, but it seems safe to conclude that they were average because his last performance IQ measured 97. This evidence suggests that developmental problems in auditory language probably are more devastating to arithmetical competence than is a deficit in any other psychological process, because it impairs inner language, conceptual growth, and incidental learning.

Cohn (1968) has provided some interesting case histories with data from neurological examinations. He concludes that developmental dyscalculia is manifested by (1) malformed, frequently reversed, or large number symbols; (2) dyslexia; (3) inability to sum single integers; (4) inability to recognize operator signs and to use linear separators; (5) failure to read accurately the correct value of multidigit numbers because of their order and spacing; (6) poor memory for basic number facts; (7) failure to "carry" numbers where appropriate; and (8) inaccurate ordering and spacing of numbers in multiplication and division. The reader will recognize the close relationship between this list of behavioral deficits and Luria's sequential examination of acalculia in traumatically brain-damaged adults.

Because most of the current neuroimaging studies (in particular PET and BEAM) of brain functions during controlled cognitive tasks have addressed problems of reading, dyslexia, spelling, and verbal ideation, investigations of brain changes during mathematical computation have so far been largely neglected. Consequently the neuropsychological literature on mathematical disorders has had limited educational use (Keller & Sutton, 1991), and this situation may remain until we know much more about specific brain functions during mathematical calculations. This situation is also a result of the fact that most writers in this field are basic research neuropsychologists, almost all without classroom experience with either normal-learning or LD students, and many of whom admit to no interest in or responsibility for educational remediation. In the past, the few researchers who also had classroom teaching experience and who combined their knowledge of both fields (i.e., research and teaching), produced publications that have been invaluable to special educators for many years (e.g., Cruickshank, 1961, 1966, 1977, 1979, 1981; Cruickshank & Hallahan, 1975; Johnson & Myklebust, 1967; Myklebust, 1965, 1967, 1971, 1973, 1983). Fortunately in the nonneuropsychological educational literature readers can learn about the contents of mathematics as recommended by the National Council of Teachers of Mathematics in the United States, and they can find some detailed material on recommended current instructional methods (Smith & Rivera, 1991). The reader can combine the neuropsychological with the purely educational literature for a better-balanced presentation, which can offer the teacher and the school clinical neuropsychologist the promise of devising a more successful remedial program.

Arithmetical Aptitude, Nonverbal Learning, and Social Adjustment

One of the first to recognize the important relationship between nonverbal learning and social adjustment was Myklebust (1975b), who produced many new insights pertaining to this reciprocal association. Because all learning implies both verbal and nonverbal processes, and because the verbal aspects of learning have attracted most attention in the past, Myklebust examined nonverbal intelligence and its relation to academic achievement. Nonverbal learning, in addition to including spatial–constructional skills, temporal estimates, knowledge of body parts, and directional sense, also implies social perceptions of oneself and of others. Competent social understanding is intimately related to personal independence and greater comprehension of the subtleties of social interactions. Myklebust has proposed that because a weak ability for social perceptions limits one's inner experience, and because this has an impoverishing effect on all deductions and adaptive learning, it is reasonable to conclude that nonverbal learning disorders "are more debilitating than verbal disabilities" (Myklebust, 1975b). He argues that although both verbal and nonverbal skills contribute simultaneously to normal information processing in social perceptions, verbal deficits may have little effect on nonverbal experiences, but nonverbal impairments can produce serious distortions in social perceptions. People so impaired may have fluent speech but may be indecisive, emotionally immature, and socially dependent. Examinations of large samples of children supported his hypotheses. Academically failing students of normal intelligence possessed significantly poorer nonverbal skills on a battery of performance tests. These children were less able to produce time concepts; to orient themselves in space; to make judgments of size, speed, height, and laterality; to identify body parts; to carry out motor activities smoothly; and to behave in a socially mature way. A discriminant function analysis showed a large number of performance tests to discriminate between LD and normal children.

As we have already seen, the cognitive functions involved in arithmetical calculations (i.e., number concept, relative value, and accurate reading of numbers) draw heavily on basic spatial skills, abilities essential to success on all or most performance tests. Strang and Rourke (1983) found that a group of children whose arithmetic scores on the Wide Range Achievement Test (Jastak & Jastak, 1965) were at least 1.8 years higher than their reading and spelling scores on the same test, had a mean performance IQ (PIQ) on the WISC (Wechsler, 1949) of 107.2 and a mean verbal IQ (VIQ) of only 92.27. Another group with the reverse pattern (i.e., reading and spelling scores more than at least 2 years higher than arithmetic) had a mean VIQ of 102.2 and a mean PIQ of 87.93. Differences in both cases were highly significant. With these findings these researchers concluded that, "It would seem clear that the deficient nonverbal concept-formation and reasoning abilities found to be characteristic of Group 3 children [those with VIQ > PIQ] contribute in some way to their social inadequacies" (Strang & Rourke, 1983). They also found that on the Halstead Category Test (a test of inductive and deductive reasoning using geometric figures in spatial relationships) the Group 2 children (those with PIQ > VIQ) tended to improve with experience, but Group 3 children did not benefit to the same extent.

Myklebust has provided a number of detailed case histories to illustrate individual examples of his group findings that led him to conclude that, "No longer is it feasible to consider deficits in learning only in psycholinguistic terms or only in any other terms that overlook the nonverbal aspects of experience" (1975b). These comprise not only social comprehension and nonverbal reasoning, but should also include emotional and motivational aspects. This means that the social behavior and learning strategies of the learner should be included in a comprehensive examination of cognitive structure and development.

Drawing on Luria's model of the functional organization of the brain (see Chapter 2, page 85), Das, a student of Luria, and his colleagues have developed a theory of intelligence that sees *coding* and *planning* as the basic cognitive functions (Das, Kirby, & Jarman, 1979). Within coding they include Luria's concepts of *simultaneous* and *successive* processing. By coding, Das, Kirby, and Jarman recognize the cognitive functions of Luria's second cerebral functional unit or block—that is, the reception, analysis, and storage of information. Physically, this block of the brain was conceived by Luria to include the post-Rolandic areas. Like Luria, Das, Kirby, and Jarman see planning and executive direction as the principal function of the frontal lobes. To summarize, "The three blocks of the brain are concerned respectively, with arousal, coding, and planful behavior" (Das, Kirby, & Jarman, 1979). Intelligent behavior is conceived as including an adequate level of arousal (Block 1), comprehensive knowledge (Block 2), and competence in creative thinking, planning, and decision making (Block 3). A weakness in any one or more of these can lead to inferior learning.

An example of simultaneous processing is looking at a map or geometric figure, where all parts of the stimulus can be perceived at once. An example of successive processing is listening to or reading human speech, where each part is perceived serially and the whole meaning is not conveyed until the end of the sentence. Serial processing has been attributed largely to left-hemisphere function and simultaneous processing mainly to the right.

This model of cognition, though not complete, has been useful for examining academic achievement because coding and planning are involved in all learning tasks, although some types of learning stress one more than the other. For example, learning a ten-word vocabulary list does not require much planning; it depends primarily on verbal memory and retrieval. Arithmetical facts are memorized and coded, but using them in problem solving requires decision making and planning (i.e., adaptive intelligence).

Kirby and Ashman (1984) have examined the possible relation between planning skills and achievement in mathematics. They see some aspects of the ability for planning as susceptible to instructions, and its weakness as one of the causes of poor academic achievement in LD children. By a factor analysis they found four types of planning that emerged from the tests that they used: a scanning factor, both visual (e.g., mazes) and verbal (e.g., word fluency); a rehearsal factor (specific to digit-span tasks); a clustering factor (specific to semantic categorizing of common objects); and a metacognition factor employed in open-ended situational problems. They compared the arithmetic scores of 121 grade 5 students with their scores on a battery of planning tests and concluded that the scanning, or selective attention factor, is the best predictor of mathematical achievement, followed perhaps by metacognition.

Social maladjustment and emotional problems have frequently been noticed more often in LD children and adults than in the general population of the same age (Spreen, 1988). A poor academic self-image is an expected result of continued school failure or a frustrating level of academic mediocrity. Failure in any field of educational achievement may contribute to feelings of frustration and inferiority, but mathematics, because it is completely uncompromising, may be more likely to undermine the self-image than reading, spelling, or writing. "It is quite possible to gain an appreciation of the gist of a sentence or passage even when a number of words have been misread or skipped over" (Strang & Rourke, 1985). But mathematics are not as forgiving. Even in simple arithmetical calculations, a mistake made at any point in the operation can result in an error in the final answer. Most teachers of mathematics are aware of the anxiety that their subject arouses in many of their students, and the best of them attempt to defuse this anxiety with explicit and lucid explanations, and comments implying success by the student.

However, there is no single LD personality type (Porter & Rourke, 1985). These investigators, using the Personality Inventory for Children and a Q-type factor analysis, found that of 77 children with learning problems the sample included four subtypes of LD children who differed from one another in socioemotional behavior. The first subtype, which made up almost half of their sample, were aware of their poor academic achievement but there were no more test signs of personality problems, on average, than their normally achieving peers. It seems that this group may represent the students who, although academically mediocre, have been able to compensate in other areas so that their school record is not disturbing to them. The second subtype, about a quarter of the sample, appeared from the results of the inventory to be the most seriously disturbed. Half of the scales measured in the high range interpreted to indicate serious personality problems, and most of the other scales were elevated enough to be considered sources of at least mild difficulty. Porter and Rourke concluded that "one would expect these children to be moody . . . with many of the symptoms of childhood depression. . . . Their self-esteem tends to be low, and they are notably more fearful, worried, anxious, and emotionally labile than are their well adjusted peers." The third subtype, comprising 13% of the sample, measured high scores on only one scale, Somatic Concern. These children provided test scores indicating roughly normal personality functioning other than overconcern for their health. It is possible that some of them had experienced serious health problems or that their mothers had been hypochondriacally overanxious and had communicated this anxiety to them. The fourth subtype, making up almost a fifth of the sample, showed high scores on the Delinquency, Hyperactivity, and other scales. These children "tend to be overactive, restless, highly distractible, and impulsive" (Porter & Rourke, 1985) and they typically have difficulty adjusting to authority and frequently are in conflict with the law. Every experienced teacher recognizes this type of child. Porter and Rourke's study has value in drawing attention to the variety of possible behavior patterns of LD children and dispels the assumption of homogeneity of behavior resulting from long-term academic frustration.

The research studies cited here point to a possible relationship between "social intelligence" and mathematical ability, and though much more study of this relationship is needed to clarify it, these studies may alert the educator to recognize much broader cognitive and behavioral attributes in mathematical competence than have been formerly and generally realized.

Piaget and Luria

Probably no one has examined the development of the child's cognitive growth in more depth than Piaget, and very few have studied in more detail the neuropsychological relationships of cerebral dysfunction than Luria, so that a comparison of their work should prove useful.

Although Piaget was not primarily concerned with establishing normative data for children, all of his studies revealed an emerging cognitive complexity determined by the biological growth of the child. "Piaget's early academic training was in zoology, and his theory of cognitive development is rooted firmly there" (Phillips, 1975). The biology of the growing human brain and its relation to learning is just beginning to be understood. As recently as 1950, Lashley admitted an inability to find any difference in brain structure following learning (Lashley, 1950), but since then histological evidence has appeared (Conel, 1939–1963) to reveal a marked change in brain structure with growth and experience. Although

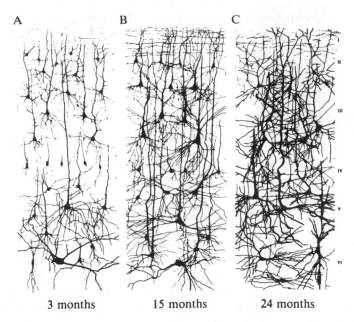

3 months   15 months   24 months

Figure 9.15. Drawings of sections from the cerebral cortex of children aged 3, 15, and 24 months. The increased growth with age of interconnections and the thickening of the dendrites can be observed. (From the work of Conel (A), 1947; (B), 1955; (C), 1959. With the permission of Dr. Karl H. Pribram.)

the total number of neurons in the central nervous system is almost complete at birth and continues to increase for only a very short period postnatally, the work of Conel has shown a marked increase in dendritic arborization at the age of 3, 15, and 24 months postnatally (see Fig. 9.15). Although it is evident that the engram or neural trace accompanying learning is not an increase in neural cell bodies, it may result from (1) neural growth of growth cones or amoeboid-like structures on the tips of dendritic branches; (2) the increase of neuroglia, nonneural tissue that supports the neurons; or (3) biochemical changes at the synapse or within the neurons, which possess some degree of permanence (Pribram, 1971).

Regardless of the physiological etiology of the neural trace, Piaget's work possesses hundreds of examples of cognitive change, from perceptual naiveté to logical abstraction, and from simplicity to mental complexity, which parallel the development of the brain and nervous system. In studying the mental imagery of the child at ages 5, 7, and 11 years and at the adult level, he found a progressive decrease in errors in copying a 20-cm rod, and after imagining rotating it 180° or seeing it in another indicated position (Piaget &

Inhelder, 1971). In studying the development of the child's concept of number, a problem particularly pertinent to the present discussion, Piaget was interested in establishing the concept of permanence (conservation) of a number or quantity. Just as he had found that the infant in the first months discovered the permanence of perceived objects when they were out of sight, the realization of a permanent number concept appears between the ages of about 4 and 7 years. This cognitive process must develop before the child can reason in arithmetic because "a number is only intelligible if it remains identical with itself, whatever the distribution of the units of which it is composed" (Piaget, 1941). Initially the child perceives quantities perceptually "in the sensible universe." At the age of 4 or 5, most children have no idea about the conservation of quantity regardless of its change in shape. If two containers of identical size and shape are filled with exactly identical quantities of liquid, the child at this age will say the two quantities are similar because he *sees* the two levels are the same. If the contents of one of these containers is poured into a tall, narrow container, however, the child will now say it contains more liquid than the other, because he can *see* the level of the liquid much higher.

By about the age of 6, children begin to become less *perceptual* and more *conceptual* and will begin to give answers that show an unresolved conflict between what they see and what they think. By age 7, most children understand that the quantities of liquid are conserved "irrespective of the number and nature of the changes made" (Piaget, 1941).

This same pattern of cognitive development can be demonstrated with continuous quantities (liquids) and discontinuous quantities (such as beads or beans). A 5-year-old confronted with two glass containers of similar size and shape filled with equal numbers of identical beads will say the quantities are similar, again because he can *see* the levels are the same. However, if the beads from one container are poured into a tall narrow one, he will say it now contains more beads than the other container. When questioned, he will say that a necklace made from the beads in the tall container will be longer than a necklace made from the beads in the other one. When the beads from the tall container are poured back into the original one, the 5-year-old will state that a necklace now would be the same length as the other one. In other words the quantities, according to the child at this stage, will increase and decrease because of their *perceived* sizes. By the time they are 6 years old, most children realize that the numbers of beads remain constant regardless of the shapes of their containers, and that necklaces made from two equal quantities of beads, regardless of the shape of their container, will be the same lengths.

Because Piaget was primarily interested in studying the intellectual growth of normal children, his experimental evidence parallels normal brain development. To examine the effects of brain dysfunctions on the pattern of cognitive growth he described, we will look at a few Piagetian experiments carried out with mentally retarded subjects.

"Piaget sees the mind as a dynamic system which, en route to maturity, passes through qualitatively different levels of integration" (Robinson & Robinson, 1976), as opposed to a view of the mind as possessing a fixed structure that acquires new knowledge and skills. The Piagetian view not only gives more hope to the retarded child but gives us more information about his intellectual development. It will be remembered that Piaget proposed four major developmental periods: (1) the sensorimotor period, extending from birth to about 2 years, is marked by reflex, sensory, and motor activity; (2) the preoperational period, extending from about 2 to 7 years, is marked by the beginning of symbolic thinking, although it is characterized by perceptual rather than conceptual processes; (3) the period of concrete operations, extending from age 7 to 11, is typified by rapid development of number and spatial processes and an understanding of mechanical cause and effect; and (4) the period of formal operations, extending from age 11 to 15, is marked by rapid expansion of symbolic thinking, abstract conceptualizing, and the improved ability to carry on inductive and deductive reasoning. Because mental life is mediated by the brain and central nervous system, brain-damaged subjects may be expected to function at a level lower than normal for their age. Research, both within Piaget's laboratory and in other centers, with mentally retarded subjects has shown this to be true. Inhelder (1968), a colleague of Piaget, found the profoundly mentally retarded adult as fixated at the sensorimotor level of intelligence. The moderately retarded adult reached the preoperational stage of intuition but usually could develop no further. The mildly retarded adult, usually a trainable and educable subject, reached the level of concrete operations, and the borderline mentally dull subject might master a limited repertoire of the simpler forms of mental abstractions. Independent work carried on in centers other than the Geneva Laboratory have been largely confirmatory, although some researchers have not found all mentally impaired subjects to fall into the stages in a clear-cut way. This is understandable in terms of present neuropsychological knowledge: Spotty or localized brain damage may impair many mental functions and leave others to function at an above-average level because the cerebral areas vital to their operation may have been spared.

The three major causes of a developmental number retardation and dyscalculia—that is, deficits in language (auditory–gnostic), reading (visual–gnostic), and/or spatial imagery, can be understood within the Piagetian model of development. Auditory language or oral speech develops mainly during the first two periods, reading and writing and automatic handling of numbers in the third period, and abstract reasoning in mathematics in the final period, during adolescence. This developmental model also fits the usual curriculum pattern of the elementary and junior high school. The first-grader arrives, at age 6, with an oral vocabulary of about 2500 words or more; he or she still is largely "magical" and subjective in thinking and is unable to deal with temporal abstractions. During the next 4 or 5 years the child learns very rapidly to read and write and to master hundreds of number and verbal facts and to understand spatial diagrams and maps. By junior high school he is learning to solve problems in arithmetic that require adaptive thinking, to manage problematic abstractions in algebra, and to resolve spatial theorems in geometry. All of this learning requires normal and healthy bilateral cerebral function; any brain damage or dysfunction, whether localized or diffuse, may impair some or all of these psychological processes.

Although most of Luria's clinical experimentation had been with brain-injured adults he drew liberally from the work of Piaget and many Russian investigators to put together his theory of the ontogenetic formation of the concept of number and of arithmetical operations. He recognized the visual, spatial, and finally conceptual aspects of number processes in that order as the child grows, but he stressed that "in the latter stages the concept of number and arithmetical operations retain their spatial components" (Luria, 1966).

If a child suffers from cerebral agenesis in the parts of the brain primarily responsible for spatial perception and spatial imagery (these parts in the traumatically brain-damaged adult are always in the temporo–parieto–occipital systems), then he may be unable to scan or imagine points in asymmetrical space "which are essential for correct calculation" (Luria, 1966). Arithmetical operations become difficult or impossible through loss of their spatial coordinates.

In our laboratory we have found significant correlations of .43 between arithmetic and sequential memory of light patterns at the grade 2 level and one of .32 at the grade 5 level (Gaddes & Spellacy, 1977). This relationship was measured by the Dynamic Visual Retention Test, a device that illuminates patterns of lights on a computer screen. To do this test successfully the child must imagine a set of spatial coordinates on the bare screen against which he or she must compare the location of the lights being illuminated. Although sequential memory may be related to arithmetical competence, it seems almost certain that the spatial skills demanded by the test are also strongly involved.

Luria's model of arithmetical acquisition parallels Piaget's. This model comes largely from his study of brain-damaged adults, but it is based on his observations of the order in which number operations disappear with brain damage. It seems reasonable to believe that they appear during normal growth in the reverse order, and clinical observation supports this. The preschool child begins with material objects, which he or she can handle, arranged in space, and later acquires the number facts from visual and manual contact with the objects. When the child learns to write numbers this knowledge leads to the formation of tabular calculation, and following this automatized learning through oral recitation and writing in a particular spatial arrangement, he finally learns to think symbolically with numbers and to reason abstractly.

This model also fits the curriculum of the elementary and junior high school. In grades 1–4 inclusive, children are mostly occupied in automatizing number facts and writing the calculations in correct spatial pattern. By grades 5 and 6 they begin to read and contend with problems the calculations of which depend on correct mechanical function but in which choice of method is not automatic but deductive. Some children who may have been adequate in arithmetic up to grade 4 may begin to have difficulties because their abilities for logical abstraction are inadequate.

In Chapter 4 the case of Will, who was born with a medial right-hemisphere lesion, was described. Although he was above average in the language arts, he had extreme difficulty with art, reading maps in geography, arithmetic, and anything demanding spatial analysis or synthesis. When he reached high school he could manage algebra at a passing grade but geometry was impossible for him. This evidence suggests that his inarithmetria was not a result of inferior reasoning abilities, otherwise he could not have succeeded in algebra, but a result of his severely impaired spatial skills. Certainly, this case can be understood in the light of Luria's model and provides a special example of normal language and reading skills but defective spatial abilities. In this case, the boy's deficit, in only one of the major etiological areas, was enough to produce a severe anarithmetria but an average calculation ability in algebra, which is a type of quantitative reasoning expressed in verbal rather than numerical symbols.

10 Remediation, Therapy, and the Learning Disabled Child

Theory provides insights that lead to effective action, which in turn keeps the theory alive and dynamic. The problem is to assure that neither dominates the other.

Landon Pearson (1990)

In remediation planning, we must recognize the ways in which the learning disability influences the child's pattern of motivation, not only the ways in which motivational factors might be influential in complicating the effects of the learning disability. This is the essence of the psychoneurologic approach to intervention.

Helmer R. Myklebust (1975a)

Although remedial measures have been described throughout this book, this chapter is devoted to a more systematic examination of possible treatment measures for the child or adult with learning problems.

Teachers are primarily practitioners and usually are more interested in what to do about a child's learning disorder than in spending time looking for causes. Whereas this approach may be admissible for the busy teacher, the school psychologist should take time to be experimental and help the teacher by suggesting new remedial alternatives. In the past, it has not been unknown for a teacher to apply the same remedial method to all his or her students. One young teacher recently said, "I find the Gillingham method the best for my children." Unfortunately, one of her students with a subtle form of receptive aphasia and auditory imperception was unable to learn to read under her energetic and well-meaning efforts. She failed to realize that a phonetic system such as the Gillingham method, though successful for most children, is almost useless for a child who cannot discriminate phonetic sounds. With more knowledge she would have had a better chance of success with this boy.

A second common pattern is the teacher who learns two or more methods of teaching reading or some other academic skill. When faced with the LD child this teacher tries every technique in his or her repertoire in a "shotgun" attack. This approach need not include any diagnostic understanding of the child's learning problem, and frequently does not; it does include a blind trial of one technique after another until the teacher's repertoire is exhausted. With luck, one of these methods may happen to mesh with the child's needs, and he or she begins to show improvement. Without this kind of luck the teacher is defeated and the child may be abandoned to "busywork," sarcasm, or neglect, all of which compound his personal problems.

A third pattern, and the one recommended here, includes an educational, psychological, and social analysis of the child, a task analysis of the skills to be taught; a choice of a remedial program; and a periodic evaluation of the possible progress. The psychological analysis should include both physiological and behavioral data in cases where neurological dysfunction is clearly indicated.

Cognitive Processes and Cerebral Organization

A knowledge of normal brain function can direct the diagnostician to examine all or most psychological processes involved in learning. In other words, we can *let the knowledge of brain structure and function direct us*. If we start with the occipital lobes, we will need a battery of tests to tap the various visual–perceptual skills such as figure–ground, form recognition, letter and word recognition, visual memory, visual sequential memory, and visual–motor speed and accuracy, to name a few. If we then move to the temporal lobes, we will want to know about auditory perception of verbal and nonverbal stimuli, auditory sequential memory, dichotic listening, oral and written language, verbal memory, spatial imagery, etc. The parietal lobes should direct us to enquire into tactile form recognition, tactile sensitivity, finger localization, directional sense, body image, tactile naming, etc. The frontal lobes should remind us to check motor speed and accuracy, hand-grip strength, motor speech, and a variety of motor, postural, and movement skills (Ayres, 1972a; de Quiros & Schrager, 1978). As we saw in Chapter 9, frontal lobe function should remind us to examine visual scanning (e.g., mazes); selective attention (e.g., cognitive scanning of the lexicon, or personal active vocabulary, in a word-fluency test);

and planning (mobilizing and organizing ideas into a useful and systematic pattern). Even a small battery of "planning" tests can be useful to indicate cognitive functions usually missed or insufficiently assessed by standard intelligence tests (Kirby & Ashman, 1984). A consideration of the two cerebral hemispheres should direct our attention to the expected balance of language and spatial–constructional skills, and the sensorimotor cortex should suggest examining kinesthetic sensations, visual–manual and auditory–manual reaction times, and any skill integrating "spatial, kinesthetic, and language information to motor formulation and movement" (Calanchini & Trout, 1971). A neuropsychological knowledge of normal brain function can direct attention to normal processes in all the various perceptual and motor skills instrumental in academic competence. In understanding abnormal behavior it is essential.

One of the most inclusive concepts of normal brain function and the relation of central processing deficiencies to children's learning problems is that of Rourke (1982). Drawing on the model of normal brain function proposed by Goldberg and Costa (1981), Rourke has presented a tentative theory to understand better "central processing deficiencies in children." Although some researchers have held that ontogenetically cerebral hemispheric organization proceeds from the left to the right hemisphere, Rourke, following Bakker (1979), Goldberg and Costa, and others, holds the reverse view. This concept seems to be supported by naturalistic observation of small children who, during their first year of life, appear to be observing and interpreting their world *nonverbally* and pictorially. Then, at about 12 months of age, when they have had time to learn some simple interpretations of their environment, they begin to code these in vocal utterances. Some observers interpret this as "filling the right hemisphere first" with broad, nonverbal concepts, and when small children have reached a certain level of simplistic understanding, they then begin to develop speech. Presumably the first process is mediated mainly by the right hemisphere and the second by the left. Rourke has explained all common forms of learning disabilities in terms of the right hemisphere subserving novel experiences that involve global, nonverbal concepts. "Right-hemisphere systems provide the content for concepts whereas left-hemisphere systems are particularly geared to their articulation, elaboration, and stereotypic application" (Rourke, 1982). Because reading is at first a novel experience, it may be mediated initially by the right hemisphere, but with practice the graphemes, which at first were unfamiliar, are related to the already established speech pattern of phonemes. As the process of reading becomes automatized, in most children it is seen as drawing less on right hemisphere function for decoding and more on the left. Rourke sees the right hemisphere as then free to analyze, organize, and synthesize the conceptual content of what is read—that is, the essence of comprehension. This model can explain why some children can decode and read orally at a normal speed for their age, but their comprehension is limited or inadequate. These children presumably have adequate left-hemisphere functions to mediate normally automatized reading, and either deficient or partially inaccessible right-hemisphere activity to provide successful conceptual understanding. Using this model of normal brain function with localized or regional dysfunctions, Rourke also accounts for the child who can learn to read by the "look–say" method but later has difficulty with phonetic decoding and resulting impaired comprehension; this same child frequently understands the same material very well when it is read to him by someone else at a normal speed. Rourke has also examined the phonetically accurate and the phonetically inaccurate spellers; various subtypes of empirically derived reading disabled children; and the acquisition of arithmetical skills, both routinized and calculable. Rourke presents his model as tentative and limited by areas of present ignorance of the detailed cerebral functions and the psychological processes involved in children's learning and its disorders. Nevertheless, it seems to be one of the most promising theoretical frameworks to explain the clinical findings of LD children, and to provide a basis for their remediation.

Luria, in his studies of brain-damaged adults, recognized (1) the *psychological structure* of an act, and (2) the organized cerebral activity mediating that particular behavior. The first is the observed behavior (e.g., the child learning to write "mat" may sound each letter singly, remember its visual form, and draw each letter laboriously). The cerebral areas subserving these various activities are becoming more accessible to observation with the appearance of the many brain-scanning and other new investigative techniques.

Remediation drills change not only the psychological structure of a given operation, and this is what concerns the remedial teacher, but also its cerebral organization. With repeated exercise, desired skills can be automatized with presumed neural traces established to enable a repetition of the skill at a desired time in the future. Luria believed that well-automatized forms of mental activity are based on a cerebral control system quite different from newly acquired ones, so that all new learning implies a reorganization of it with the old learning, and a parallel reorganization of the various cerebral structures underlying these different skills.

The neuropsychological model of diagnosis and remediation as practiced by Luria, Reitan, Myklebust, and many others is summarized in Table 10.1. Columns A and B include the neuropsychological information obtained on a particular child or adult. The

Table 10.1. The Neuropsychological Model of Diagnosis and Remediation

Neuropsychological Information

Neurological Data	Psychological Structure of the Child	Task Analysis
A	B	C
Information from neurologist *re* locus, intensity, and nature of identifiable brain dysfunction, or lack of such evidence	Information from neuropsychological test battery *re* which perceptual, cognitive, and motor skills are normal and which defective	List of perceptual, cognitive, and motor skills needed for successful achievement of the academic skill under consideration (e.g., reading, spelling, arithmetic)
Brain function or dysfunction	Learning disability	

school psychologist may use his or her broad knowledge of the discipline to relate the neurological information in A with the behavioral evidence in B, and to judge the possible chronicity of the learning disability and its response to remediation. Column C contains a detailed task analysis of the desired academic skill, and the discrepancies between specific points in B and C will provide the clues for the choice of an appropriate therapeutic procedure by the teacher and the school psychologist.

Any learning task can be analyzed by observing systematically and in detail how an "expert" completes the task. An expert, in this case, is anyone who performs the task efficiently and successfully. "Task analysis has very little to do with instructional methodology. It has everything to do with figuring out how people go about doing certain tasks" (Johnson & Morasky, 1977, p. 272). Of course, it may provide the basis for directing the teacher to include the skills, decisions, and strategies necessary for success.

However, while it is highly likely that chronic perceptual, cognitive, or motor deficits are the most common causes for failure to learn in school–age children, the factors described in Table 10.1 do not account for all underachievers. Some children fail because of ineffective learning strategies (Torgesen, 1977), inattention, weak self-confidence, poor motivation, and a lack of a strong intent to learn. Others fail because of a mixture of perceptual deficits and motivational weaknesses. Other students, with neither of these deficiencies, may perform at a mediocre level because they lack originality or creative imagination. Students of this type may be able to perform well enough on tests of highly structured material that they have mastered, but they may feel defeated when faced with an open-ended problem that requires mental procedures of trial-and-error, independent choice and decision, and restructuring and reorganization of present knowledge. These students may be able to master the routinized number facts, but be intimidated by arithmetical problem solving that demands a flexible interaction of several conceptual processes operating simultaneously and sequentially. Such students may lack adequate adaptive intelligence either because of inheritance or unimaginative teaching.

This means that the school psychologist must exercise a sensitive insight in his or her interpretation of the test findings in column B, Table 10.1. The psychologist can guard against diagnostic invalidities by testing the possible chronicity or transience of a deficit symptom (e.g., repeating the test at another time) or being aware of those behavioral skills that are more vulnerable to the effects of anxiety or less appealing or more threatening to the testee (e.g., a finger-tapping test as the first test in a battery is usually more interesting to the academically underachieving subject, and also more reliable than a problem-solving task designed to measure an ability for deductive or inductive reasoning). As Torgesen has pointed out, a better understanding of these motivational factors in learning will be useful in deciding on remedial measures.

What Is Meant by Remediation?

Remediation implies a controlled balance between the impaired learner's abilities and the demands of his environment, and this is true whether the learner is a child or an adult. If this balance is finely tuned, the learner can be led to acquire new academic and social skills and to continue to be stimulated and satisfied. If the demands are too easy, the balance is too lax and the learner becomes bored; if the demands are too difficult, the balance is too strained and the learner is frustrated, distracted, and increasingly disinterested. A strong disturbing force in either the learner or his environment will shift the balance of diagnostic attention by demanding more understanding in devising compensatory treatment of the source of disturbance. Two examples should clarify this. A 10-year-old boy is referred because of failing grades in school and an uncontrolled temper at home and at school. Analysis of the problem shows a stable, supporting family, but medical evidence of a marked EEG dysrhythmia in the boy's left temporal lobe. This electrical disturbance very likely may be related to his temper outbursts and his poor achievement in the language arts. These findings can lead to a medical consultation, a prescription of an appropriate medication to reduce the temper outbursts, and a psychoeducational treatment of the boy's aphasoid symptoms. Another case may show normal physical health but a family pattern of emotional conflict and marital strife. Here attention is directed more to the environmental side of the equation, and a balance is sought by attempting to resolve the disturbing family situation and to train the child to understand the problems and to learn some compensatory skills.

Assessment and Diagnosis

A careful diagnostic analysis of the child's perceptual, cognitive, motor, and educational skills precedes any consideration of a remedial program. If there are strong behavioral indications of possible cerebral dysfunctions, a complete neurological and neuropsychological examination is carried out. Even without such indications, a neuropsychological test battery may still be useful because of its thorough coverage of the child's psychological abilities. Also, it might reveal some soft signs not previously detected, or in their absence it can provide evidence of the child's cognitive strengths and confirm the purely motivational nature of his learning problems.

Neuropsychological assessment may contain two levels of examination: (1) Screening. This includes the evaluation of groups of children on a brief battery of tests shown to have a high level of predictive validity for selecting "at risk" LD children. Such a test battery is only a scanning instrument, and "scanning does not imply diagnosis" (Silver, 1978); at best, it will select only those subjects with the deficit that the battery is designed to identify, and having done that, the learning-impaired children so designated may be referred for in-depth diagnosis. It has a number of methodological problems that should be observed by anyone planning to construct or use a screening battery (de Hirsch, 1971; Hynd, Hayes, & Snow, 1982; Jansky & de Hirsch, 1972; Satz & Fletcher, 1979; Silver, 1978). (2) Diagnosis. Most referrals of children for diagnostic study come from parents or school personnel concerned about the child's obvious learning problems. LD adults who come (they are usually severe developmental dyslexics) are either self-referred or urged by a concerned spouse. This means that only a minority are referred from screening programs. Clinical assessment programs vary and will reflect the clinician's theoretical preferences and applied training. For children, the most commonly used test batteries are the Halstead–Reitan tests (Reitan & Davison, 1974; Reitan & Wolfson, 1992a,b; Selz, 1981), the Spreen–Benton tests

(Benton, Hamsher, Varney, & Spreen, 1983; Gaddes & Crockett, 1975; Spreen & Benton, 1977; Spreen & Strauss, 1991), and composite batteries of well-established tests. Composite batteries frequently lack a systematic conceptual framework but have the advantage of flexibility. New tests may be added with the discovery of new insights, and modified batteries can be adapted to differing behavioral patterns of specific children. This approach is recommended by Obrzut (1981, p. 249) and is used in our own laboratory. Golden (1981) began in 1980 to adapt the Luria tests for children, and in the past decade considerable research has investigated its validity, reliability, and clinical usefulness. Tramontana and Hooper (1988) provide a useful summary account of the major studies carried out between 1980 and 1988, with a discussion and evaluation of the Luria-Nebraska Neuropsychological Battery—Children's Revision (LNNB–CR, 1988, pp. 13–16). Useful discussions of assessment methods for children can be found in Obrzut & Hynd, Part II, 1986; Obrzut & Hynd, Part Two, 1991; Reitan & Davison, 1974; Reitan & Wolfson, 1992a,b; Reynolds & Fletcher-Janzen, 1989; Rourke, Bakker, Fisk, & Strang, 1983, Ch. 5; Spreen & Strauss, 1991; Tramontana & Hooper, 1988.

Assessments of adults, though sometimes directed to developmental learning disorders, are more frequently concerned with the study and rehabilitation of brain-damaged patients, monitoring the course of progressive neurological diseases and the effects of traumatic damage or neurosurgery, providing information on psychiatric patients with and without underlying neurological disorders, and detecting neurological dysfunctions in their early stages of development. For further discussions, the reader is referred to Benton, Hamsher, Varney, and Spreen (1983) for an instruction manual for the Spreen-Benton tests; to Lezak (1983) for an updated and comprehensive discussion of the whole field and to Reitan and Wolfson (1992c) for explanations of the Halstead–Reitan battery.

Interventionist Theory

The neuropsychological literature contains numerous attempts to identify and classify the various subtypes of LD, but few studies explore the validity of different forms of intervention (Obrzut & Hynd, 1991, pp. 513–518). Academic remedial procedures in the past have come from current educational practices, from trial-and-error attempts by teachers, and from discoveries and theories derived from medicine, neurology, social philosophy, psychology, and religion. Many theoretical models have been proposed (e.g., perceptual processing, multisensorimotor training, language facilitation, direct and indirect methods of training the brain, and so on), but most of these models are descriptive. Their causal aspects are implied but difficult or impossible to demonstrate empirically.

The teacher and the educational administrator are satisfied if the student's directed learning has occurred. But for the researcher in the field of interventionist theory, that is not enough. That specialist will want to know (1) how much learning has taken place in the material being taught, as well as (2) how much transfer of training has directly resulted from the remedial model being scrutinized. Shayer (1987) has reported three research studies designed to examine the effectiveness of Piagetian methods for improving formal operational thinking in early adolescents (ages 12–14). All three studies demonstrated that Piagetian methods achieve substantial positive effects in relation to control groups. Shayer has pointed out, however, that the improvement was shown by using psychological tests of specific cognitive skills as posttests, and these correlate with and predict learning; they do not indicate a metacognitive or general mental improvement in formal operational thinking. "Until a study carries out a post-intervention comparison of fresh learning by experimental and control groups we will not know how much transfer of training has taken place" (Shayer, 1987).

Training the Brain: A Direct Approach

The influence of Luria's impressive clinical assessments and treatment of severely brain-damaged patients; the notable work of Benton, Reitan, Teuber, Geschwind, and others in the United States; and Penfield, Hebb, and Milner in Canada during the 1950s and 1960s preceded the adoption of neuropsychological ideas and practices in special education by Cruickshank, Myklebust, Kephart, and others. And as more knowledge about brain–behavior relationships appeared, some researchers applied this knowledge in an attempt to improve academic learning with *direct training* of the brain.

One of the more impressive attempts of this type is that of Bakker and his associates in Amsterdam. Bakker bases his training practices on a theory that beginning readers tend to process their visual input of print or script more in their right hemispheres, and after a year or so, because cerebral processing becomes less form–perceptual and more verbal–conceptual, they normally shift their linguistic processing to the left hemisphere (Bakker, 1973, 1979). However, if the left hemisphere becomes overdeveloped in this process, presumably through overuse, there may be a poor balance between the functioning of the two hemispheres and the child may become dyslexic. Bakker calls this type of reading disorder L-type (for linguistic) dyslexia. Children with overdeveloped right-hemisphere function during reading may also have difficulties, and Bakker calls this disorder P-type (for perceptual) dyslexia. Bakker reports that dichotic listening, visual half-field stimulation, and electrophysiological evidence support this theory. By prolonged visual presentation of words in the right visual field, he was able to improve the word and sentence reading of P-type boys, and the improvement correlated with increased left-hemisphere activity, as indicated in electrophysiological measures (Bakker, 1981, 1985).

One of us (W.H.G.) was associated professionally for 10 years with a residential school for neurologically impaired and severely learning disabled children, where remedial procedures were based on neuropsychological knowledge of each child's brain. On admission, all the children were examined by a neurologist, providing the school's clinical neuropsychologist with current data on the status of the brain of any child whom he wished to study. Each child was assessed individually and received all remedial procedures designed specifically for him or her. Three examples will illustrate how knowledge of the brain facilitated the invention of the remedial plan that was designed to make the best use of the healthier parts of each child's brain.

1. Some mentally retarded children with neurological evidence of bilateral cerebral dysfunction and retarded language use may have their vocabularies increased and their communicative abilities improved by the use of Bliss Symbols, provided that their right hemisphere is less affected than their left. Presumably their better right hemisphere can process the picture-writing forms, in place of the damaged left hemisphere's inability to respond to printed and written letters and words.

2. Some children with severe difficulty in learning the alphabet may learn it easily by singing it first and then learning to write it. This may happen with a child who has better right-hemisphere function than left. Such a case (Pearson Morsby) was described earlier in Chapter 9. This mechanism appears to be the same that enables congenital stutterers to sing the words in a song completely fluently.

3. A child with a mild or severe hemiparesis will alert the informed teacher not to be surprised if a marked split in verbal and spatial abilities occurs. Understanding the neuropsychological relationships in these types of cases improves the knowledge of the teacher and/or the school psychologist to *predict* the student's possible learning problems and to deal with them remedially. An ignorance by the teacher of these types of cases can lead to frustration and unhappiness on the part of the student; knowledge can

lead to the reverse situation (see case of Will in the Addendum, Chapter 4).

Training the Brain: Indirect Approaches

Every time a learner pronounces a new word correctly with attention to each syllable in order to learn to spell it, every time the piano student repeats a line or phrase of music with awareness of the movement of each finger, or every time a person striving to learn a new verbal or motor skill does it with self-awareness and determination, some type of alteration (the neural engram) is believed to take place in the CNS. The method used by Bakker to improve reading, described above, was specified as "direct training of the brain" because he was using knowledge of brain–behavior relationships to direct the influence of his remedial efforts to specific areas of the cerebral cortex. Our attempts to help impaired children were also designed to stimulate one hemisphere or the other. Most learning and most habilitative approaches, however, are more general in their effects; their neural changes are fortuitous results of cognitive exercises primarily designed to improve a particular academic or intellectual skill. Consequently, this type of brain training has been categorized as "indirect."

An influential proponent of indirect brain training to enhance learning is A. Jean Ayres, whose method to do this is through sensorimotor training. Ayres is both an occupational therapist and psychologist, and has developed a detailed battery of perceptual, motor, and psycholinguistic tests (1976), the findings of which she uses to infer CNS dysfunctions. She strives to improve neuromuscular function with exercises to increase sensorimotor integration at all levels of the nervous system. "If the brain develops the *capacity* to perceive, remember, and motor plan, the ability can then be applied toward mastery of all academic and other tasks, regardless of the specific content" (Ayres, 1972a). Interestingly, in the chapter "The Art of Therapy" in her book on learning disorders, no mention is ever made of specific academic remedial measures. The whole discussion centers on the improvement of sensorimotor accuracy and efficiency. Her book has had a considerable influence on occupational and physiotherapists in clinics with orthopedically and mentally handicapped children, where these therapists' chief responsibility is to improve brain function and motor skills. It is for someone else, presumably a special teacher, to teach the child to read and write.

Another example of indirect brain training are the many programs of "cognitive retraining." These programs grew out of the need for neuropsychological treatment of traumatically brain-injured patients following traffic accidents, and began to appear in the past 20 years in rehabilitation hospitals and outpatient clinics. They include sensory and motor training designed to train the brain and nervous system, as well as mental exercises to recover lost academic and intellectual skills.

An example is Reitan's REHABIT program (Reitan & Wolfson, 1992b), which "has been designed to remediate specific neuropsychological deficits and impairment related to brain damage and dysfunction" (p. 132). It involves assessing the brain-injured child or adult with the Halstead–Reitan Neuropsychological Test Batteries to provide a profile of the "subject's impaired or deficient neuropsychological functions in the framework of a model of brain–behavior relationships, thereby producing an evaluation on which a remediation program can be developed and prescribed" (p. 129). The retraining program is organized around five groups of cognitive abilities with "five tracks" of remediation materials. All five tracks stress abstract reasoning, with emphasis differing from track to track in verbal, spatial, and left- and right-hemisphere function. Diagnostic assessment will indicate which of the five areas are more deficient and which are stronger, and the rationale of the REHABIT program is to provide remediation in the needed areas. Reitan has found that to retrain cognitive functions of persons with cerebral damage, "it is frequently necessary to begin training in the area of abstraction, reasoning, and logical analysis" (p. 114). The reader will remember that Halstead established this approach with his concept of "biological intelligence" 50 years ago; his plan was to compensate for the weaknesses in measures of psychometric intelligence that included too much weight on habituated verbal memory.

Train the Brain or Teach the Child What You Want Him to Learn?

To teach the retarded reader to read, do you only improve brain function, or do you drill the child in the specific perceptual and cognitive skills needed to read? Proponents of both views are equally enthusiastic in recommending their theoretical and remedial beliefs. Let us look at the evidence.

The view that recommends exercising the brain and sensorimotor systems to improve their capacity to learn has a highly respectable history. It grew from an awareness of the integration of neuromuscular functions and cognitive ideas. Maria Montessori, as we have already seen, 90 years ago produced a theory and practice based on motor training, self-direction of the child during learning, and the integration of cognitive development with the "education of the senses" (Montessori, 1964). More recently Kephart, Barsch, Cruickshank, Johnson, Myklebust, and many others have made perceptual and motor training a keystone in their practices of treating LD children. In some extreme cases, poor readers have been removed from regular instruction in reading to crawl around a gymnasium and engage in an intensive motor-training program, with the unfortunate consequence that at the end of the training period, because of educational neglect, they are frequently even further retarded in reading. Such abuses of sensorimotor training are practiced by teachers or others with no real understanding of its functions and potential educational value.

Teach the Child What You Want Him to Learn. The proponents of this view range from some who minimize the value of sensorimotor training to those who encourage training in both basic behavioral skills *and* academic skills. Critchley and Critchley (1978) have used neurological knowledge to throw doubt on the usefulness of sensorimotor integration training for alleviating dyslexia. They take the stand that "there is no logical place in the curriculum for elaborate systems of motor training," on the grounds that reading and writing are functions of the whole brain, whereas motor skills principally involve the limited cortical areas of the sensory and motor strips. Anatomically and functionally their statements are true, but they do not necessarily disprove the value of sensory and motor training as a preparation for academic learning.

Although most remedial programs include drilling the requisite skills for successful academic achievement (e.g., Cruickshank, 1961, 1975, 1977; Downing, 1964; Fernald, 1943; Frostig, 1975; Gillingham, 1965; Gillingham & Stillman, 1936; McGinnis, 1963; Myklebust, 1965; Strauss & Lehtinen, 1947), many, if not most, special educators believe there is value in perceptual and motor training and teaching cognitive and verbal skills.

Some studies suggest that improving sensory integration improves academic scores (Ayres, 1972b), and that at kindergarten and first-grade level it is superior to academic remediation (Serwer, Shapiro, & Shapiro, 1973). A study comparing the relative effectiveness of the Distar II Program with a color-coding system (Scull, 1978) and a traditional phonics approach, found a combination of the Distar and the color coding superior either to the Distar alone or to an achromatic phonics program with second-grade children (Wright, 1978). If color coding improves visual–language integration, as it seems to do, then all of these studies suggest real value in perceptual and sensorimotor training. Unfortunately, all three studies (Ayres, Serwer, and Wright) failed to control for the effects of different remedial teachers and therapists across groups.

Our own clinical experience suggests that some cases of sub-cortical brain damage may not necessarily impair academic skills of adults with traumatic brain injuries. A woman with a benign and progressive brain tumor, seen in our laboratory, gradually developed double vision and difficulty in reading, arithmetic, and mental concentration. The tumor was located centrally just above the thalamus and as it grew it imposed pressure on the optic tracts. Although the woman was depressed and complained that she felt as though "a black cloud of fog" was on her mind, we found that she could read accurately, although slowly, and she could answer the arithmetic questions on the Wechsler (WAIS) if we encouraged her. This performance suggested that her perceptual and motor integrating functions were not defective and that she was not truly learning disabled. Within 24 hours of surgical removal of the tumor, which was about 2 inches long and a half-inch thick, this lady could read, write, and do arithmetic perfectly normally, and her thinking was clear.

A 30-year-old man, seen in our laboratory, sustained a serious head injury in a traffic accident. His car was struck on the driver's side, the door was crushed in, and he was ejected through the front of the car. As a result, he suffered a fractured skull and severe cerebral concussion. He was unconscious for 6 days and then regained his faculties gradually over the next 5 days.

There were neurological and neuropsychological signs of sub-cortical and brainstem damage with cortical sparing. There was no permanent interference with his oral speech or his reading and writing, all of which were normal, but he did develop marked emotional and personality changes in the form of depression and apathy. He lost his former enthusiasm for sports, boating, skiing, and even girls, all of which suggested thalamic damage. His scores on perception, sensorimotor integration, and abstract reasoning were all above average.

These two cases were studied in detail both neurologically and psychologically. Both cases sustained severe brainstem damage or dysfunction with no cortical damage, and both cases suffered no primary academic impairment. This evidence suggests that the cortical levels of integration are essential to academic learning, and that the subcortical levels (in these two cases, the thalamus and brainstem) can sustain rather severe injury or dysfunction without destroying academic ability, so long as the cortical integration is still functional.

It will probably be most useful for teachers to know that sensorimotor and perceptual training appear to improve the possibilities of successful academic learning *especially in young children*, but that remedial drills must also include language and academic content. Much more research is needed in this area to clarify the neuropsychological processes affected by indirect (sensorimotor training) and direct remediation (academic skill training). This question reduces itself to what is *relevant*; the evidence appears to indicate that both direct and indirect remediation are needed, the relative proportions being indicated by the age of the child and the severity of the learning problem.

Motivation to Learn

The remedial procedure recommended here is a "success model" of learning, which implies that a desire to learn must precede learning. White (1959) considered the child's level of competence in dealing with the environment essential to total motivation, and the desire to interact with the environment to be neurogenic. Directing the child into appealing activities at a level he or she can manage with satisfaction is the first step in remedial teaching and in improving the child's self-evaluation.

Incentives

A detailed explanation of the principles of delivering reinforcement in behavior therapy is beyond the scope of the present discussion, but it is important to recognize that because the LD child will be asked to try to master skills that will be difficult for him or her, the child will need to be motivated. In adult behavior, activities that are intrinsically pleasurable are usually done with no extrinsic reward (e.g., recreation). If adult society wants a particularly unpleasant or dangerous task done, however, it is usually necessary to pay someone to do it.

Any one teaching method, no matter how successful with a majority of students, will be inappropriate and even detrimental for children constitutionally unsuited to it. This is true of behavior-modification techniques as well as of other methods, and this should serve as a caution to educators who consider any method, including behavior modification, a cure-all for all learning problems. For example, the Distar method for teaching reading is motivationally well designed, using a behavioral approach, but it is not suited to a child with a serious or moderate auditory imperception. The Gillingham method, like any other phonics procedure, although successful with most children, is also ineffective with the same type of child. Motivating a child to try to do something he or she is neurologically unable to achieve can only lead to frustration and a lack of interest in learning. Motivational methods, using behavior therapy, are desirable and useful with most children, but they must be used diagnostically and selectively.

Bos and Van Reusen (1991) have drawn attention to "the emerging importance of self-concept and intrinsic motivation in the effectiveness of academic interventions." Because LD students tend to have a lower academic self-concept than their image of general self-worth, they usually are less confident and less able to deal with loosely structured problems than academically self-assured students. By providing more structured problems and teaching specific learning strategies to improve general thinking processes, and by promoting skills related to the acquisition of and proficiency in meeting academic demands, a teacher may improve a student's self-confidence in facing academic problems and at the same time provide improved skills for resolving them.

Experimental Teaching

Once a program of remediation has been chosen on the basis of the neuropsychological and personal analysis of the child, as well as a task analysis of the skills to be taught, its effectiveness should be checked periodically. If, after 2 or 3 weeks, the child is making little or no progress, a critical reexamination should be made of his measured potential and the teaching methods. If the teacher has exhausted all diagnostic hypotheses and has no further useful ideas, then help should be sought from the school psychologist, speech therapist, language specialist, or other professional who may possess better diagnostic skills. If that person is unable to offer any improvement to what is already being done and the child is still showing no progress, then a referral to a research center or university learning laboratory may be indicated. In fact, some of the best remedial teaching programs are research-based and experimentally monitored. This procedure demands a knowledgeable and imaginative psychologist, a back-up group of specialists, and a teacher willing to adapt and try new methods; and all of these people must be experimentally oriented. Leong (1982), drawing on Critchley, has recommended a number of requisites for effective teaching of reading disabilities, but these are applicable to any areas of learning and teaching problems: (1) early and efficient diagnosis; (2) study of speech and language development; (3) in-depth case studies and follow-ups; (4) studies of theory-based programs and remediation; (5) research on brain–behavior mechanisms in disabled readers; and (6) research on information processing in disabled readers.

The best program evaluation comes from a multidisciplinary team approach. The teacher, if supplied with information from the child, the parents, the neurologist and other medical practitioners, the social worker or child-care worker (if involved), the school psychologist, and other teachers of the child, is better equipped to devise an effective remediation program. This regime may include remedial exercises that exploit the child's perceptual, motor, and cognitive strengths; that encourage an integration of his perceptual and motor functions; and that motivate him to learn through use of skilled behavior modification techniques.

Social Skills Enhancement in LD Students

Social and emotional problems have been observed more frequently among LD children and adolescents than in the general population of the same age. Theories to account for this (Spreen, 1988, 1989a) have included (1) Secondary reaction theories: children develop poor self-concepts as a result of their continual school failure; (2) Primary disorder theories: LD is a result of inherent personality traits or emotional problems that interfere with the child's ability to attend and to learn. (3) Cerebral dysfunction theories: LD and an emotional disorder "are related to a third factor which is either genetic/constitutional or based on brain dysfunction" (Spreen, 1989a). It seems probable that all three of these determinants are involved.

The first definition of learning disabilities formulated in the United States by the National Advisory Commission on Handicapped Children (1968) excluded children with "emotional disturbance." But it soon became evident that emotional and social behavior was an integral part of all forms of learning, and the NJCLD's new definition (1987) allowed that "LD may occur *concomitantly* with [among other conditions] serious emotional disturbance." This perception of LD made it necessary to provide remedial programs to address *all* of its aspects.

The early Behaviorists had shown (J.B. Watson, 1924) that phobias could be conditioned without conscious awareness of the learning process. With subsequent research into the acquisition of various forms of social behavior, however, it was concluded that "cognitive processes play a prominent role in the acquisition and retention of new behavior patterns," that "cognitive events are induced and altered most readily by experience of mastery arising from effective performance," and that "self-efficacy," or the conviction that one can successfully cope with the demands of a particular situation, is the essential precursor to successful learning of behavior change (Bandura, 1977; Bandura et al., 1977).

Because LD students are less accepted as friends and more frequently rejected by their classmates, and because they tend to have an unrealistically high self-perception of their social acceptance (Vaughn et al., 1990) there is a pressing need to address their behavioral problems as an essential part of remediating their academic deficits. "To limit our concern in LDs to the acquisition of reading and math skills and to ignore thinking, listening, and speaking in interpersonal relations limits the likelihood that we can help children, or grow in our understanding of the nature of LDs" (Bryan, 1991).

Expectations of personal efficacy result from four main sources of information: (1) experiences of personal mastery, (2) vicarious experience, (3) verbal persuasion, and (4) emotional arousal (Bandura et al., 1977). Drawing on the work of Bandura and others, Ladd and Mize (1983) have proposed a cognitive–social learning model of social-skill training for children that is designed to improve and clarify the child's social knowledge (i.e., knowledge of appropriate goals for social interaction, of successful strategies, and of the appropriate social situations in which these strategies may be applied). This training is done by (1) enhancing skill concepts (e.g., establishing an intent to learn the skill concept), (2) promoting skill performance (e.g., providing guided rehearsal), and (3) fostering skill maintenance and generalization (e.g., providing self-directed rehearsal). Training includes (1) instruction that may be verbal or modeled by an actor, a peer, or a teacher; (2) rehearsal, which may include overt behavioral actions, and covert (imagining a response, and reciting skill information); and (3) feedback from observing one's own performance and feedback from others.

To supplement this brief review of some important ideas and concepts in social-skills training, the reader is urged to read some of the original sources (e.g., Bandura, 1977; Bandura et al., 1977; Ladd & Mize, 1983; etc.) and comprehensive reviews of the nature of nonverbal and social-skills deficits in LD children (Semrud-Clikeman & Hynd, 1991) and social-skills training programs (Vaughn, 1991).

The Child's Social Environment

The Role of the Parents

The parents of a chronically learning disabled child may find themselves in a painfully conflicting situation. Living with their child on a daily basis, they are usually the first to become aware of his subtle and largely invisible disabilities. Because the child is usually but not always of average or above-average intelligence, the sensitive parent may hesitate to report the problem to anyone. If the parents do consult the family doctor, they are usually told that the child is normally healthy (which he probably is) and will "grow out of" the symptoms reported by the parent. This may result in parental feelings of embarrassment or frustration, and a belief by the doctor that he is dealing with an overanxious parent.

Parents of LD children during interviews provide an intriguingly similar type of information. They all report a disturbing suspicion that their child is different from their other children and a persistent assurance by all the professionals not to worry. Many family doctors have a pat response that "he will grow out of it," and many teachers deny there is anything wrong, other than inattention or laziness, until the problem becomes so complex that it can no longer be ignored. By this time, there are so many compounded problems of a perceptual, motor, cognitive, emotional, and social nature that the school staff members find they are not adequately equipped to deal with them. Let us listen to some of these parents.

Mrs. Wallace is an intelligent woman who was a successful nurse prior to her marriage. Mr. Wallace holds an honors degree in biology and chemistry and works in a government fisheries station. The Wallaces have three children: Donald, age 20, an honors science student at a university; Peter, age 17, who has always suffered with a specific language disability; and Mary, age 10, who has no learning problems. Her nurse's training alerted Mrs. Wallace to the possibility of a problem with Peter as early as his third year. Because he was slow to walk and talk, was clumsy, and had unusual feeding habits, she consulted their family doctor, who told her not to worry because there were lots of slow kids. "That was my first putdown," she said. In first grade the teacher was sarcastic and intolerant, and within a month Peter learned to hate school. By the time he was in grade 3, the parents consulted the school principal, who refused to believe there was any real problem. Peter was quiet and amenable to control at school, and so the visit to the principal made the Wallace's feel as if they were trying to fabricate a problem where one did not exist. The principal and Peter's teacher did not know that Peter frequently stormed into the house after a particularly frustrating day and smashed toys, dishes, and other things. One day, while telling his mother about especially unpleasant and unjust treatment at school, he picked up a cutting of material she was sewing and unconsciously pulled it to shreds as he talked.

Another mother, also a trained nurse, felt her son Carl was immature and not ready to enter first grade when he was 5 years 9 months old. Her family pediatrician reported he could find nothing wrong, but Carl's teacher, after 1 month of school, informed the parents, "He isn't seeing right." He was sent to an ophthalmologist, who reported that everything was okay. However, everything was not okay, so Carl was sent to see a child psychiatrist, who also could find nothing wrong. Because Carl was a healthy and cheery little boy, the psychiatrist advised the mother not to be over-anxious. Carl had entered school with real enthusiasm, but by October 1, he came home dejected and told his mother, "I know I'm not dumb, but I can't see what the teacher wants us to do. The other kids don't seem to have any difficulty doing it, but it makes no sense to me." A few months later he was referred to the university clinic, where a neuropsychologist identified Carl's per-ceptual problems and communicated them to his parents. His audi-tory language skills were good but he had severe difficulties in the visual and tactile perceptual spheres. On tests of visual memory, figure–ground perception, tactile form recognition (stereognosis), finger localization, visual–motor skills, and right–left orientation, Carl's scores were below average. These perceptual problems in-terfered seriously with his attempts to read, spell, and do arith-metic, because he was unable to remember and transcribe his auditory language into the correct visual–graphic symbols.

At the beginning of grade 2, Carl's mother explained his prob-lems to his new teacher, but because the teacher was not impressed with this important information, or did not understand it, or for some other reason, it was never recorded anywhere and not com-municated to anyone else at the school. As a result, each suc-ceeding September, Carl's mother found herself faced with the same discouraging and repetitive task of explaining the details of Carl's perceptual and cognitive difficulties.

Not all LD children are as fortunate as Carl in having such a loyal, loving, responsible, and persistent parent, and children who do not have an advocate are frequently neglected. All LD children need a persuasive backer to protect them from the onslaughts of teachers, parents, physicians, and others with little or no know-ledge of the subtleties of sensorimotor and neurolinguistic func-tions in learning. Unfortunately, many of them possess no such protector.

Although teachers need training in understanding the LD child, so do parents. Mittler (1970) believes that "the involvement of parents in the treatment of the child is probably one of the most important developments of the future." This training includes know-ledge of their child's strengths and weaknesses in learning. They should get this information from the school psychologist, the child's teachers, the family doctor, and anyone else involved in assessing and teaching him. Many intelligent parents, active in a local ACLD

(Association for Children with Learning Disabilities) chapter, are better informed about the subtleties of learning disabilities than their child's teacher or school principal.

So far, we have described cases of parents who were intelligent, responsible, and persistent advocates for their LD children. When told not to worry, they continued to look for answers and improved remedial programs for their disabled children. The frustrations and injustices that they and their children were constantly experiencing were infuriating, but they learned to curb their anger, knowing that to alienate anyone who might help is to threaten constructive action. Such behavior requires unusual courage, insight, and patience, and many parents have shown these admirable qualities.

However, a few parents are not so objective. They are angry and resentful that their child does not have an equal chance academically with other children and they project their anger to the school, physician, or psychologist. This reaction is unfortunate not only for them but also for their child, because their negative attitudes may undermine much of the help that a well-meaning teacher or psychologist is trying to give.

Only the parents of an LD child are aware of the family tensions that the child's presence generates. One mother described it as "living with a volcano." Marriage counsellors frequently report that breakdowns in the family unit usually occur following the arrival of children. Children with no specific problems are likely to restrict their parents' activities, frustrate their ambitions, and increase their anxieties. If both parents understand all this and agree to tolerate the pressures for the advantages of having children, then the marriage is likely to survive or even strengthen. However, when one or more of their children is learning disabled, all of these parental pressures are intensified. The father or the mother may gain knowledge and understand something of the child's genuine difficulties, but the other parent may refuse to read "all this modern nonsense" and deny the child is anything but incorrigible. In time, violent arguments may arise and drive the child closer to one parent and away from the other, while both parents drift apart. Likewise, both parents may have informed themselves of the child's problem but disagree about how to treat it. One parent wants the child seen by a child psychiatrist and the other refuses because such a move is an admission of certain weakness. One parent favors a special school for the child and the other opposes this on the grounds that the child should be educated in a normal environment. Even if the parents are reasonably agreed on the child's treatment they are constantly faced with exposure to his emotional outbursts resulting from daily frustrations at school and the chance callous remarks of those around him. The child is the helpless target of any child or teacher who wish to express their hostility by drawing attention to his academic incompetence.

To summarize, the parents need to be informed about the nature of their child's learning disability. This information can come from professional consultations, reading, study, and active participation in the ACLD and other parents' groups.

The Role of the School

Not too many years ago schools commonly expelled a child for not conforming to their satisfaction. Most psychoeducational clinics have seen children subjected to such professional mishandling. Cruickshank has described the case of Jeff, who, by the age of 8, had been permanently excluded from the Boys' Club facilities in his city and expelled from the public school. Fortunately for Jeff, he was admitted to the university clinic–school, where he made progress "through careful nurturing, a highly structured teaching program, parent involvement, and well-prepared teachers" (Cruickshank, 1977). Well-trained teachers for the neurologically handicapped child are in short supply, and until our schools are adequately staffed in this special area, many LD children are likely to be mistreated and their families to be frustrated and angry.

Interviews with parents repeatedly reveal a lack of confidence in the public school's ability to deal adequately with the education of children with subtle learning problems. A mother recently reported that after her LD son had been in a junior high school for 2 months, "It was evident that his teachers had no knowledge of his problems," even though she had explained them to the principal when enrolling him. The art teacher had put sarcastic remarks on the boy's report, and when his mother explained the visual–perceptual and visual-motor problems he had, the teacher replied naively, "Oh, I didn't know he wasn't normal." Parents are frequently wounded by such insensitive remarks.

A high-school teacher of a "modified English course" designed for the poorer students insisted that a dyslexic 16-year-old boy read five novels and write a lengthy book report on each. With help from his parents he composed and wrote out the first book report, which because of misspellings was returned for correction. On the fourth rewrite, the boy's mother, a past president of the local ACLD chapter, tried to explain to the teacher that it was impossible for this boy to read five novels and that because of his perceptual deficits it was highly likely he would continue to misspell some words no matter how many times he was asked to rewrite the report. The teacher refused to believe the boy had a problem; to her he was just lazy and careless.

In Chapters 2 and 8 we described the case of a girl who, at the age of 6, suffered a spontaneous hemorrhage in the left posterior part of her brain. To stop the bleeding, brain surgery was required. Following this trauma to her brain she experienced chronic visual–perceptual difficulties, although many of her high-school teachers denied her disabilities. They thought her overprotective mother was making excuses for an academically mediocre student.

Such reports are meant not to put down teachers but to draw attention to the limited knowledge of some of them about the nature of learning disabilities. Had the junior high school principal, in the first case, really understood what the boy's mother was telling him during the initial interview, he would have alerted his teachers and suggested an appropriate remedial program. Had the teachers been knowledgeable about perceptual deficits and learning disorders, they would have provided a suitable remedial teaching plan rather than resorting to sarcasm and stereotyping the boy as "abnormal."

The high school teacher, in the second case, had she understood the nature of dyslexia, would have provided the boy with suitable remedial drills and demanded realistic responses, instead of projecting her own prejudices by labeling him lazy and careless.

Ignorance about learning disabilities usually leads to a denial and nonacceptance of the problem. Understanding leads to an acceptance and recognition of the problem, which is the first step to successful remediation.

When parents are asked their opinion of how to improve the prospects of their LD children, the most common answer is, "The teachers need more training in special education." Many government departments of education and universities, aware of this need, are planning improved training programs, not only for teachers, but also specially designed orientation courses in learning disabilities for school superintendents, principals, and other administrators. Many educators believe that postservice training in special education (after the teacher has had a year or two of successful classroom teaching) is more effective than preservice training (during a teacher-training course prior to employment). Then only the most competent teachers should be selected for further training, which may be formal (a higher degree or diploma) or informal (an extra course or courses covering a topic the teacher needs and wants, workshops, conferences, and visits to other classrooms or experimental clinics).

How the teacher may gain better training is a problem of professional education and is beyond the limits of this discussion other than to draw attention to its importance. There is a huge literature in this field that the interested reader may consult. Attempting to understand subtle learning problems in children, whether they are neurogenic or have no known cause, is stimulating and challenging for the teacher. Because of the gaps in our knowledge and also the rapid increase in new scientific insights, successful teachers will need to continue to upgrade their knowledge and maintain an experimental view of the child. Much more is to be gained by studying the child's types of cognitive difficulties, perceptual errors, and abnormal learning strategies than by berating him or her for hyperactive or restless behavior, which may very well be a secondary result of the primary nature of his disabilities. *The child has the clues to his own remediation* if the teacher is knowledgeable and sensitive enough to recognize them.

But academic understanding by itself is not enough. The teacher still needs a number of social and pedagogical skills that enable an easy communication with the student. "There is little reason to doubt that the dominant factor in successful teaching is and will always remain the teacher's skill in nourishing, and sometimes even arousing, the child's curiosity and interest and in providing a rich and challenging intellectual environment in which the child can find his own unique way toward understanding, knowledge, and skill" (N. Chomsky, 1970).

The Role of the Physician

The reader will have recognized from the discussions throughout this book that contributions by the medical doctor are essential in the diagnosis of and decisions on remediation for the severely LD child. In making a neuropsychological study of such a child, a referral to a neurologist is the first step. Frequently referrals are made directly by a neurologist or neurosurgeon for neuropsychological assessment prior to brain surgery. Where testing is done following brain surgery, much information can be obtained about (1) the differences between pre- and post-surgery mental skills, and (2) the new pattern of mental skills with which the patient may have to adapt, although testing about a year later will also be needed before any reliable predictions can be made about the permanence of any mental deficits.

Although diagnostic information usually comes from the pediatric neurologist, it may also include the neurosurgeon, the radiologist, the orthopedic surgeon, the internist, the ophthalmologist, the audiologist, the psychiatrist, the general practitioner, or any other medically trained person involved in the case.

An early diagnosis is desirable in cases of neurogenic learning problems because "research indicates that the earlier the diagnosis, the better the prognosis" (Tarnopol, 1971). However, sometimes the less experienced physician may obstruct such a move by assuring the child's parents they have nothing to worry about. If the request has been recommended to the mother by a psychologist, some general practitioners have been known to refuse it on the basis of its being a nonmedical referral. Fortunately for the children who need this medically diagnostic help, however, the defensive medical doctor is in the minority, and most doctors are happy to cooperate on a diagnostic team that includes medical, psychological, and educational personnel.

Masland (1969) himself a physician, has drawn attention to the other extreme response by a medical doctor. With no neurological examination and no real knowledge of learning disabilities, the parents are told that because the child is hyperactive he or she is brain damaged, and because he did not respond to the doctor's questions during the examination, the doctor may add another superficial diagnosis that the child is mentally dull or retarded. The implication is that the case is hopeless. Some years ago a medical doctor referred a boy to our laboratory because, he reported in his referral letter, the boy was incorrigible in school, was brain damaged (his diagnosis was made purely on observing the boy's restless behavior), and was mentally retarded (because the boy was reluctant to answer the doctor's questions). When the lad arrived at our laboratory, he was a bright-looking and alert boy who was cautious at first, but who was soon enjoying the variety of tests. He measured a WISC verbal IQ of 128 (superior), and on both a standard neurological examination and on our 5-hour battery of neuropsychological tests he showed no signs of brain damage or CNS dysfunction. His "incorrigible" behavior at school was his reaction to being told by the family doctor that he was brain damaged, to being expelled from school by the school principal, and from sensing his parents' feelings of panic regarding the whole situation. Careless medical examinations and superficial diagnostic reports are better ignored; the parent can be advised to consult a competent physician.

Many teachers and some psychologists insist that "Learning disabilities are an *educational* problem, *not* a *medical* one." It is certainly true that the definition and treatment of learning deficits is psychoeducational, but the diagnosis, if it is to be thorough and comprehensive, must include the findings of a medical examination, whether positive or negative. If the child suffers from a cerebral lesion or dysfunction, a biochemical imbalance, a nutritional problem, or a genetic defect, we need to know. If he is *free* of any or all of these, we will also need to know.

Educators who insist that their responsibilities are exclusively educational should be reminded that some of the most valuable knowledge and practices in special education have come from medically trained scholars concerned about how children learn. Broca, Hughlings Jackson, Maria Montessori, and Alfred Binet all made significant contributions to our knowledge. Currently, Elena Boder, Macdonald Critchley, Marcel Kinsbourne, Orlando Schrager, Sylvia Richardson, Drake Duane, and the late Julio de Quiros (all medically trained), to name just a few, are or have been in constant demand at conferences and through their writings by ACLD groups and others striving to improve their knowledge of learning disabilities.

Once the teacher or school psychologist is persuaded of the value of the medical input (and this is particularly important for the multihandicapped child) he or she will still need to establish some reliable channels of communication. How this is done will vary with the size of the school and the city and the skills of the people involved. Frequently, the psychologist is in a favored position to organize a meeting of the parents, the child's teacher(s), and the family doctor. The doctor may agree to have this meeting at his or her office to save time, and its essential value is to enhance each member's respect for the other. The doctor may not be willing to provide time for more than one meeting, so matters of interdisciplinary communication regarding medical findings and medication therapies should be discussed. Sometimes a one-paragraph summary of the child's medical problems is adequate and can be dictated by the doctor very quickly immediately following the conference. If the child's diet is radically altered or if he is put on medication designed to have behavioral effects, this should be reported to the school so that the child's teachers can provide observational feedback regarding his behavior.

One of the significant influences of the neuropsychological approach to learning disabilities in the last 30 years is its tendency to reduce the professional isolation of medical doctors and school personnel, and to include important medical knowledge in decisions on remedial treatment.

The Role of the Clinical or School Psychologist

The psychologist's chief function is to adopt and develop improved diagnostic and treatment facilities for the LD child, and he or she does this through research and careful therapeutic procedures. The role of the clinical neuropsychologist has emerged within the last 30 years, and because of its recency it is still taking shape. However, in most applied settings, in our experience , he or she is the liaison on the team between the neurologist or other medical person and the teacher and/or parent. This seems to be a spontaneous result of the psychologist's training in research methods and clinical procedures that leads to communication with medical personnel, teachers, and parents. The psychologist can reserve time to observe a child in depth, to confer with the parents periodically, and to be available to the child's teacher. The skillful psychologist will create experimental clinical tasks specifically to investigate the learning strategies of the child being assessed. The busy teacher and the active physician may not be able to devote as much time to one case. As well as developing unique testing activities to study a particular child, the school psychologist should have an ongoing group study to investigate the validity of some concept or test technique in the rapidly expanding field of neuropsychology.

The psychologist's relation with the LD child should be warm and nonthreatening and can be measured by his or her success in communicating with the child. Teachers are frequently put off by the psychologist's report, which, they will tell you, indicates nothing that they did not already know about the child and may be couched in a smoke-screen of professional jargon. Parents can also be put off by abstruse language and what appears to them to be a preoccupation with a professional role quite remote from the needs of their child. Many excellent clinical researchers have failed to be very effective in a parent consultation because of their inability to communicate clearly and easily, and in some cases by a lack of personal warmth and concern.

If the psychologist hopes that his or her findings are to be used in the remedial treatment of the child, then he or she must be careful not to pose as an "expert" directing the teacher, but as a colleague on a professional team on which the teacher enjoys equal input. In our experience, remedial prescriptions made unilaterally by the clinical or school psychologist usually end up ignored in a filing cabinet. If the psychologist, in consultation with the teacher, shares his or her findings and listens to the teacher explain the types of remedial procedures that she could use based on these findings, they can then produce a joint prescription that is more likely to be used because the teacher has been involved in producing it.

Because of the rapid advances and discoveries in neuropsychology and its influence on neurolinguistics and learning generally, the successful clinical psychologist will need to cultivate a program of continuing professional development. Personal contact with an active group of referring neurologists, neurosurgeons, psychiatrists, and special educators can provide a constant source of stimulation, refinement, correction, and development of the psychologist's knowledge of neuropsychology and its relation to learning. The complexity of this relationship demands constant study if the clinical psychologist is to stay abreast of new knowledge and remain competent in understanding how to use it.

The above has been a description of the plan of professional collaboration that has been practised in our laboratory for the past 35 years. For teachers, medical practitioners, and psychologists to consult regularly on a case was unusual at first, and the practice needed to be cultivated. It was the neurological input that made this cooperation necessary, and the neuropsychologist became the obvious person to promote and maintain interprofessional communication. This liaison was done by an exchange of professional reports from all members of the group, and with group consultations with all or most of the members. Periodic follow-up checks were made on the child's response to the recommended treatment of the group, and further decisions were made if necessary.

Within the last 25 years, because of the growth of mainstreaming in the general school population there has been an increased need for inter-communication among regular teachers, special educators, psychologists, and other professional specialists, in meeting the needs of the most seriously impaired LD students. At the classroom level this cooperation may include group teaching, which is designed to make a better use of the special talents of the participating teachers. Within the school it may include resource teachers (McLoughlin & Kass, 1978) and the school psychologist. In the community it will involve the child's parent(s) and any medical or other professional person participating in the assessment and decisions affecting the child's future. In recent years in the professional educational literature this group approach to dealing with the assessment and treatment needs of the LD student has been labeled "Collaborative Consultation" (Robinson, 1991). Essentially it is the application of sound administrative principles to special education.

The Role of the Speech and Language Specialist[1]

Because most learning problems include some aspect of language impairment it is important that the professional team include someone with special knowledge and skills in the diagnosis and treatment of linguistic problems. The qualifications of this person may

[1] We are indebted to Brenda Costa, M.A., Speech Pathologist, for preparing the original discussion in the 1st and 2nd Editions, and to Sherri McIntyre, M.A. for up-dating the present discussion. Ms. McIntyre is the Director of Communication Disorders at the Queen Alexandra Hospital for Children, the G.R. Pearkes Centre for Children, and the Jack Ledger Child and Adolescent Psychiatric Unit of the Queen Alexandra Centre for Children's Health in Victoria, British Columbia.

be quite variable in school systems where certification is not required. It may range from a research/clinical speech-language pathologist, an audiologist or linguist, to a classroom teacher with no special training in language development or diagnostic skills. In the United States, speech and hearing specialists are required to have a masters degree and supervised clinical training to be certified by the American Speech-Hearing-Language Association. This A.S.H.A. certification is not required by all states because some of them have individual licensing requirements. In Canada similar standards are required for membership in the Canadian Association of Speech-Language Pathologists and Audiologists, but at present professional licensing or registration is required by some provincial governments, but not all.

The chief areas of expertise cover the use of audiological screening, diagnosis, and interpretation of the nature of hearing loss and/or auditory imperception; analysis and explanation of a communication disorder; knowledge of normal language development and the hierarchical structure of language, psycholinguistics, diagnosis, and treatment of speech and language problems; and skills in interpreting all of this so that the teacher will want to make use of it. In cases of known brain damage or neuromuscular dysfunction where receptive and/or expressive language processes are impaired, the speech-language specialist must be familiar with the many new technical aids that assist in communication and education. These are computerized electronic devices for improving language understanding and use by students with slow language development, and for severely impaired students who, because of brain damage or severe neuromuscular dysfunction are unable to speak, or whose speech is severely impaired. The large variety and commercial sources of these devices may be obtained by consulting the nearest language-speech clinic.

Only rarely would one person be professionally qualified to supply all of these services, so the speech and language specialist in different school systems will have greater strengths and professional qualifications in some of these skills and less in others.

Most school systems carry out group screening tests for hearing in kindergarten or first grade. These usually are administered by the school or public health nurse. Any severe or unusual hearing cases from this initial screening may be referred to an audiologist in a local hospital, clinic, or research center. Children who happen to live in a rural area where none of these facilities is available, will have to travel some distance for professional assessment.

The professional team to deal with language and speech problems will vary in size and level of expertise in different school systems. In a large urban center it may include, besides the child's teacher, an occupational therapist, a physiotherapist, the school psychologist, and the speech and hearing specialist. However in many remote rural areas the teacher may have none of these disciplines for regular support and may have to depend on reading, summer courses, and intermittent professional advice. Between these extremes, only a psychologist or reading specialist may be available to aid the teacher, and in this situation it is hoped that he or she will develop many of the diagnostic competencies and remedial skills of the language specialist. No profession possesses "territorial rights" on language because it is central to all academic learning, so that the most successful use of professional expertise is to encourage all members of the team to assume an experimental approach and to broaden their knowledge and skills in treating language learning disorders.

Where school systems are fortunate enough to have professionally qualified speech and language specialists on their staffs, the teachers can seek continued help in learning more about perceptual deficits, cognitive retardation, and the diagnostic rationale of particular cases. A continued interaction may be maintained between the teacher and the language specialist, so that the results of the speech therapy sessions may be included in the classroom teacher's teaching methods.

Throughout the United States and Canada the speech-language pathologists (SLPs) are attempting to work more closely with teachers in the classroom setting. This current practice differs from the more traditional model of service delivery in which the child is removed from the classroom to spend a therapy session with "the expert". This new approach recognizes that both teachers and SLPs have the same professional goal as facilitators of learning (Hoskins, 1990). It stresses therapeutic collaboration between the SLP and the teacher in working with the child, rather than the former situation in which teacher and SLP were practicing parallel professional roles. In theory it is similar to the linguistic practice of Pragmatics in stressing the contextual and social aspects of language (see Chapter 8).

Like any successful applied scientist, the speech and language specialist will make experimental investigations of the language disabled child, assess deficits in the light of normal language development, and discuss with the teacher what seems to be the best remedial measures for the child. This information will be communicated not only to the child's teacher but to the other members of the professional team in their ongoing evaluation of the pedagogical efficacy of their remedial activities.

The Role of the Child

In a brief discussion of personality development, we can only refer to its importance in the growth of all children and the added obstacles that the LD child encounters. The development of the ego or self-concept is a longitudinal process that begins at birth and reaches maturity in late adolescence or young adulthood, although superficial changes in it no doubt continue all through life.

Many personality theorists have included the bodily sense of body image as basic to a sound personality structure (Allport, 1955; Maslow, 1955). Others have recognized it as basic to cognitive development (Piaget, 1952), and numerous special educators have accepted sensorimotor performance as essential to learning (Ayres, 1972; Barsch, 1966; Kephart, 1966; Montessori, 1964). The child with no specific learning disabilities may still suffer problems in developing a poised and secure self-image because of a poor complexion, lack of feminine beauty in the girl, lack of adequate height or muscular development in the boy, etc. If we add to these common developmental frustrations poor sensorimotor coordination or clumsiness, perceptual deficits, defective directional sense, or some type of language impairment, we have some idea of the increased developmental problems of the LD child. It is particularly difficult for such a child to feel sure of his footing, his manual dexterity, his body image, and himself. It is also difficult for him to feel competent in relation to the environment; because his ego structure is frail, he is poorly equipped to identify strongly with things and people around him. Intellectual development is hindered by his learning disabilities, and all of these frustrations can be magnified by hostile or insensitive treatment by others.

To try to understand how such a child feels, let us look at the verbal account of a child who, at the age of 6 years, encountered brain surgery in the left posterior part of his brain just prior to entering first grade. His account is a recollection written at the age of 21.

> I remember the first week of school, better yet the first day. I remember being scared and not wanting to walk into the large strange classroom with strange people. Everything was dark and dismal, at least that is what it seemed like to me. I walked around like a zombie, completely in my own world, and always a mad look on my face. No wonder most of my friends lost interest in me.
>
> I remember my teacher's sarcastic ways. In my first week she wouldn't let me wear the knitted skull cap my mother had knitted to cover my shaved head. She made a fool of me in front of the class. I was scared of that teacher all year, and even today I shake at loud noises and being yelled at.

In grade 2 my teacher was young and attractive, but an old grouch like the first one. I was still up in the air (tense and anxious). I just wish I had been old enough to express my point of view instead of being pushed around by every one. No wonder I was so uptight, I was on tranquilizers. The worst part was that I took my yelling and screaming home to my family who didn't deserve it or want it. The trouble was that so much was ticking around in my head and I couldn't express myself logically so that others could understand what was wrong. I wish that I had had help.

This excerpt reveals many significant points that are important to the teacher of the brain-injured child. Traumatic brain damage in the initial stages pervades the patient's thinking. It is both frightening and depressing and tends to color the child's perceptions. The classroom was modern, bright, and colorful, but it seemed "dark and dismal" to this child. His first two teachers sound like ogres from his description, but again it is possible that he perceived them in a more frightening role than they appeared to the other children. It is interesting that he still remembers he had a "mad face." It is a common symptom for brain-damaged patients to have less tolerance to loud noises. For small children it is frightening. He remembers displacing his anger from school to home, and the unhappy confusion of a mild receptive aphasia.

Although most learning disabled children may not have to endure as intense intellectual deficits as this traumatically damaged boy, their emotional frustrations from their inability to compete evenly may be just as acute. Their disabilities, although "minimal," may be just enough to promote nasty name calling and social exclusion from a peer group . Many LD children are made to suffer these personal attacks by other children, and they often report, as adults, that their elementary school teachers either were oblivious to these interpersonal occurrences or they made no attempt to stop them. Although it is important to encourage the independence of all children, the neurologically impaired child usually needs help in understanding his or her deficits and in adjusting successfully to them. Because some parents are unable to provide this help, it is desirable that special teachers recognize the common signs of language reduction, intolerance to noise, heightened anxiety, and difficult social adjustment.

Classifications for Remediation

The young or inexperienced teacher may feel confused or overwhelmed when faced with a child with a complex pattern of intellectual and emotional disabilities. A classification model may help to clarify one's thinking and direct one's knowledge systematically. The following is a classification of groups of children who will need special help.

1. Primary learning disabilities
   a. Traumatically brain damaged
   b. Congenital brain dysfunction
   c. Congenital learning disability with no clear neurological signs (e.g., developmental dyslexia)
2. Secondary learning disabilities: Emotional disturbance
3. Attention deficit disorder
   a. With hyperactivity
   b. Without hyperactivity

Primary Learning Disabilities

Traumatically Brain Damaged

Throughout this book, detailed cases of traumatic brain damage in both adults and children have been presented. The reader will recognize that remediation may include both training the brain and training an academic skill. Choice of drills may be selected to stress the child's perceptual strengths; the visually impaired child may have drills that emphasize auditory and tactile input (e.g., Gillingham or Distar) and the child with a phonetic imperception will do better with a system stressing visual and tactile–kinesthetic activities (e.g., color coding with a tactile alphabet and kinesthetic involvement). The language impaired learner may profit by increasing his or her skills in task-specific strategies (i.e., cognitive training) and by acquiring techniques to monitor and appraise the progress in their own learning (i.e., metacognitive training) (Flavell, 1979; Loper, 1982). Neurologically impaired learners (the BD and MBD groups in Table 1.1) will usually require more analysis of the verbal material to be learned than the normal learner, and more help in the auditory, visual, tactile, and kinesthetic perceptual spheres. The LD learner with no hard or soft neurological signs may or may not require as much analysis; that can be learned by experimental teaching. The reader will remember that Luria's methods of teaching brain-damaged subjects, McGinnis's approaches to teaching aphasic children, and Montessori's procedures with retarded children all used a language system "from the bottom up" (i.e., from letters to words to phrases to sentences). Proponents of the whole-language approach to teaching reading (i.e., from the top down) contend that because the child learns to speak with no effort and no formal training, reading should be acquired in the same way with a minimum of analytical instruction and with emphasis on extracting meaning from words the child already knows or is helped to recognize. But this approach assumes that speech and reading are similar processes, and the reader will remember from Chapter 8 that they are not. Reading requires the acquisition of an alphabetical code, and though most children may acquire it without formal instruction, possibly "20 to 25% will *not* discover the point of the alphabet except as it is made apparent to them by appropriate instruction" (Liberman & Liberman, 1990). Children with known brain dysfunctions and those with severe verbal learning problems will most likely be in the minor segment who need instruction in phonological awareness and the acquisition of the alphabetic code. The whole-language approach may be used with the majority of children who can master it without difficulty. Anyone who tries to use the method with a child with marked left-hemisphere damage and/or dysfunction will likely find that it will not work.

Congenital Brain Dysfunction

At this stage in our knowledge it is probable that remedial measures similar to those above will succeed with the child or adult learner with neurological soft signs because of the likelihood of neurological damage or dysfunction. In any event, an experimental approach with careful monitoring should indicate the best methods.

Congenital Learning Disabled Child with No Abnormal Physiological Signs

The developmental dyslexic child frequently is normally healthy and presents negative findings on a neurological examination. Nevertheless he or she is abnormally retarded in reading and writing and does not respond to normal teaching procedures.

A complete neuropsychological examination is still useful because it provides a more complete inventory of the child's perceptual, intellectual, and motor strengths. Frequently the child measures normally on all perceptual and motor skills singly but has difficulty integrating them. In such cases, remediation may include exercises to integrate two perceptual skills, then three, and then these three with the required motor response. If any perceptual or cognitive deficits are discovered, therapeutic treatment may be directed to exercise the weaknesses in company with the child's strengths.

Secondary Learning Disabilities

Emotionally Disturbed Personality

Children with abnormal forms of behavior involving marked mood swings, poor social adaptability, or inappropriate social response may be primarily a psychiatric problem. Referral to a competent medical specialist might turn up an abnormal blood chemistry level, poor nutrition, or an unhealthy family environment. In such cases these children may be intellectually bright as measured by an intelligence test, but their learning problems are secondary to their emotional distress. Academic remediation normally will not be resumed until the child's medical problems are reasonably resolved.

Attention Deficit Disorder (with and without Hyperactivity)

Although a small percentage of children diagnosed as ADHD appear to outgrow their hyperactivity, most find their problems, including impulsivity, restlessness, low self-esteem, and poor social skills, persisting into the adult years (Gittleman et al., 1985). The ADHD disorder, then, needs to be managed throughout the school years and is not cured. As the child matures physiologically, emotionally, and socially, support services and management techniques will vary. The teacher presented with such a child in the classroom will require support from parents and a number of professionals to maximize the child's learning potential. A variety of treatment techniques, including medication, behavior modification, cognitive modeling, EEG biofeedback, and dietary changes will need to be evaluated and investigated for appropriateness. (These treatment techniques are reviewed in Chapter 7). As many as 30% to 40% of ADHD children also have learning problems (Lambert & Sandoval, 1980), and these too will need to be addressed following full neuropsychological investigation of the child's cognitive strengths and weaknesses. Accordingly, the child with ADHD may require not only management and support for the disorder, but also specialized remedial instruction to address any specific learning disability. Supportive counseling services, family counseling, training in social skills, play therapy, and individual psychotherapy may also be warranted, depending upon the child's and family's adjustment at home and in school.

A Proposed Remedial Program

In proposing any method or model of remedial education, one is compelled at the outset to recognize the complete lack of any conclusive validity studies of any current programs. But because clinical neuropsychologists are constantly faced with the need to counsel their brain-damaged patients about possible methods of rehabilitation, and to give their LD child-clients recommendations for improving their academic competence, a remedial program is proposed in an attempt to meet this need.

Whether the clinical neuropsychologist likes it or not, he or she, as an applied researcher, is faced with the professional responsibility for delivering to the parents and teachers of the LD children whom they assess useful and practical remedial suggestions. As Shayer (1987) has pointed out, in proposing a model of educational practice "the touchstone . . . is that of *utility*."

The stages in arriving at any remedial decisions include (1) assessment; (2) a study of the assessment findings from which to infer a conceptual image of the subject's perceptual, motor, and cognitive strengths and weaknesses; (3) a choice of a remedial program based on this knowledge; (4) periodic measures of the subject's cognitive status to measure the possible effectiveness of the remediation; and (5) a second look, if necessary, and a decision to alter the remediation in the event that there is little or no academic progress.

Assessment. Any comprehensive battery of tests should provide information on sensation and perception (visual, auditory, tactile, and kinesthetic), motor response, cross-modal speed and competence, cognitive and linguistic skills (memory, spatial imagery, verbal conceptualizing, reasoning, and adaptive intelligence), and academic achievement. Any recognized neuropsychological batteries, because they are designed to scan the cerebral cortex, include all of these measures, and as a result they are the most useful in diagnosing, not only brain-damaged and neurologically dysfunctioning subjects, but also any children or adults with complex learning problems.

Diagnostic Picture. The test profiles will provide a comprehensive and detailed set of data. The clinical neuropsychologist will form a conceptual picture of the subject's behavioral and cognitive strengths and weaknesses as well as the mental level of functioning, the home background, emotional status, the level of competence in spoken, read, and written language, and anything relevant in the child's health history (Johnson & Myklebust, 1967). A remedial program that makes use of the subject's strengths and avoids the weaknesses as much as possible is more likely to be successful. If it is possible to improve any of the weaknesses (e.g., speech perception or short-term or long-term memory) then a program of perceptual or cognitive training might be carried out in practice periods just long enough not to be frustrating or boring. In cases of brain damage some perceptual–cognitive disabilities may be impossible to improve, and in that case the training must be designed to circumvent it (e.g., Mrs. Stanley could perceive words auditorily, but because of her stroke practice had no effect in training her to read visually).

Models of Intervention

1. Perceptual and Perceptual–Motor Processing: An aspect of LD that has had considerable research attention and applied use since the early work of Strauss and Werner with mentally retarded and brain-damaged children is perception (Cruickshank, 1961; Strauss & Lehtinen, 1947). For many special-education researchers it became the central cause of LD. Cruickshank conceived of LD children as "children with perceptual processing deficits" (Cruickshank, 1981) and its use in remediation was based on the assumption that training exercises in visual (Frostig, 1966; Werner & Strauss, 1941); auditory (Myklebust, 1954); tactile (Reitan, 1959); kinesthetic perception (Barsch, 1966; Kephart, 1966); and/or perceptual-motor performance will enhance academic competence by remediating basic processing deficits. These concepts developed from studies and attempts to improve intellectual functioning in mentally retarded and brain-damaged children and adults (Werner & Strauss, 1940; Goldstein, 1939). Using differential diagnostic information to develop a remedial program to assist and improve underlying ability weaknesses has had wide use in the past 50 years, although more recently it has been criticized as largely ineffective (Arter & Jenkins, 1979). The evidence against the method, however, has been derived from group studies that, because of the neurological and environmental variability of LD subjects, include determining forces many of which are unknown and most of which cannot be controlled. And more important, the results of validity studies on LD children with no neurological signs are highly suspect in judging the validity of their use with brain-damaged and/or cerebrally dysfunctioning subjects. As Johnson and Myklebust have emphasized, "Teaching of children with learning disabilities must be strikingly individualized" (1967, p. 58). Many researchers have used this model but have arrived "at their particular viewpoints by different routes" (Myers and Hammill, 1990, 373–449).

   2. Multisensorimotor–Language Approach: This model also includes perceptual–motor activities, but they are used to help the child to read and write rather than to develop sensorimotor integration *per se.* One of the best known of these methods is that of Grace Fernald, developed at the University of California at Los Angeles between 1921 and 1948. Her VAKT method makes use of simultaneous visual, auditory, kinesthetic, and tactile experiences to learn to read and spell. Words are learned in their whole form rather than broken into parts, and they are reinforced by VAKT input (Fernald, 1943).

The Gillingham and Stillman Alphabetic Method is also a multi-sensorimotor–language approach (Gillingham & Stillman, 1965) that uses tactile and kinesthetic exercises to reinforce the visual learning of language. The method draws on the theory of cerebral dominance of Samuel Orton and it stresses the function of auditory processes in language. Multisensorimotor–language methods probably have been used more frequently than any other in the last 60 years, and that is still true. The Gillingham and Stillman method is the recommended therapeutic approach of the Orton Dyslexia Society.

3. Psychoneurological Approach: The first well-developed neuropsychological theory of learning was that of Helmer R. Myklebust, whose preparatory training included professional education, audiology, and the study and education of the deaf, clinical neurology, and experimental psychology. For many years Myklebust was director of the Institute for Language Disorders at Northwestern University in Evanston, Illinois, where he studied all types of sensory, perceptual, and language deficits in children. He and his colleagues were interested in studying intersensory and intrasensory processes in behavior and examining how they are related to learning (Johnson & Myklebust, 1967).

Another well-known approach making use of the knowledge of brain function and language is that of Samuel A. Kirk and his colleagues, who developed the Illinois Test of Psycholinguistic Abilities (ITPA). Like Myklebust, who examined the various neurosensory systems that may function almost independently of one another, may complement one another, or may act in an integrated or interrelated fashion, Kirk included, in his analysis of language, the functions of receptive processes (auditory and visual), association processes (auditory and visual), expressive processes (verbal and manual), closure (auditory and visual), and sequential memory (auditory and visual) (Kirk & Kirk, 1971).

4. Applied Behavior Analysis: This model includes a number of techniques that are based on operant learning principles (Skinner, 1957, 1968) to improve academic learning and classroom management (Hewett, 1967; Lovitt, 1975). More recently, Horton (1981,

1989; Horton & Puente, 1986) has been an articulate proponent of the applied integration of neuropsychological assessment methods for the diagnostic understanding of the LD child, and treatment methods based on learning theory (i.e., behavior modification) to direct the child's learning. Horton has called this approach "behavioral neuropsychology," and it is the remedial model that we support as the most useful because of its detailed diagnostic and motivational aspects.

5. Cognitive and Metacognitive Methods: Poor readers have had their reading improved by being taught specific skills (cognitive training) such as verbal rehearsal and the use of mnemonic strategies (Torgeson, 1977; Torgeson & Goldman, 1977). Improvement may also result from training children to become more aware of their own cognitive strengths and study methods by training them in self-monitoring and self-appraisal (metacognitive training). Such training may lead to more efficient learning, greater consistency and accuracy of performance, and greater understanding (Loper, 1982) because it may transfer to all learning situations.

6. Technical Aids: Any learning may be enriched and aided by the use of one or more of the many technical aids now available. Radio programs for enrichment have been used in some schools since the 1930s, and television, both inside and outside the classroom, has been used to enrich the child's imagination and knowledge. Taped books, tape recorders, calculators, speech-pacs, biofeedback, and microcomputers have their uses, the latter being especially effective in programs of language learning (Cochran & Bull, 1991; Steiner & Larson, 1991).

Summary

The most frequent reason for referral of children to most clinical neuropsychologists is a school-related problem involving academic performance or problem social behavior or both. For this reason the psychologist's training and professional experience must include more than just assessment and diagnosis. Neither of these is of any use to the child, the parents, or the child's teachers unless they lead to some intelligent suggestions for dealing with the child's problem. The best clinicians assessing LD have also been creative teachers in the clinic; Luria, Myklebust and Johnson, Cruickshank, Frostig, and Kephart are a few examples. Unless clinicians learn a large repertoire of useful remedial procedures and test these methods directly on many subjects, or through supervision by some other diagnostic teacher, and unless they learn how to use their large body of neuropsychological data for designing successful remedial programs, their efforts will meet only half of the problem. The other half, the real reason for the referral in the first place, will be neglected because of professional inability or disinterest.

11 Postscript

We find it a clinical and scientific advantage to acknowledge that there is both a neurology and psychology of learning . . . when we combine psychologic and neurologic constructs, we gain new insights into the differing types of learning disabilities.
Helmer R. Myklebust (1975a)

We now have a wealth of material to indicate the principles of functional organization of the brain, to identify the principal units of the working brain, and to indicate the role of individual brain systems in the organization of mental processes.
A.R. Luria (1973)

The following discussion attempts to clarify and summarize the thesis of this book by presenting the basic assumptions underlying the neuropsychological approach to understanding and treating learning disabilities.

Basic Assumptions

1. All behavior—including cognitive processes, which essentially are psychological—is mediated by the brain and central nervous system and their integrated and supporting physiological systems. All behavior has two aspects, the psychological and the physiological.
2. When all supporting and mediating organic subsystems are functioning normally they usually can be ignored. The perception, understanding, and treatment of behavior, in this case, can deal successfully with behavior exclusively at the psychological or behavioral level.
3. When one or more of the physiological subsystems is dysfunctioning so as to impede normal perception, cognition, or motor response, then a consideration of behavior only at the psychological level is inadequate. In such cases both psychological and physiological processes and their interactions will need to be recognized for successful diagnosis and treatment.

4. The neuropsychological concept of behavior acknowledges all physiological subsystems (e.g., respiratory, circulatory, digestive) as essential to vegetative life, but the brain and central nervous system provide the most subtle, the most important, and the most remarkable aspects of human behavior. These are cortical function and creative mental life.

5. All behavior and neural function are perfectly correlated; one is caused by the other. "Each kind of mental activity has a distinct psychological structure and is effected through the joint activity of discrete cortical zones" (Luria, Simernitskaya, & Tubylevich, 1970). Clinical neuropsychological research, especially in the past 50 years, has revealed many brain–behavior relationships and is continuing to increase our knowledge of many areas not yet understood.

6. The physiologist, neurologist, neurosurgeon, and neuropsychologist frequently have direct access to data of genuine importance to the special educator, who will never be aware of this commanding information unless it is made available in a form relevant to educational theories and practices.

7. There is a systematic development and function of the human brain that reveals lawful relationships between its normal function and specific patterns of behavior; also, systematic relationships exist between deficit functioning of the brain when it is damaged and specific behavior deficits. Clinical neurological studies of brain function and dysfunction have provided, and continue to provide, a large body of empirically established knowledge that can supply a useful level of predictive validity to the neurosurgeon, neurologist, and neuropsychologist. This knowledge can be invaluable to the special educator who will take the time to understand and use it.

8. Because of the unity of nature and its systematic and lawful functions, it is logical to conclude that brain functions among large samples or populations vary from perfect structural integrity and normal, healthy function to severe structural damage and inferior cerebral action. In the extreme cases of localized damage, deficits in both the brain and behavior can frequently be identified unequivocally with the presence of hard neurological signs. In the borderline cases, the behavior deficit may be obvious, but the neurological dysfunction, when there is one, may have to be inferred through scientific speculation until more sensitive neurological test procedures are developed, or until neuropsychological knowledge is more nearly complete.

9. Since the adoption of the concept of learning disabilities in 1963, various definitions have been proposed, and they continue to be produced. The main reasons for this confusion are (1) the incomplete understanding of the nature of LD at present,

and (2) the variability among the professional groups attempting to define it. This situation is likely to continue until etiological knowledge is complete, and the various professional groups agree on a definition. It is certain that that time is not in the near future.

10. Brain-damaged patients and cerebrally dysfunctioning subjects are not a homogeneous group and must be understood differentially in terms of the type of lesion (whether it is evolving, resolving, or static), of its locus, intensity, extent, and history. Similarly, LD children or adults are not a homogeneous group and must be understood diagnostically according to the *nature* of their learning problems. A detailed neuropsychological battery of tests can provide information on perception (visual, auditory, and tactile–kinesthetic), both intramodally and intermodally; on language development (both understanding and expression); on mental imagery (both verbal and nonverbal); on reasoning (both inductive and deductive); on memory (both short-term and habitual); on sequencing (both verbal and nonverbal); on motor speed and accuracy; on cerebral dominance and handedness; on sensorimotor integration; and on academic achievement.

11. Chronic localized lesions in critical parts of the language circuits, usually in the left hemisphere, or in critical parts of the cortex mediating spatial perception, usually in the right hemisphere, are permanent and have an established negative effect on perception and cognition. Research of others (Calanchini & Trout, 1971, especially pp. 215–219) and our own (e.g., cases of Sam and Will in Chapter 4) have shown a permanence of learning deficit. The learning profiles of these children do not alter significantly with time; "the intact and deficient areas remain the same" (Calanchini & Trout, 1971). These same authors, in describing one of these cases, wrote, "His method of learning is unique for his brain." In such cases a neuropsychological assessment provides a better basis for understanding and *predicting* the child's possible learning in the future.

12. Chronic brain lesions, though they mean that the cerebral deficit is permanent, do not mean that the child cannot improve in learning achievement. Even though the child's learning profile may show the same "lows" and "highs" over time, he can be taught, with skilled remedial teaching, to make better use of intrinsic strengths. In brief, the child's intellectual "capacity" remains fixed but learning strategies can improve.

13. Children with several neurological "soft signs" also are likely to retain most of them, and "many show additional and different signs in adulthood that were not seen in childhood" (Hern,

1984). Most of these children are learning impaired in school and tend to retain these disabilities in adulthood, although by then they may have learned compensatory strategies.

14. Minimal "soft signs" in children tend to present various cognitive and behavioral deficits in adulthood that restrict their training and vocational opportunities (Spreen, 1983, 1988). But again, they may learn compensatory strategies that can lead to occupational success and personal satisfaction. Many years ago, Somerset Maugham wrote a charming and amusing short story, "The Verger" (Maugham, 1953), about an adult dyslexic who amassed a fortune in business but who could neither read nor write. Such cases are not uncommon but they seldom come to public notice because successful dyslexics, understandably prefer to conceal their disability.

Neuropsychological Principles

The clinical responsibility of neuropsychological assessment is a serious one, and to reach a level of clinical competence requires several years of training under experienced supervision. Because it is beyond the scope of this book to explain this very complex subject, only some of the most reliable and tested principles are listed here. Each principle may stimulate a number of clinical investigating techniques, and a few examples of these are listed for purposes of illustration.

1. A left-hemisphere lesion or dysfunction, if in the area of the language circuits, may impede the understanding and expression of spoken and/or written language, and/or result in an inability to repeat oral material on command. Such a dysfunction, if severe, results in some form of aphasia and, if minimal, in a specific language retardation. Such students will typically have poor achievement and difficulty in learning all verbal academic subjects, but they may be superior in mechanical design and invention and all visual–spatial tasks such as geometry, cartography, and graphic and industrial arts.

   A few of the behavioral signs of left-hemisphere dysfunction include: a markedly lower verbal IQ relative to a performance IQ; the presence of language retardation (or aphasic symptoms) along with average or superior spatial–constructional skills; poor tactile form recognition in the right hand coupled with normal stereognosis in the left; poor finger localization in the right hand with normal awareness for the left; a right visual field defect with normal vision on the left; slow finger tapping in the right hand accompanying normal or fast tapping in the left hand; tactile suppression in the right hand when both hands are touched simultaneously, with habitual reporting of tactile stimulation in the left hand; tactile insensitivity in the right hand when stimulated with graded fine nylon hairs along with normal sensitivity in the left hand; and poor sequential perception and memory. Such symptoms are never used singly to indicate a neuropsychological diagnosis; they are evaluated in constellations (Reitan included a composite of 10 signs for his Impairment Index) and they are correlated with medical data (e.g., brain-scan indications of abnormal functions in the left hemisphere with none in the right).

2. A right-hemisphere lesion or dysfunction, if in the medial and posterior cortical areas, typically impedes spatial perception and imagery and may result in inferior achievement in arithmetic, geometry, map drawing, graphic arts, and all types of mechanical and constructional skills. This is the pattern of the child with a nonverbal learning disability (Myklebust, 1975b; Rourke, 1989). Such students may be competent in learning and achieving successfully in the language arts.

   Sensory and motor signs of right-hemisphere dysfunction appear on the side opposite to the signs listed above in item 1. Although an educator will not use these signs for a neuropsychological diagnosis, they can be used as invaluable information in understanding the nature of a child's learning problem, in terms of perception, cognition, motor response, and language competence.

3. Throughout this book we have attempted to observe the various behaviors that appear to be dominated by one cerebral hemisphere or the other. Although knowledge of hemispheric functional asymmetry is a first step in our understanding of brain function, the essence of this understanding is how the two differentially functioning hemispheres *interact*. As Rourke (1982) has shown, during the past 35 years we have progressed through a "static" phase where behavioral deficits and localized brain lesions were related by performance on fixed batteries of psychological tests. Then followed a phase of cognitive neuropsychology, in which attempts were made to identify the tasks that the tests were alleged to measure. The third and present phase is an attempt to escape the rigidity of the first two by examining the development of the human brain and its dynamic interactions in determining human behavior.

   The successful school psychologist will need to be aware of the knowledge emanating from the first two phases and will need to follow the current and lively discussions of dynamic cerebral organization. If neuropsychological knowledge is to be used successfully in deciding on remediation programs, a complete and accurate model of brain function and behavior is a basic requisite. Such a model is not yet available, nor is there general agreement on how the two cerebral hemispheres interact. Although there is much segmental empirical evidence to enable us to use our knowledge of brain–behavior relationships, there is still much speculation on how these segments fit together in a functional model. Some theorists propose that the brain develops first from the left to the right side and that this left–right maturational gradient results in the leading side (usually the left) exerting an inhibitory influence on the lagging side (usually the right) (Corballis & Morgan, 1978). There are others who, using histological evidence of greater sensory and motor representation in the left hemisphere and greater areas of associative cortex in the right, have proposed a right-to-left shift in learning new material (Goldberg & Costa, 1981; Rourke, 1982). All of these theories, though enjoying much empirical support, still are somewhat speculative and have only a tentative status, because none of them accounts completely for cognition and behavior.

4. Intramodal analysis is profitable for analyzing learning problems, particularly when they involve a specific sense mode. For example, if visual–perceptual deficits seem to be related to a child's academic underachieving, the diagnostician will want to know about the level of functioning of the child's visual form recognition, letter and word form recognition, pictorial sequential memory, nonverbal visual sequential memory, verbal visual sequential memory, figure–ground perception, visual–manual reaction time, visual–motor accuracy and speed, and the relation of visual perception to cerebral dominance. A similar detailed analysis may need to be carried out in the auditory and tactile–kinesthetic sense modes if deficit functioning is detected in either of them.

5. Intermodal integration must be evaluated. Ayres (1976) has developed a detailed battery of tests suitable for measuring sensorimotor integration, and Geschwind, Luria, Myklebust, Reitan, Satz, Spreen and Benton, Aaron Smith, and many others have written about intermodal sensory, motor, and language integration at the cortical and subcortical levels.

It is sometimes found that a child is competent in perceptual–motor functions when the various sense modes are viewed separately. However, this child's inability to integrate visual, auditory, tactile, and motor expression may impede his or her learning to read, write, and spell.

Although cross-modal integration is essential to perception and understanding, as demonstrated by earlier researchers (Birch, 1964; Myklebust, 1963), the various channels of sensory input, though semiautonomous in function, are also able to interact and to process verbal contents at one time and nonverbal ones at other times (Johnson & Myklebust, 1967). In reading research, there is evidence to suggest that "letter and word perception and reading comprehension are affected by the visual, semantic, syntactic, and pragmatic environments in which the reading occurs" (Chase & Tallal, 1991). This implies that interaction can occur among all the sensorimotor and cognitive processes involved in a particular perceptual–learning event.

6. The LD child's cerebral dominance and handedness need to be known, and in the past this information has usually been unknown or ignored.

7. Learning disabilities, as we have seen, may be either verbal (mainly left hemisphere) and/or nonverbal (mainly right hemisphere). Myklebust (1975a,b), using a cognitive model, has shown that imagery may be weak because the original perceptual input may be distorted or partial. To develop a mental image of a chair (and this must precede the development of the concept of it), the child must re-create in his or her imagination the visual form and the tactile feel of sitting in a chair. The child whose nonverbal or spatial perceptions are accurate, vivid, and facile may be better equipped to produce a mental image, a symbol, and ultimately a concept of a class of objects known as "chair." Myklebust (1975b) thinks that nonverbal learning disturbances may be more debilitating than the verbal. They may include "deficiencies in ability to judge time, size, distance, and weight, to acquire spatial orientation, to learn right from left, and to learn directions" (p. 90).

The Knowledge of Brain Structure and Function

A study of brain structure and function has led most neuropsychologists to "accept that at least the basic skills such as perception, movement and language are separately organized within the cortex" (Warrington, 1970). Luria (1973) has attributed attention to the brainstem; perception (including spatial interpretation) to the post-Rolandic cerebrum; and motor, sequential, planning, and temporal behavior to the frontal lobes. Whether it is all as simplistically related as this is not certain, but it is true that a detailed knowledge of brain functions will lead the school psychologist in a systematic and thorough hunt for the possible attentional, perceptual, linguistic, motor, or sequential deficits that an academically or socially under-achieving child may have. The teacher, with at least a gross or practical understanding of the regional functions of the brain, will make a better use of the knowledge supplied by the school psycho-logist and should, because of this systematic functional knowledge of the brain, be able to produce more testable hypotheses in choosing a successful plan for remediation. The child has the clues to the causes of his or her learning problems if the diagnostician has the understanding and knowledge to recognize them; and a knowledge of the structure and function of the child or adult's brain can help to direct the search for causes. It must be remembered that *not all LD is caused by brain damage or cerebral dysfunction*. Because neuropsychology grew out of the study of patients with localized brain lesions, most of the early knowledge of brain behavior relationships was gained from such cases, but throughout this book we have introduced many other possible causes. It is highly likely that brain damage is responsible for a minority of the cases of LD. The educator using neuropsychological data in assessing and treating an LD child should be constantly reminded of the many other possible physiological and psychosocial influences.

A Cautionary Note

A concentration on neuropsychological factors in behavior may cause a neglect of other equally important etiological variables. Because all human behavior results from a delicate and complex interaction between organic and psychosocial forces, any deviation in behavior or learning must be understood in this multicausal model. We have examined only the neuropsychological causes in this book, but there are, in addition to the psychosocial forces, many other physiological determiners, such as genetic defects, glandular dysfunctions, malnutrition, lead poisoning, neural maldevelopment, and atypical growth.

To avoid a wrong diagnosis it will be useful to remember:

1. In examining the academically underachieving learner, the school psychologist or educational diagnostician (and this includes the teacher) must guard against searching for pathology and as-suming that something must be organically wrong with the re-ferred child or adult. It is important to keep an open mind and assess the empirical evidence to decide how much of the

learner's deficits are organically caused (if, in fact, they are), and how much they are sociogenically produced.
2. The diagnostic decision about the quality of underachievement may be carefully or superficially carried out. In the latter case it may be inaccurate and misleading. Ysseldyke and his colleagues (1983) have made a number of detailed studies of this process. Some of their findings have shown that:
   a. Team meetings of professionals to assess children's academic underachievement frequently include no input, or very little, from teachers.
   b. Sometimes decisions are made that ignore the collected data.
   c. Achievement and intelligence tend to be emphasized by educational team members, but most participants base their acceptance of a child's IQ on only *one* test. More than a third of them base their opinions of achievement on only *one* test, and frequently inadequate tests are used.
   d. In one study (Algozzine & Ysseldyke, 1981), about half of a group of decision makers (n > 200) identified *normal* students as needing special educational help.
   e. Depending on which current criteria are used to select under-achievers, most *normal* students can be classified as LD.
   Such studies show clearly that the decision making process is too often inconsistent and unreliable, and to improve it, better trained professionals are needed on the team. To translate diagnostic test data into successful remedial treatment is probably the most difficult professional demand in special education. Collecting large masses of test data is a waste of time unless the remedial measures they suggest are monitored regularly, edited, and continually readjusted to provide successful results.
3. Even if it is obvious or highly probable that the person we are studying is suffering from a chronic brain dysfunction, this is not *the* single cause of his or her learning problems. Its effect on the learner's behavior (is he discouraged, indifferent, or hostile?) and relationships with his family and peers will still need to be considered.
4. If a neurological dysfunction is obvious or highly probable we must remember that, despite a fairly large body of tested knowledge in neuropsychology, there are still many gray areas, ranging from partial or confused understanding to complete ignorance. Aaron Smith, in his presidential address to the International Neuropsychological Society (A. Smith, 1979) told a charming story which, in essence, indicated that at least half of what is taught in medical schools eventually turns out to be false. But the irony of the situation is that *we don't know which half!* This is likely true in clinical neuropsychology and special education

as well, for both of these disciplines are applied studies, in which practices and principles evolve unevenly, and frequently in situations of practical need.

5. To protect ourselves from serious mistakes that may have damaging effects on students, the diagnostician is wise to assume the view of the experimental scientist. He or she must not rely only on a favorite diagnosis or recommend a standard or simplistic remedial program but must study the child or adult systematically and in depth and look there for clues. A profile of standard scores is not enough; we also need to know in detail the child's strengths, weaknesses, learning strategies, and relations with his or her social environment.

6. Pet theories, pet diagnoses, and pet remedial plans should be avoided. These are probably signs of a superficial knowledge of the whole field of learning disabilities and indications of a set of simplistic beliefs based on emotion and desire rather than on diagnostic understanding.

7. Special education includes many people with an "either–or" approach. Some support behavior modification or environmental causes exclusively and deny that organic factors are either relevant or appropriate. Others refuse to have behavior modification practices in their schools because they are too mechanistic and impersonal. To view the LD child or adult scientifically and objectively we cannot afford to exclude any area of tested knowledge or any form of remediation that promises possible help to the learner. No doubt the "either–or" approach could soon be erased if all school psychologists and LD specialists were required, in their graduate training, to spend an intensive supervised practicum stressing applied behavior analysis, and an equally intensive supervised practicum working with LD subjects, where neuropsychological assessment methods were used. Unfortunately, at present, only a few graduate training programs for school psychologists include neuropsychological assessment in their curricula (Hynd, Quackenbush, & Obrzut, 1979; Hynd & Obrzut, 1980; Hynd, 1992).

As we have seen throughout this book, the influence of neuropsychology, first on experimental psychology in the 1940s and 1950s, then on clinical psychology in the 1960s, and finally on school psychology, has resulted in changes at an alarming speed. Such rapid growth has meant that practices have preceded theory, and molar hypotheses have come into use before they have been justified by all of the necessary microinvestigations. But "neurophysiological methods do not allow one to understand function instantly" (Barlow, 1980); it is a slow process of continuous experimental microinvestigations of exact or nearly accurate understanding of small segments of knowledge. However, knowledge in this fractionated form is useless to the clinician unless it is integrated and related to the practical problems faced by the practitioner (in this case, the clinical psychologist, the school psychologist, and the special educator). Knowing all this, these professionals will understand that they are practicing a treatment procedure with limited knowledge and remedies yet to be fully related to theory. The 1980s and 1990s have already seen important advances in behavioral neurology; it is hoped that this trend will continue so that our knowledge of the brain−behavior relationships will be significantly advanced and special education can boast of remedial measures more closely based on sound theory.

Appendix

Neuropsychological Tests

In Chapter 3, the use of neuropsychological tests is discussed as being useful for making a differential diagnosis of brain damage versus non-brain-damage in detecting cognitive deficits in brain-damaged and MBD subjects, and for assessing the pattern of behavioral and mental strengths, and weaknesses in both neurologically impaired and normal subjects. The trained clinical neuropsychologist may be competent to make all of these diagnoses, but in cases where an educational diagnostician has had no training in clinical neuropsychology, it is important that he or she avoid making neuropsychological statements and instead use the test results for understanding the child's pattern of cognitive competencies and deficits. This knowledge is essential for the preparation of an effective remedial program.

1. The Victoria Test Battery
   The collection of tests, or flexible battery, used in the University of Victoria Neuropsychology Laboratory and its associated test facilities has been developed and expanded during the past 30 years since the establishment of the center in the early 1960s. The first battery was formed from a selection of tests which appeared to possess the highest level of theoretical validity and clinical usefulness, as reported in various research papers in the professional literature. It included the Wechsler tests of intelligence, the adult tests of the Halstead-Reitan battery (the children's tests were still being developed by Reitan and were added later), and a collection of the many tests being developed by Arthur Benton and Otfried Spreen at the University of Iowa. This choice meant that the Victoria Laboratory was introducing, as part of its test program, subtests from a "fixed" battery (Reitan) and tests from a flexible battery that was problem-centered (Benton and Spreen). Each approach has its advantages. The Reitan model provides large numbers of subjects for study, all of whom have been tested by the same comprehensive selection of tests. Reitan's research was designed to test a large sample of medically documented patients with some degree of brain damage or dysfunction on the same large battery of tests. This

enabled him to accumulate a huge library of files with the same comprehensive pattern of psychometric data, to provide a basis for producing basic deductions about human brain function and behavior. Reitan produced his first summary of brain-behavior conclusions in mimeographed form in 1959. This model produces a large data base of clinically homogeneous findings, but it is expensive in testing time.

The approach in Benton's Laboratory, by contrast, was problem-centered. Each problem to be studied (e.g., facial agnosia, finger localization, auditory perception, or language deficit) used available tests appropriate to the problem, or new and original tests developed specifically for that purpose. This approach makes a more efficient use of tests and testing time, and can be maintained with fewer psychometricians, but it does not provide as large samples of clinically-tested subjects as the Reitan model. The practice in the Victoria Neuropsychology Laboratory from the beginning has been to make use of the best features of both models.

With the arrival of Otfried Spreen in 1966 as the Director of the Victoria Laboratory, the Victoria battery has been developed and expanded to include a large variety of sensory, motor, neuropsychological, neurological, intelligence, and academic achievement tests. Many of these have been psychometrically revised to improve their clinical validity and their practical usefulness. A detailed discussion of all of these tests has been published by Spreen and Strauss (1991) in a useful compendium or clinical reference book. It includes explanatory discussions of history taking; general intellectual ability and the assessment of premorbid intelligence; the method of profiling test results (including the Victoria revision of the Halstead Category Test, the Mattis Dementia Rating Scale, the North American Adult Reading Test, Raven's Progressive Matrices, the Stroop Test, the Wechsler Intelligence Tests, and the Wisconsin Card Sorting Test); three cognitive tests for children (Bayley, Kaufman, and Stanford-Binet); five widely used academic achievement tests; 10 attention and memory tests; four language tests that include the Spreen-Benton Aphasia Battery; 11 visual, visuomotor and auditory tests; five tactile, tactile-visual, and tactile-motor tests; four motor tests; and seven adaptive behavior and personality tests. Generous tables of normative data are included for most of the tests.

The book, besides describing the current Victoria test collection, is a useful reference book for the experienced clinical neuropsychologist or the graduate student pursuing training in the field.

2. The Halstead-Reitan Neuropsychological Test Batteries

The Halstead-Reitan Neuropsychological Test Battery for Adults (15 years and older), for older children (ages 9–14 years), and for younger children (ages 5–8 years) are available from Dr. R. M.

Reitan, Neuropsychology Laboratory, 2920 S. 4*th* Avenue, South Tucson, Arizona 85713-4819. These batteries, as well as being used for diagnosing learning disorders, are used by clinical neuropsychologists to assess brain functions and dysfunctions and adaptive abilities.

3. Aphasia Testing
   (1) Goodglass, H., and Kaplan, E. *The assessment of aphasia and related disorders*. Philadelphia: Lea & Febiger, 1972.
   (2) Spreen, O., and Benton, A.L. *Neurosensory center comprehensive examination for aphasia* [also known as the Spreen-Benton aphasia battery]. Produced and distributed by the Neuropsychology Laboratory, University of Victoria, Victoria, B.C., Canada, 1968 and 1977 (revised). It is also discussed in detail by Spreen and Strauss (1991).

4. Description of the five nonverbal sequential tests used in the study of serial order (see Chapter 4, p. 165)
   (1) Visual Receptive Serial Order Test
       This is the Dynamic Visual Retention Test (DVRT; Gaddes, 1988), which shows sequential patterns of lights on a display screen. The subject is asked to watch a standard pattern of lights and a test pattern in which one light is in a different position. The subject is asked to state which light in the sequence is different. This is a visual version of the Seashore Tonal Memory Test. The patterns of lights have recently been transferred to a disk for use on a microcomputer at two speeds.
       (a) Slow speed: Light exposure 1 second; interlight interval 1 second.
       (b) Fast speed: Light exposure 0.1 second; interlight interval 0.4 second.
   This test, on microcomputer disk Apple and IBM compatible, is available through the Neuropsychology Laboratory, University of Victoria, P.O. Box 1700, Victoria, B.C., Canada, V8W 2Y2
   (2) Visual Expressive Serial Order Test
       The apparatus for this test can be made in any technical shop. The device includes a telegrapher's key connected to a battery-powered 14-volt lamp. The experimenter taps out a serial pattern of lights while the subject watches. The subject is asked to remember the sequential pattern and to tap it out immediately.
   (3) Auditory Receptive Serial Order Test
       The subject listens to two serial patterns of taps presented on a tape recorder and is required to say whether the second pattern is the same or different from the first.
   (4) Auditory Expressive Serial Order Test
       Following the perception of a pattern of taps presented on a tape recorder, the subject is required to remember and imitate them with a drumstick on the edge of the table.

5. Technical Aids in Remediation

Technical aids for improving the language development of the deaf, brain-damaged, and language-impaired child, also may be useful in teaching the LD child. In recent years there has been a major increase in the variety of these techniques available to speech therapists and remedial teachers.

Children with receptive language deficits may be helped by the visual identification of pictures on a computer screen. Identification may be by oral response or by touching the picture on the screen. Learning all parts of speech can be assisted by this procedure.

FM auditory trainers can help any classification of language-impaired child. An FM auditory trainer system consists of a wireless microphone and transmitter that sends a frequency-modulated (FM) signal to an FM receiver. The teacher may wear the transmitter and microphone unit, and each student wears a receiver and headset that enables him or her to hear the teacher's speech more clearly. Blake *et al.* (1991) found this procedure successful in improving the attending behavior of LD children.

A tactile response may be used in pressing a computer key to select words in forming a sentence.

Children with expressive speech-language problems may be helped with synthetic speech devices, and those with severe motor problems may control their computerized equipment with a puff switch.

Parents of language-impaired children, teachers, graduate students and interested others should consult a speech-language pathologist (SLP) at the nearest children's hospital or audiological clinic to learn more about the available technical aids in this field and to learn names and addresses of current commercial suppliers.

6. Student Membership in I.A.R.L.D.

The International Academy for Research in Learning Disabilities (I.A.R.L.D.) invites applications from "individuals who are in the beginning stages of a career in learning disabilities research and/or to clinically oriented students who as future professionals may very well contribute to the field of learning disabilities through publications, service, and/or policy making activities". A Newsletter informs members of meetings and current publications in the field of LD, and research papers by senior members and fellows are published periodically. Student membership fees are reduced from full membership.

Interested graduate students or others may write for further information to:

Dr. Doris Johnson
Executive Director, I.A.R.L.D.
Northwestern University
2299 North Campus Drive
Evanston, IL 60208, USA

Glossary

A

Å. Also called Angstrom unit, the unit of electromagnetic wavelength equal to 10^{-7} mm.

Ablation. Cutting and removing a section of tissue. Cerebral ablation: surgical removal of a part of the brain.

Acalculia. An inability to carry out simple arithmetical calculations.

Agenesis. Failure of tissue or an organ to grow and develop normally.

Agnosia. A perceptual deficit; the inability to recognize the meaning of sensory stimuli.

Allergy. A specific and hypersensitive reaction to a particular substance to which most people show a normal reaction.

Anesthesia. Sensory loss; a loss or reduction of feeling of any of the senses.

Aneurysm. The dilatation of the wall of an artery.

Angiogram. X-ray studies of the cerebral blood vessel system following injection of radiopaque material into the arterial system.

Angiography. The practice of studying the circulatory system with angiograms.

Angular Gyrus. A convolution located in the parietal cortices believed to be involved in cross-modal integration; a "tertiary" cortical zone in Luria's brain model.

Anomia. The inability to name an object that one recognizes and understands. A symptom of receptive aphasia.

Anosmia. An absence or reduction of the sense of smell.

Anoxia. A lack or reduction of oxygen in the body.

Aphasia. An inability, partial or complete, to understand or express language whether written or spoken, because of injury or disease of the language centers in the brain.

Aphasoid. A mild or moderate retardation in language development and competence; minimal aphasic symptoms.

Aplasia. Failure to grow and develop normally; agenesis.

Apraxia. A defective ability in the absence of severe sensory or motor loss for carrying out neuromuscular acts normally, even though the patient understands what is expected of him.

Arteriovenous Malformation. An abnormal space-occupying tangle of arteries and veins; a benign tumor of abnormally developed blood vessels; hemangioma.

Astereognosis. An impaired ability to recognize objects by touch alone.

Ataxia. Impaired neuromuscular coordination in voluntary muscular movements.

Athetoid. A reduced degree of athetosis.

Athetosis. Involuntary neuromuscular movements and facial grimaces as in cerebral palsy, caused by brain lesion(s).

Atrophy. Wasting away of live tissue.

Audiology. The study and treatment of hearing.

Auditory–Gnostic. The perception and understanding of auditory stimuli.

Avascular. Lacking in sufficient blood vessels, resulting in an inadequate blood supply.

B

Babinski Reflex. Extension and fanning of the toes when the plantar surface of the foot is stroked.

Basal Ganglia (or Striatum). A cluster of nuclei located in the brainstem near the thalamus and concerned with various motor activities.

Behavioral Model. A concept of behavior stressing environmental influences.

Betz Cells. Large neurons in the deep layers of the motor cortex.

Bilateral. Pertaining to both sides of the body or both cerebral hemispheres.

Biochemistry. The chemical study of living tissue.

Biofeedback. A technique using operant conditioning to alter the brain waves of a patient. Clinically this may be used to reduce pulse rate, lower temperature, and alter other autonomic functions.

Brain Scan. A technique for detecting pathological brain tissue using radioactive material injected into the bloodstream. A radiation detector picks up the gamma rays emitted by the damaged tissue and produces a type of X-ray picture of the brain structure.

Brain Tumor. A swelling or abnormal enlargement of brain tissue; a space-occupying lesion; the abnormal tissue may be benign or malignant.

Brodmann's Cerebral Areas. The cortical areas numbered by Brodmann, a German neurologist; see Fig. 2.10, p. 88

C

Calcarine Fissure. A fissure on the mesial surface of the occipital lobe.

Callosal. Pertaining to the corpus callosum.

Carotid Artery. The large artery on each side of the neck that supplies blood to the brain.

Cathode Ray Oscilloscope. A vacuum tube; an electronic device that acts as an electron gun and serves as an instrument for detecting and measuring changes in a magnetic field; the basic design of a television picture tube.

Cerebellum. A division of the central nervous system situated on the posterior surface of the brain stem and involved in neuromuscular coordination.

Cerebral Vascular Accident (CVA) or "Stroke". Cerebral bleeding resulting in linguistic and/or other behavioral deficits.

Cervical. Pertaining to the neck. The cervical level of the spinal cord is at the level of the neck.

Choreiform. Mild, jerky, involuntary movements, frequently involving the hands; somewhat like chorea.

Clonic. Rapid alternate spasms of contraction and relaxation as in epileptic seizures.

CNS. Abbreviation for central nervous system.

Commissurotomy. A surgical procedure by which the commissures or neural fibers of the corpus callosum are severed. In some cases the complete corpus callosum may be cut and in others only part, frequently the anterior commissures. This procedure, frequently referred to as the "split-brain" technique, may be used for relief of intractible epilepsy. It incidentally provides split- and half-brain models with which to study various forms of human behavior and behavior change.

Concurrent Validity. Correlating a new test with the results of an established test known to be valid may provide a measure of concurrent validity for the new test if the measure correlating the two tests is high.

Construct Validity. If the correlation is positive and high between test scores and a particular type of hypothesized behavior in a theory (e.g., anxiety), the test is said to have construct validity.

Contre-coup Effect. A sudden blow on one side of the head may produce damage to the opposite side of the brain.

Contralateral. Pertaining to the opposite side of the body or brain. Antonym for ipsilateral.

Convolution. An irregular convex formation in the brain; a gyrus.

Corpora Quadrigemina. Four rounded protuberances on the posterior surface of the midbrain. The two upper ones (the superior colliculi) are involved in vision; the two lower ones (the inferior colliculi) are involved in audition.

Corpus Callosum. Wide band of neural fibers interconnecting the two cerebral hemispheres.

Cortex. The convoluted outer layer of gray neural tissue that covers the brain. For convenience it is divided in frontal, parietal, temporal, and occipital lobes by the fissure of Rolando and the fissure of Sylvius. Both the left and right cerebral hemispheres are similarly divided.

Cortical Electrostimulation. During brain surgery a conscious patient may report specific experiences following electrostimulation of particular areas of the cerebral cortex. Stimulation of the motor strips may temporarily interfere with volitional motor activity or cause involuntary movements.

Cortices. Plural of cortex.

Craniotomy. Any operation on the cranium. In neurology it usually refers to brain surgery.

Cutaneous. The skin senses, usually thought to include touch, cold, warm, and pain.

CVA. Cerebral vascular accident.

Cyanosed. The skin takes on a blue color because of inadequate oxygen content in the blood.

Cyst. A liquid-filled sac; in abnormal form it shows as a swelling.

Cytology. The study of living cells.

D

Decussation. A crossing over from one side to the other. Neural decussation refers to the bodily sensory and motor tracts that cross over and connect to the contralateral cerebral hemisphere.

Dextral. Pertaining to the right side of the body.

Diaschisis. A localized brain lesion may impair the function of healthy tissue at some distance from it. These "distance effects" can be misleading if only behavioral signs are used for diagnosis.

Dichotic Listening. A technique for stimulating simultaneously both ears of a subject with different words, usually with similar initial sounds and lengths. This is used to investigate cerebral dominance for language.

Diplopia. Double vision.

Dorsal. Posterior, back part or surface.

Dynamometer. A device for measuring hand-grip strength.

Dysarthria. Defective articulation.

Dyscalculia. Faulty calculation ability; a mild or moderate acalculia.

Dysgraphia. Impaired ability to express ideas in writing.

Dysphasia. An impairment of speech; sometimes used as a synonym for aphasia.

Dysnomia. Faulty word-finding ability; a mild or moderate anomia.

Dysrhythmia. Abnormal rhythm of electrical changes in the brain; detected by the electroencephalogram.

E

Echoencephalogram. A device that directs high-frequency sound waves through the skull and brain tissue to detect brain tissue abnormalities. It is particularly used to detect shift of the midline in the brain resulting from a space-occupying lesion on one side.

EEG. Abbreviation for electroencephalogram.

Electrode Implantation in the Brain. Surgical insertion of metal electrodes to record the electrical changes in the cerebral locus of the electrode during specific behaviors.

Electroencephalogram. A tracing recorded on a moving graph showing the changes in electrical potential in various parts of the brain.

Electromyogram (EMG). A recording device that provides graphic information on the electrical activity of the muscles, as well as the correlated electrical changes in the peripheral nerves.

Empirical Validity. This refers to validating a test or a function by reference to real facts.

Encephalitis. Infection or inflammation of brain tissues.

Endocrine. Pertaining to the glands that secrete their hormones directly into the bloodstream.

Engram. The hypothesized neural trace; the concept that neural tissue manifests permanent change following learning.

Epilepsy. A seizure condition resulting from intense and abnormal electrical activity in the brain.

Epileptogenic Foci. Focal areas of pathological brain tissue that appear to be related to the occurrence of epileptic seizures.

Epithelial. Pertaining to the skin or outer covering.

Equipotentiality. The idea that within large areas of the cerebral cortex one part is equally as potent as another part for determining a particular type of behavior, e.g., Lashley's theory of mass action.

Esophagus. The membraneous tube connecting the throat with the stomach.

Euclidean. Two dimensional; spatial as in Euclidean geometry.

Evoked Potential. The measurement of electrical changes in the brain or central nervous system following environmental stimulation; e.g., light flashes in a subject's eyes will evoke sharp electrical changes in the posterior parts of the brain, and staccato sound patterns will evoke sequentially similar electrical changes in the temporal lobes.

Extremities. An arm, leg, hand, or foot; body parts distal from the brain.

F

Face Validity. A test that seems suitable for measuring a certain phenomenon purely on a logical basis but without any empirical testing is said to have face validity.

False Negatives. Those cases wrongly excluded from a category because of error in the selection instrument.

False Positives. Those cases wrongly included in a category because of error in the selection instrument.

Falx. A part of the brain deep in the longitudinal fissure that divides the cerebral hemispheres.

Familial. A family pattern; a syndrome that appears in several members of the same family (e.g., developmental dyslexia).

Feature Detecting Cells. Cortical cells that respond to a specific feature of the environment and not to other features, e.g., some cortical cells in the cat's striate cortex respond to vertical lines of light but not to horizontal or sloping ones.

Flicker Fusian Rate. When two visual stimuli are presented sequentially at a comfortable speed they are seen as two separate stimuli with a time interval between them. As the interval is reduced there comes a time when the two lights appear to fuse, or are seen as one continuous light stimulus. The flicker fusion rate for a particular subject is the fastest speed that two stimuli can be seen by that subject.

Foramen. An opening or passage.

G

Galvanic Skin Response. Electrical changes of the skin following certain stimuli; sometimes used as an indicator of emotion.

Ganglia. A group of nerve cells forming a sort of nerve center; usually located outside the brain and spinal cord.

Genetic Defects. Abnormal or subnormal physical or psychological symptoms resulting from a defective gene or chromosome pattern.

Gerstmann Syndrome. A configuration of behavioral symptoms stated by Gerstmann, a German neurologist, to result from a lesion of the parietal lobe on the dominant side. The syndrome includes finger agnosia, defective right-left orientation, agraphia, and acalculia.

Gestalt Psychology. A school of psychology that originated in Germany in 1912 and that stressed perception and a holistic view of behavior.

Granule Cells. In the cortex, the fourth layer contains many granular cells with short axons.

Gray Matter. The layman's term for the cortex made up largely of cell bodies that are gray in color.

Gyrus. A convolution or convex fold of tissue.

H

Haptic. Sense of touch; recognition of three-dimensional objects; stereognosis.

Hard Signs. These refer to unequivocal, medically documented signs of brain damage, such as brain surgery, cerebral bleeding, hemiplegia, brain tumor, or penetrating head injury.

Hemangioma. A tumor formed of a tangle of blood vessels.

Hematoma. A mass of effused blood following a hemorrhage.

Hemianopia. A half visual field defect; blindness or impaired vision in the left or right visual field.

Hemianopsia. Same as hemianopia.

Hemiasomatognosia. Being aware of only one half or one side of the body; the side contralateral to the brain lesion is neglected or ignored.

Hemiparesis. Partial paralysis of one side of the body.

Hemiplegia. Paralysis of one side of the body.

Heschl's Gyrus. Convolution on the floor of the fissure of Sylvius.

Hippocampus. A structure of the brain located subcortically below the anterior area of the temporal lobes. Along with the temporal lobes and other parts of the brain it is essential in mediating memory.

Histology. Microscopic study of the structure of bodily tissues.

Homeostasis. A principle of physiology describing the tendency of a dynamic energy system to seek a state of equilibrium or normality.

Hyperthyroidism. A condition in which the thyroid gland secretes too much thyroxin and the subject's behavior is marked by hyperactivity, irritability, and restlessness.

Hypothalamus. A portion of the thalamus contiguous to the optic chiasm; is related to the control of many visceral processes and emotional behavior.

Hypothyroidism. An underfunctioning of the thyroid gland often marked by apathy, overweight, and slow mentation.

I

Idiopathic. Of unknown cause.

Imperception. Impaired ability to understand environmental stimuli; agnosia.

Inferior colliculi. The two lower protuberances of the corpora quadrigemina; conduction centers in the auditory tracts.

Insult. In neurology, refers to a lesion or neurological tissue damage.

Internuncial neurons. Interconnecting neurons between sensory and motor neurons.

Intracerebral. Inside the brain or cerebrum.

Invaginated. An infolding of tissue.

Ipsilateral. On the same side; antonym for contralateral.

K

Kinesthesis. Awareness of the body and body parts in space; it includes awareness of balance and motion.

L

Lateral Geniculate Bodies. Two neural bodies, located in the thalamus, that are interconnecting centers for the visual tracts.

Lesion. Any tissue that is damaged or abnormal, e.g., by infection, trauma, or tumor.

Lexicon. Of or belonging to words; their particular meanings, as in a dictionary.

Limbic System. A set of cerebral structures, inside the brain and above the brainstem, believed to be involved in emotional behavior and short-term memory. It may include the cingulate gyrus, isthmus, hippocampal gyrus, and uncus.

Loci. Plural of locus.

Locus. Place, site, or location; used in medicine to indicate a specific area or point in the body.

M

Mass Action. See equipotential.

MBD. Abbreviation of minimal brain dysfunction.

Medulla Oblongata. The part of the brainstem above the spinal cord and below the pons; a neural center for many vital functions.

Meningioma. A slowly growing tumor in the meninges or membranes covering the brain.

Mesial. Situated in the middle; at or near the middle line of the body.

Monaural Listening. Auditory stimulation of one ear alone, or one ear more strongly than the other.

Monotonic. Literal meaning, attracting in one direction. In statistics it is used to describe curvilinear relationships that are markedly skewed.

N

Neoplasm. New and abnormal growth of tissue; tumor.

Nucleus Centralis Lateralis. A neural center connecting the lateral surface of the thalamus and the parietal lobes.

Nystagmus. Involuntary oscillating movements of the eyeballs.

O

Obscuration. A phenomenon, during double or simultaneous stimulus (e.g., both hands or cheeks), in which a patient with a unilateral brain lesion reports that a stimulus is sensed weaker, but not completely extinguished, when applied to the side of the body contralateral to the lesion. It is a form of partial extinction.

Occlusion. The state of closure; e.g., blood flow through an artery might be obstructed or occluded.

Ontogenetic. Pertaining to the origin, growth, and development of a living organism.

Ophthalmology. Medical study and treatment of the eye.

Optic Chiasm. The point of decussation of the optic tracts.

Optic Chiasma. See optic chiasm.

P

Paralexia. Unintended misreading of words. They may occur in patients whose reading is seriously impaired as in alexia or dyslexia.

Paraphasia. Spontaneous substitutions of unintended syllables, words, or phrases during speech. It is characteristic of aphasic speech.

Patellar Reflex. Knee jerk; response to sudden pressure on the tendon below the knee cap.

Perisylvian Region. The cortical areas contiguous to the fissure of Sylvius.

Phylogenetic. Pertaining to the origin and development of a phylum or species of living organism.

Planum Temporale. An area of differentiated nerve tissue on the floor of the Sylvian fissure. It is larger in the left temporal lobe in most people.

Pleasure Centers of the Brain. An area of the brain near the hypothalamus; when it is electrostimulated it produces sensations pleasurable to the animal or person.

Plethysmograph. Instrument for measuring changes in volume of parts of the body; usually involves changes in blood volume.

Pneumoencephalogram. X-ray study of the brain following injection of air into the lumbar subarachnoid space. The air passes into the ventricles or system of cavities in the brain and spinal column and appears black on the X-ray. It may enable the detection of ventricular abnormalities

Pons. A connecting center of the brain stem for sensory and motor nerves.

Pontine. To do with the pons.

Positivistic View of Behavior. A model of behavior based on empirical evidence and avoiding untested speculation.

Post-Rolandic Area. The area just posterior to the fissure of Rolando; the sensory strips, parietal, occipital, and temporal lobes.

Primary Visual Cortex. Posterior area of the occipital lobes where the elements of vision are registered; Brodmann's Area 17.

Proactive Inhibition. Impaired memory for learned material because of recent learning of different material.

Prognosis. A prediction of the probable nature and course of a disease or impaired condition.

Proprioceptor. A sense organ in the tissues of the body providing information about body functions or kinesthesia.

Purkinje Cells. A large cell with numerous dendrites located in the cerebellum.

R

Receptive Aphasia. Impaired understanding of language, whether spoken or written.

Reticular System. A network of fibers in the brainstem that alerts the cortex to incoming stimuli.

Retroactive Inhibition. Impaired memory because of the disturbing effects of interpolated activity between original learning and recall.

Retrograde Amnesia. The inability to remember events for a fixed period prior to a traumatic event.

S

Sacral. Lower end of the backbone.

Scotoma. A blind spot or area of decreased vision in the visual fields.

Secondary Visual Cortex. Cortical area contiguous to Brodmann's Area 17; believed to be the visual association area; it provides "meaning" to visual sensation.

Simultagnosia. A form of visual agnosia; the inability to see two or more things at the same time.

Sinistral. Pertaining to the left side of the body.

Soft Signs. Refer to minimal behavioral deviations in a child, reported by the neurologist, where the traditional neurological examination shows no clear signs of brain damage or dysfunction. These indications, such as neuromuscular clumsiness, involuntary twitching movements in the hands, and poor directional sense, are strongly suggestive of abnormal functioning of the central nervous system, but such a diagnosis is not supported by the usual neurological examination techniques. Consequently, these are suspected neurological signs.

Somatic Cells. Bodily cells, e.g., bone cells, blood cells, tissue cells, muscle cells.

Somesthesis. Bodily awareness.

Spasticity. The result of muscle spasm or rigidity in which certain muscles are in a state of contraction that may result in paralysis or partial paralysis.

Specific Learning Disability. A difficulty in learning despite normal intelligence and usual opportunities for academic instruction; it may result from a genetic defect or a subtle and localized brain dysfunction.

Stereognosis. Tactile form recognition.

Strabismus. A failure of normal convergence of the two eyes because of incoordination of the eye muscles (commonly called squint or cross-eyed).

Striate Cortex. Primary visual cortex in the occipital lobes, so named because of a white stripe formed by the connecting nerve fibers.

Striatum. See basal ganglia.

Striped Muscles. The skeletal muscles, so named because of striated cellular structure.

Subarachnoid Hemorrhage. The arachnoid is the middle layer of the meninges (thin sheets of tissue) that cover the brain and spinal cord. The space between it and one layer below it is filled with cerebrospinal fluid. In case of brain injuries, a hemorrhage occurring in this space is called a subarachnoid hemorrhage.

Subdural Hematoma. Bleeding in the membranes covering the brain; i.e., a collection of blood between the dura and the arachnoid.

Subliminal. Below a threshold of activation (*limen*, threshold).

Subthalamus. A division of the thalamus.

Sulcus. A fissure or depression.

Superior Colliculi. The two upper protuberances of the corpora quadrigemina; conduction centers in the visual tracts.

Suprasylvian. The area of the human cortex immediately above the fissure of Sylvius.

Syntax. The study of the grammatical arrangement of words in a sentence that provides meaning.

T

Topological. Refers to topology, a form of geometry that deals with spaces with flexible boundaries. Kurt Lewin in the 1930s proposed using topology to apply to psychology so that both time and space would be included.

Toxic. Pertaining to poison or a poisonous condition.

Tumor. A new growth or neoplasm, which may be malignant or benign. A mass of tissue that grows independently of its surrounding structures and that has no physiological use.

Turner's Syndrome. A genetic condition in which a female has only a single X chromosome, and may result in severe spatial problems.

U

Unilateral Brain Damage. Damage in either the left or the right hemisphere.

V

Ventral. Toward the front; anterior.

Ventricles. Fluid-filled cavities in the brain.

Visual-Gnostic. The perception and understanding of visual stimuli.

W

Wada Carotid Amytal Test. Refers to the test of speech dominance first developed by Dr. Juhn Wada in 1949. When amytal is injected into the left carotid artery it is carried to the left cerebral hemisphere in a matter of seconds, where it has an anesthetizing effect. In most patients this produces temporary interference with all language processes. When injected into the right carotid artery amytal usually interferes with the patient's ability for pictorial interpretation and spatial perception.

Wernicke's Aphasia. Receptive aphasia.

Wernicke's Area. The cerebral cortical area, usually in the left temporal area, believed to be involved in the understanding of language. It is believed to include one-third of the left superior temporal gyrus and part of the middle temporal gyrus.

Within-Child Model. A concept of child behavior that includes internal psychological and physiological variables, as opposed to a purely behavioral model.

References

Abrams, J.C. The National Joint Committee on Learning Disabilities: History, mission, process. *Journal of Learning Disabilities*, 1987, *20*(2), 102–106.

Ackerman, P.T., Dykman, R., & Peters, J. Teenage status of hyperactive and nonhyperactive learning disabled boys. *American Journal of Orthopsychiatry*, 1977, *47*, 577–596.

Adams, J. Clinical neuropsychology and the study of learning disorders. *Pediatric Clinics of North America*, 1973, *20*, 587–598.

Adams, J. Visual and tactile integration and cerebral dysfunction in children with learning disabilities. *Journal of Learning Disabilities*, 1978, *11*, 197–204.

Alavi, A., Reivich, M., Greenberg, J., Hand, P., Rosenquist, A., Rintelmann, W., Christman, D., Fowler, J., Goldman, A., MacGregor, R., & Wolf, A. Mapping of functional activity in brain with ^{18}F-Fluoro-Deoxyglucose. *Seminars in Nuclear Medicine*, 1981, XI(1), 24–31.

Algozzine, B., & Ysseldyke, J.E. Special education services for normal students; better safe than sorry? *Exceptional Children*, 1981, *48*, 238–243.

Allport, G.W. *Becoming, basic considerations for a psychology of personality*. New Haven: Yale University Press, 1955.

Aman, N.G., & Sprague, R.L. The state dependent effect of methylphenidate and dextroamphetamine. *Journal of Nervous and Mental Diseases*, 1974, *158*, 268–279.

American Psychiatric Association. *Diagnostic and statistical manual of mental disorders*. (2nd ed.). American Psychiatric Association, Washington, DC: Author, 1968.

American Psychiatric Association. *Diagnostic and statistical manual of mental disorders—DSM III*. American Psychiatric Association, Washington, DC: Author, 1980.

American Psychiatric Association. *Diagnostic and statistical manual of mental disorders—DSM III-R*. (3rd ed., revised). American Psychiatric Association, Washington, DC: Author, 1987.

Annett, M. A model of the inheritance of handedness and cerebral dominance. *Nature* (London), 1964, *204*, 59–60.

Annett, M. The growth of manual preference and speed. *British Journal of Psychology*, 1970a, *61*, 545–558.

Annett, M. Handedness, cerebral dominance and the growth of intelligence. *In* Bakker. D.J., & Satz, P. (Eds.), *Specific reading disability, advances in theory and method*. Rotterdam: Rotterdam University Press, 1970b, 61–79.

Annett, M. The distribution of manual asymmetry. *British Journal of Psychology*, 1972, *63*, 343–358.

Annett, M. Handedness in the children of two left-handed parents. *British Journal of Psychology*, 1974, *65*, 129–131.

Annett, M. Left, right, hand and brain: The right shift theory. London: Erlbaum, 1985.

Annis, L.F. *The child before birth*. New York: Cornel University Press, 1978.

Arter, J.A., & Jenkins, J.R. Differential diagnosis—Prescriptive teaching: A critical appraisal. *Review of Educational Research*, 1979, *49*(4), 517–555.

Atkinson, J. Vision in dyslexics: Letter recognition acuity, visual crowding, contrast sensitivity accomodation, convergence and sight reading music. In *Studies in visual information processing*. North Holland: Elsevier (in press, 1992).

Atkinson, R., & Shiffrin, R. Human memory: A proposed system and its control processes. *In* Spence, K.W., & Spence, J.T. (Eds.), *The psychology of learning and motivation*. New York: Academic Press, 1968, Vol. 2.

Ayers, D., & Downing, J. The development of linguistic concepts and reading achievement. Invited paper presented at the International Reading Research Seminar on Linguistic Awareness and Learning to Read, University of Victoria, Victoria, B.C., Canada, June 26–30, 1979.

Ayres, A.J. Sensory integrative processes and neuropsychological learning disabilities. *In* Hellmuth, J. (Ed.), *Learning disorders*, Vol. 3. Seattle: Special Child Publications, 1968, 41–58.

Ayres, A.J. *Sensory integration and learning disorders*. Los Angeles: Western Psychological Services, 1972a.

Ayres, A.J. Improving academic scores through sensory integration. *Journal of Learning Disabilities*, 1972b, *6*, 338–343.

Ayres, A.J. Sensorimotor foundations of academic ability. *In* Cruickshank, W.M., & Hallahan, D.P. (Eds.), *Perceptual and learning disabilities in children*, Vol. 2. Syracuse: Syracuse University Press, 1975, 300–358.

Ayres, A.J. *Interpreting the Southern California Sensory Integration Tests*. Los Angeles: Western Psychological Services, 1976.

Baddeley, A. *Working memory*. Oxford: Clarendon Press, 1986.

Bakker, D.J. *Temporal order in disturbed reading*. Rotterdam: Rotterdam University Press, 1972.

Bakker, D.J. Hemispheric specialization and stages in the learning-to-read process. *Bulletin of the Orton Society*, 1973, *23*, 15–27.

Bakker, D.J. Hemispheric differences and reading strategies: Two dyslexias? *Bulletin of the Orton Society*, 1979, *29*, 84–100.

Bakker, D.J. Perceptual asymmetries and reading proficiency. *In* Bortner, M. (Ed.), *Cognitive growth and development: Essays in memory of Herbert G. Birch*. New York: Brunner/Mazel, 1979, 134–152.

Bakker, D.J. The brain as a dependent variable. *Journal of Clinical Neuropsychology*, 1984, *6*, 1–16.

Bakker, D.J., & Satz, P. *Specific reading disability, advances in theory and method*. Rotterdam: Rotterdam University Press, 1970.

Bakker, D.J., Teunissen, J., & Bosch, J. Development of laterality-reading patterns. *In* Knights, R.M., & Bakker, D.J. (Eds.), *The neuropsychology of learning disorders*. Baltimore: University Park Press, 1976, 207–220.

Bakker, D.J., & Van Rijnsoever, R. Language proficiency and lateral position in the classroom. *Bulletin of the Orton Society*, 1977, XXVII, 37–53.

Bakker, D.J., Moerland, R., & Goekoop-Hoefkens, M. Effects of hemisphere-specific stimulation on the reading performance of dyslexic boys: A pilot study. *Journal of Clinical Neuropsychology*, 1981, *3*(2), 155–159.

Bakker, D.J., & Vinke, J. Effects of hemisphere-specific stimulation on brain activity and reading in dyslexics. *Journal of Clinical and Experimental Neuropsychology*, 1985, *7*(5), 505–525

Balow, B., Rubin, R., & Rosen, J.J. Perinatal events as precursors of reading disability. *Reading Research Quarterly*, 1975–1976, *11*(1), 36–71.

Bandura, A. Self-efficacy: Toward a unifying theory of behavior change. *Psychological Review*, 1977, *84*, 191–215.

Bandura, A., Adams, N., & Beyer, J. Cognitive processes mediating behavioral change. *Journal of Personality and Social Psychology*, 1977, *35*(3), 125–139.

Bannatyne, A. *Language, reading, and learning disabilities, psychology, neuropsychology, diagnosis and remediation*. Springfield, IL: Charles C Thomas, 1971.

Barkley, R.A. *Hyperactive children: A handbook for diagnosis and treatment*. New York: Guilford Press, 1981.

Barkley, R.A. Attention deficit hyperactivity disorder. *In* Mash, E., & Barkley, R.A. (Eds.), *Treatment of childhood disorders*. New York: Guilford Press, 1988, 39–72.

Barkley, R.A. *Attention-deficit hyperactivity disorder: A handbook for diagnosis and treatment*. New York: Guilford Press, 1990.

Barlow, H.B. Cortical function: A tentative theory and preliminary tests. *In* McFadden, D. (Ed.), *Neural mechanisms in behavior*. New York: Springer-Verlag, 1980, 143–171.

Barnes, G.T., & Lakshminarayanan, A.V. Computed tomography: Physical principles and image quality considerations. *In* Lee, K.T.L., Sagel, S.S., & Stanley, R.J. (Eds.), *Computed body tomography with MRI correlation, 2nd edition*. New York: Raven Press, Chapter 1, 1989.

Barnsley, R.H., & Rabinovitch, M.S. Handedness: proficiency versus stated preference. *Perceptual and Motor Skills*, 1970, *30*, 343–362.

Barsch, R.H. Six factors in learning. *In* Hellmuth, J. (Ed.), *Learning disorders*, Vol. 1. Seattle: Special Child Publications, 1965, 328–343.

Barsch, R.H. Teacher needs—motor training. *In* Cruickshank, W.M. (Ed.), *The teacher of brain-injured children*. Syracuse: Syracuse University Press, 1966, 183–195.

Barsch, R.H. *Achieving perceptual-motor efficiency: A space-oriented approach to learning*. Seattle: Special Child Publications, 1967.

Bateman, B. Learning disabilities—yesterday, today, and tomorrow. *Exceptional Children*, 1964, *31*(4), 167–177.

Bateman, B.C. *Interpretation of the 1961 Illinois Test of Psycholinguistic Abilities*. Seattle: Special Child Publications, 1968.

Bauer, R.H. Memory processes in children with learning disabilities: Evidence for a deficient rehearsal. *Journal of Experimental Child Psychology*, 1979, *24*, 415–430.

Bay, E. Principles of classification and their influence on our concepts of aphasia. *In* de Reuck A.V.S., & O'Connor, M. (Eds.), *CIBA Foundation symposium: Disorders of language: Proceedings*. Boston: Little, Brown, 1964.

Beery, K.E. *Developmental test of visual-motor integration*. Chicago: Follett Educational Corporation, 1967.

Bender, L. Post encephalitic behavior disorders in children. *In* Neal, J.B. (Ed.), *Encephalitis: A clinical study*. New York: Grune & Stratton, 1942.

Bender, L. Problems in conceptualization and communication in children with developmental alexia. *In* Hoch, P.H., & Zubin, J. (Eds.), *Psychopathology of communication*. New York: Grune & Stratton, 1958.

Benson, D.F. Graphic orientation disorders of left handed children. *Journal of Learning Disabilities*, 1970, *3*, 126–131.

Benson, D.F. Aphasia. *In* Heilman, K.M., & Valenstein, E. (Eds.), *Clinical neuropsychology*. New York: Oxford University Press, 1979, 22–58.

Benson, D.F., & Denckla, M.B. Verbal paraphasia as a source of calculation disturbance. *Archives of Neurology*, 1969, *21*, 96–102.

Benson, D.F., & Geschwind, N. Cerebral dominance and its disturbances. *Pediatric Clinics of North America*, 1968, *15*(3), 759–769.

Benson, D.F., & Geschwind, N. The alexias. *In* Vinken, P.J., & Bruyn, B.W. (Eds.), *Handbook of clinical neurology*, Vol. 4. Amsterdam: North-Holland Publishing Co., 1969, 112–140.

Benson, D.F., & Greenberg, J.P. Visual form agnosia. *American Medical Association Archives of Neurology*, 1969, *2*, 82–89.

Benton, A.L. Significance of systematic reversal in right-left discrimination, *Acta Psychiatrica et Neurologica Scandinavica*, 1958, *33*(2), 129–137.

Benton, A.L. *Right-left discrimination and finger localization*. New York: Hoeber-Harper, 1959.

Benton, A.L. The fiction of the Gerstmann syndrome. *Journal of Neurology, Neurosurgery, and Psychiatry*, 1961, *24*, 176–181.

Benton, A.L. The visual retention test as a constructional praxis task. *Confinia Neurologica*, 1962a, *22*, 141–155.

Benton, A.L. Behavioral indices of brain injury in school children. *Child Development*, 1962b, *33*, 199–208.

Benton, A.L. Developmental aphasia and brain damage. *In* Kirk, S.A., & Becker, W. (Eds.), *Conference on children with minimal brain impairment*. Urbana, IL: University of Illinois, 1963a, 71–91.

Benton, A.L. *The revised visual retention test*. 3rd Ed. New York: The Psychological Corporation, 1963b.

Benton, A.L. Developmental aphasia and brain damage. *Cortex*, 1964, *1*, 40–52.

Benton, A.L. The problem of cerebral dominance. *The Canadian Psychologist*, 1965, *6a*(4), 332–346.

Benton, A.L. Problems of test construction in the field of aphasia. *Cortex*, 1967, *3*, 42–46.

Benton, A.L. Differential behavioral effects in frontal lobe disease. *Neuropsychologia*, 1968, *6*, 53–60.

Benton, A.L. Disorders of spatial orientation. *In* Vinken, P.J., & Bruyn, G.W. (Eds.), *Handbook of clinical neurology*, Vol. 3. Amsterdam: North-Holland Publishing Co., 1969a.

Benton, A.L. *The three dimensional praxis test: Manual of instructions*. Victoria: Neuropsychology Laboratory, University of Victoria, Victoria, B.C., Canada, 1969b.

Benton, A.L. *Stereognosis test*. Victoria: Department of Psychology, University of Victoria, Victoria, B.C., Canada, 1969c.

Benton, A.L. *Der Benton-Test, Handbuch* (Multiple Choice Form). Bern: Hans Huber, 1972.

Benton, A.L. Developmental dyslexia: Neurological aspects. *In* Friedlander, W.J. (Ed.), *Advances in Neurology*. New York: Raven Press,
1975, 1–47.

Benton, A.L. Reflections on the Gerstmann Syndrome. *Brain and
Language*, 1977, *4*, 45–62

Benton, A.L. Child neuropsychology: Retrospect and prospect. *In* Wit,
de. J., & Benton, A.L. (Eds.), *Perspectives in child study*. Lisse,
Netherlands: Swets & Zeitlinger, 1982, 41–61.

Benton, A.L. Dyslexia and spatial thinking. *Annals of Dyslexia*, 1984, *34*,
69–85.

Benton, A.L., & Blackburn, H.L. Practice effects in reaction time tasks
in brain-injured patients. *Journal of Abnormal and Social Psychology*,
1957, *54*(1), 109–113.

Benton, A.L., Hamsher, K. deS., Varney, N.R., & Spreen, O. *Contributions to neuropsychological assessment, a clinical manual*. New York:
Oxford University Press, 1983.

Benton, A.L., Levin, H.S., & Varney, N.R. Tactile perception of direction in normal subjects. *Neurology*, 1973, *23*, 1248–1250.

Bereiter, C. Development in writing. *In* Gregg, L.W., & Steinberg, E.R.
(Eds.), *Cognitive processes in writing*. Hillsdale, NJ: L. Erlbaum, 1980,
73–93.

Berger, H. Uber das elektren kephalagram des menschen, VI. *Archiv
Psychiatrie und Nervenkrankheiten*, 1929, *87*, 527–510.

Berger, N.S. Why can't John read? Perhaps he's not a good listener.
Journal of Learning Disabilities, 1978, *11*(10), 633–638.

Berlin, C.I., Lowe-Bell, S.S., Cullen, J.K., Thompson, C.L., & Stafford,
M.R. Is speech "special"? Perhaps the temporal lobectomy patient can
tell us. *Journal of the Acoustical Society of America*, 1972, *52*(2),
702–705.

Berlin, C.I., Lowe-Bell, S.S., Janetta, P.J., & Kline, D.G. Central
auditory deficits after temporal lobectomy. *Archives of Otolaryngology*,
1972, *96*, 4–10.

Berlucchi, G., & Buchtel, H.A. Some trends in the neurological study of
learning. *In* Gazzaniga, M.S., & Blakemore, C. (Eds.), *Handbook of
psychobiology*. New York: Academic Press, 1975, 481–498.

The Bible. King James version, 1605.

Bigler, E.D. Radiological techniques in neuropsychological assessment.
In Reynolds C.R., & Fletcher-Janzen, E. (Eds.), *Handbook of clinical
child neuropsychology*. New York: Plenum Press, 1989, 247–264.

Binet, A., & Simon, T. Langage et Pensée. *Année Psychologie*, 1908,
14, 284–339. [Quoted in Myklebust, H.R. Childhood aphasia: an
evolving concept. *In* Travis, L.E. (Ed.), *Handbook of speech pathol-*

ogy and audiology. New York: Appleton-Century-Crofts, 1971, 1181–1202.]

Bingol, N., Fuchs, M., Diaz, V., Stone, R.K., & Grimisch D.S. Terotegenicity of cocaine in humans. *Journal of Pediatrics*, 1987, *10*, 93–96.

Birch, H.G. (Ed.). *Brain damage in children, the biological and social aspects.* Baltimore: Williams & Wilkins, 1964.

Birch, H.G. Nutritional factors in mental retardation. Paper presented at Fifth Annual Neuropsychology Workshop, University of Victoria, Victoria, B.C., Canada, 1970.

Bjørgen, I.A., Undheim, J.O., Nordvik, K.A., & Romslo, I. Dyslexia and hormone deficiencies. *European Journal of Psychology and Education*, 1987, II(3), 283–295.

Black, F.W. Neurological dysfunction and reading disorders. *Journal of Learning Disabilities*, 1973, *6*, 313–316.

Blackburn, H.L. Effects of motivating instructions on reaction time in cerebral disease. *Journal of Abnormal and Social Psychology*, 1958, *56*(3), 359–366.

Blackburn, H.L., & Benton, A.L. Simple and choice reaction time in cerebral disease. *Confinia Neurologica*, 1955, *15*(6), 327–338.

Blackwell, R., & Chang, A. Video display terminal and pregnancy: A review. *Obstetrical and Gynecological Survey*, 1988, *44*, 128–129.

Blake, R., Field, B., Foster, C., Platt, F., & Wertz, P. Effect of FM auditory trainers on attending behaviors of learning-disabled children. *Language, Speech, and Hearing Services in Schools*, 1991, Vol. *22*, 111–114.

Blakemore, C., & Cooper, G.F. Development of the brain depends on the visual environment. *Nature*, 1970, *228*, 477–478.

Blakemore, C., & Mitchell, D.E. Environmental modification of the visual cortex and the neural basis of learning and memory. *Nature*, 1973, *241*, 467–468.

Blau, A. Mental changes following head trauma in children. *Archives of Neurology & Psychiatry*, 1936, *35*, 722–769.

Blau, T.H. Unusual measures for the spelling invalid. *In* Arena, J.I. (Ed.), *Building spelling skills in dyslexic children.* San Rafael: Academic Therapy Publications, 1968, 1–3.

Blumstein, S.E. *A phonological investigation of aphasic speech.* The Hague: Mouton, 1973.

Boder, E. Developmental dyslexia: prevailing diagnostic concepts and a new diagnostic approach. *In* Myklebust, H.R. (Ed.), *Progress in learning disabilities*, Vol. II. New York: Grune & Stratton, 1971, 293–321.

Boder, E. Developmental dyslexia: A diagnostic approach based on three atypical reading-spelling patterns. *Developmental Medicine and Child Neurology*, 1973, *15*, 663–687.

Bogen, J.E. Some educational aspects of hemispheric specialization. *U.C.L.A. Educator*, 1975, *17*, 24–32.

Bogen, J.E. The callosal syndrome. *In* Heilman, K.M., & Valenstein, E. (Eds.), *Clinical neuropsychology*. New York: Oxford University Press, 1979, 308–359.

Boll, T.J. Behavioral correlates of cerebral damage in children aged 9 through 14. *In* Reitan, R.M., & Davison, L.A. (Eds.), *Clinical neuropsychology: Current status and applications*. Washington, DC: Winston & Sons, 1974, 91–120.

Boring, E.G. *A history of experimental psychology*. 2nd Ed., New York: Appleton-Century-Crofts, 1957.

Bos, C.S., & Van Reusen, A.K. Academic interventions with learning disabled students: A cognitive/metacognitive approach. *In* Obrzut, J.E., & Hynd, G.W. (Eds.), *Neuropsychological foundations of learning disabilities*. San Diego: Academic Press, 1991, 659–683.

Bower, G.H., & Morrow, D.G. Mental models in narrative comprehension. *Science*, 1990, *247*, 44–48.

Boyd, T.A. Clinical assessment of memory in children: A developmental framework for practice. *In* Tramontana, M.G., & Hooper, S.R. (Eds.), *Assessment issues in child neuropsychology*. New York: Plenum Press, 1988, 137–201.

Bradley, W. The behavior of children receiving benzedrine. *American Journal of Psychiatry*, 1937, *94*, 577–585.

Bradshaw, J.L. Peripherally presented and unreported words may bias the perceived meaning of a centrally-fixated homograph. *Journal of Experimental Psychology*, 1974, *103*, 1200–1202.

Bradshaw, J.L., & Nettleton, N.C. *Human cerebral asymmetry*. Englewood Cliffs, NJ: Prentice-Hall, 1983.

Brady, J.V. Ulcers in "executive" monkeys. *Scientific American*, October 1958, 3–6.

Brain, Sir Russell. *Clinical neurology*. London: Oxford University Press, 1960.

Brain, W.R. *Speech disorders: Aphasia, apraxia and Agnosia*. London: Butterworths, 1961.

Brenner, M.W., Gillman, S., Zangwill, O.L., & Farrell, M. Visuo-motor disability in school children. *British Medical Journal*, 1967, *4*, 259–262.

Briggs, G.G., Nebes, R.D., & Kinsbourne, M. Intellectual differences in relation to personal and family handedness. *Quarterly Journal of Experimental Psychology*, 1976, *28*, 591–601.

Britton, J.F. *Language and learning*. Harmondsworth, England: Penguin Books, 1970.

Broadbent, D.E. The role of auditory localization in attention and memory span. *Journal of Experimental Psychology*, 1954, *47*, 191–196.

Broadbent, D.E., & Gregory, M. Effects of noise and of signal rate upon vigilance analyzed by means of decision theory. *Human Factors*, 1965, *7*, 155–162.

Brodmann, K. Verleichende Lokalisationslehre der Grosshirnrinde in ihren Prinzipien dergestellt auf Grund des Zellenbanes. Leipzig: Barth, 1909.

Brooks, T.C. Spatial & verbal components of the act of recall. *Canadian Journal of Psychology*, 1968, *22*, 349–368.

Brown, J. Some tests of the decay theory of immediate memory. *Quarterly Journal of Experimental Psychology*, 1958, *10*, 12–21.

Brown, R.T., Abramowitz, A.J., Mada-Swain, A., Eckstrand, D., & Dulcan, M. *ADHD gender differences in a clinic referred sample*. Paper presented at the annual meeting of the American Academy of Child & Adolescent Psychiatry, New York. October, 1989.

Brunekreef, B., Noy, D., Biersteker, K., & Boleij, J. Blood lead levels of Dutch city children and their relationship to lead in the environment. *Journal of the Air Pollution Control Association*, 1983, *33*, 872–876.

Bryan, T. Social problems and learning disabilities. *In* Wong, B.Y.L. (Ed.), *Learning about learning disabilities*. San Diego: Academic Press, 1991, 195–229.

Bryden, M.P. "Tachistoscopic perception and serial order." Unpublished Ph.D. thesis, McGill University, 1960a.

Bryden, M.P. Tachistoscopic recognition of non-alphabetical material. *Canadian Journal of Psychology*, 1960b, *14*, 78–86.

Bryden, M.P. Order of report in dichotic listening. *Canadian Journal of Psychology*, 1962, *16*, 291–299.

Bryden, M.P. Left-right differences in tachistoscopic recognition. *Journal of Experimental Psychology*, 1963, *66*(6), 568–571.

Bryden, M.P. The manipulation of strategies of report in dichotic listening. *Canadian Journal of Psychology*, 1964, *18*, 126–138.

Bryden, M.P. Accuracy and order of report in tachistoscopic recognition. *Canadian Journal of Psychology*, 1966, *20*, 262–272.

Bryden, M.P. A model for the sequential organization of behavior. *Canadian Journal of Psychology, Revue Canadienne de Psychologie*, 1967, *21*(1), 37–56.

Bryden, M.P. Laterality effects in dichotic listening: relations with handedness and reading ability in children. *Neuropsychologia*, 1970, *8*, 443–450.

Bryden, M.P. Perceptual asymmetry in vision: Relation to handedness, eyedness, and speech lateralization. *Cortex*, 1973, *9*, 418–435.

Bryden, M.P. Measuring handedness with questionnaires. *Neuropsychologia*, 1977, *15*, 617–624.

Bryden, M.P., & Allard, F.A. Do auditory perceptual asymmetries develop? *Cortex*, 1981, *17*, 313–318.

Bryden, M.P. *Laterality, functional asymmetry in the intact brain*. New York: Academic Press, 1982.

Bryden, M.P., Hécaen, H., & DeAgostini, M. Patterns of cerebral organization. *Brain and Language*, 1983, *20*, 249–262.

Bryden, M.P., & Steenhuis, R. The assessment of handedness in children. *In* Obrzut, J.E., & Hynd, G.W. (Eds.), *Neuropsychological foundations of learning disabilities*. San Diego: Academic Press, 1991, 411–436.

Buffery, A.W.H. Sex differences in the neuropsychological development of verbal and spatial skills. *In* Knights, R.M., & Bakker, D.J. (Eds.), *The neuropsychology of learning disorders, theoretical approaches*. Baltimore: University Park Press, 1976, 187–205.

Buffery, A.W.H., & Gray, J.A. Sex differences in the development of spatial and linguistic skills. *In* Ounsted, C., & Taylor, D.C. (Eds.), *Gender differences: Their ontogeny and significance*. Edinburgh: Churchill Livingstone, 1972, 123–157.

Burg, C., Rappaport, J., Bartley, L., Quinn, P., & Timmins, P. Newborn minor abnormalities and problem behavior at age 3. *American Journal of Psychiatry*, 1980, *137*, 791–796.

Butters, N., Barton, M., & Brody, B.A. Role of the right parietal lobe in the mediation of crossmodal associations and reversible operations in space. *Cortex*, 1970, *6*, 174–190.

Butters, N., & Brody, B.A. The role of the left parietal lobe in the mediation of the intra- and cross-modal associations. *Cortex*, 1968, *4*, 328–343.

Calanchini, P.R., & Trout, S.S. The neurology of learning disabilities. *In* Tarnopol, L. (Ed.), *Learning disorders in children, diagnosis, medication, education*. Boston: Little, Brown, 1971, 207–251.

Call, J.D. Psychological and behavioral development in infants and children. *In* Kelley, V.C. (Ed.), *Practice of Pediatrics*. Philadelphia: Harper & Row, 1985.

Calvin, W.H. *The throwing madonna, essays on the brain*. New York: McGraw-Hill, 1983.

Calvin, W.H., & Ojemann, G.A. *Inside the brain*. New York: Mentor Books, 1980.

Canadian Association for Children and Adults with Learning Disabilities, Kildare House, 323 Chapel Street, Ottawa, Ontario, Canada K1N 7Z2.

Cantwell, D.P. Psychiatric illness in the families of hyperactive children. *Archives of General Psychiatry*. 1972, *27*, 414–417.

Cantwell, D.P., & Baker, L. Psychiatric and learning disorders in children with speech and language disorders: A descriptive analysis. *Advances in Learning & Behavioral Disabilities*, 1985, *4*, 29–47.

Caramazza, A. The logic of neuropsychological research and the problem of patient classification in aphasia. *Brain and Language*, 1984, *21*, 9–20.

Carmon, A., & Benton, A.L. Tactile perception of direction and number in patients with unilateral cerebral disease. *Neurology* (Minneapolis), 1969, *19*, 525–532.

Carter, J.L., & Russell, H.L. Use of EMG biofeedback procedures with learning disabled children in a clinical setting. *Journal of Learning Disabilities*, 1985, *18*(4), 213–216.

Catlin, J. Chapter 13 in Millar, G.A., & Lenneberg, E. *Psychology and biology of language and thought*. New York: Academic Press, 1978, 271–280.

Cawley, J.F. Commentary on whole issue devoted to mathematics. *Topics in Learning and Learning Disabilities*, 1981, *1*(3), 89–93.

Chalfant, J.C., & Scheffelin, M.A. *Central processing dysfunctions in children: A review of research*. NINDS Monograph No. 9. Bethesda, MD: U.S. Department of Health, Education, and Welfare, 1969.

Chall, J.S., & Mirsky, A.F. *Education and the brain* (The Seventy-seventh Yearbook of the National Society for the Study of Education, Part II). Chicago: The University of Chicago Press, 1978.

Chapman, R.M., & Bragdon, H.R. Evoked responses to numerical and nonnumerical visual stimuli while problem solving. *Nature*, September 12, 1964, 1155–1157.

Chase, C.H., & Tallal, P. A developmental, interactive activation model of the word superiority effect. *Journal of Experimental Child Psychology*, 1990, *49*, 448–487.

Chase, C.H., & Tallal, P. Cognitive models of developmental reading disorders. *In* Obrzut, J.E., & Hynd, G.W. (Eds.). *Neuropsychological foundations of learning disabilities*. San Diego: Academic Press, 1991, 199–240.

Chédru, F., & Geschwind, N. Writing disturbances in acute confusional states. *Neuropsychologia*, 1972, *10*, 343–353.

Chelune, G.J., Ferguson, W., Koon, R., & Dickey, T.O. Frontal lobe disinhibition in attention deficit disorder. *Child Psychiatry & Human Development*, 1986, *16*, 221–234.

Cherry, E.C. Some experiments on the recognition of speech, with one and with two ears. *Journal of the Acoustic Society of America*, 1953, *25*, 975–979.

Chomsky, N. *Syntactic structures*. The Hague: Mouton, 1957.

Chomsky, N. *Language and mind*. New York: Harcourt, Brace and World, 1968.

Chomsky, N. Phonology and reading. *In* Levin, H., & Williams, J.P. (Eds.), *Basic studies on reading*. New York: Basic Books, 1970, 3–18.

Chomsky, N. *Language and mind* (enlarged edition). New York: Harcourt, Brace and the World, 1972.

Chomsky, N. On the biological basis of language capacities. *In* Miller, G.A., & Lenneberg, E. (Eds.), *Psychology and biology of language and thought*. New York: Academic Press, 1978, Chapter *11*, 199–220.

Clark, C. "The reliability of ear advantage and attentional capacity in dichotic listening." Unpublished Ph.D. dissertation, University of Victoria, B.C., Canada, 1981.

Clarke, E., & Dewhurst, K. *An illustrated history of brain function*. Oxford: Sandford, 1972.

Clark, R.W. *Einstein: The life and times*. New York: The World Publishing Co., 1971.

Clements, S.D. *Minimal brain dysfunction in children*. NINDB Monograph No. 3. Washington, DC: U.S. Depart. of Health, Education, and Welfare, 1966.

Cochran, P.S., & Bull, G.L. Integrating word processing into language intervention. *Topics in Language Disorders*, 1991, 31–48.

Cohen, N., Douglas, V.I., & Morgenstern, G. The effect of methylphenidate on attention deficit and autonomic activity in hyperactive children. *Psychopharmacologia*, 1971, *22*, 282–294.

Coren, S., Porac, C., & Ward, L.M. *Sensation and perception*. New York: Academic Press, 1978.

Cohn, R. Developmental dyscalculia. *Pediatric Clinics of North America*, 1968, *15*(3), 651–668.

Cohn, R. Arithmetic and learning disabilities. *In* Myklebust, H.R. (Ed.), *Progress in learning disabilities*, Vol. II. New York: Grune & Stratton, 1971, 322–389.

Colbourn, C.J. Can laterality be measured? *Neuropsychologia*, 1978, *16*, 283–289.

Coleman, J.C. *Abnormal psychology and modern life*, 2nd Ed. Chicago: Scott, Foresman, 1956.

Coles, G.S. The learning-disabilities test battery: empirical and social issues. *Harvard Educational Review*, 1978, *48*(3), 313–340

Collins, A., & Gentner, D. A framework for a cognitive theory of writing. *In* Gregg, L.W., & Steinberg, E.R. (Eds.), *Cognitive processes in writing*. Hillsdale, NJ: L. Erlbaum, 1980, 51–72.

Coltheart, M. Disorders of reading and their implications for models of normal reading. *Visible Language*, 1981, XV(3), 245–286.

Coltheart, M., Patterson, K., & Marshall, J.C. (Eds.) *Deep dyslexia*. London: Routledge & Kegan Paul, 1980.

Cone, T.E., & Wilson, L.R. Quantifying a severe discrepancy: A critical analysis. *Learning Disability Quarterly*, 1981, *4*, 359–371.

Conel, J.L. *Postnatal development of the human cerebral cortex*. Vols. I–VI. Cambridge: Harvard University Press, 1939–1963. [Quoted in Pribram, K.H. *Languages of the brain*. Englewood Cliffs, NJ: Prentice-Hall, 1971, p. 27.]

Conners, C.K. A teacher rating scale for use in drug studies with children. *American Journal of Psychiatry*, 1969, *126*, 884–888.

Conners, C.K. Learning disabilities and stimulant drugs in children: theoretical implications. *In* Knights, R.M., & Bakker, D.J. (Eds.), *The neuropsychology of learning disorders*. Baltimore: University Park Press, 1976, 389–401.

Conners, C.K. *Food additives & hyperactive children*. New York: Plenum Press, 1980.

Conners, C.K., Eisenberg, L., & Sharpe, L. Effects of methylphenidate (ritalin) on paired-associate learning and porteus maze performance in emotionally disturbed children. *Journal of Consulting Psychology*, 1964, *28*, 14–22.

Conners, C.K., & Wells, K.C. *Hyperkinetic children: A neuropsychosocial approach*. Beverly Hills: Sage, 1986.

Conte, R. Attention Disorders. *In* Wong, B.Y.L. (Ed.), *Learning about learning disabilities*. New York: Academic Press, 1991, 60–96.

Conte, R., Kinsbourne, M., Swanson, J., Zirk, H., & Samuels, M. Presentation rate effects on paired associate learning by attention deficit disordered children. *Child Development*, 1986, *57*, 681–687.

Corballis, M.C., & Morgan, M.J. On the biological basis of human laterality: I. Evidence for a maturational left-right gradient. *The Behavioral and Brain Sciences*, 1978, *2*, 261–336.

Coren, S., & Porac, C. Fifty centuries of right-handedness: The historical record. *Science*, November 1977, *198*, 631–632.

Coren, S., Porac, C., & Ward, L.M. *Sensation and perception*. New York: Academic Press, 1978.

Coulter, D.L. *Hypoconnection syndromes in learning-disabled children*. Paper presented at Child Neurology Society Meeting, Minneapolis, 1981.

Courchesne, E., Yeung-Courchesne, R., Press, G.A., Hesselnik, J.R., & Jernigan, T.L. Hypoplasia of cerebellar vermal lobules VI and VII in autism. *New England Journal of Medicine*, 1988, *318*, 1349–1354.

Coyle, J.T., Price, D.L., & DeLong, M.H. Alzheimer's disease: A disorder of central cholinergic innervation. *Science*, 1983, *219*, 1184–1189.

Craik, F.I.M., & Tulving, E. Depth of processing & the retention of words in episodic memory. *Journal of Experimental Psychology: General*, 1975, *104*, 268–294

Cratty, B.J. *Developmental sequences of perceptual-motor tasks*. Baldwin, NY: Educational Activities, 1967.

Cratty, B.J. Movement and the intellect. *In* Hellmuth, J. (Ed.), *Learning disorders*, Vol. 3. Seattle: Special Child Publications, 1968, 524–536.

Cratty, B.J. *Some educational implications of movement*. Seattle: Special Child Publications, 1970.

Cratty, B.J., & Martin, M.M. *Perceptual-motor efficiency in children*. Philadelphia: Lea & Febiger, 1969.

Cravioto, J., De Licardie, E.R., & Birch, H.G. Nutrition, growth and neurointegrative development: An experimental and ecologic study. *Pediatrics*, 1966, *38*(Suppl. 2), 319–372.

Critchley, M. *The dyslexic child*. London: William Heinemann, 1970.

Critchley, M., & Critchley, E.A. *Dyslexia defined*. London: William Heinemann Medical Books Ltd., 1978.

Cromwell, R., Baumister, A., & Hawkins, W. Research in activity level. *In* Ellis, N. (Ed.), *Handbook of mental deficiency*. New York: McGraw-Hill, 1963, 632–663.

Crook, W.G. The allergic-fatigue syndrome. *In* Speer, F., (Ed.), *The allergic child*. New York: Paul, B. Hoeber, Inc., 1963, 329–341.

Crovitz, H.F., & Zener, K.A. A group test for assessing hand- and eye-dominance. *American Journal of Psychology*, 1962, *75*, 271–276.

Crowhurst, M., & Piche, G.L. Audience and mode of discourse effects on syntactic complexity in writing at two grade levels. *Research in the Teaching of English*, 1979, *13*(2), 101–109.

Cruickshank, W.M. *A teaching method for brain-injured and hyperactive children*. Syracuse: Syracuse University Press, 1961.

Cruickshank, W.M. (Ed.). *The teacher of brain-injured children*. Syracuse: Syracuse University Press, 1966.

Cruickshank, W.M. The problem of delayed recognition and its correction. *In* Keeney, A.H., & Keeney, V.T. (Eds.), *Dyslexia: Diagnosis and treatment of reading disorders*. St. Louis: C.V. Mosby, 1968.

Cruickshank, W.M. The psychoeducational match. *In* Cruickshank, W.M., & Hallahan, D.P. (Eds.), *Perceptual and learning disabilities in children*, Vol. 1. Syracuse: Syracuse University Press, 1975a, 71–112.

Cruickshank, W.M. *Learning disabilities in home, school, and community*. Syracuse: Syracuse University Press, 1977.

Cruickshank, W.M. Learning disabilities: a definitional statement. *In* Polak, E. (Ed.), *Issues and initiatives in learning disabilities: Selected papers from the First National Conference on Learning Disabilities*.

Ottawa: Canadian Association for Children with Learning Disabilities, 1979.

Cruickshank, W.M. The interdisciplinary model for manpower development for mental retardation. *Indian Journal of Mental Retardation*, 1972, *5*, 44–57. Reprinted in Cruickshank, W.M., *Concepts in special education, Selected writings, Vol. I*. Syracuse: Syracuse University Press, 1981, 81–92.

Cruickshank, W.M. Learning disabilities: Perceptual or other? *Tijdschrift voor Orthopedagogiek*, 1978, *9*, 421–431. Reprinted in Cruickshank, W.M. *Concepts in learning disabilities: Selected writings, Vol. 2*. Syracuse: Syracuse University Press, 1981, 111–122.

Cruickshank, W.M. Learning disabilities: A charter for excellence. *In* Kirk, S.A., & McCarthy, J. (Eds.), *Learning disabilities: Selected ACLD papers*. Boston: Houghton-Mifflin, 1975, 103–117. Also reprinted in Cruickshank, W.M. *Concepts in learning disabilities: Selected writings, Vol. 2*. Syracuse: Syracuse University Press, 1981, 223–238.

Cruickshank, W.M. *Concepts in learning disabilities, Selected writings, Vol. 2*. Syracuse: Syracuse University Press, 1981.

Cruickshank, W.M. Learning disabilities: An international overview. *Paedoperisse*, 1987, *1*(1), 1–15.

Cruickshank, W.M. Straight is the bamboo tree. *Journal of Learning Disabilities*, 1983, *16*(4), 191–197.

Cruickshank, W.M., Bice, H.V., Wallen, N.E., & Lynch, K.S. *Perception and cerebral palsy: Studies in figure-background relationship*. Syracuse: Syracuse University Press, 1957.

Cruickshank, W.M., & Haring, N.G. *Assistants for teachers of exceptional children: A demonstration*. Syracuse: Syracuse University Press, 1957.

Cruickshank, W.M., & Hallahan, D.P. (Eds.). *Perceptual and learning disabilities in children, Vols. 1 & 2*. Syracuse: Syracuse University Press, 1975.

Dabbs, J.M., & Choo, G. Left-right carotid blood flow predicts specialized mental ability. *Neuropsychologia*, 1980, *18*, 711–713.

Damico, J. A clinical approach to discourse analysis in school age children. Paper presented at a miniseminar at the American Speech-Language-Hearing Association Convention, Detroit, MI., 1980. Quoted in McCord, J.S., & Haynes, W.O. *Journal of Learning Disabilities*, 1988, *21*(4), 237–243.

Darwin, C.J., Turvey, M.T., & Crowder, R.G. An auditory analogue of the Sperling partial report procedure. *Cognitive Psychology*, 1972, *3*, 255–267.

Das, J.P., Kirby, J.R., & Jarman, R.F. *Simultaneous and successive cognitive processes*. New York: Academic Press, 1979.

Davis, A.E., & Wada, J.A. Hemispheric asymmetries of visual and auditory information processing. *Neuropsychologia*, 1977, *15*, 799– 806.

De Ajuriaguerra, J., & Tissot, R. The apraxias. *In* Vinken, P.J., & Bruyn, G.W. (Eds.), *Handbook of clinical neurology*, Vol. 4. Amsterdam: North-Holland Publishing Co., 1969, 48–66.

Decety, J., Ryding, E., Sjoholm, H., Stenberg, G., & Ingvar, D.H. The cerebellum participates in mental activity: tomographic measurements of regional cerebral blood flow. *Brain Research*, 1990.

DeFries, J.C., & Gillis, J.J. Etiology of reading deficits in learning disabilities: Quantitative genetic analysis. *In* Obrzut, J.E., & Hynd, G.W. (Eds.), *Neuropsychological foundations of learning disabilities*. San Diego: Academic Press, 1991, 29–47.

de Hirsch, K. Prediction in reading disability: A review of the literature. *In* Hayes, A., & Silver, A. (Eds.), *Report of the interdisciplinary committee on reading disability*. Washington, DC: Center for Applied Linguistics, 1971.

de Hirsch, K., Jansky, J.J., & Langford, W.S. *Predicting reading failure*. New York: Harper & Row, 1966.

Déjerine, J. 1892. His famous case is described and discussed by Norman Geschwind, in "The anatomy of acquired disorders of reading." *In* Money, J. (Ed.), *Reading disability*. Baltimore: The Johns Hopkins Press, 1962, 115–129.

Delacato, C.H. *The treatment and prevention of reading problems*. Springfield, Ill.: Thomas, 1959.

Delacato, C.H. *The diagnosis and treatment of speech and reading problems*, 6th Ed. Springfield, IL: Charles C. Thomas, 1963.

De La Cruz, F.F., Fox, B.H., & Roberts, R.H. (Eds.). "Minimal Brain Dysfunction." *Annals of the New York Academy of Sciences*, 1973, *205* (whole volume).

Delgado, J.M.R. *Physical control of the mind*. New York: Harper-Colophon Books, 1971.

Delgado, J.M.R, Roberts, W.W., & Miller, N.E. Learning motivated by electrical stimulation of the brain. *American Journal of Physiology*, 1954, *179*, 587–593.

Denckla, M.B. Minimal brain dysfunction and dyslexia: Beyond diagnosis by exclusion. *In* Blaw, M.E., Rapin, I., & Kinsbourne, M. (Eds.), *Child neurology*. New York: Spectrum Publications, 1977.

Denckla, M.B. Minimal brain dysfunction. *In* Chall, J.S., & Mirsky, A.F. (Eds.), *Education and the brain* (The Seventy-Seventh Yearbook of the National Society for the Study of Education). Chicago: The University of Chicago Press, 1978, 223–268.

Denckla, M.B. Childhood learning disabilities. *In* Heilman, K.M., & Valenstein, E. (Eds.), *Clinical neuropsychology*. New York: Oxford University Press, 1979, 535–573.

Denckla, M.B. Learning for language and language for learning. *In* Kirk, U. (Ed.), *Neuropsychology of language, reading, and spelling*. New York: Academic Press, 1983, 33–43.

Denckla, M.B., & Rudel, R.G. Rapid "automatized" naming (R.A.N.): Dyslexia differentiated from other learning disabilities. *Neuropsychologia*, 1976, *14*, 471–479.

Denkla, M.B., & Rudel, R.G. Naming & object-drawings by dyslexic & other learning disabled children. *Brain & Language*, 1976, *3*, 1–15.

Dennis, M. Capacity and strategy for syntactic comprehension after left and right hemi decortication. *Brain and Language*, 1980, *10*, 287–317.

Dennis, M., & Kohn, B. Comprehension of syntax in infantile hemiplegics after cerebral hemidecortication: left hemisphere superiority. *Brain and Language*, 1975, *2*, 472–482.

Dennis, M., & Whitaker, H.A. Language acquisition following hemidecortication: Linguistic superiority of the left over the right hemisphere. *Brain and Language*, 1976, *3*, 404–433.

de Quiros, J.B., & Schrager, O.L. *Neuropsychological fundamentals in learning disabilities*. San Rafael: Academic Therapy Publications, 1978.

DeRenzi, E., Pieczuro, A., & Vignolo, L.A. Ideational apraxia: A quantitative study. *Neuropsychologia*, 1968, *6*, 41–52.

DeRenzi, E., & Vignolo, L.A. The Token Test: a sensitive test to detect receptive disturbances in aphasics. *Brain*, 1962, *85*, 665–678.

Dimond, S.J., & Beaumont, J.G. (Eds.). *Hemisphere functions of the human brain*. London: Elek Science, 1974.

Dingman, H.F., & Tarjan, G. Mental retardation and the normal distribution curve. *American Journal of Mental Deficiency*, 1960, *64*, 991–994.

Dobbing, J. Vulnerable periods in developing brain. *In* Davison, A.N., & Dobbing, J. (Eds.), *Applied neurochemistry*. Oxford: Blackwell, 1968.

Dodwell, P. Some factors affecting the hearing of words presented dichotically. *Canadian Journal of Psychology*, 1964, *18*, 72–79.

Doehring, D.G. *Patterns of impairment in specific reading disability*. Bloomington: Indiana University Press, 1968.

Dolch, E.W. *A manual for remedial reading*. New Canaan: Garrard Publishing Co., 1945.

Douglas, V.I. Higher mental processes in hyperactive children: Implications for training. *In* Knights, R.M., & Bakker, D.J. (Eds.). *Rehabilitation, treatment, & management of learning disorders*. Baltimore: University Park Press, 1980, 65–91.

Douglas, V.I. Attention and cognitive problems. *In* Rutter, M. (Ed.), *Developmental neuropsychiatry*. New York: Guilford Press, 1983, 280–329.

Douglas, V.I. Cognitive deficits in children with attention deficit disorder with hyperactivity. *In* Bloomingdale, L.M., & Sergeant, J. (Eds.), *Attention deficit disorder: Criteria, cognition, intervention*. A book supplement of the Journal of Child Psychology and Psychiatry (No. 5). New York: Pergamon Press, 1988.

Douglas, V.I., & Peters, K.B. Toward a clear definition of the attentional deficit of hyperactive children. *In* Hale, G.A., & Lewis, M. (Eds.), *Attention & the development of cognitive skills*. New York: Plenum, 1978, 173–248.

Dow, R.S. Contributions of electrophysiological studies to cerebellar physiology. *Journal of Clinical Neurophysiology*, 1988, *5*, 307–323

Dowling, J.E. Elements of retinal function. *In* Schmitt, F.O., & Worden, F.G. (Eds.), *The neurosciences, fourth study program*. Cambridge: The M.I.T. Press, 1979, 161–181.

Downing, J.A. *The initial teaching alphabet reading experiment*. Chicago: Scott, Foresman, 1964.

Downing, J.A., & Leong, C.K. *Psychology of reading*. New York: Macmillan, 1982.

Drake, W.E. Clinical and pathological findings in a child with a developmental learning disability. *Journal of Learning Disabilities*, 1968, *1*(9), 486–502.

Drew, A.L. A neurological appraisal of familial congenital word blindness. *Brain*, 1956, *79*, 440.

Duane, D.D. Toward a definition of dyslexia: A summary of views. *Bulletin of the Orton Society*, 1979, *29*, 56–64.

Duane, D.D. Neurodiagnostic tools in dyslexic syndromes in children: Pitfalls and proposed comparative study of computed tomography, nuclear magnetic resonance, and brain electrical activity mapping. *In* Pavlidis, G.Th., & Fisher, D.F. (Eds.), *Dyslexia: Its neuropsychology and treatment*. New York: John Wiley & Sons, 1986, 65–84.

Duara, R., Kushch, A., Gross-Glenn, K., Barker, W.W., Jallad, B., Pascal, S., Loewenstein, D.A., Sheldon, J., Rabin, M., Levin, B., & Lubs, H. Neuroanatomic differences between dyslexic and normal readers on magnetic resonance imaging scans. *Archives of Neurology*, 1991, *48*, 410–416.

Dudley-Marling, C. The pragmatic skills of learning disabled children: A review. *Journal of Learning Disabilities*, 1985, *18*(4), 193–199.

Duffy, F.H. Topographic display of evoked potentials: clinical applications of brain electrical activity mapping (BEAM). *Annals of the New York Academy of Sciences*, 1982, *388*, 183–196.

Duffy, F.H., Burchfiel, J.L., & Lombroso, C.T. Brain electrical activity mapping (BEAM): a method for extending the clinical utility of EEG and evoked potential data. *Annals of Neurology*, April 1979, *5*(4), 309–321.

Duke, W.W. Mental & neurologic reactions of the asthma patient. *Journal of Laboratory & Clinical Medicine*, 1927, *13*, 20–23.

Dunn, H.G., McBurney, A., Ingram, S., & Hunter, M. Maternal cigarette smoking during pregnancy and the child's subsequent development. II. Neurological and intellectual maturation to the age of $6\frac{1}{2}$. *Canadian Journal of Public Health*. 1977, Vol. *68*, 43–50.

Dunn, L.M. *Expanded manual for the Peabody Picture Vocabulary Test*. Circle Pines, MN: American Guidance Service, 1965.

DuPaul, G.J., Guevremont, D.C., & Barkley, R.A. Attention deficit disorder. *In* Kratochwill, T.R., & Morris, R.J. (Eds.), *The practice of child therapy*. New York: Pergamon Press, 1991, 115–144.

Durbrow, H.C. Children who cannot write. *Bulletin of the Orton Society*, 1963, XIII, 115–118.

Dykman, R.A., & Gantt, H. A case of experimental neurosis and recovery in relation to the orienting response. *Journal of Psychology*, 1960, *50*, 105–110.

Eaves, L.C., Kendall, D.C., & Crichton, J.U. The early detection of minimal brain dysfunction. *Journal of Learning Disabilities*, 1972, *5*(8), 454–462.

Ebbinghaus, H. *Memory*. New York: Teacher's College, 1913. (Originally published in 1885). Reprinted by Dover, New York, 1964.

Eccles, J.C. *The Understanding of the Brain*. New York: McGraw-Hill, 1973.

Efron, R. Temporal perception, aphasia and déjà vu. *Brain*, 1963, *86*, 403–424.

Ehrenhaft, P.M., Wagner, J.L., & Herdman, R.C. Changing prognosis for very low birth weight infants. *Obstetrics and Gynecology*, 1989, *74*, 528–535.

Eisenberg, L. Reading retardation. I. Psychiatric and sociologic aspects. *Pediatrics*, 1966, *37*(2), 352–365.

Elbert, J.C. Short-term memory encoding and memory search in the word recognition of learning-disabled children. *Journal of Learning Disabilities*, 1984, *17*, 342–345.

Emmerich, D., Goldenbaum, D., Hayden, D., Hoffman, L., & Treffets, J. Meaningfulness as a variable in dichotic hearing. *Journal of Experimental Psychology*, 1965, *69*, 433–436.

Engelmann, S., & Bruner, E.C. *Distar reading II, Teacher's guide*. Chicago: Science Research Associates, 1975.

Epstein, W. Temporal schemata in syntactically structured material. *Journal of Genetic Psychology*, 1963, *68*, 157–164.

Fantz, R.L. The origin of form perception. *Scientific American*, 1961, *204*, 66–72.

Fedio, P., & Mirsky, A.F. Selective intellectual deficits in children with temporal lobe or centrencephalic epilepsy. *Neuropsychologia*, 1969, *7*, 287–300.

Fedio, P., & Van Buren, J.M. Memory deficits during electrical stimulation of the speech cortex in conscious man. *Brain and Language*, 1974, *1*, 29–42.

Feingold, B.F. *Why your child is hyperactive*. New York: Random House, 1974.

Feingold, B.F. Recognition of food additives as a cause of symptoms of allergy. *Annals of Allergy*, 1986, *26*, 309–313.

Felton, R.H., & Woods, F.B. Cognitive deficits in reading disability & attention deficit disorder. *Journal of Learning Disabilities*, 1989, *22*, 3–13.

Ferguson, J.H., & Boller, F. A different form of agraphia: Syntactic writing errors in patients with motor speech and movement disorders. *Brain and Language*, 1977, *4*, 382–389.

Ferguson, R., & Munson, P.A. The effects of artificial illumination on the behavior of elementary school children. *Final report to extramural research programs directorate, Health Sciences & Welfare Canada*, 1987.

Fernald, G.M. *Remedial techniques in basic school subjects*. New York: McGraw-Hill, 1943.

Filskov, S.B., & Boll, T.J. (Eds.). *Handbook of clinical neuropsychology*. New York: John Wiley, 1981.

Finucci, J.M., Isaacs, S.D., Whitehouse, C.C., & Childs, B. Classification of spelling errors and their relationship to reading ability, sex, grade placement, and intelligence. *Brain and Language*, 1983, *20*, 340–355.

Firestone, P., Kelly, M.J., Goodman, J.T., & Davey, J. Differential effects of parent training & stimulant medication with hyperactives. *Journal of the American Academy of Child Psychiatry*, 1981, *20*, 135–147.

Flavell, J. Metacognition and cognitive monitoring: A new area of cognitive-developmental inquiry. *American Psychologist*, 1979, *34*, 906–911.

Flechsig, P. Meine myelogenetische Hirnlehre mit biographischer Einleitung, 1927. Described in Nash, *Journal of Developmental Psychology*. Englewood Cliffs, NJ: Prentice-Hall, 1970, 98.

Fletcher, J.M., Satz, P., & Scholes, R.J. Developmental changes in the linguistic performance correlates of reading achievement. *Brain and Language*, 1981, *13*, 78–90.

Flowers, F., Wood, F.B., & Naylor, C.E. Regional cerebral blood flow correlates of language processes in reading disability. *Archives of Neurology*, 1991, *48*, 637–643.

Folsom, A.T. The epilepsies. *In* Haywood, H.C. (Ed.), *Brain damage in school age children*. Washington, DC: The Council for Exceptional Children, 1968, 62–86.

Fontenot, D.J., & Benton, A.L. Tactile perception of direction in relation to hemispheric locus of lesion. *Neuropsychologia*, 1971, *9*, 83–88.

Forehand, R., & McMahon, R.J. *Helping the non-compliant child: A clinician's quide to effective parent training*, New York: Guilford Press, 1981.

Frauenheim, J.G., & Heckerl, J.R. A longitudinal study of psychological and achievement test performance in severe dyslexic adults. *Journal of Learning Disabilities*, 1983, *16*(5), 339–347.

Frederiks, J.A.M. The agnosias. *In* Vinken, P.J., & Bruyn, G.W. (Eds.), *Handbook of clinical neurology*, Vol. 4. Amsterdam: North-Holland Publishing Co., 1969a, 13–47.

Frederiks, J.A.M. Disorders of the body schema. *In* Vinken, P.J., & Bruyn, G.W. (Eds.), *Handbook of clinical neurology*, Vol. 4. Amsterdam: North-Holland Publishing Co., 1969b, 207–240.

Freidus, E. Methodology for the classroom teacher. *In* Hellmuth, J. (Ed.), *The special child in Century 21*. Seattle: Special Child Publications, 1964, 303–321.

Freidus, E. The needs of teachers for specialized information on number concepts. *In* Cruickshank, W.M. (Ed.), *The teacher of brain-injured children*. Syracuse: Syracuse University Press, 1966, 111–128.

Friederici, A.D., Schoenle, P.W., & Goodglass, H. Mechanisms underlying writing and speech in aphasia. *Brain and Language*, 1981, *13*, 212–222.

Frith, C.D., Friston, K.J., Liddle, P.F., & Frackowiak, R.S.J. A PET study of word finding. *Neuropsychologia*, 1991, *29*(12), 1137–1148.

Frostig, M. The needs of teachers for specialized information on reading. *In* Cruickshank, W.M. (Ed.), *The teacher of brain-injured children*. Syracuse: Syracuse University Press, 1966, 89–109.

Frostig, M. The role of perception in the integration of psychological functions. *In* Cruickshank, W.M., & Hallahan, D.P. (Eds.), *Perceptual and learning disabilities in children*, Vol. 1. Syracuse: Syracuse University Press, 1975, 115–146.

Frostig, M., & Maslow, P. *Movement education: Theory and practice*. Chicago: Follett, 1970.

Frostig, M., & Maslow, P. *Learning problems in the classroom: Prevention and remediation*. New York: Grune & Stratton, 1973.

Fry, D.B. The development of the phonological system in the normal and the deaf child. *In* Smith, F., & Miller, G.A. (Eds.), *The genesis of language*. Cambridge: The M.I.T. Press, 1966, 187–206.

Fulton, M., Thomson, G., Hunter, R., Raab, G., Laxen, D., & Hepburn, W. Influence of blood lead on the ability and attainment of children in Edinburgh. *The Lancet*, May 30, 1987, 1221–1226.

Gaddes, W.H. The mental effects of pellagra. Unpublished Master's Thesis, University of British Columbia, 1946.

Gaddes, W.H. The performance of normal and brain-damaged subjects on a new dynamic visual retention test. *The Canadian Psychologist*, 1966a, *7a*, Inst. Suppl., 313–323.

Gaddes, W.H. The needs of teachers for specialized information on handedness, finger localization, and cerebral dominance. *In* Cruickshank, W.M. (Ed.), *The teacher of brain-injured children*. Syracuse: Syracuse University Press, 1966b, 207–221.

Gaddes, W.H. Neuropsychological approach to learning disorders. *Journal of Learning Disabilities*, 1968, *1*(9), 523–534.

Gaddes, W.H. Can educational psychology be neurologized? *Canadian Journal of Behavioral Science*, 1969a, *1*(1), 38–49.

Gaddes, W.H. *Dynamic visual retention test, manual of instructions and norms*. Victoria: Neuropsychology Laboratory, University of Victoria, Victoria, B.C., Canada, 1969b.

Gaddes, W.H. Learning disorders in the neurologically handicapped. *British Columbia Medical Journal*, 1972, Vol. *14*(1), 13–16.

Gaddes, W.H. Neurological implications for learning. *In* Cruickshank, W.H. & Hallahan, D.P. (Eds.), *Perceptual and learning disabilities in children*, Vol. 1. Syracuse: Syracuse University Press, 1975, 148–194,

Gaddes, W.H. Prevalence estimates and the need for definition of learning disabilities. *In* Knights, R.M., & Bakker, D.J. (Eds.), *The neuropsychology of learning disorders*. Baltimore: University Park Press, 1976, 3–24.

Gaddes, W.H. Learning disabilities: The search for causes. *In Bell Canada Monograph on Learning Disabilities*, Canadian Association for Children with Learning Disabilities, 4820 Van Horne Avenue, Montreal, Quebec, Canada, 1978.

Gaddes, W.H. *Learning disabilities and brain function*. New York: Springer-Verlag, 1980/1985.

Gaddes, W.H. An examination of the validity of neuropsychological knowledge in educational diagnosis and remediation. *In* Hynd, G.W., & Obrzut, J.E. (Eds.), *Neuropsychological assessment and the school-age child; issues and procedures*. New York: Grune & Stratton, 1981a, 27–85.

Gaddes, W.H. Neuropsychology, fact or mythology, educational help or hindrance? *School Psychology Review*, 1981b, X(3), 322–330.

Gaddes, W.H. Serial order behavior: to understand it, a scientific challenge, an educational necessity. *In* Cruickshank, W.M., & Lerner, J.W. (Eds.), *Coming of Age, Vol. 3, The best of ACLD*. Syracuse: Syracuse University Press, 1982, 87–107.

Gaddes, W.H. Applied educational neuropsychology: Theories and problems. *Journal of Learning Disabilities*, 1983, *16*(9), 511–514.

Gaddes, W.H. *Manual of instructions for the Dynamic Visual Retention Test, Revised Form (1988, Apple and IBM Versions)*. Victoria, B.C.: Neuropsychology Laboratory, University of Victoria, 1988.

Gaddes, W.H., & Crockett, D.J. *The Spreen-Benton Aphasia tests, normative data as a measure of normal language development*, Research Monograph No. 25. Department of Psychology, University of Victoria, Victoria, B.C., Canada, 1973.

Gaddes, W.H., & Crockett, D.J. The Spreen-Benton Aphasia tests, normative data as a measure of normal language development. *Brain and Language*, 1975, 2, 257–280. [This is a shorter version of the departmental monograph of the same name, 1973. The Monograph contains a complete set of all the graphs and tables. The text is essentially similar.]

Gaddes, W.H., & Spellacy, F.J. *Serial order perceptual and motor performances in children and their relation to academic achievement*. Research Monograph No. 35. Victoria, B.C., Canada: Department of Psychology, University of Victoria, 1977.

Gaddes, W.H., & Tymchuk, A.J. *A validation study of the dynamic visual retention test in functional localization of cerebral damage and dysfunction*. Research Monograph No. 38, Victoria, B.C., Canada: Department of Psychology, University of Victoria, 1967.

Galaburda, A.M. Developmental dyslexia: current anatomical research. *Annals of Dyslexia*, 1983, XXXIII, 41–53.

Galaburda, A.M. Anatomical asymmetries. *In* Geschwind, N., & Galaburda, A.M. (Eds.), *Cerebral dominance*. Cambridge, MA: Harvard University Press, 1984, 11–25.

Galaburda, A.M., & Eidelberg, D. Symmetry and asymmetry in the human posterior thalamus. II. Thalamic lesions in a case of developmental dyslexia. *Archives of Neurology*, 1982, *39*, 333–336.

Galaburda, A.M., & Kemper, T.L. Cytoarchitectonic abnormalities in developmental dyslexia: A case study. *Annals of Neurology*, 1979, *6*(2), 94–100.

Galaburda, A.M., Sherman, G.F., Rosen, G.D., Aboitiz, F., & Geschwind, N. Developmental dyslexia: Four consecutive patients with cortical anomalies. *Annals of Neurology*, 1985, *18*, 222–233.

Galton, F. *Inquiries into human faculty and its development*. London: J.M. Dent & Sons, 1907.

Gardner, E. *Fundamentals of neurology*. Philadelphia: W.B. Saunders, 1968 (5th Ed.)/1975 (6th Ed.).

Gazzaniga, M.S., Bogen, J.E., & Sperry, R.W. Observations on visual perception after disconnection of the cerebral hemispheres in man. *Brain*, 1965, *88*, 221–236.

Gazzaniga, M.S., & Hillyard, S.A. Language and speech capacity of the right hemisphere. *Neuropsychologia*, 1971, *9*, 273–280.

Geffen, G., Traub, E., & Stierman, I. Language laterality assessed by unilateral ECT and dichotic monitoring. *Journal of Neurology, Neurosurgery & Psychiatry*, 1978, *41*, 354–359.

Geldard, F.A. *The human senses*, 2nd Ed. New York: John Wiley, 1972.

Gellner, L. *A neurophysiological concept of mental retardation and its educational implications*. Chicago: The Dr. Julian D. Levinson Research Foundation, 519 South Wolcott Street, 1959.

Geschwind, N. The anatomy of acquired disorders of reading. *In* Money, J. (Ed.), *Reading disability*. Baltimore: The Johns Hopkins Press, 1962, 115–129.

Geschwind, N. Disconnexion syndromes in animals and man. *Brain*, 1965, *88*, Part II, 237–294, and Part III, 585–644.

Geschwind, N. Language and the brain. *Scientific American*, 1972, *226*(4), 76–83.

Geschwind, N. The apraxias: Neural mechanisms of disorders of learned movement. *American Scientist*, 1975, *63*, 188–195.

Geschwind, N. Asymmetries of the brain—New developments. *Bulletin of the Orton Society*, 1979a, *29*, 67–73.

Geschwind, N. Anatomical foundations of language and dominance. *In The neurological bases of language disorders in children: Methods and directions for research*. NINCDS Monograph #22, 1979b, 145–157.

Geschwind, N. Why Orton was right. *Annals of Dyslexia*. Baltimore: The Orton Dyslexia Society, 1982, XXXII, 13–30.

Geschwind, N. Biological associations of left-handedness. *Annals of Dyslexia*, 1983, XXXIII, 29–40.

Geschwind, N., & Levitzky, W. Human brain: Left-right asymmetries in temporal speech region. *Science*, 1968, *161*, 186–187.

Geschwind, N., Quadfasel, F.A., & Segarra, J.M. Isolation of the speech area. *Neuropsychologia*, 1968, *6*, 327–340.

Getman, G.N. The needs of teachers for specialized information on the development of visuomotor skills in relation to academic performance. *In* Cruickshank, W.M. (Ed.), *The teacher of brain-injured children*. Syracuse: Syracuse University Press, 1966, 153–168.

Gibson, E.E. Learning to read. *Science*, 1965, *148*, 1066–1072.

Gillingham, A. *Remedial training for children with specific disability in reading, spelling, and penmanship*, 7th Ed. Cambridge, MA: Educators Publishing Service, 1965.

Gillingham, A., & Stillman, B. *Remedial work for reading, spelling, and penmanship*. New York: Hackett & Wilhelms, 1936.

Gillingham, A., & Stillman, B. *Remedial training for children with specific disability in reading spelling and penmanship*. Cambridge, MA: Educators Publishing Service, 1965.

Gittelman, R., Manunuzza, S., Shenker, R., & Bonagura, N. Hyperactive boys almost grown up: I. Psychiatric status. *Archives of General Psychiatry*, 1985, *42*, 937–947.

Glasser, W. *Schools without failure*. New York: Harper & Row, 1969.

Goldberg, E., & Costa, L.D. Hemisphere differences in the acquisition and use of descriptive systems. *Brain and Language*, 1981, 14, 144–173.

Golden, C.J. The Luria-Nebraska children's battery: Theory and formulation. *In* Hynd, G.W., Obrzut, J.E. (Eds.), *Neuropsychological assessment and the school-age child: Issues and procedures*. New York: Grune & Stratton, 1981, 277–302.

Goldscheider, A. Unrersuchungen uber den Muskelsinn. II. Ueber die Empfindung der Schwere und des Widerstandes. *In Gesammelte Abhandlungen von A. Goldscheider, Vol. II.* Leipzig: Barth, 1898. Cited by Geldard, F.A. *The Human Senses, 2nd Ed*. New York: John Wiley, 1972.

Goldstein, K. *The organism*. New York: American Book Co., 1939.

Goldstein, K. *Human nature in the light of psychopathology*. New York: Schocken Books, 1940.

Goldstein, K. *Aftereffects of brain-injuries in war*. New York: Grune & Stratton, 1942.

Goldstein, S., & Goldstein, M. *Managing attention disorders in children*. New York: J. Wiley & Sons, 1990.

Goodglass, H., & Kaplan, E. *The assessment of aphasia and related disorders*. Philadelphia: Lea and Febiger, 1972.

Goodman, D.M., Beatty, J., & Mulholland, T.B. Detection of cerebral lateralization of function using EEG alpha contingent visual stimulation. *Electroencephalography and Clinical Neurophysiology*, 1980, *48*, 418–431.

Goodman, R., & Stevenson, J.A. A twin study of hyperactivity-II. The etiological role of genes, family relationships and perinatal adversity. *Journal of Child Psychology & Psychiatry*, 1989, *5*, 691–709.

Goodyear, P., & Hynd, G.W. Attention deficit disorder with (ADD/H) and without (ADD/WO) hyperactivity. *Journal of Clinical Child Psychology*, in press.

Gordon, H. Left-handedness and mirror writing especially among defective children. *Brain*, 1920, *43*, 313–368.

Gottlieb, G. Ontogenesis of sensory function in birds and mammals. *In* Tobach, E., Aronson, L.R., & Shaw, E. (Eds.), *The biopsychology of development*. New York: Academic Press, 1971, 67–128.

Gottschalk, J.A. Temporal order in the organization of children's behavior. Unpublished M.A. Thesis, McGill University, 1962.

Gottschalk, J.A. Spatiotemporal organization in children. Unpublished Ph.D. Thesis, McGill University, 1965.

Gray, J., & Wedderburn, A. Grouping strategies with simultaneous stimuli. *Quarterly Journal of Experimental Psychology*, 1960, *12*, 180–184.

Gray, J.W., & Dean, R.S. Approaches to the cognitive rehabilitation of children with neuro-psychological impairment. *In* Reynolds, C.R., & Fletcher-Janzen, E. (Eds.), *Handbook of clinical child neuropsychology*. New York: Plenum, 1989, 397–408.

Grieser, D.L., & Kuhl, P.K. Maternal speech to infants in a tonal language: Support for universal prosodic features in Motherese. *Developmental Psychology*, 1988, *24*, 14–20.

Gross-Glenn, K., Duara, R., Barker, W.W., Loewenstein, D., Chang, J.Y., Yoshii, F., Apicella, A.M., Pascal, S., Boothe, T., Sevush, S., Jallad, B.J., Novoa, L., & Lubs, H.A. Positron emission tomographic studies during serial word-reading by normal and dyslexic adults. *Journal of Clinical and Experimental Neuropsychology*, 1991, *13*(4), 531–544.

Guetzkow, H.S., & Bowman, P.H. *Men and hunger*. Elgin, IL: Brethren Publishing House, 1946.

Gur, R.C., Gur, R.E., Rosen, A.D., Warach, S., Alavi, A., Greenberg, J., & Reivich, M. A cognitive-motor network demonstrated by positron emission tomography. *Neuropsychologia*, 1983, *21*(6), 601–606.

Guthrie, E.R. The status of systematic psychology. *The American Psychologist*, 1950, *5*(4), 97–101.

Hagan, J. The effects of distraction on selective attention. *Child Development*, 1967, *38*, 685–694.

Hallahan, D.P., & Cruickshank, W.M. *Psychoeducational foundations of learning disabilities*. Englewood Cliffs, NJ: Prentice-Hall, 1973.

Hallgren, B. Specific dyslexia: A clinical and genetic study. *Acta Psychiatrica et Neurologica*, Suppl., 1950, *65*, 1.

Halstead, W.C. Brain and intelligence. Chicago: University of Chicago Press, 1947.

Halstead, W.C. Biological intelligence. *Journal of Personality*, 1951, *20*, 118–130.

Hammill, D.D., Leigh, J.E., McNutt, G., & Larsen, S.C. New definition of learning disabilities, *Journal of Learning Disabilities*, 1987 *20*(2), 109–113.

Hanson, J.W., & Smith, D.W. The fetal hydantoin syndrome. *Journal of Pediatrics*, 1975, *87*, 285.

Harcherick, D.F., Cohen, D.J., Ort, S., Paul, R., Shaywitz, B.A., Volkman, F.R., Rotham, S.L.G., & Leckerman, T.F. Computerized tomographic brain scanning of four neuropsychiatric disorders of childhood. *American Journal of Psychiatry*, 1985, 731–737.

Harley, J.P., Ray, R.S., Tomasi, L., Eichman, P.L., Matthews, C.G., Chun, R., Cleeland, C.S., & Traisman, E. Hyperkinesis & food additives: Testing the Feingold Hypothesis. *Pediatrics*, 1981, *61*, 818–828.

Harris, A.J. *Harris tests of lateral dominance: Manual of directions for administration and interpretation*, 3rd Ed. New York: Psychological Corporation, 1958.

Harris, L.J. Left-handedness: Early theories, facts, and fancies. *In* Herron, J. (Ed.), *Neuropsychology of left-handedness*. New York: Academic Press, 1980, 3–78.

Harris, T.L., & Hodges, R.W. (Eds.). *A dictionary of reading and related terms*. Newark, DE: International Reading Association, 1981.

Hartlage, L.C. Neuropsychological approaches to predicting outcome of remedial strategies for learning disabled children. *Pediatric Psychology*, 1975, *3*, 23.

Hartlage, L.C. Management of common clinical problems: Learning disabilities. *School Related Health Care*, 1979, (Ross Laboratories Monograph #9), 29–33.

Hartlage, L.C., & Hartlage, P.L. Application of neuropsychological principles in the diagnosis of learning disabilities. *In* Tarnopol, L., & Tarnopol, M. (Eds.), *Brain function and reading disabilities*. Baltimore: University Park Press, 1977, 111–146.

Hartlage, L.C., & Reynolds, C.R. Neuropsychological assessment and the individualization of instruction. *In* Hynd, G.W., Obrzut, J.E. (Eds.), *Neuropsychological assessment and the school-age child: Issues and procedures*. New York: Grune & Stratton, 1981, 355–378.

Harvey, J.E. The effects of permanent and temporary occlusion of the middle cerebral artery in the monkey. Unpublished Ph.D. Dissertation, Department of Surgery, The University of Chicago, 1950.

Harvey, J.E., & Rasmussen, T. Occlusion of the middle cerebral artery. *American Medical Association Archives of Neurology and Psychiatry*, 1951, *66*, 20–29.

Hasher, L., & Zachs, R.T. Automatic & effortful processing in memory. *Journal of Experimental Psychology: General*, 1979, *108*, 365–388.

Haslam, R.H.A. Teacher awareness of some common pediatric neurologic disorders. *In* Haslam, R.H.A., & Valletutti, P.J.(Eds.), *Medical problems in the classroom*. Baltimore: University Park Press, 1975, 51–74.

Head, H., & Holmes, G. Sensory disturbances from cerebral lesions. *Brain*, 1911, *34*, 102–254. [Described by J.A.M. Frederiks *In* Vinken, P.J., & Bruyn, G.W. (Eds.), *Handbook of clinical neurology*, Vol. 4. Amsterdam: North-Holland Publishing Co., 1969, 208.]

Heath, C.P., & Kush, J.C. Use of discrepancy formulas in assessment of learning disabilities. *In* Obrzut, J.E., & Hynd, G.W. (Eds.). *Neuropsychological foundations of learning disabilities: A handbook of issues, methods and practice*. New York: Academic Press, 1991, 287–304.

Hebb, D.O. Intelligence in man after large removals of cerebral tissue: Report of four left frontal lobe cases. *Journal of Genetic Psychology*, 1939, *21*, 73–87.

Hebb, D.O. The effect of early and late brain injury upon test scores, and the nature of normal adult intelligence. *Proceedings of the American Philosophical Society*, 1942a, *85*, 275–292.

Hebb, D.O. Verbal test material independent of special vocabulary difficulty. *Journal of Educational Psychology*, 1942b, *33*, 691–696.

Hebb, D.O. Man's frontal lobes: A critical review. *Archives of Neurology and Psychiatry*, 1945, *54*, 10–24.

Hebb, D.O. *Organization of behavior*. New York: Wiley, 1949.

Hebb, D.O. *A textbook of psychology*. Philadelphia: Saunders, 1958 (1st Ed)/1966 (2nd Ed)/1972 (3rd Ed).

Hebb, D.O., & Morton, N.W. The McGill Adult Comprehension Examination: "Verbal situation" and "picture anomaly" series. *Journal of Educational Psychology*, 1943, *34*, 16–25.

Hebb, D.O., & Penfield, W. Human behavior after extensive bilateral removal from the frontal lobes. *Archives of Neurology and Psychiatry*, 1940, *44*, 421–438.

Hebb, D.O., & Thompson, W.R. The social significance of animal studies. *In* Lindzey, G. (Ed.), *Handbook of social psychology*. Cambridge, MA: Addison-Wesley, 1954, 532–561.

Hécaen, H. Acalculia. *In* Mountcastle, V.B. (Ed.), *Interhemispheric relations and cerebral dominance*. Baltimore: The Johns Hopkins University Press, 1962, 235–237.

Hécaen, H. Aphasic, apraxic and agnosic syndromes in right and left hemisphere lesions. *In* Vinken, P.J., & Bruyn, G.W. (Eds.), *Handbook of clinical neurology*, Vol. 4. Amsterdam: North-Holland Publishing CO., 1969, 291–311.

Hécaen, H., & de Ajuriaguerra, J. *Left-handedness, manual superiority and cerebral dominance*. New York: Grune & Stratton, 1964.

Hécaen, H., & Sauget, J. Cerebral dominance in left-handed subjects. *Cortex*, 1971, *7*, 19–48.

Heilman, K.M., Kytja, K.S., Voeller, M.D., & Nadeau, S.E. A possible pathophysiologic substrate of Attention Deficit Hyperactivity Disorder. *Journal of Child Neurology*, Supplement, 1991, *6*, S76-S81.

Heilman, K.M., & Valenstein, E. (Eds.). *Clinical neuropsychology*. New York: Oxford University Press, 1979.

Hermann, K. *Reading disability*. Springfield, IL: Charles C Thomas, 1959.

Hern, A. Neurological signs in learning disabled children: persistence over time, and incidence in adulthood compared to normal learners. Unpublished Ph.D. Dissertation, University of Victoria, 1984.

Hernández-Peón, R. Psychiatric implications of neuropsychological research. *Bulletin of the Menninger Clinic*, 1964, *28*, 165–185.

Hernández-Peón, R., Scherrer, H., & Jouvet, M. Modification of electric activity in cochlear nucleus during "attention" in unanesthetized cats. *Science*, 1956, *123*, 331–332.

Hernández-Peón, R., & Sterman, M.B. Brain functions. *Annual Review of Psychology*, 1966, *17*, 363–395.

Heron, W. Perception as a function of retinal locus and attention. *American Journal of Psychology*, 1957, *70*, 38–48.

Herrick, C.J. *Brains of rats and men*. Chicago: University of Chicago Press, 1926.

Herrick, C.J. Apparatus of optic and visceral correlation in the brain of amblystoma. *The Journal of Comparative Psychology*, 1944, *37*(2), 97–105.

Herron, J. Two hands, two brains, two sexes. *In* Herron, J.(Ed.), *Neuropsychology of left-handedness*. New York: Academic Press, 1980, 233–260.

Hertzig, M. Stability and change in nonfocal neurologic signs. *Journal of the American Academy of Child Psychiatry*, 1982, *21*, 231–236.

Hess, R. *EEG handbook, Sandoz monographs*. Zurich: Sandoz, 1966.

Hewett, F.M. Educational engineering with emotionally disturbed children. *Exceptional Children*, 1967, *33*, 459–467.

Higenbottam, J.A. An investigation of lateral and perceptual preference relationship. Unpublished Ph.D. Dissertation, University of Victoria, 1971.

Hilgard, E.R. *Theories of learning*. New York: Appleton-Century-Crofts, 1948.

Hirsch, H.V.B., & Jacobson, M. The perfectible brain: Principles of neuronal development. *In* Gazzaniga, M.S., & Blakemore, C. (Eds.), *Handbook of psychobiology*. New York: Academic Press, 1975, 107–137.

Hiscock, M. Language lateralization in children: Dichotic listening studies. Paper presented at the Symposium on Hemispheric Specialization in the Developing Brain, International Neuropsychological Society, New York, January 31-February 3, 1979.

Hobson, J. Sex-differences in primary mental abilities. *Journal of Educational Psychology*, 1947, *41*, 126–132.

Hodes, R.L. The biofeedback treatment of neurological and neuropsychological disorders of childhood and adolescence. *In* Reynolds, C.R., & Fletcher-Janzen, E. (Eds.). *Handbook of clinical child neuropsychology*. New York: Plenum Press, 1989, 377–396.

Hohman, L.B. Post-encephalitic behavior disorder in children. *Johns Hopkins Hospital Bulletin*, 1922, *33*, 372–375.

Hordijk, W. Epilepsie en links-handigheid. *Nederlands Tijdschrift voor Geneeskunde*, 1952, *96*(5), 263–269. Cited in Hécaen, H. & de Ajuriaguerra, J. *Left-handedness*. New York: Grune & Stratton, 1964.

Horton, A.M. Behavioral neuropsychology in the schools. *School Psychology Review*, 1981, *10*(3), 367–372.

Horton, A.M. Child behavioral neuropsychology. *In* Reynolds, C.R., & Fletcher-Janzen, E. (Eds.), *Handbook of clinical child neuropsychology*. New York: Plenum, 1989, 521–533.

Horton, A.M., & Puente, A.E. Behavioral neuropsychology with children. *In* Obrzut, J.E., & Hynd, G.W. (Eds.), *Child neuropsychology: Clinical practice, Vol. 2*. New York: Academic Press, 1986, 299–314.

Hoskins, B. Collaborative consultation: Designing the role of the speech-language pathologist in a new educational context. *In* Secord, W.A., & Wiig, E.H. (Eds.), *Best practices in school speech-language pathology*. San Antonio, TX: Harcourt Brace Jovanovich, 1990, 29–36

Hounsfield, G.N. Computerized axial scanning (tomography): Part 1: Description of system. *British Journal of Radiology*, 1973, *46*, 1016–1022.

Houselander, J., Hatcher, R., Burns, W., & Chasnoff, I. Infants born to narcotic addicted mothers. *Psychological Bulletin*, 1982, *2*, 453–468.

Hubel, D.H. The visual cortex of the brain. *Scientific American*, 1963, *209*(5), 54–62.

Hubel, D.H., & Wiesel, T.N. Receptive fields of single neurones in the cat's striate cortex. *Journal of Physiology*, 1959, *148*, 574–591.

Huheey, J.E. Concerning the origin of handedness in humans. *Behavior Genetics*, 1977, *7*(1), 29–32.

Hundleby, G.D. Effectiveness of the Benton Right-Left discrimination test in identifying children with reading disabilities. Unpublished Master's Thesis, Faculty of Education, University of Victoria, 1969.

Hunter, J., & Jasper, H.H. Effects of thalamic stimulation in unanesthe-tised animals. *Electroencephalography and Clinical Neurophysiology*, 1949, *1*, 305–324.

Hynd, C.R. Educational intervention in children with developmental learning disorders. *In* Obrzut, J.E., & Hynd, G.W. (Eds.), *Child neuropsychology: Clinical practice, Vol. 2*. New York: Academic Press, 1986, 265–293.

Hynd, G.W. Training the school psychologist in neuropsychology; pers-pectives, issues, and models. *In* Hynd, G.W., & Obrzut, J.E. (Eds.), *Neuropsychological assessment and the school-age child: Issues and procedures*. New York: Grune & Stratton, 1981, 379–404.

Hynd, G.W. Personal communication, 1992.

Hynd, G.W., Hayes, F., & Snow, J. Neuropsychological screening with school-age children: Rationale and conceptualization. *Psychology in the Schools*, 1982, *19*, 446–451.

Hynd, G.W., Hern, K.L., Novey, E.S., Eliopulos, D., Marshall, R., & Gonzales, J.J. Attention deficit hyperactivity disorder (ADHD) and asymmetry of the caudate nucleus. Submitted for publication to the *Journal of Child Neurology*, 1992.

Hynd, G.W., & Hynd, C.R. Dyslexia: Neuroanatomical/neurolinguistic perspectives. *Reading Research Quarterly*, 1984, *19*, 482–498.

Hynd, G.W., Hynd, C.R., Sullivan, H.G., & Kingsbury, T.B. Regional cerebral blood flow (rCBF) in developmental dyslexia: Activation during reading in a surface and deep dyslexic. *Journal of Learning Disabilities*, 1987, *20*, 294–300.

Hynd, G.W., Lorys, A.R., Semrud-Clikeman, M., Nieves, N., Hyettner, M.I.S., & Lahey, B.B. Attention deficit disorder without hyperactivity: A distinct behavioral and neurocognitive syndrome. *Journal of Child Neurology*, 1991a, Supplement 6, S37–S42.

Hynd, G.W., & Obrzut, J.E. Neuropsychological assessment and consul-tation in the public schools. Paper presented at the annual convention of the National Association of School Psychologists, Washington, DC, April, 1980.

Hynd, G.W., & Obrzut, J.E. (Eds.). *Neuropsychological assessment and the school-age child: Issues and procedures*. New York: Grune & Stratton, 1981.

Hynd, G.W., Quackenbush, R., & Obrzut, J.E. Training school psychol-ogists in neuropsychological assessment: Current practices and trends. Paper presented at the Annual Convention of the National Association of School Psychologists, San Diego, CA, March 1979.

Hynd, G.W., & Semrud-Clikeman, M. Dyslexia and neurodevelopmental pathology: Relationships to cognition, intelligence, and reading skill acquisition. *Journal of Learning Disabilities*, 1989, *22*, 204–216.

Hynd, G.W., & Semrud-Clikeman, M. Dyslexia and brain morphology. *Psychological Bulletin*, 1989, *106*, (3), 447–482.

Hynd, G.W., Semrud-Clikeman, M., Lorys, A.R., Novey, E.S., & Eliopulos, D. Brain morphology in developmental dyslexia and attention deficit disorder/hyperactivity. *Archives of Neurology*, 1990, *47*, 919–926.

Hynd, G.W., Semrud-Clikeman, M., Lorys, A.R., Novey, E.S., Eliopulos, D., & Lyytinen, H. Corpus callosum morphology in Attention Deficit-Hyperactivity Disorder: Morphometric Analysis of MRI. *Journal of Learning Disabilities*. 1991b, *24*, 141–146.

Hynd, G.W., Semrud-Clikeman, M., & Lyytinen, H. Brain imaging in learning disabilities. *In* Obrzut J.E., & Hynd, G.W. (Eds.), *Neuropsychological foundations of learning disabilities*. San Diego: Academic Press, 1991c, 475–511.

Hynd, G.W., & Willis, W.G. *Pediatric neuropsychology*. New York: Grune & Stratton, 1988.

Ingvar, D.H. Serial aspects of language and speech related to prefrontal cortical activity: A selective review. *Human Neurobiology*, 1983, *2*, 177–189.

Ingvar, D.H. Ideography: Mapping ideas in the brain. *In* Lassen, N.A., Ingvar, D.H., Raichle, M.E., & Friberg, L. (Eds.), *Brain work and mental activity, Alfred Benzon Symposium 31*. Copenhagen: Munksgaard, 1991, 346–359.

Ingvar, D.H. Language functions related to prefrontal cortical activity. Paper presented to the New York Academy of Sciences Conference, New York, September 10–16, 1992.

Ingvar, D.H., & Risberg, J. Increase of regional cerebral blood flow during mental effort in normals and in patients with focal brain disorders. *Experimental Brain Research*, 1967, *3*, 195–211.

Ingvar, D.H., & Schwartz, M.S. Blood flow patterns induced in the dominant hemisphere by speech and reading. *Brain*, 1974, *97*(II), 273–288.

Inhelder, B. *The diagnosis of reasoning in the mentally retarded*, 2nd Ed. New York: Chandler Publishing, 1968.

Iosub, S., Bamji, M., Stone, R.K., Gromisch, D.S., & Wasserman, E. More on human immunodeficiency virus embryopathy. *Pediatrics*, 1987, *80*, 512–516.

Jackson, J.H. *Selected writings of John Hughlings Jackson*, Vol. II. London: Staples Press, 1958.

Jacobs, J. Experiments on "prehension." *Mind*, 1887, *12*, 75–79.

Jacobson, J.L., Jacobson, S.W., Fein, G.G., Schwartz, P.M., & Dowler, J.K. Prenatal exposure to an environmental toxin: A test of the multiple effects model. *Developmental Psychology*, 1984, *20*, 523–533.

Jacobson, M. Development, specification and diversification of neuronal circuits. *In* Schmidt, F.O. (Ed.), *The neurosciences: Second study program.* New York: Rockefeller University Press, 1970, 116–129.

James, W. *The principles of psychology.* New York: Henry Holt & Co., 1890.

Jan, J.E., Ziegler, R.G., & Erba, G. *Does your child have epilepsy?* Baltimore: University Park Press, 1983.

Jansky, J., & de Hirsch, K. *Preventing reading failure.* New York: Harper & Row, 1972.

Janz, D., Bossi, L., Dam, M., Helge, H., Richens, A., & Schmidt, D. *Epilepsy, pregnancy & the child.* New York: Raven Press, 1982.

Jasper, H.H., Solomon, P., & Bradley, C. Electroencephalographic analysis of behavior problems in children. *American Journal of Psychiatry,* 1938, *95,* 641–658.

Jastak, J.F., & Jastak, S.R. *The Wide Range Achievement Test.* Wilmington, DE: Guidance Associates, 1965.

John, E.R. Switchboard versus statistical theories of learning and memory. *Science,* 1972, *177,* 850–864.

Johnson, D.A., & Roethig-Johnson, K. Life in the slow lane: Attentional factors after head injury. *In* Johnson, D.A., Uttley, D., & Wyke. M.A. (Eds.), *Children's head injury: who cares?* London: Taylor & Francis, 1989, 80–95.

Johnson, D.J., & Myklebust, H.R. Dyslexia in childhood. *In* Hellmuth, J. (Ed.), *Learning disorders,* Vol. 1. Seattle: Special Child Publications, 1965, 259–292.

Johnson, D.J., & Myklebust, H.R. *Learning disabilities: Educational principles and practices.* New York: Grune & Stratton, 1967.

Johnson, S.W., & Morasky, R.L. *Learning disabilities.* Boston: Allyn & Bacon, 1977.

Jorm, A.F. The cognitive and neurological basis of developmental dyslexia: A theoretical framework and review. *Cognition,* 1979, *7,* 19–33.

Kabat, H., & Dennis, C. Decerebration in the dog by complete temporary anemia. *Proceedings of the Society for Experimental Biology and Medicine,* 1938, *38,* 864.

Kabat, H., Dennis, C., & Baker, A.B. Recovery of function following arrest of the brain circulation. *American Journal of Physiology,* 1941, *132,* 737.

Kahn, E., & Cohen, L.H. Organic driveness: A brain stem syndrome and an experience. *New England Journal of Medicine,* 1934, *210,* 748–756.

Kail, R., & Hagen, J.W. Memory in childhood. *In* Wolman, B.B. (Ed.), *Handbook of Developmental Psychology.* New Jersey: Prentice-Hall, Inc., 1982, 350–366.

Kalverboer, A.F. A neurobehavioural study in preschool children. *Clinics in Developmental Medicine*, No. 54. London: Heinemann, 1975.

Kalverboer, A.F. Neurobehavioral relationships in young children: Some remarks on concepts and methods. *In* Knights, R.M., & Bakker, D.J. (Eds.), *The neuropsychology of learning disorders*. Baltimore: University Park Press, 1976, 173–183.

Kaplan, B., McNicol, J., Conte, R., & Moghadam, H.K. Dietary replacement in preschool-aged hyperactive boys. *Pediatrics*, 1989, *83*, 7–17.

Karpov, B.A., Luria, A.R., & Yarbuss, A.L. Disturbances of the structure of active perception in lesions of the posterior and anterior regions of the brain. *Neuropsychologia*, 1968, *6*, 157–166.

Kashani, J., Chapel, J.L., Ellis, J., & Shekim, W.O. Hyperactive girls. *Journal of Operational Psychiatry*, 1979, *10*, 145–148.

Kaspar, J.C., Millichap, J.C., Backus, D.C., Child, D., & Schulman, J. A study of the relationship between neurological evidence of brain damage in children with hyperactivity and distractibility. *Journal of Consulting Clinical Psychology*, 1971, *36*, 329–337

Kaufman, A.S., & Kaufman, N.L. *K-ABC interpretive manual*. Circle Pines, MN: American Guidance Service, 1983.

Kee, D.W., Bathurst, K., & Hellige, J.B. Lateralized interference of repetitive finger tapping: Influence of familial handedness, cognitive load and verbal production. *Neuropsychologia*, 1983, *21*(6), 617–624.

Keller, C.E., & Sutton, J.P. Specific mathematics disorders. *In* Obrzut, J.E., & Hynd, G.W. (Eds.), *Neuropsychological foundations of learning disabilities*, 1991, 549–571.

Kendall, D., & Wong, B. Canadian policies, practices, and programs related to learning disabilities: An overview. *Paedoperisse*, 1987, *1*(1), 29–44.

Kendall, P.C., & Braswell, L. *Cognitive behavioral therapy for impulsive children*. New York: Guilford Press, 1984.

Kephart, N.C. *The slow learner in the classroom*. Columbus, OH: Merrill, 1960 (1st Ed.)/1971 (2nd Ed.).

Kephart, N.C. The needs for teachers for specialized information on perception. *In* Cruickshank, W.M. (Ed.), *The teacher of brain-injured children*. Syracuse: Syracuse University Press, 1966, 169–180.

Kephart, N.C. The perceptual-motor match. *In* Cruickshank, W.M., & Hallahan, D.P. (Eds.), *Perceptual and learning disabilities in children*, Vol. 1. Syracuse: Syracuse University Press, 1975, 63–69.

Kertesz, A., Lesk, D., & McCabe, P. Isotope localization of infarcts in aphasia. *Archives of Neurology*, 1977, *34*, 590–601.

Kertesz, A., & McCabe, P. Recovery patterns and prognosis in aphasia. *Brain*, 1977, *100*, 1–18.

Kess, J.F. *Psycholinguistics: Introductory perspectives*. New York: Academic Press, 1976.

Kimble, D.P., & Pribram, K.H. Hippocampectomy and behavior sequences. *Science*, 1963, *139*, 824–825.

Kimura, D. The effect of letter position on recognition. *Canadian Journal of Psychology*, 1959, *13*(1), 1–10.

Kimura, D. Some effects of temporal-lobe damage on auditory perception. *Canadian Journal of Psychology*, 1961a, *15*(3), 156–165.

Kimura, D. Cerebral dominance and the perception of verbal stimuli. *Canadian Journal of Psychology*, 1961b, *15*(3), 166–171.

Kimura, D. Left-right differences in the perception of melodies. *Quarterly Journal of Experimental Psychology*, 1964, *16*, 355–358.

Kimura, D. Dual functional asymmetry of the brain in visual perception. *Neuropsychologia*, 1966, *4*, 275–285.

Kimura, D. Functional asymmetry of the brain in dichotic listening. *Cortex*, 1967, *3*, 163–178.

Kimura, D. Spatial localization in left and right visual fields. *Canadian Journal of Psychology*, 1969, *28*(6), 445–458.

Kimura, D. The asymmetry of the human brain. *Scientific American*, 1973a, *228*(3), 70–78.

Kimura, D. Manual activity during speaking—I. Right-handers. *Neuropsychologia*, 1973b, *11*, 45–50.

Kimura, D. Manual activity during speaking—II. Left-handers. *Neuropsychologia*, 1973c, *11*, 51–55.

Kimura, D. The neural basis of language qua gesture. *In* Avakian-Whitaker, H., & Whitaker, H.A. (Eds.), *Studies in neurolinguistics*, Vol. 2. New York: Academic Press, 1976.

Kimura, D., & Durnford, M. Normal studies on the function of the right hemisphere in vision. *In* Dimond, S.J., & Beaumont, J.G. (Eds.), *Hemisphere function in the human brain*. London: Elek Science, 1974, 25–47.

Kinkel, P.R. Nuclear magnetic resonance imaging in clinical neurology. *Clinical Neurology*, 1987, *1*, 4A.

Kinney, G.C., Marsetta, M., & Showman, D.J. Studies in display symbol legibility. Part 12. The legibility of alpha numeric symbols for digitalized television. Bedford, Mass.: The Mitre Corporation ESD-TR-66-1117, 1966.

Kinsbourne, M. The neuropsychology of learning disabilities. Paper presented at *Seventh Annual Neuropsychology Workshop*, University of Victoria, Victoria, B.C., Canada, 1972.

Kinsbourne, M. Mechanisms of hemispheric interaction in man. *In* Kinsbourne, M., & Smith, W.L. (Eds.), *Hemispheric disconnection and cerebral function*. Springfield, IL: Charles C. Thomas, 1974.

Kinsbourne, M. Minor hemisphere language and cerebral maturation. *In* Lenneberg, E.H., & Lenneberg, E. (Eds.), *Foundations of Language Development*, Vol. 2. New York: Academic Press, 1975a, 107–116.

Kinsbourne, M. The ontogeny of cerebral dominance. *Annals of the New York Academy of Sciences*, 1975b, *263*, 244–250.

Kinsbourne, M. The mechanism of hemispheric control of the lateral gradient of attention. *In* Rabbitt, P.M.A., & Dornic, S. (Eds.), *Attention and performance V*. London: Academic Press , 1975c.

Kinsbourne, M. Mechanisms and development of hemisphere specialization in children. *In* Reynolds, C.R., & Fletcher-Janzen, E. (Eds.), *Handbook of clinical child neuropsychology*. New York: Plenum Press, 1989, 69–83.

Kinsbourne, M., & Cook, J. Generalized and lateralized effects of concurrent verbalization on a unimanual skill. *Quarterly Journal of Experimental Psychology*, 1971, *23*, 341–345.

Kinsbourne, M., & Hiscock, M. Cerebral lateralization and cognitive development. *In* Chall, J., & Mirsky, A.F. (Eds.), *Education and the brain* (Seventy-seventh Yearbook of the National Society for the Study of Education). Chicago: The University of Chicago Press, 1978, 169–222.

Kinsbourne, M., & McMurray, J. The effect of cerebral dominance on time sharing between speaking and tapping by preschool children. *Child Development*, 1975, *46*, 240–242.

Kinsbourne, M., & Smith, W.L. (Eds.). *Hemispheric disconnection and cerebral function*. Springfield, IL: Charles C. Thomas, 1974.

Kinsbourne, M., & Warrington, E.K. Disorders of spelling. *Journal of Neurology, Neurosurgery and Psychiatry*, 1964, *27*, 224–228.

Kirby, J.R., & Ashman, A.F. Planning skills and mathematics achievement: Implications regarding learning disability. *Journal of Psychoeducational Assessment*, 1984, *2*, 9–22.

Kirk, S.A. *The diagnosis and remediation of psycholinguistic disabilities*. Urbana: University of Illinois Press, 1966.

Kirk, S.A., & Bateman, B. Diagnosis and remediation of learning disabilities. *Exceptional Children*, 1962, *29*, 73–78.

Kirk, S.A., & Becker, W., (Eds.). *Conference on Children with Minimal Brain Impairment*. Urbana: University of Illinois, 1963. (mimeo.)

Kirk, S.A., & Kirk, W.D. *Psycholinguistic learning disabilities: Diagnosis and remediation*. Urbana: University of Illinois Press, 1971.

Kirk, S.A., McCarthy, J., & Kirk, W. *The Illinois test of psycholinguistic abilities (revised edition)*. Urbana: Illinois University Press, 1968.

Kirk, U. Introduction: Toward the understanding of the neuropsychology of language, reading and spelling. *In* Kirk, U. (Ed.), *Neuropsychology of language, reading, and spelling*. New York: Academic Press, 1983a, 3–31.

Kirk, U. (Ed.). *Neuropsychology of language, reading, and spelling*. New York: Academic Press, 1983b.

Kitchen, W., Ford, G., Orgill, A., Rickards, A., Astbury, J., Lissenden, J., Bajuk, B., Yu, V., Drew, J., & Campbell, N. Outcome of infants of birth weight 500–900 g: A continuing regional study of 5 year-old survivors. *Journal of Pediatrics*, 1987, *111*, 761–766.

Klonoff, H. Factor analysis of a neuropsychological battery for children aged 9 to 15. *Perceptual and Motor Skills*, 1971, *32*, 603–616.

Kløve, H. The relationship of differential electroencephalographic patterns to the distribution of Wechsler-Bellevue scores. *Neurology*, 1959, *9*, 871–876.

Kløve, H. Clinical neuropsychology. *Medical Clinics of North America*, 1963, *11*, 1647–1658.

Kløve, H., & Matthews, C.G. Psychometric and adaptive abilities in epilepsy with differential etiology. *Epilepsia*, 1966, *7*, 330–338.

Kløve, H., & Reitan, R.M. The effect of dysphasia and spatial distortion on Wechsler-Bellevue results. *American Medical Association Archives of Neurology and Psychiatry*, 1958, *80*, 708–713.

Knights, R.M. *Normative data on tests for evaluating brain damage in children from 5 to 14 years of age*. London, Ontario: Department of Psychology, The University of Western Ontario, Research Bulletin #20, June, 1966.

Knights, R.M. A review of the neuropsychological research program. *Special Education*, 1970 (Nov.), 9–27.

Knights, R.M. Battery of neuropsychological tests. Department of Psychology, Carleton University, Ottawa, Ontario, Canada, 1971. (mimeo.)

Knights, R.M. The effects of cerebral lesions on the psychological test performance of children. Final Report, March, 1973, Carleton University, Ottawa, Ontario, Canada.

Knights, R.M., & Bakker, D.J. (Eds.). *The neuropsychology of learning disorders, theoretical approaches*. Baltimore: University Park Press, 1976.

Knights, R.M., & Ogilvie, R.M. Comparison of Test Results from Normal and Brain Damaged Children. *Research Bulletin* No. 53, Department of Psychology, University of Western Ontario, London, Ontario, Canada, July, 1967.

Knott, J.R., Platt, E.B., Ashby, M.C., & Gottlieb, J.S. A familial evaluation of the electroencephalogram of patients with primary disorder and psychopathic personality. *Electroencephalography and Clinical Neurophysiology*, 1953, *5*, 363–370.

Kolb, B., & Whishaw, I.Q. *Fundamentals of human neuropsychology*. San Francisco: W.H. Freeman & Co., 3nd Ed., 1990.

Koorland, M.A., & Wolking, W.D. Effect of reinforcement on modality of stimulus control in learning. *Learning Disability Quarterly*, 1982, *5*, 264–273.

Krashen, S.D. Lateralization, language learning, and the critical period: Some new evidence. *Language and Learning*, 1973, *23*, 63–74.

Kuhl, P.K. Perception, cognition, and the ontogenetic and phylogenetic emergence of human speech. *In* Brauth, S.E., Hall, W.S., & Dooling, R.J. (Eds.). *Plasticity of development*. Cambridge, MA: The MIT Press, 1991, 73–106.

Kuhl, P.K., Williams, K.A., Lacerda, F., Stevens, K.N., & Lindblom, B. Linguistic experience alters phonetic perception in infants by 6 months of age. *Science*, 1992, *255*, 606–608.

Kushner, M.J., Rosenquist, A., Alavi, A., Rosen, M., Dann, R., Fazekas, F., Bosley, T., Greenberg, J., & Reivich, M. Cerebral metabolism and patterned visual stimulation: A positron emission tomographic study of the human visual cortex. *Neurology*, 1988, *38*, 89–95.

Ladd, G.W., & Mize, J. A cognitive-social learning model of social-skill training. *Psychological Review*, 1983, *90*(2), 127–157.

Lahey, B.B., Schaughency, E.A., Frame, C.C., & Straus. C.C. Teacher ratings of attention problems in children experimentally classified as exhibiting attention deficit disorders with and without hyperactivity. *Journal of the American Academy of Child and Adolescent Child Psychiatry*, 1984, *23*, 302–309.

Lambert, N., & Sandoval, J. The prevalence of learning disabilities in a sample of children considered hyperactive. *Journal of Child Psychology*, 1980, *8*, 33–50.

Landau, W.M., Goldstein, R., & Kleffner, F.R. Congenital aphasia, a clinicopathologic study. *Neurology*, 1960, 915–921.

Landis, T., Regard, M., Graves, R., & Goodglass, H. Semantic paralexia: A release of right hemispheric function from left hemispheric control? *Neuropsychologia*, 1983, *21*(4), 359–364.

Lansdell, H. A sex difference in effect of temporal-lobe neurosurgery on design preference. *Nature*, 1962, *194*, 852–854.

Lashley, K.S. Studies in cerebral function in learning. *Psychobiology*, 1920, *2*, 55–136.

Lashley, K.S. *Brain mechanisms and intelligence: A quantitative study of injuries to the brain*. Chicago: University of Chicago Press, 1929.

Lashley, K.S. In search of the engram. In *Society of Experimental Biology Symposium No. 4: Physiological Mechanisms in Animal Behavior*. Cambridge, England: Cambridge University Press, 1950, 478–505.

Lashley, K.S. The problem of serial order in behavior. *In* Jeffress, L.A. (Ed.), *Cerebral mechanisms in behavior, the Hixon symposium*. New York: Wiley, 1951.

Lassen, N.A., & Ingvar, D.H. The blood flow of the cerebral cortex determined by radioactive Krypton-85. *Experimentia*, 1961, *17*, 42–43.

Laufer, M.W., & Denhoff, E. Hyperkinetic impulse disorder in children. *Journal of Pediatrics*, 1957, *50*, 463–474.

Lawrence, D. Personal communication, 1992

Lee, J.K.T., Koehler, R.E., & Heiken, J.P. MR imaging techniques. *In* Lee, J.K.T., Sagel, S.S., & Stanley, R.J. (Eds.), *Computed body tomography with MRI correlation, 2nd edition*. New York: Raven Press, 1989, 61.

Lee, S.W. Biofeedback as a treatment for childhood hyperactivity: A critical review of the literature. *Psychological Reports*, 1991, *68*, 163–192.

Lehman, E.B., & Brady, K.M. Presentation modality and taxonomic category as encoding dimensions from good and bad readers. *Journal of Learning Disabilities*, 1982, *15*, 103–105.

Leiner, H.C., Leiner, A.L., & Dow, R.S. Does the cerebellum contribute to mental skills? *Behavioral Neuroscience*, 1986, *100*(4), 443–454.

Leiner, H.C., Leiner, A.L., & Dow, R.S. Reappraising the cerebellum: What does the hindbrain contribute to the forebrain? *Behavioral Neuroscience*, 1989, *103*(5), 998–1008.

Leiner, H.C., Leiner, A.L., & Dow, R.S. The human cerebro-cerebellar system: its computing, cognitive, and language skills. *Behavioral Brain Research*, 1991, *44*, 113–128.

Lenneberg, F.H. Speech as a motor skill with special reference to non-aphasic disorders. *In* Beelugi, U., & Brown, R. (Eds.), *Acquisition of Language*. Monograph of the Society for Research in Child Development. Ser. No. 92, Vol. 29, No. 1, 1964.

Lenneberg, E.H. The natural history of language. *In* Smith, F., & Miller, G.A. (Eds.), *The genesis of language, a psycholinguistic approach*. Cambridge, MA: The M.I.T. Press, 1966, 219–252.

Lenneberg, E.H. *Biological foundations of language*. New York: Wiley, 1967.

Lenneberg, E.H. The effect of age on the outcome of central nervous system disease in children. *In* Isaacson, R.L. (Ed.), *The neuropsy-*

chology of development, a symposium. New York: Wiley, 1968, 147–170.

Leong, C.K. Dichotic listening with related tasks for dyslexics—Differential use of strategies. *Bulletin of the Orton Society*, 1975, XXV, 111–126.

Leong, C.K. Lateralization in severely disabled readers in relation to functional cerebral development and synthesis of information. *In* Knights, R.M., & Bakker, D.J. (Eds.), *The neuropsychology of learning disorders*. Baltimore: University Park Press, 1976, 221–231.

Leong, C.K. Promising areas of research into learning disabilities with emphasis on reading disabilities. *In* Das, J.P., Mulcahy, R.F., & Wall, A.E. (Eds.), *Theory and research in learning disabilities*. New York: Plenum Press, 1982, 3–26.

Leong, C.K. *Children with specific reading disabilities*. Amsterdam: Swets & Zeitlinger, 1987.

Leong, C.K. Neuropsychological models of learning disabilities. *In* Reynolds, C.R., & Fletcher-Janzen, E. (Eds.), *Handbook of clinical child neuropsychology*. New York: Plenum, 1989a, 335–355.

Leong, C.K. The locus of so-called IQ test results in reading disabilities. *Journal of Learning Disabilities*, 1989b, *22*(8), 507–512.

Levin, H.S. Evaluation of the tactile component in a proprioceptive feedback task. *Cortex*, 1973, *9*, 197–203.

Levin, H.S. The acalculias. *In* Heilman, K.M., & Valenstein, E. (Eds.), *Clinical Neuropsychology*. New York: Oxford University Press, 1979, 128–140.

Levin, P.M. Restlessness in children. *Archives of Neurology and Psychiatry*, 1938, *39*, 764–770.

Levine, D. Prosopagnosia and visual object agnosia: A behavioral study. *Brain and Language*, 1978, *5*, 341–365.

Levy, F., & Hobbes, G. The action of stimulant medication in attention deficit disorder with hyperactivity: Dopaminergic, noradrenergic, or both? *Journal of the American Academy of Child & Adolescent Psychiatry*, 1988, *27*, 808–805.

Levy, J. Psychobiological implications of bilateral asymmetry. *In* Dimond, S.J., Beaumont, J.G. (Eds.), *Hemisphere function in the human brain*. London: Elek Science, 1974, 121–183.

Lezak, M.D. *Neuropsychological assessment*. New York: Oxford University Press, 1976/1983.

Lezak, M.D. IQ: R.I.P. *Journal of Clinical and Experimental Neuropsychology*, 1988, *10*(3), 351–361.

Lhermitte, F., & Gautier, J.-C. Aphasia. *In* Vinken, P.J., & Bruyn, B.W. (Eds.), *Handbook of clinical neurology*, Vol. 4. Amsterdam: North-Holland Publishing Co., 1969, 84–104.

Liberman, I.Y., & Liberman, A.M. Whole language vs. code emphasis: Underlying assumptions and their implications for reading instruction. *Annals of Dyslexia*, 1990, *40*, 51–76.

Liberman, I.Y., & Shankweiler, D. Phonology and the problems of learning to read and write. *Remedial and Special Education*, 1985, *6*(6), 8–17.

Litowitz, B.E. Developmental issues in written language. *Topics in Language Disorders*, 1981, *1*, 73–89.

Livingstone, M.S., Rosen, G.D., Drislane, F.W., & Galaburda, A.M. Physiological and anatomical evidence for a magnocellular defect in developmental dyslexia. *Proceedings of the National Academy of Science, USA*, 1991, *88*, 7943–7947.

Lockey, S.D., Sr. Allergic reactions due to FD C dyes used in coloring and identifying agents in various medications. *Bulletin of Lancaster General Hospital.* Lancaster, Pa., 1948.

Loper, A.B. Metacognitive training to correct academic deficiency. *Topics in learning and learning disabilities*, 1982, *2*, 61–68.

Lotz, J. How language is conveyed by script. *In* Kavanagh, J.F., & Mattingly, I.G. (Eds.), *Language by ear and by eye.* Cambridge, MA: The MIT Press, 1972, 117–124.

Lou, H.C., Henriksen, L., & Bruhn, P. Focal cerebral hypofusion in children with dysplasia and/or attention deficit. *Archives of Neurology*, 1984, *41*, 825–829.

Lou, H.C., Henriksen, L., Bruhn, P., Borner, H., & Nielsen, J.B. Striatal dysfunction in attention deficit and hyperkinetic disorder. *Archives of Neurology*, 1989, *46*, 48–52.

Lovitt, T.C. Characteristics of applied behavior analysis, general recommendations, and methodological limitations (Part 1). *Journal of Learning Disabilities*, 1975, *8*, 432–443.

Lowe, A.D., & Campbell, R.A. Temporal discrimination in aphasoid and normal children. *Journal of Speech and Hearing Research*, 1965, *8*, 313–314.

Lubar, J.F. Discourse on the development of EEG diagnostics and biofeedback for Attention-deficit/Hyperactivity Disorders. *Biofeedback and Self-regulation*, 1991, *16*(3), 201–225.

Lubar, J.O., & Lubar, J.F. Electroencephalographic biofeedback of SMR and beta for treatment of attention deficit disorders in a clinical setting. *Biofeedback and Self-Regulation* 1984, *9*, 1–23.

Lubs, H.A., Rabin, M., Carland-Saucier, K., Wen, X.L., Gross-Glenn, K., Duara, R., Levin, B., & Lubs, M.L. Genetic bases of developmental dyslexia: Molecular studies. *In* Obrzut, J.E., & Hynd, G.W. (Eds.), *Neuropsychological foundations of learning disabilities.* San Diego: Academic Press, 1991, 49–77.

Lundberg, I., Olofsson, A., & Wall, S. Reading and spelling skills in the first school years predicted from phonemic awareness skills in kindergarten. *Scandinavian Journal of Psychology*, 1980, *21*, 159–173.

Luria , A.R. Neuropsychology in the local diagnosis of brain damage. *Cortex*, 1964, *1*, 3–18.

Luria, A.R. *Higher cortical functions in man*. New York: Basic Books, 1966.

Luria, A.R. *The mind of the mnemonist: A little book about a vast memory*. Henry Regenery Co., 1968.

Luria, A.R. *Traumatic aphasia, its syndromes, psychology and treatment*. The Hague: Mouton, 1970.

Luria, A.R. *The working brain*. Harmondsworth: Penguin Books, 1973.

Luria, A.R., Simernitskaya, E.G., & Tubylevich, B. The structure of psychological processes in relation to cerebral organization. *Neuropsychologia*, 1970, *8*, 13–19.

Lyon, G.R. IQ is irrelevant to the definition of learning disabilities: A position in search of logic and data. *Journal of Learning Disabilities*, 1989, *22*(8), 504–506, 512.

Lyon, G.R., Newby, R.E., Recht, D., & Caldwell, J. Neuropsychology and learning disabilities. *In* Wong, B.Y.L. (Ed.), *Learning about learning disabilities*. San Diego: Academic Press, 1991, 375–406.

Maccoby, E.E., & Jacklin, C.N. *The psychology of sex differences*. Stanford: Stanford University Press, 1974.

Mackworth, N.H. Researches on the measurement of human performance. *Medical Research Council (Great Britain) Special Report, Series*, 1950, SRS–268.

MacLean, P.D. The limbic system with respect to two basic life principles. In Brazier, M.A.B. (Ed.), *The central nervous system and behavior*. Washington, DC: National Science Foundation, 1959.

Mahl, G.F., Rothenberg, Λ., Delgado, J.M.R., & Hamlin, H. Psychological responses in the human to intracerebral electrical stimulation. *Psychosomatic Medicine*, 1964, *26*(4), 337–368.

Malatesha, R.N., & Dougan, D.R. Clinical subtypes of developmental dyslexia: Resolution of an irresolute problem. *In* Malatesha, R.N., & Aaron, P.G. (Eds.). *Reading disorders: Varieties and treatments*. New York: Academic Press, 1982, 69–92.

Manter, J.T., & Gatz, A.J. *Essentials of clinical neuroanatomy and neurophysiology*, 2nd Ed. Philadelphia: F.A. Davis Co., 1961.

March of Dimes Birth Defects Foundation. *Drugs, alcohol, tobacco use during pregnancy*. White Plains, New York: Author, 1983a.

Marcie, P., Hécaen, H. Agraphia: writing disorders associated with unilateral cortical lesions. *In* Heilman, K.M., & Valenstein, E. (Eds.),

Clinical neuropsychology. New York: Oxford University Press, 1979, 92–127.

Marshall, J.C., & Newcombe, F. Patterns of paralexia: A Psycholinguistic approach. *Journal of Psycholinguistic Research*, 1973, *2*(3), 175–199.

Marshall, J.C., & Newcombe, F. The conceptual status of deep dyslexia: An historical perspective. *In* Coltheart, M., Patterson, K., & Marshall, J.C. (Eds.), *Deep dyslexia*. London: Routledge & Kegan Paul, 1980, 1–21.

Marshall, P. Attention deficit & allergy: A neurochemical model of the relation between the illnesses. *Psychological Bulletin*, 1989, *106*, 434–446.

Martin, F., & Lovegrove, W. Flicker contrast sensitivity in normal and specifically disabled readers. *Perception*, 1987, *16*(2), 215–221.

Martin, J.H., Brust, J.C.M., & Hilal, S. Imaging the living brain. *In* Kandel, E.R., Schwartz, J.H., & Jessell, T.M. (Eds.), *Principles of neural science, 3rd edition*. New York: Elsevier, 1991, 309–324.

Masland, R.L. Children with minimal brain dysfunction; a national problem. *In* Tarnopol, L. (Ed.), *Learning disabilities: Introduction to educational and medical management*. Springfield, IL: Charles C. Thomas, 1969.

Maslow, A.H. Deficiency motivation and growth motivation. *In* Jones, M.R. (Ed.), *Nebraska symposium on motivation*. Lincoln, NE: University of Nebraska Press, 1955.

Maspes, P.E. Le syndrome expérimental chez l'homme de la section du splénium du corps calleux alexie visuelle pure hemianopsique. *Revue Neurologique (Paris)*, 1948, *80*(2), 100–112.

Masserman, J.H. Is the hypothalamus a center of emotion? *Psychosomatic Medicine*, 1941, *3*, 3–25.

Masserman, J.H. Experimental neuroses. *Scientific American*, 1950, *182*(3), 38–43.

Matazow G.S., & Hynd, G.W. *Right hemisphere deficit syndrome: Similarities with subtypes of children with Attention deficit Disorder (ADD)*. Poster presented at the 20th Annual Convention of the International Neuropsychological Society at San Diego, CA, Feb. 8, 1992.

Mateer, C., & Kimura, D. Impairment of nonverbal oral movements in aphasia. *Brain and Language*, 1976, *4*, 262–276.

Mateer, F. *Glands and efficient behavior*. New York: Appleton-Century-Crofts, 1935.

Mattes, J.A. The role of frontal lobe dysfuntion in childhood hyperkinesis. *Comprehensive Psychiatry*, 1980, *21*, 358–369.

Matthews, C.G., & Folk, E.D. Finger localization, intelligence, and arithmetic in mentally retarded subjects. *American Journal of Mental Deficiency*, 1964, *69*(1), 107–113.

Matthews, C.G., & Kløve, H. Differential psychological performances in major motor, psychomotor, and mixed seizure classifications of known and unknown etiology. *Epilepsia*, 1967, *8*, 117–128.

Mattis, S. Dyslexia syndromes: A working hypothesis that works. *In* Benton, A.L., & Pearl, D. (Eds.), *Dyslexia, an appraisal of current knowledge*. New York: Oxford University Press, 1978, 45–58.

Mattis, S., French, J.H., & Rapin, I. Dyslexia in children and young adults: three independent neuropsychological syndromes. *Developmental Medicine and Child Neurology*, 1975, *17*, 150–163.

Maugham, W.S. The verger. *In The complete short stories of W. Somerset Maugham, Vol. II*. New York: Doubleday & Co., 1953, 572–578.

Mayron, L.W. Allergy, learning & behavior problems. *Journal of Learning Disabilities*, 1979, *12*, 41–51.

McCarthy, R.A., & Warrington, E.K. *Cognitive neuropsychology: A clinical introduction*. New York: Academic Press, 1990.

McCord, J.S., & Haynes, W.O. Discourse errors in students with learning disabilities and their normally achieving peers: Molar versus molecular views. *Journal of Learning Disabilities*, 1988, *21*(4), 237–243.

McGee, R., Williams, S., & Silva, P. A comparison of girls & boys with teacher-identified problems of attention. *Journal of the American Academy of child & Adolescent Psychiatry*, 1987, *26*, 711–717.

McGeer, P.L., McGeer, E.G., & Innanen, V.T. Dendro axonic transmission. I. Evidence from receptor binding of dopaminergic and cholinergic agents. *Brain Research*, 1979, *169*, 433–441.

McGinnis, M.A. *Aphasic children: Identification and education by the association method*. Washington, DC: Volta, 1963.

McGlone, J., & Davidson, W. The relation between cerebral speech laterality and spatial ability with special reference to sex and hand preference. *Neuropsychologia*, 1973, *11*, 105–113.

McGlone, J., & Kertesz, A. Sex differences in cerebral processing of visuospatial tasks. *Cortex*, 1973, *9*, 313–320.

McGuire, W.J. Attitudes and opinions. *Annual Review of Psychology*, 1966, *17*, 474–514.

McLaughlin, J.P., Dean, P., & Stanley, P. Aesthetic preference in dextrals and sinistrals. *Neuropsychologia*, 1983, *21*(2), 147–153.

McLeod, J. *Psychometric identification of children with learning disabilities*. Saskatoon: University of Saskatchewan, 1978.

McLoughlin, J.A., & Kass, C. Resource teachers: Their role. *Learning Disability Quarterly*, 1978, *1*, 56–62.

McMahon, S.A., & Greenberg, L.M. Serial neurologic examination of hyperactive children. *Pediatrics*, 1977, *59*, 585–587.

McRae, D.L., Branch, C.L., & Milner, B. The occipital horns and cerebral dominance. *Neurology*, 1968, *18*, 95–98.

Meadows, S.R. Anticonvulsant drugs and congenital anomalies *Lancet*, 1968, *2*, 1296.

Meichenbaum, D. *Cognitive behavior modification*, New York: Plenum Press, 1977.

Mesulam, M.-M. A cortical network for directed attention and unilateral neglect. *Annals of Neurology*, 1981, *38*, 501–506.

Mesulam, M.-M. *Principles of behavioral neurology*. Philadelphia: F.A. Davis, 1985.

Meyer, A. The frontal lobe syndrome, the aphasias and related conditions, a contribution to the history of cortical localization. *Brain*, 1974, *97*, 565–600.

Meyer, V., & Yates, H.J. Intellectual changes following temporal lobectomy for psychomotor epilepsy. *Journal of Neurosurgery and Psychiatry*, 1955, *18*, 44–52.

Milberg, W.P., Hebben, N., & Kaplan, E. The Boston process approach to neuropsychological assessment. *In* Grant, I., & Adams, K.M. (Eds.), *Neuropsychological assessment of neuropsychiatric disorders*. New York: Oxford University Press, 1986.

Miller, G.A. The magical number seven, plus or minus two: Some limits on our capacity for information processing. *Psychological Review*, 1956, *63*, 81–87.

Miller, G.A., & Lenneberg, E. *Psychology and biology of language and thought*. New York: Academic Press, 1978.

Miller, R.W. Susceptibility of the fetus and child to chemical pollutants. *Science*, 1974, *184*, 812–813.

Milner, B. Intellectual function of the temporal lobes. *Psychological Bulletin*, 1954, *51*, 42–62.

Milner, B. Psychological defects produced by temporal lobe excision. *In The brain and human behavior*, Vol. 36, Proceedings of the Association for Research in Nervous and Mental Disease. Baltimore: Williams & Wilkins, 1958, *36*, 244–257.

Milner, B. Laterality effects in audition. *In* Mountcastle, V.B. (Ed.), *Interhemispheric relations and cerebral dominance*. Baltimore: The Johns Hopkins University Press, 1962, 177–195.

Milner, B. Effects of different brain lesions on card sorting. *Archives of Neurology*, 1963, *9*, 90–100.

Milner, B. Amnesia following operation on the temporal lobes. *In* Whitty, C.W.M., & Zangwill, O.L. (Eds.), *Amnesia*. London: Butterworth & Co., 1966, 109–133.

Milner, B. Brain mechanisms suggested by studies of temporal lobes. *In* Darley, F.L. (Ed.), *Brain mechanisms underlying speech and language.* New York: Grune & Stratton, 1967, 122–145.

Milner, B. Visual recognition and recall after right temporal—lobe excision in man. *Neuropsychologia*, 1968, *6*, 191–209.

Milner, B. Evidence of bilateral speech. Paper presented at Tenth Annual Neuropsychology Workshop, University of Victoria, Victoria, B.C., 1975.

Milner, B., Branch, C., & Rasmussen, T. Observations on cerebral dominance. *In* de Reuck, A.V.S., & O'Connor, M. (Eds.), *Ciba Foundation symposium on disorders of language.* London: J. & A. Churchill, 1964, 200–214.

Milner, B., Branch, C., & Rasmussen, T. Evidence for bilateral speech representation in some non-right handers. *Transactions of the American Neurological Association*, 1966, *91*, 306–308.

Milner, P.M. A neural mechanism for the immediate recall of sequences. *Kybernetick*, 1961, *1*, 76–81.

Milner, P.M. *Physiological psychology.* New York: Holt, Rinehart and Winston, 1970.

Mishkin, M., & Forgays, D.G. Word recognition as a function of retinal locus. *Journal of Experimental Psychology*, 1952, *43*, 43–48.

Mittler, P. (Ed.). *The psychological assessment of mental and physical handicaps.* London: Methuen, 1970.

Moely, B.E., Hart, S.S., Santulli, K., Leal, L., Johnson, T., & Rao, N. How do teachers teach memory skills? *Educational Psychology*, 1986, *21*, 55–57.

Money, J. Dyslexia: A postconference review. *In* Money, J. (Ed.), *Reading disability, progress, and research needs in dyslexia.* Baltimore: The Johns Hopkins University Press, 1962, 9–33.

Montessori, M. *The Montessori method: Scientific pedagogy as applied to child education in the "children's houses."* (Translated by Anne E. George.) New York: F.A. Stokes, 1912.

Montessori, M. *The Montessori method.* New York: Schocken Books, 1964.

Montessori, M. *Spontaneous activity in education.* New York: Schocken Books, 1965.

Morrell, F. Electrophysiological contributions to the neural basis of learning. *Physiological Reviews*, 1961, *41*(3), 443–494.

Morrell, F. Colloquium presentation, Massachusetts Institute of Technology, Cambridge, MA, 1967.

Morrison, S.R., & Siegal, L.S. Learning disabilities: A critical review of definitional and assessment issues. *In* Obrzut, J.E., & Hynd, G.W.

(Eds.), *Neuropsychological foundations of learning disabilities*. San Diego: Academic Press, 1991, 79–97.

Moruzzi, G., & Magoun, H.W. Brain stem reticular formation and activation of the EEG. *Electroencephalography and clinical neurophysiology*, 1949, *1*, 455–473.

Moscovitch, M. Information processing and the cerebral hemispheres. *In* Gazzaniga, M.S. (Ed.), *Handbook of behavioral neurobiology, Vol. 2, Neuropsychology*. New York: Plenum Press, 1979.

Moscovitch, M. A model of hemispheric organization based on studies of hemispheric specialization in normal and brain-damaged people. Invited paper presented at Fifteenth Annual Neuropsychology Workshop, University of Victoria, Victoria, B.C., Canada, 1980.

Moss, J.W. Neuropsychology: One way to go. *The Journal of Special Education*, 1979, *13*(1), 45–49.

Mountcastle, V.B. (Ed.). *Interhemispheric relations and cerebral dominance*. Baltimore: The Johns Hopkins University Press, 1962.

Muehl, S., & Forell, E.R. A follow-up study of disabled readers: variables related to high school reading performance. *Reading Research Quarterly*, 1973, *9*, 110–123.

Myers, P.I., & Hammill, D.D. *Learning disabilities, basic concepts, assessment practices, and instructional strategies, Fourth edition*. Austin, TX: Pro-ed, 1990.

Myklebust, H.R. *Auditory disorders in children: A manual for differential diagnosis*. New York: Grune & Stratton, 1954.

Myklebust, H.R. Psychoneurological learning disorders in children. *In* Kirk, S.A., & Becker, W. (Eds.), *Conference on children with minimal brain impairment*. Urbana: University of Illinois, 1963.

Myklebust, H.R. Personal communication, 1963.

Myklebust, H.R. *The psychology of deafness*. New York: Grune & Stratton, 1964.

Myklebust, H.R. *Development and disorders of written language*, Vol. I. New York: Grune & Stratton, 1965.

Myklebust, H.R. Learning disabilities: Definition and overview. *In* Myklebust, H.R. (Ed.), *Progress in learning disabilities*, Vol. I. New York: Grune & Stratton, 1967a, 1–15.

Myklebust, H.R. (Ed.). *Progress in learning disabilities*, Vol. I. New York: Grune & Stratton, 1967b.

Myklebust, H.R. (Ed.). *Progress in learning disabilities*, Vol. II. New York: Grune & Stratton, 1971a.

Myklebust, H.R. Childhood aphasia: An evolving concept: and Childhood aphasia: Identification, diagnosis, remediation. Chapters 46 and 47 *in*

Travis, L.E. (Ed.), *Handbook of speech pathology and audiology*. New York: Appleton-Century-Crofts. 1971b, 1181–1217.

Myklebust, H.R. *Development and disorders of written language*, Vol. II. New York: Grune & Stratton, 1973a.

Myklebust, H.R. Identification and diagnosis of children with learning disabilities: An interdisciplinary study of criteria. *In* Walzer, S., & Wolff, P.H. (Eds.), *Minimal cerebral dysfunction in children*. New York: Grune & Stratton, 1973b.

Myklebust, H.R. (Ed.), *Progress in learning disabilities*. Vol. III. New York: Grune & Stratton, 1975a.

Myklebust, H.R. Nonverbal learning disabilities: assessment and intervention. *In* Myklebust, H.R. (Ed.), *Progress in learning disabilities*, Vol. III. New York: Grune & Stratton, 1975b, 85–121.

Myklebust, H.R. Preface in Myklebust, H.R. (Ed.), *Progress in learning disabilities, Vol. V*. New York: Grune & Stratton, 1983.

Myklebust, H.R., & Boshes, B. *Final report, minimal brain damage in children*. Washington, DC: U.S. Department of Health, Education, and Welfare, 1969.

Myklebust, H.R., & Brutten, M.A. study of the visual perception of deaf children. *Acta Oto-laryngolica*, 1953, Supplementum 105. Whole Monograph, 126 pp.

Näätänen, R. Evoked potential, EEG, and slow potential correlates of selective attention. *Acta Psychologica*, 1970, *33*, 178–192.

Naeye, R.L., & Peters, E.C. Mental development of children whose mothers smoked during pregnancy. *Obstetrics and Gynecology*, 1984, *64*, 301.

National Advisory Committee on Handicapped Children, *Special Education for Handicapped Children*, First Annual Report. Washington, DC: U.S. Dept. of Health, Education, and Welfare, Office of Education, 1968.

National Conference on Learning Disabilities. *In* Kavanaugh, J.F., & Truss, T.J., (Eds.), *Proceedings of the National Conference on Learning Disabilities*. Parkton Maryland; Yorkton Press, 1988.

National Joint Committee on Learning Disabilities, A position paper. *Journal of Learning Disabilities*, 1987, *20*(2), 107–108.

Needleman, H.L., Gunnoe, C., Leviton, A., Reed, R., Peresie, H., Maher, C., & Barrett, P. Deficits in psychologic and classroom performance of children with elevated dentine lead levels. *New England Journal of Medicine*, 1979, *300*, 689–695.

Neisser, U. *Cognitive psychology*, New York: Appleton-Century-Crofts, 1967.

Netter, F.H. *The CIBA Collection of Medical Illustrations, Vol. I, Nervous System*. New York: CIBA, 1972.

Newcombe, F., & Marshall, J.C. On psycholinguistic classifications of the acquired dyslexias. *Bulletin of the Orton Society*, 1981, *31*, 29–46.

Newell, A. Reasoning, problem-solving, and decision processes: The problem space as a fundamental category. *In* Nickerson, R. (Ed.), *Attention & performance VIII*. New Jersey: Lawrence Erlbraum, 1980.

Newman, S., Wright, S., & Fields, H. Identifying subtypes of reading and spelling disorders by discrepancy scores. *The Irish Journal of Psychology*, 1989, *10*(4), 647–656.

Nieburg, P., Marks, J.S., McLaren, N.M., & Remington, P.L. The fetal tobacco syndrome. *Journal of the American Medical Association*, 1985, *253*, 2998–2999.

Nodine, B.F., Barenbaum, E., & Newcomer, P. Story composition by learning disabled, reading disabled, and normal children. *Learning Disability Quarterly*, 1985, *8*, 167–179.

Nolan, K.A., & Caramazza, A. An analysis of writing in a case of deep dyslexia. *Brain and Language*, 1983, *20*, 305–328.

Nolte, J. *The human brain: An introduction to its functional anatomy*. St. Louis: C.V. Mosby, 2nd ed., 1988.

Obrzut, J.E. Neuropsychological procedures with school-age children. *In* Hynd, G.W., & Obrzut, J.E. (Eds.). *Neuropsychological assessment and the school-age child: Issues and procedures*. New York: Grune & Stratton, 1981, 237–275.

Obrzut, J.E., & Hynd, G.W. (Eds.). *Child Neuropsychology: Theory and Research, Vol. I*. New York: Academic Press, 1986a.

Obrzut, J.E., & Hynd, G.W. (Eds.). *Child Neuropsychology: Clinical Practice, Vol. 2*. New York: Academic Press, 1986b.

Obrzut, J.E., & Hynd, G.W. (Eds.). *Neuropsychological foundations of learning disabilities: A handbook of issues, methods, and practice*. San Diego: Academic Press, 1991.

O'Donnell, J.P. Neuropsychological assessment of learning disabled adolescents and young adults. *In* Obrzut, J.E., & Hynd, G.W. (Eds.). *Neuropsychological foundations of learning disabilities*. San Diego: Academic Press, 1991, 331–353.

Ojemann, G.A. Mental arithmetic during human thalamic stimulation. *Neuropsychologia*, 1974, *12*, 1–10.

Ojemann, G.A. Language and the thalamus: Object naming and recall during and after thalamic stimulation. *Brain and Language*, 1975, *2*, 101–120.

Ojemann, G.A. Individual variability in cortical localization of language. *Journal of Neurosurgery*, 1979, *50*, 164–169.

Ojemann, G.A. Interrelationships in the brain organization of language-related behaviors: Evidence from electrical stimulation mapping. *In* Kirk, U. (Ed.), *Neuropsychology of language, reading, and spelling.* New York: Academic Press, 1983, 129–152.

Ojemann, G.A., & Mateer, C. Human language cortex: Localization of memory, syntax, and sequential motor-phoneme identification systems. *Science*, 1979, *205*, 1401–1403.

Ojemann, G.A., & Whitaker, H.A. Language localization and variability. *Brain and Language*, 1978, *6*, 239–260.

Oldfield, R.C. The assessment and analysis of handedness: The Edinburgh inventory. *Neuropsychologia*, 1971, *9*, 97–113

Orton, S.T. "Word-blindness" in school children. *Archives of Neurology and Psychiatry*, 1925, *14*, 581–615.

Orton, S.T. Reading disability. *Genetic Psychology Monographs*, 1926, *14*, 335–453.

Orton, S.T. Specific reading disability—Strephosymbolia. *Journal of the American Medical Association*, 1928, *90*, 1095–1099.

Orton, S.T. *Reading, writing and speech problems in children.* New York: W.W. Norton, 1937.

Osler, W. *Aequanimitas, with other addresses to medical students, nurses and practitioners of medicine, 2nd ed.* London: H.K. Lewis, 1906.

Osofsky, J.D. *Handbook of infant development.* New York: Wiley, 1979.

Ott, J.N. *Health and light.* New York: Pocket Books, 1976.

Ounsted, C., & Taylor, D.C. (Eds.). *Gender differences: Their ontogeny and significance.* Edinburgh: Churchill Livingstone, 1972.

Paine, R.S. Minimal chronic brain syndromes in children. *Developmental Medicine and Child Neurology*, 1962, *4*, 21–27.

Paivio, A., & te Linde, J. Imagery, memory, and the brain. *Canadian Journal of Psychology*, 1982, *36*(2), 243–272.

Parks, R.W., Loewenstein, D.A., Dodrill, K.L., Barker, W.W., Yoshii, F., Chang, J.Y., Emran, A., Apicella, A., Sheramata, W.A., & Duara, R. Cerebral metabolic effects of a verbal fluency test: A PET scan study. *Journal of Clinical and Experimental Neuropsychology*, 1988, *10*(5), 565–575.

Pavlidis, G.Th. How can dyslexia be objectively diagnosed? *Reading*, 1979, *13*(3), 3–15.

Pavlidis, G.Th. Erratic sequential eye movements in dyslexics: Comments and reply to Stanley *et al. British Journal of Psychology*, 1983, *74*, 189–193.

Pavlidis, G.Th. The role of eye movements in the diagnosis of dyslexia. *In* Pavlidis, G.Th., & Fisher, D.F. (Eds.), *Dyslexia: Its neuropsychology and treatment.* New York: John Wiley & Sons, 1986, 97–110.

Pavlov, I.P. *Lectures on conditioned reflexes*. New York: International Publishers, 1928.

Pearson, L. *Children of glasnost*. Toronto: Lester & Orpen Dennys, 1990.

Pelham, W.E. The effects of psychostimulant drugs on learning & academic achievement in children with attention-deficits disorders & learning disabilities. *In* Torgesen, J., & Wong, B.Y.L. (Eds.), *Psychological & Educational Perspectives on Learning Disabilities*. New York: Academic Press, 1986, 259–295.

Pelham, W.E., & Murphy, H.A. Attention deficit and conduct disorders. *In* Hersen, M. (Ed.), *Pharmacological & behavioral treatment: An integrative approach*. New York: J. Wiley & Sons, 1986, 108–148.

Penfield, W. The cerebral cortex in man: I. The cerebral cortex and consciousness. *Archives of Neurology and Psychiatry*. Chicago. 1938, *40*, 417–442.

Penfield, W. Some observations of the cerebral cortex of man. Ferrier Lecture. *Proceedings of the Royal Society*, 1947, *134*, 329–347.

Penfield, W. *No man alone, a neurosurgeon's life*. Boston: Little, Brown, 1977.

Penfield, W., & Roberts, L. *Speech and brain mechanisms*. Princeton: Princeton University Press, 1959.

Pennington, B. *Diagnosing learning disorders*. New York: Guilford Press, 1991.

Pennington, H., Galliani, C.A., & Voegele, G.E. Unilateral electroencephalographic dysrhythmia and children's intelligence. *Child Development*, 1965, *36*, 539–546.

Petersen, L.R., & Petersen, M.J. Short-term retention of individual items. *Journal of Experimental Psychology*, 1959, *91*, 341–343.

Petersen, S.E., Fox, P.T., Posner, M.I., Mintun, M.A., & Raichle, M.E. Positron emission tomographic studies of the cortical anatomy of single word processing. *Nature*, 1988, *331*, 585–589.

Phillips, J.L. *The Origins of Intellect: Piaget's Theory*. San Francisco: W.H. Freeman, 1969 (1st Ed.)/1975 (2nd Ed.).

Piaget, J. *The child's conception of number*. London: Routledge & Kegan Paul, 1941.

Piaget, J. *The origins of intelligence in children*. New York: International Universities Press, 1952.

Piaget, J. *The language and thought of the child*. New York: Humanities Press, 1965.

Piaget, J., & Inhelder B. *The child's conception of space*. London: Routledge & Kegan Paul, 1956.

Piaget, J., & Inhelder, B. *Mental imagery in the child*. London: Routledge & Kegan Paul, 1971.

Pierson, J.M., Bradshaw, J.L., & Nettleton, N.C. Head and body space to left and right, front and rear—I. Unidirectional competitive auditory stimulation. *Neuropsychologia*, 1983, *21*(5), 463–473.

Pihl, R.O. Learning disabilities: programs in the schools. *In* Myklebust, H.R. (Ed.), *Progress in learning disabilities*, Vol. III. New York: Grune & Stratton, 1975, 19–48.

Pirozzolo, F.J. *The neuropsychology of developmental reading disorders*. New York: Praeger Publishers, 1979.

Pirozzolo, F.J. Language and brain: Neuropsychological aspects of developmental reading disability. *School Psychology Review*, 1981, X(3), 350–355.

Pisterman, S., McGrath, P., Firestone, P., Goodman, J., Webster, I., & Mallory, R. Outcome of parent-mediated treatment for preschoolers with attention deficit disorder with hyperactivity. *Journal of Consulting & Clinical Psychology*, 1989, *57*, 628–635.

Plato, *The Republic*. Great Books of the Western World, Vol. 7. Toronto: Encyclopaedia Britannica, 1952, 295–441.

Poeck, K. What do we mean by "Aphasic Syndromes?": A neurologist's view. *Brain and Language*, 1983, *20*, 79–89.

Poeck, K., & Orgass, B. The concept of the body schema: A critical review and some experimental results. *Cortex*, 1971, *7*(3), 254–277.

Porges, S.W., Walter, G.F., Korb, R.J., & Sprague, R.L. The influence of methylphenidate on heart rate and behavioral measures of attention. *Child Development*, 1975, *46*, 727–733.

Porter, J.E., & Rourke, B.P. Socioemotional functioning of learning disabled children: A subtypal analysis of personality patterns. *In* Rourke, B.P. (Ed.), *Neuropsychology of learning disabilities: Essentials of subtype analysis*. New York: The Guilford Press, 1985, 257–280.

Posner, M.I., & Boies, S.J. Components of attention. *Psychological Review*, 1971, *78*, 391–408.

Posner, M.I., & Peterson, S.E. (in press). The attention system of the human brain. *Annual Review of Neuroscience*.

Posner, M.I., Petersen, S.E., Fox, P.T., & Raichle, M.E. Localization of cognitive operations in the human brain. *Science*, 1988, *240*, 1627–1631.

Prechtl, H.F.R. Minimal brain dysfunction syndrome and the plasticity of the nervous system. *Advances in Biological Psychiatry*, 1978, *1*, 95–105.

Pribram, K.H. Neurological notes on the art of educating. *In* Hilgard, E.R. (Ed.), *Sixty-third Yearbook, National Society for the Study of Education*. Chicago: University of Chicago Press, Part I, 1964, 78–110.

Pribram, K.H. *Languages of the brain*. Englewood Cliffs, NJ: Prentice-Hall, 1971.

Prout, H.T. Behavioral intervention with hyperactive children: A review. *Journal of Learning Disabilities*, 1977, *10*(3), 141–146.

Provins, K.A. Motor skills, handedness, and behaviour. *Australian Journal of Psychology*, 1967, *19*, 137–150.

Prutting, C.A., & Kirchner, D.M. A clinical appraisal of the pragmatic aspects of language. *Journal of Speech and Hearing Disorders*, 1987, *52*, 105–119.

Quadfasel, F.A., & Goodglass, H. Specific reading disability and other specific disabilities. *Journal of Learning Disabilities*, 1968, *1*(10), 590–600.

Raab, G.M., Fulton, M., Laxen, D.P.H., & Thomson, G.O.B. The Edinburgh lead study; aspects of design and progress. *The Statistician*, 1985, *34*, 45–57.

Raab, G.M., Thomson, G.O.B., Boyd, L., Fulton, M., & Laxen, D.P.H. Blood lead levels, reaction time, inspection time and ability in Edinburgh children. *British Journal of Developmental Psychology*, 1990, *8*, 101–118.

Raczkowski, D., Kalat, J.W., & Nebes, R. Reliability and validity of some handedness questionnaire items. *Neuropsychologia*, 1974, *12*, 43–47.

Rapcsak, S.K., Fleet, W.S., Verfaellie, M., & Heilman, K.M. Selective attention in hemispatial neglect. *Archives of Neurology*, 1989, *4*, 1863–1874.

Rapp, D.J. Does diet affect hyperactivity? *Journal of Learning Disabilities*, 1978, *11*, 383–389.

Rapport, J.L., Buchsbaum, M., Weingartner, H., Zahn, T., Ludlow, C., & Mikkelson, E.J. Dextroamphetamine: Cognitive & behavior effects in normal & hyperactive boys & normal men. *Archives of General Psychiatry*, 1980, *37*, 933–934.

Ratcliff, G., Dila, C., Taylor, L., & Milner, B. The morphological asymmetry of the hemispheres and cerebral dominance for speech: A possible relationship. *Brain and Language*, 1980, *11*, 87–98.

Raven, J.C. *The Coloured Progressive Matrices Test*. London: Lewis, 1965.

Reed, D.W. A theory of language, speech, and writing. *In* Singer, H., & Ruddell, R.B. (Eds.), *Theoretical models and processes of reading*. Newark, DE: International Reading Association, 1970, 219–238.

Reed, J.C., & Reitan, R.M. Verbal and performance differences among brain-injured children with lateralized motor deficits. *Perceptual and Major Skills*, 1969, *29*, 747–752.

Regehr, S.M. The genetic aspects of developmental dyslexia. *Canadian Journal of Behavioural Science*, 1987, *19*(3), 239–253.

Reitan, R.M. Certain differential effects of left and right cerebral lesions in human adults. *Journal of Comparative and Physiological Psychology*, 1955a, *48*, 474–477.

Reitan, R.M. Investigation of the validity of Halstead's measures of biological intelligence. *American Medical Association Archives of Neurology and Psychiatry*, 1955b, *73*, 28–35.

Reitan, R.M. Investigation of relationships between "psychometric" and "biological" intelligence. *Journal of Nervous and Mental Disease*, 1956, *123*, 536–541.

Reitan, R.M. The validity of the Trail Making Test as an indicator of organic brain damage. *Perceptual and Motor Skills*, 1958, *8*, 271–276.

Reitan, R.M. *The effects of brain lesions on adaptive abilities in human beings*. Indianapolis: Indiana University Medical Center, 1959. (mimeo.)

Reitan, R.M. *The effects of brain lesions on adaptive abilities in human beings*. Tucson, AZ: Neuropsychology Press, 1959.

Reitan, R.M. *Manual for administering and scoring the Reitan–Indiana Neuropsychological Battery for Children (aged 5 through 8)*. Indianapolis: University of Indiana Medical Center, 1964a.

Reitan, R.M. Psychological deficits resulting from cerebral lesions in man. *In* Warren, J.M., & Akert, K.A. (Eds.), *The frontal granular cortex and behavior*. New York: McGraw-Hill, 1964b, 301.

Reitan, R.M. The needs of teachers for specialized information in the area of neuropsychology. *In* Cruickshank, W.M. (Ed.), *The teacher of brain-injured children*. Syracuse: Syracuse University Press, 1966a, 225–243.

Reitan, R.M. Diagnostic inferences of brain lesions based on psychological test results. *The Canadian Psychologist*, 1966b, *7a*(4), Inst. Suppl., 368–388.

Reitan, R.M. Psychological effects of cerebral lesions in children of early school age. *In* Reitan, R.M., & Davison, L.A. (Eds.), *Clinical neuropsychology: Current status and applications*. Washington, DC: Winston, 1974, 53–89.

Reitan, R.M., & Boll, T.J. Neuropsychological correlates of minimal brain dysfunction. *Annals of the New York Academy of Sciences*, 1973, *205*, 65–88.

Reitan, R.M., & Davison, L.A. *Clinical neuropsychology: Current status and applications*. Washington, DC: Winston, 1974.

Reitan, R.M., & Wolfson, D. *Neuropsychological evaluation of young children*. Tucson, AZ: Neuropsychology Press, 1992a.

Reitan, R.M., & Wolfson, D. *Neuropsychological evaluation of older children*. Tucson, AZ: Neuropsychology Press, 1992b.

Reitan, R.M., & Wolfson, D. *The Halstead-Reitan neuropsychological test battery, 2nd edition.* Tucson, AZ: Neuropsychology Press, 1992c.

Reitan, R.M., & Wolfson, D. Conventional intelligence measurements and neuropsychological concepts of adaptive abilities. *Journal of Clinical Psychology*, 1992d, *48*, 521–529.

Rennie, J. Defining dyslexia. *Scientific American*, July 1992, 31–32.

Reschly, D.J., & Gresham, F.M. Current neuropsychological diagnosis of learning problems: A leap of faith. *In* Reynolds, C.R., & Fletcher-Janzen, E. (Eds.), *Handbook of clinical child neuropsychology.* New York: Plenum, 1989, 503–519.

Restak, R.M. *The brain.* New York: Bantam Books, 1984.

Reynolds, C.R. The fallacy of "two years below grade level for age" as a diagnostic criterion for reading disorders. *Journal of School Psychology*, 1981a, *19*(4), 350–358.

Reynolds, C.R. Neuropsychological assessment and the habilitation of learning: considerations in the search for the aptitude x treatment interaction. *School Psychology Review*, 1981b, *10*(3), 343–349.

Reynolds, C.R. Critical measurement issues in learning disabilities. *The Journal of Special Education*, 1984–1985, *18*(4), 451–475.

Reynolds, C.R. Measuring the aptitude-achievement discrepancy in learning disability diagnosis. *Remedial and Special Education*, 1985, *6*(5), 37–55.

Reynolds, C.R., & Fletcher-Janzen, E. (Eds.). *Handbook of Clinical Child Neuropsychology.* New York: Plenum, 1989.

Richards, G.P., Samuels, S.J., Turnure, J., & Ysseldyke, J. Sustained and selective attention in children with learning disabilities. *Journal of Learning Disabilities & Reading Disorders*, 1990, *23*, 129–136.

Riese, W. Kurt Goldstein—The Man and His Work. *In* Simmel, M.L. (Ed.), *The reach of mind, essays in memory of Kurt Goldstein.* New York: Springer Publishing Co., 1968.

Risberg, J., Halsey, J.H., Wills, E.L., & Wilson, E.M. Hemispheric specialization in normal man studied by bilateral measurements of the regional cerebral blood flow—a study with the 133-Xe inhalation technique. *Brain*, 1975, *98*, Pt. III, 511–524.

Robb, P. *Epilepsy, a manual for health workers.* Bethesda, MD: NIH Publication, No. 82–2350, September 1981.

Roberts, L. Childhood aphasia and handedness. *In* West, R. (Ed.), *Childhood aphasia.* San Francisco: California Society for Crippled Children and Adults, 1962, 45–46.

Robinson, N.M., & Robinson, H.B. *The mentally retarded child, a psychological approach*, 2nd Ed. New York: McGraw-Hill, 1976, 255.

Robinson, S.M. Collaborative consultation. *In* Wong, B.Y.L. (Ed.), *Learning about learning disabilities*. San Diego: Academic Press, 1991, 441–463.

Rockel, A.J., Hiorns, R.W., & Powell, T.P.S. Numbers of neurons through full depth of neocortex. *Proceedings of the Anatomy Society of Britain and Ireland*, 1974, *118*, 371.

Rosen, B.R., & Brady, T.J. Principles of nuclear magnetic resonance for medical application, *Seminars in Nuclear Medicine*, 1983, XIII(4), 308–318.

Rosen, G.D., Sherman, G.F., & Galaburda, A.M. Biological interactions in dyslexia. *In* Obrzut, J.E., & Hynd, G.W. (Eds.), *Child neuropsychology: Theory and research, Vol. 1*. New York: Academic Press, 1986, 155–173.

Rosenblith, J.F., & Sims-Knight, J.E. *In the beginning: development in the first two years*. Monterey: Brooks-Cole, 1985.

Rosenzweig, M.R. Auditory localization. *Scientific American*, 1961, *205*, 132–142.

Rosenzweig, M.R. Environmental complexity, cerebral change, and behavior. *American Psychologist*, 1966, *21*(4), 321–332.

Rosenzweig, M.R., Krech, D., Bennett, E.L., & Diamond, M.C. Modifying brain chemistry and anatomy by enrichment or impoverishment of experience. *In* Newton, G., & Levine, S. (Eds.), *Early experience and behaviour*. Springfield, IL: Charles C. Thomas, 1968.

Rosett, H.L., & Sander, L.W. Effects of maternal drinking on neonatal morphology & state regulation. *In* Osofsky, J. (Ed.). *Handbook of infant development*. New York: Wiley & Sons, 1979, 809–836.

Rosner, J. *Helping children overcome learning difficulties*, 2nd Ed. New York: Walker & Co., 1979.

Ross, D.M., & Ross, S.A. *Hyperactivity, research, theory, action*. New York: Wiley, 1976.

Ross, D.M., & Ross, S.A. *Hyperactivity: Current issues, research, and theory, 2nd Edition*. New York: Wiley, 1982.

Rourke, B.P. Brain-behavior relationships in children with learning disabilities: A research program. *American Psychologist*, 1975, *30*, 911–920.

Rourke, B.P. Neuropsychological assessment of children with learning disabilities. *In* Filskov, S.B., & Boll, T.J. (Eds.), *Handbook of clinical neuropsychology*. New York: Wiley-Interscience, 1981.

Rourke, B.P. Central processing deficiencies in children: Toward a developmental neuropsychological model. *Journal of Clinical Neuropsychology*, 1982, *4*(1), 1–18.

Rourke, B.P. (Ed.). *Neuropsychology of learning disabilities: Essentials of subtype analysis*. New York: Guilford Press, 1985.

Rourke, B.P. *Nonverbal learning disabilities*. New York: Guilford Press, 1989.

Rourke, B.P., Bakker, D.J., Fisk, J.L., & Strang, J.D. *Child neuropsychology, an introduction to theory, research, and clinical practice*. New York: Guilford, 1983.

Rourke, B.P., & Finlayson, M.A.J. Neuropsychological significance of variations in patterns of academic performance: verbal and visual-spatial abilities. *Journal of Abnormal Child Psychology*, 1978, *6*, 121–133.

Rourke, B.P., & Gates, R.D. Neuropsychological research and school psychology. *In* Hynd, G.W., & Obrzut, J.E. (Eds.), *Neuropsychological assessment and the school-age child*. New York: Grune & Stratton, 1981, 3–25.

Rourke, B.P., & Orr, R.R. Prediction of the reading and spelling performances of normal and retarded readers: a four year follow-up. *Journal of Abnormal Child Psychology*, 1977, *5*(1), 9–20.

Russell, W.R., & Espir, M.L.E. *Traumatic aphasia, a study of aphasia in war wounds of the brain*. London: Oxford University Press, 1961.

Rutter, M. Brain damage syndrome in childhood: Concepts & findings. *Journal of Child Psychology & Psychiatry*, 1977, *18*, 1–21.

Rutter, M., Graham, P., & Yule, W. *A Neuropsychiatric Study in Childhood*. Philadelphia: Lippincott, 1970.

Rutter, M., Tizard, J., & Whitmore, K. (Eds.). *Education, health and behaviour*. London: Longmans, 1970.

Safer, D.J., & Krager, J.M. A survey of medication treatment for hyperactive/inattentive students. *Journal of the American Medical Association*, 1988, *260*, 2256–2258.

Sagal, R., Rosenbaum, P., Stotskopf, B., & Milner, R. Follow-up of infants 501–1500 gm birth weight delivered to residents of a geographically defined region with perinatal intensive care facilities. *Journal of Pediatrics*, 1982, *100*, 606–613.

Salame, P., & Baddeley, A. Disruption of short-term memory by unattended speech: Implications for the structure of working memory. *Journal of Verbal Learning & Verbal Behavior*, 1982, *21*, 150–164.

Salk, L. The role of the heart beat in the relations between mother and infant. *Scientific American*, 1973, *228*(5), 24–29.

Samuels, S.J. Automatic decoding and reading comprehension. *Language Arts*, 1976, *53*, 323–325.

Sandström, C. Sex differences in localization and orientation. *Acta Psychologica*, 1953, *9*, 82–96.

Sanides, F. Comparative neurology of the temporal lobe in primates including man with reference to speech. *Brain and Language*, 1975, *2*, 396–419.

Satterfield, J.H., Cantwell, D.P., Saul, R.E., Lesser, L.I., & Podosin, R.L. Response to stimulant drug treatment in hyperactive children: Prediction from EEG & neurological findings. *Autism & Childhood Schizophrenia*, 1973, *3*, 36–48.

Satterfield, J.H., & Dawson, M.E. Electrodermal correlates of hyperactivity in children. *Psychophysiology*, 1971, *8*, 191–197.

Satz, P. Pathological left-handedness: An explanatory model. *Cortex*, 1972, *8*, 121–135.

Satz, P. Left-handedness and early brain insult: An explanation. *Neuropsychologia*, 1973, *11*, 115–117.

Satz, P., Achenbach, K., & Fennell, E. Correlations between assessed manual laterality and predicted speech laterality in a normal population. *Neuropsychologia*, 1967, *5*, 295–310.

Satz, P., & Bullard-Bates, C. Acquired aphasia in children. *In* Sarno, M.T. (Ed.), *Acquired aphasia*. New York: Academic Press, 1981, 399–426.

Satz, P., & Fletcher, J.M. Early screening tests: Some uses and abuses. *Journal of Learning Disabilities*, 1979, *12*, 43–50.

Satz, P., Taylor, H.G., Friel, J., & Fletcher, J.M. Some developmental and predictive precursors of reading disabilities: A six year follow-up. *In* Benton, A.L., & Pearl, D. (Eds.), *Dyslexia: An appraisal of current knowledge*. New York: Oxford University Press, 1978.

Sauerwein, H., & Lassonde, M.C. Intra- and interhemispheric processing of visual information in callosal agenesis. *Neuropsychologia*, 1983, *21*(2), 167–171.

Sawrey, W.L., & Sawrey, J.M. Conditioned fear and restraint in ulceration. *Journal of Comparative and Physiological Psychology*, 1964, *57*(1), 150–151.

Sawrey, W.L., & Sawrey, J.M. UCS effects on ulceration following fear conditioning. *Psychonomic Science*, 1968, *10*(3), 85–86.

Sawrey, W.L., & Wiesz, J.D. An experimental method of producing gastric ulcers. *Journal of Comparative and Physiological Psychology*, 1956, *49*, 269–270.

Schacter, D.L. Memory, amnesia, and frontal lobe dysfunction. *Psychobiology*, 1987, *15*, 21–36.

Schain, R.J. *Neurology of childhood learning disorders*. Baltimore: Williams & Wilkins, 1972.

Schmahmann, J.D. An emerging concept: The cerebellar contribution to higher function. *Archives of Neurology*, 1991, *48*(11), 1178–1187.

Schmidt, R.F. (Ed.). *Fundamentals of sensory physiology*. New York: Springer-Verlag, 1978a.

Schmidt, R.F. (Ed.). *Fundamentals of neurophysiology*, 2nd Ed. New York: Springer-Verlag, 1978b.

Schmitt, B.D. The minimal brain dysfunction myth. *American Journal of Diseases of Children*, 1975, *129*, 1313–1318.

Schmitt, F.O., & Worden, F.G. (Eds.) *The neurosciences, fourth study program*. Cambridge, MA: The M.I.T. Press, 1979.

Schoemaker, M.M., & Kalverboer, A.F. Treatment of clumsy children. *In* Kalverboer, A.F. (Ed.). *Developmental biopsychology*. Ann Arbor: The University of Michigan Press, 1990, 241–255.

Schwartz, M.F. What the classical aphasia categories can't do for us, and why. *Brain and Language*, 1984, *21*, 3–8.

Scoville, W.B., & Milner, B. Loss of recent memory after bilateral hippocampal lesions. *Journal of Neurology, Neurosurgery, and Psychiatry*, 1957, *20*(11), 11–19.

Scrimshaw, N.S., & Gordon, J.E. (Eds.). *Malnutrition, learning and behavior*. Cambridge, MA: The M.I.T. Press, 1968.

Scull, J.W. *The Cedar Lodge colour reading project*. Cobble Hill, B.C., Canada: Cedar Lodge Centre, 1978.

Seashore, C.E., Lewis, D., & Saetveit, J.G. *Seashore measures of musical talents, manual, revised 1960*. New York: The Psychological Corporation, 1960.

Segalowitz, S.J. (Ed.). *Language functions and brain organization*. New York: Academic Press, 1983.

Segalowitz, S.J., & Bryden, M.P. Individual differences in hemispheric representation of language. *In* Segalowitz, S.J. (Ed.), *Language functions and brain organization*. New York: Academic Press, 1983, 341–372.

Segalowitz, S.J., & Gruber, F.A. (Eds.). *Language development and neurological theory*. New York: Academic Press, 1977.

Seifert, A.R., & Lubar, J.F., Reduction of epileptic seizures through EEG feedback training. *Biological Psychology*, 1975, *3*, 157–184.

Seino, M., & Wada, J.A. Chronic focal cortical epileptogenic lesion and behavior. *Epilepsia*, 1964, *5*, 321–333.

Selz, M. Halstead-Reitan neuropsychological test batteries for children. *In* Hynd, G.W., & Obrzut, J.E. (Eds.), *Neuropsychological assessment and the school-age child: Issues and procedures*. New York: Grune & Stratton, 1981, 195–235.

Semmes, J. A non-tactual factor in astereognosis. *Neuropsychologia*, 1965, *3*, 295–315.

Semrud-Clikeman, M., & Hynd, G.W. Specific nonverbal and social-skills deficits in children with learning disabilities. *In* Obrzut, J.E., & Hynd, G.W. (Eds.). *Neuropsychological foundations of learning disabilities*. San Diego: Academic Press, 1991, 603–629.

Semrud-Clikeman, M., Hynd, G.W., Novey, E.S., & Eliopulos, D. Dyslexia and brain morphology: Relationships between neuroanatomical variation and neurolinguistic tasks. *Learning and Individual Differences*, 1991, *3*(3), 225–242.

Senden, M.v. Raum- und Gestaltauffasung bei operierten Blindgeborenen vor und nach der Operation. Leipzig: Barth, 1932. Described in D.O. Hebb, *Organization of Behavior*, 1949.

Senf, G.M. Development of immediate memory for bisensory stimuli in normal children and children with learning disorders. *Developmental Psychology Monograph*, 1969, *6*, 1–29.

Senf, G.M. Can neuropsychology really change the face of special education? *The Journal of Special Education*, 1979, *13*(1), 51–56.

Serwer, B.L., Shapiro, B.J., & Shapiro, P.P. The comparative effectiveness of four methods of instruction on the achievement of children with specific learning disabilities. *Journal of Special Education*, 1973, *7*(3), 241–249.

Shallice, T. *From neuropsychology to mental structure*. New York: Cambridge University Press, 1988.

Shankweiler, D., & Liberman, I.Y. Exploring the relations between reading and speech. *In* Knights, R.M., & Bakker, D.J. (Eds.). *The neuropsychology of learning disorders: Theoretical approaches*. Baltimore: University Park Press, 1976, 297–313.

Shankweiler, D., Liberman, I.Y., Marks, S.L., & Fischer, F.W. The speech code and learning to read. *Journal of Experimental Psychology: Human Learning & Memory*, 1984, *4*, 531–545.

Shankweiler, D., & Studdert-Kennedy, M. A continuum of lateralization for speech perception. *Brain and Language*, 1975, *2*(2), 212–225.

Shannon, W.R. Neuropathic manifestations in infants & children as a result of anaphylactic reactions to foods contained in their dietary. *American Journal of Diseases of Children*, 1922, *24*, 89–94.

Shapley, R. Visual sensitivity and parallel retinocortical channels. *Annual Review of Psychology*, 1990, *41*, 635–658.

Shayer, M. Neo-Piagetian theories and educational practice. *International Journal of Psychology*, 1987, *22*, 751–772.

Shaywitz, B.A., Cohen, D.J., & Bowers, M.B. CSF monoamine metabolites in children with minimal brain dysfunction: Evidence for alteration of brain dopamine. *Journal of Pediatrics*, 1977, *1*, 67–71.

Shaywitz, S.E., Escobar, M.D., Shaywitz, B.A., Fletcher, J.M., & Makuch, R. Evidence that dyslexia may represent the lower tail of a normal distribution of reading ability. *The New England Journal of Medicine*, 1992, *326*(3), 145–150.

Shaywitz, S.E., Hunt, R.D., Jatlow, P., Cohen, D.J., Young, J.G., Pierce, R.N., Anderson, G.M., & Shaywitz, B.A. Psychopharmacology of attention deficit disorder: Pharmacokinetic neuroendocrine & behavioral measures following acute & chronic treatment with methylphenidate. *Pediatrics*, 1982, *69*, 688–694.

Shaywitz, S.E., & Shaywitz, B.A., Attention deficit disorder: Current perspectives. *In* Kavanaugh, J.F., & Truss, T.J., (Eds.), *Learning disabilities: Proceedings of the national conference*. Parkton, MD: York Press, 1988, 369–523.

Shaywitz, S.E., & Shaywitz, B.A., Introduction to the special series on attention deficit disorder. *Journal of Learning Disabilities*. 1991, *24*, 68–71.

Sherrington, C.S. *The integrative action of the nervous system*. New Haven: Yale University Press, 1906.

Shetty, T., & Chase, T.N. Central monoamines and hyperkinesis of childhood. *Neurology*, 1976, *26*, 1000–1002.

Sidtis, J.J. On the nature of the cortical function underlying right hemisphere auditory perception. *Neuropsychologia*, 1980, *18*, 321–330.

Sidtis, J.J., & Bryden, M.P. Asymmetrical perception of language and music: Evidence for independent processing strategies. *Neuropsychologia*, 1978, *16*, 627–632.

Siegel, L.S. Evidence that IQ scores are irrelevant to the definition and analysis of reading disability. *Canadian Journal of Psychology*, 1988, *42*(2), 201–215.

Siegel, L.S. IQ is irrelevant to the definition of learning disabilities. *Journal of Learning Disabilities*, 1989, *22*(8), 469–478, 486.

Siegel, L.S., & Linder, B.A. Short-term memory processing in children with reading and arithmetic learning disabilities. *Developmental Psychology*, 1984, *20*, 200–207.

Silver, A.A. Prevention. *In* Benton, A.L., & Pearl, D. (Eds.), *Dyslexia, an appraisal of current knowledge*. New York: Oxford University Press, 1978, 351–376.

Silver, A.A., & Hagin, R.A. *Search*. New York: Bellevue Medical Center, 1975.

Silverman, L.J., & Metz, A.S. Number of pupils with specific learning disabilities in local public schools in the United States: Spring 1970. *Annals of the New York Academy of Sciences*, 1973, *205*, 146–157.

Skinner, B.F. *The behavior of organisms*. New York: Appleton-Century, 1938.

Skinner, B.F. *Verbal behavior*. New York: Appleton-Century-Crofts, 1957.

Skinner, B.F. *The technology of teaching*. Englewood Cliffs, NJ: Prentice-Hall, 1968.

Sladen, B.K. Inheritance of dyslexia. *Bulletin of the Orton Society*, 1970, XX, 30–40.

Smart, R.G. Conflict and conditioned aversive stimuli in the development of experimental neuroses. *Canadian Journal of Psychology*, 1965, *19*(3), 208–223.

Smith, A. Neuropsychological testing in neurological disorders. *In* Friedlander, W.J. (Ed.), *Advances in neurology*, Vol. 7. New York: Raven Press, 1975, 49–110.

Smith, A. Focusing on the hole rather than the doughnut. Presidential Address, International Neuropsychological Society, 1979. *The INS Bulletin*, March 1979.

Smith, D.D., & Rivera, D.P. Mathematics. *In* Wong, B.Y.L. (Ed.), *Learning about learning disabilities*. San Diego: Academic Press, 1991, 345–374.

Smith, F. *Understanding Reading*. New York: Holt, Rinehart & Winston, 1971.

Smith, F. *Reading*. Cambridge: Cambridge University Press, 1978.

Smith, M. Recent work on low level lead exposure and its impact on behavior, intelligence, and learning: A review. *Journal of the American Academy of Child Psychiatry*, 1985, *24*(1), 24–32.

Smith, M., Delves, T., Lansdown, R., Clayton, B., & Graham, P. The effects of lead exposure on urban children. *Developmental Medicine and Child Neurology*, 1983, *25*, (suppl. 47).

Smith, M.E. *In* Thompson, G.G., *Child Psychology*, 2nd Ed. Boston: Houghton Mifflin Co., 1962, 368.

Smith, S.D., Kimberling, W.J., Pennington, B.F., & Lubs, H.A. Specific reading disability: Identification of an inherited form through linkage analysis. *Science*, 1983, *219*, 1345–1347.

Soper, H.V., & Satz, P. Pathological left-handedness and ambiguous handedness: A new explanatory model. *Neuropsychologia*, 1984, *22*(4), 511–515.

Speer, F. The allergic-fatigue syndrome. *In* Speer, F. (Ed.), *Allergy of the Nervous System*. Springfield, Ill., Charles C. Thomas, Pub., 1970, 14–27.

Speidel, B.D., & Meadow, S.R. Maternal epilepsy & abnormalities of the fetus & newborn. *Lancet*, 1972, *2*, 839.

Spellacy, F.J. Ear preference in the dichotic presentation of patterned nonverbal stimuli. Unpublished Ph.D. Dissertation, University of Victoria, Victoria, B.C., Canada, 1969.

Spellacy, F.J. Lateral preferences in the identification of patterned stimuli. *Journal of the Acoustical Society of America*,1970, *47*[2(2)], 574–578.

Spellacy, F.J., & Blumstein, S. Ear preference for language and non-language sounds: A unilateral brain function. *Journal of Auditory Research*, 1970, *10*, 349–355.

Spellacy, F.J., & Spreen, O. A short form of the Token Test. *Cortex*, 1969, *5*, 390–397.

Sperling, G. The information available in brief visual presentations. *Psychological Monographs*, 1960, 11.

Sperry, R.W. The great cerebral commissure. *Scientific American*, 1964, *210*, 240–250.

Sperry, R.W. Lateral specialization of cerebral function in the surgically separated hemispheres. *In* McGuigan, F.J. (Ed.), *The psychophysiology of thinking*. New York: Academic Press, 1973.

Sperry, R.W. Lateral specialization in the surgically separated hemispheres. *In* Schmitt, F.O., & Worden, F.G. (Eds.), *The neurosciences, third study program*. Cambridge, MA: The M.I.T. Press, 1974, 5–19.

Sprague, R.L., & Sleator, E.K. Drugs and dosages: Implications for learning disabilities. *In* Knights, R.M., & Bakker, D.J. (Eds.), *The neuropsychology of learning disorders*. Baltimore: University Park Press, 1976, 351–366.

Spreen, O. *Sound recognition test*. Victoria, B.C., Canada: Department of Psychology, University of Victoria, 1969.

Spreen, O. Neuropsychology of learning disorders: Post-conference review. *In* Knights, R.M., & Bakker, D.J. (Eds.), *The neuropsychology of learning disorders, theoretical approaches*. Baltimore: University Park Press, 1976, 445–467.

Spreen, O. Prediction of school achievement from kindergarten to grade five: Review and report of a follow-up study. *Research Monograph No. 33*. Victoria, B.C., Canada: Department of Psychology, University of Victoria, 1978.

Spreen, O. *Learning disabled children growing up: A follow-up into adulthood*. Victoria, B.C.: Department of Psychology, University of Victoria, 1983.

Spreen, O. *Learning disabled children growing up: A follow-up into adulthood*. New York: Oxford University Press, 1988.

Spreen, O. The relationship between learning disability, emotional disorders, and neuropsychology; Some results and observations. *Journal of Clinical and Experimental Neuropsychology*, 1989a, *11*(1), 117–140.

Spreen, O. Learning disability, neurology, and longterm outcome: Some implications for the individual and for society. *Journal of Clinical and Experimental Neuropsychology*, 1989b, *11*(3), 389–408.

Spreen, O., & Benton, A.L. *Neurosensory Center Comprehensive Examination for Aphasia*. Victoria, B.C., Canada: Department of Psychology, University of Victoria, 1969 and 1977 (Revised Edition).

Spreen, O., Benton, A.L., & Fincham, R.W. Auditory agnosia without aphasia. *Archives of Neurology*, 1965, *13*, 84–92.

Spreen, O., & Gaddes, W.H. Developmental norms for 15 neuropsychological tests age 6 to 15. *Cortex*, 1969, *5*, 171–191.

Spreen, O., & Strauss, E. *A compendium of neuropsychological tests: Administration, norms and commentary*. New York: Oxford University Press, 1991.

Spreen, O., Tupper, D., Risser, A., Tuokko, H., & Edgell, D. *Human developmental neuropsychology*. New York: Oxford University Press, 2nd ed. (in press).

Squire, L. *Memory & the brain*. New York: Academic Press, 1987.

Staller, J., Buchanan, D., Singer, M., Lappin, J., & Webb, W. Alexia without agraphia: An experimental case study. *Brain and Language*, 1978, *5*, 378–387.

Standing, E.M. *Maria Montessori, her life and work*. New York: Mentor Books, 1962.

Stanovich, K.E. Individual differences in the cognitive processes of reading: I. Word decoding. *Journal of Learning Disabilities*, 1982a, *15*, 485–493.

Stanovich, K.E. Individual differences in the cognitive processes of reading: II. Text-level processes. *Journal of Learning Disabilities*, 1982b, *15*(9), 549–554.

Stanovich, K.E. Explaining the variance in reading ability in terms of psychological processes: What have we learned? *Annals of Dyslexia*, 1985, *35*, 67–96.

Stanovich, K.E. Has the learning disabilities field lost its intelligence? *Journal of Learning Disabilities*, 1989, *22*(8), 487–492.

Steiner, S., & Larson, V.L. Integrating microcomputers into language intervention with children. *Topics in Language Disorders*, 1991, *11*(2), 18–30.

Sterman, M.B., & Friar, L. Suppression of seizures in an epileptic following sensorimotor EEG feedback training. *Electroencephalography & Clinical Neurophysiology*, 1972, *33*, 89–95.

Sternberg, S. High speed scanning in human memory. *Science*, 1966, *153*, 652–654.

Stevenson, J., & Richman, N. The prevalence of language delay in a population of three-year-old children and its association with general retardation. *Developmental Medicine and Child Neurology*, 1976, *18*, 431–441.

Stewart, R.J.C., & Platt, B.S. Nervous system damage in experimental protein-calorie deficiency. *In* Scrimshaw, N.S., & Gordon, J.E. (Eds.), *Malnutrition, learning and behavior*. Cambridge, MA: The M.I.T. Press, 1968, 168–180.

Sticht, T.G. Learning by listening. *In* Freedle, R.O., & Carroll, J.B. (Eds.), *Language comprehension and the acquisition of knowledge*. New York: Wiley, 1972.

Sticht, T.G. The acquisition of literacy by children and adults. *In* Murray, F.B., & Pikulski, J.J. (Eds.), *The acquisition of reading: Cognitive, linguistic and perceptual prerequisites*. Baltimore: University Park Press, 1978.

Still, G.F. The Coulstonian Lectures on some abnormal physical conditions in children. *Lancet*, 1902, *1*, 1008–1012.

Stoch, M.B., & Smythe, P.M. Undernutrition during infancy, and subsequent brain growth and intellectual development. *In* Scrimshaw, N.S., & Gordon, J.E. (Eds.), *Malnutrition, learning and behavior*. Cambridge, MA: The M.I.T. Press, 1968, 278–289.

Stominger, A.Z., & Bashir, A.S. A nine-year follow-up of 50 language delayed children. Paper presented at the annual meeting of the American Speech and Hearing Association, 1977, Chicago. (Quoted by D.B. Tower in NINCDS Monograph No. 22, p. vii.)

Stott, D.H., Moyes, F.A., & Henderson, S.E. *Test of motor impairment*. Guelph, Ontario: Educational Publishing Ltd., 1984.

Strang, J.D., & Rourke, B.P. Concept formation/non-verbal reasoning abilities of children who exhibit specific academic problems with arithmetic. *Journal of Clinical Child Psychology*, 1983, *12*(1), 33–39.

Strang, J.D., & Rourke, B.P. Arithmetic disability subtypes: The neuropsychological significance of specific arithmetical impairment in children. *In* Rourke, B.P. (Ed.), *Neuropsychology of learning disabilities: Essentials of subtype analysis*. New York: The Guilford Press, 1985, 167–183.

Strauss, A.A., & Kephart, N.C. *Psychopathology and education of the braininjured child*, Vol. II. New York: Grune & Stratton, 1955.

Strauss, A.A., & Lehtinen, L.E. *Psychopathology and education of the braininjured child*. New York: Grune & Stratton, 1947.

Strauss, A.A., & Werner, H. Deficiency in the finger schema in relation to arithmetic disability (finger agnosia and acalculia). *American Journal of Orthopsychiatry*, 1938, *8*, 719–725.

Strauss, E., Gaddes, W.H., & Wada, J. Performance on a free-recall verbal dichotic listening task and cerebral dominance determined by the carotid amytal test. *Neuropsychologia*, 1987, *25*(5), 747–753.

Strauss, E., Satz, P., & Wada, J. An examination of the crowding hypothesis in epileptic patients who have undergone the carotid amytal test. *Neuropsychologia*, 1990, *28*, 1221–1227.

Strauss, E., & Wada, J. Lateral preferences and cerebral speech dominance. *Cortex*, 1983, *19*, 165–177.

Strauss, E., Wada, J., & Hunter, M. Sex-related differences in the cognitive consequences of early left hemisphere lesions. *Journal of Clinical and Experimental Neuropsychology*, 1992, *14*, 687–697.

Strother, F.C. Minimal cerebral dysfunction: A historical overview. *Annals of the New York Academy of Sciences*, 1973, *205*, 6–17.

Stuart, M., & Coltheart, M. Does reading develop in a sequence of stages? *Cognition*, 1988, *30*, 139–181.

Subirana, A. The prognosis in aphasia in relation to cerebral dominance and handedness. *Brain*, 1958, *81*, 415–425.

Subirana, A. Handedness and cerebral dominance. *In* Vinken, P.J., & Bruyn, G.W. (Eds.), *Handbook of clinical neurology*, Vol. 4. Amsterdam: North-Holland Publishing Co., 1969, 248–272.

Swanson, H.L. Relations among metamemory, rehearsal activity and word recall in learning disabled and nondisabled readers. *British Journal of Educational Psychology*, 1983a, *53*, 186–194.

Swanson, H.L. A developmental study of vigilance in learning disabled and non-learning disabled children. *Journal of Abnormal Child Psychology*, 1983b, *11*, 415–429.

Swanson, H.L. Do semantic differences underlie disabled readers encoding processes? *Journal of Experimental Child Psychology*, 1986, *41*, 461–488.

Swanson, H.L. Information processing theory and learning disabilities: An overview. *Journal of Learning Disabilities*, 1987, *20*, 3–7.

Swanson, H.L., Cochrane, K., & Ewers, C. Working memory & reading disabilities. *Journal of Abnormal Child Psychology*, 1989, *17*, 745–756.

Swanson, H.L., & Cooney, J.B. Learning disabilities. *In* Wong, B.Y.L. (Ed.), *Learning about learning disabilities*. New York: Academic Press, 1991, 104–127.

Sykes, D.H., Douglas, V.I., & Morgenstern, G. Sustained attention in hyperactive children. *Journal of Child Psychology and Psychiatry*, 1973, *14*, 213–220.

Szatmari, P., Offord, D.R., & Boyle, M.H. Ontario child health study: Prevalence of attention deficit disorder with hyperactivity. *Journal of Child Psychology & Psychiatry*, 1989, *30*, 219–230.

Tallal, P., & Piercy, M. Developmental aphasia: Impaired rate of non-verbal processing as a function of sensory modality. *Neuropsychologia*, 1973a, *11*, 389–398.

Tallal, P., & Stark, R. Perceptual prerequisites for language development. *In* Kirk, U. (Ed.), *Neuropsychology of language, reading, and spelling.* New York: Academic Press, 1983, 97–106.

Tansey, M.A. Brainwave signatures: An index reflective of the brain's functional neuroanatomy: Further findings on the effect of EEG sensorimotor rhythm biofeedback training on the neurologic precursors of learning disabilities. *Psychophysiology*, 1985, *3*, 85–99.

Tant, J.L., & Douglas, V.I. Problem-solving in hyperactive, normal & reading disabled boys. *Journal of Abnormal Child Psychology*, 1982, *10*, 285–306.

Tarnopol, L. Introduction to neurogenic learning disorders. *In* Tarnopol, L. (Ed.), *Learning disorders in children, diagnosis, medication, education.* Boston: Little, Brown, 1971.

Tarnowski, K.J., Prinz, R.J., & Nay, S.M. Comparative analysis of attentional deficits in hyperactive and learning disabled children. *Journal of Abnormal Psychology*, 1986, *95*, 341–345.

Taylor, L.B. Psychological assessment of neurosurgical patients. *In* Rasmussen, T., & Marino, R. (Eds.), *Functional neurosurgery.* New York: Raven Press, 1979.

Teuber, H.-L. Some alterations in behavior after cerebral lesions in man. *In Evolution of Nervous Control.* Washington, DC: American Association for the Advancement of Science, 1959, 157–194.

Teuber, H.-L. The riddle of frontal lobe function in man. *In* Warren, J.M., & Akert, K.A. (Eds.), *The frontal granular cortex and behavior.* New York: McGraw-Hill, 1964, 410–444.

Teuber, H.-L. Somatosensory disorders due to cortical lesions. Preface: Disorders of higher tactile and visual functions. *Neuropsychologia*, 1965, *3*, 287–294.

Teuber, H.-L. Why two brains? *In* Schmitt, F.O., & Worden, F.G. (Eds.), *The neurosciences: Third study program.* Cambridge: MIT Press, 1974, 71–74.

Teuber, H.-L. Evidence of neural plasticity. Major invited speaker, Tenth Annual Neuropsychology Workshop, University of Victoria, Victoria, B.C., Canada, March 1975.

Teuber, H.-L., Battersby, W., & Bender, M. *Visual field defects after penetrating missile wounds of the brain.* Cambridge, MA: Harvard University Press, 1960.

Teuber, H.-L., & Weinstein, S. Ability to discover hidden figures after cerebral lesions. *American Medical Association Archives of Neurology and Psychiatry*, 1956, *76*, 369–379.

The Random House college dictionary, revised edition. New York: 1988.

Thomas, C.C., Englert, C.S., & Gregg, S. An analysis of errors and strategies in the expository writing of learning disabled students. *Remedial and Special Education*, 1987, *8*, 21–30, 46.

Thomson, G.O.B., Raab, G.M., Hepburn, W.S., Hunter, R., Fulton, M., & Laxen, D.P.H. Blood-lead levels and children's behavior-results from the Edinburgh lead study. *Journal of Child Psychology and Psychiatry*, 1989, *30*(4), 515–528.

Thompson, G.G. *Child Psychology*, 2nd Ed. Boston: Houghton Mifflin, 1962.

Thompson, R.F., Berger, T.W., & Berry, S.D. An introduction to the anatomy, physiology, and chemistry of the brain. *In* Wittrock, M.C. (Ed.), *The brain and psychology*. New York: Academic Press, 1980, 3–32.

Thompson, R.F., Berger, T.W., Berry, S.D., & Hoehler, F.K. The search for the engram, II. *In* McFadden, D. (Ed.), *Neural mechanisms in behavior*. New York: Springer-Verlag, 1980.

Thorndike, E.L. *The original nature of man*, Vol. I. New York: Teachers College, Columbia University, 1913.

Thorndike, R.L. *The concepts of over-and-under-achievement*. Bureau of Publications, Teachers College, Columbia University, New York, 1963.

Tizard, B. Theories of brain localization from Flourens to Lashley. *Medical History*, 1959, *3*, 132–145.

Torgesen, J.K. The role of nonspecific factors in the task performance of learning disabled children: A theoretical assignment. *Journal of Learning Disabilities*, 1977, *10*(1), 33–40.

Torgesen, J.K. Why IQ is relevant to the definition of learning disabilities. *Journal of Learning Disabilities*, 1989, *22*(8), 484–486.

Torgesen, J.K., & Goldman, T. Rehearsal & short-term memory in second grade disabled students. *Child Development*, 1977, *48*, 56–61.

Touwen, B.C.L. The relationship between minor neurological dysfunction and learning disabilities. *Thalamus*, 1981, *1*(2), 2–14.

Townes, B.D., Trupin, E.W., Martin, D.C., & Goldstein, D. Neuropsychological correlates of academic success among elementary school children. *Journal of Consulting and Clinical Psychology*, 1980, *48*(6), 675–684.

Tramontana, M.G., & Hooper, S.R. (Eds.). *Assessment issues in child neuropsychology*. New York: Plenum, 1988.

Trites, R.L. *Neuropsychological test manual*. Montreal: Ronalds Federated, 1977.

Trites, R.L., Ferguson, H.B., & Tryphonas, H. Diet treatment for hyperactive children with food allergies. *In* Knights, R.M., & Bakker,

D.J. (Eds.), *The rehabilitation, treatment & management of learning disabilities*. Baltimore: University Park Press, 1980, 151–163.

Trites, R.L., & Fiedorowicz, C. Follow-up study of children with specific (or primary) reading disability. *In* Knights, R.M., & Bakker, D.J. (Eds.), *The neuropsychology of learning disorders*. Baltimore: University Park Press, 1976, 41–50.

Tryphonas, H., & Trites, R.L. Food allergy in children with hyperactivity, learning disabilities, and/or minimal brain dysfunction. *Annals of Allergy*, 1979, *42*, 22–27.

Tulving, E. Episodic & semantic memory. *In* Tulving, E., & Donaldson, W. (Eds.), *Organization of memory*. New York: Academic Press, 1973, 382–404.

Tulving, E., & Pearlstone, Z. Availability versus accessibility of information in memory for words. *Journal of Verbal Learning & Verbal Behavior*, 1966, *5*, 381–391.

Tupper, D.E. *Soft neurological signs*. Orlando, FL: Grune & Stratton, 1987.

Umilta, C., Bagnara, S., & Simion, F. Laterality effects for simple and complex geometrical figures, and nonsense patterns. *Neuropsychologia*, 1978, *16*, 43–49.

U.S. Government Printing Office, *Neurotoxicity, Identifying and controlling poisons of the nervous system*. Washington, D.C.: 1990.

Vaessen, W., & Kalverboer, A.F. Clumsy children's performance on a double task. *In* Kalverboer A.F. (Ed.), *Developmental biopsychology*. Ann Arbor: The University of Michigan Press, 1990, 223–240.

Valett, R.E. *Learning disabilities, diagnostic-prescriptive instruments*. Belmont, CA: Lear Siegler-Fearon, 1973.

Valk, J. Neuroradiology and learning disabilities. *Tÿdschrift voor Orthopedagogiek*, 1974 (Nov.), *NR 11*, 303–323.

Vallar, G., & Perani, D. The anatomy of unilateral neglect after right-hemisphere stroke lesions. A clinical CT-scan correlation study in man. *Neuropsychologia*, 1986, *24*, 609–622.

Van Bergeijk, W.A., & David, E.E. Delayed handwriting. *Perceptual and Motor Skills*, 1959, *9*, 347–357.

Vanden-Abeele, J. Comments on the functional asymmetries of the lower extremities. *Cortex*, 1980, *16*, 325–329.

Van Dellen, T., Vaessen, W., & Schoemaker, M.M. Clumsiness: Definition and selection of subjects. *In* Kalverboer, A.F. (Ed.), *Developmental biopsychology*. Ann Arbor: The University of Michigan Press, 1990, 135–152.

Van Duyne, H.J., Bakker, D., & de Jong, W. Development of ear-asymmetry related to coding processes in memory in children. *Brain and Language*, 1977, *4*(2), 322–334.

Vaughn, S. Social skills enhancement in students with learning disabilities. *In* Wong, B.Y.L. (Ed.), *Learning about learning disabilities*. San Diego: Academic Press, 1991, 407–440.

Vaughn, S., Hogan, A., Kouzekanani, K., & Shapiro, S. Peer acceptance, self-perceptions, and social skills of learning disabled students prior to identification. *Journal of Educational Psychology*, 1990, *82*(1), 101–106.

Vellutino, F.R. Toward an understanding of dyslexia: Psychological factors in specific reading disability. *In* Benton, A.L., & Pearl, D. (Eds.), *Dyslexia, an appraisal of current knowledge*. New York: Oxford University Press, 1978, 63–111.

Vellutino, F.R. *Dyslexia: Theory and research*. Cambridge: MIT Press, 1979.

Vellutino, F.R. Dyslexia. *Scientific American*, 1987, *256*(3), 34–41.

Von Bonin, G. Anatomical asymmetries of the cerebral hemispheres. *In* Mountcastle, V.B. (Ed.), *Interhemispheric relations and cerebral dominance*. Baltimore: The Johns Hopkins University Press, 1962, 1–6.

Von Economo, C., & Horn, L. *Zeitschrift fur die gesamte neurologie und psychiatrie*, 1930, *130*, 678 (Quoted by Wada, Clarke & Hamm, 1975).

Vygotsky, L.S. *Thought and Language*. Cambridge: MIT Press, 1962.

Wada, J.A. What's new on epilepsy? *Proceedings of the Vancouver epilepsy international symposium*. Vancouver: University of British Columbia, 1978.

Wada, J.A., Clarke, R., & Hamm, A. Cerebral hemispheric asymmetry in humans. *Archives of Neurology*, 1975, *32*, 239–246.

Wada, J.A., & Rasmussen, T. Intracarotid injection of sodium amytal for the lateralization of cerebral speech dominance. *Journal of Neurosurgery*, 1960, *17*, 266–282.

Wagner, R.K., & Torgesen, J.K. The nature of phonological processing and its causal role in the acquisition of reading skills. *Psychological Bulletin*, 1987, *101*(2), 192–212.

Walsh, K.W. *Neuropsychology, a clinical approach*. Edinburgh: Churchill Livingstone, 1987.

Walzer, S., & Richmond, J.B. The epidemiology of learning disorders. *Pediatric Clinics of North America*, 1973, *20*(3), 549–565.

Wann, T.W. *Behaviorism and phenomenology*. Chicago: The University of Chicago Press, 1964.

Warrington, E.K. Neurological deficits. *In* Mittler, P. (Ed.), *The psychological assessment of mental and physical handicaps*. London: Methuen & Co., 1970, 261–288.

Warrington, E.K., James, M., & Kinsbourne, M. Drawing disability in relation to laterality of cerebral lesion. *Brain*, 1966, *89*, 53–82.

Warrington, E.K., & Taylor, A.M. The contribution of the right parietal lobe to object recognition. *Cortex*, 1973, *60*, 152–164.

Watson, J.B. *Psychology from the standpoint of a behaviorist*. Philadelphia: J.B. Lippincott, 1919 (1st Ed.)/1924 (2nd Ed.).

Watson, J.B. *Behaviorism*. New York: W.W. Norton, 1924.

Watson, R.I. *The great psychologists from Aristotle to Freud*. Philadelphia: Lippincott, 1963.

Webb, T.E., & Berman, P.H. Stereoscopic form disappearance in temporal lobe dysfunction. *Cortex*, 1973, *9*, 239–245.

Webster's New Twentieth Century Dictionary, 2nd Ed. New York: The World Publishing Company, 1968.

Webster's New World Dictionary, 3rd Ed. New York: Simon & Schuster, 1988.

Wechsler, D. *The measurement of adult intelligence*. Baltimore: The Williams & Wilkins Co., 1939.

Wechsler, D. *Wechsler Intelligence Scale for Children*. New York: Psychological Corporation, 1949.

Wechsler, D. *Measurement and appraisal of adult intelligence*, 4th Ed. Baltimore: Williams & Wilkins, 1958.

Wechsler, D., & Hagin, R.A. The problem of axial rotation in reading disability. *Perceptual and Motor Skills*, 1964, *19*, 319–326.

Weinberger, L.M., Gibbon, M.H., & Gibbon, J.H., Jr. Temporary arrest of the circulation to the central nervous system. *Archives of Neurology and Psychiatry*, 1940, *43*, 961.

Weinstein, S., & Teuber, H.-L. Effects of penetrating brain injury on intelligence test scores. *Science*, 1957, *125*, 1036–1037.

Weisenburg, T., & McBride, K.E. *Aphasia, a clinical and psychological study*. New York: The Commonwealth Fund, 1935; reprinted by Hafner, New York, 1964.

Weiss, G., & Hechtman, L. *Hyperactive children grown up*. New York: Academic Press, 1979.

Weiss, P. Autonomous versus reflexogenous activity of the central nervous system. *Proceedings of the American Philosophical Society*, 1941, *84*, 53–64.

Wender, P.H. *Minimal brain dysfunction in children*. New York: Wiley, 1971.

Wender, P.H. Minimal brain dysfunction in children: Diagnosis and management, *Pediatric Clinics of North America*, 1973, *20*(1), 187–202.

Wender, P.H. Hypothesis for a possible biochemical basis of minimal brain dysfunction. *In* Knights, R.M., & Bakker, D.J. (Eds.), *The neuropsychology of learning disorders, theoretical approaches*. Baltimore: University Park Press, 1976, 111–122.

Werner, H., & Strauss, A.A. Causal factors in low performance. *American Journal of Mental Deficiency*, 1940, *45*, 213–218.

Werner, H., & Strauss, A.A. Pathology of figure-background relation in the child. *Journal of Abnormal and Social Psychology*, 1941, *36*, 236–248.

Werry, J.S. Developmental hyperactivity. *The Pediatric Clinics of North America*, 1968, *15*(3), 581–599.

Werry, J.S., Delano, J.G., & Douglas, V. Studies on the hyperactive child. I. Some preliminary findings. *Canadian Psychiatric Association Journal*, 1964, *9*, 120–130.

Wertheim, N. The amusias. *In* Vinken, P.J., & Bruyn, G.W. (Eds.), *Handbook of Clinical Neurology*, Vol. 4. Amsterdam: North-Holland Publishing Co., 1969, 195–206.

West, R. (Ed.). *Childhood Aphasia*. San Francisco: California Society for Crippled Children and Adults, 1962.

Wexler, B.E., Halwes, T., & Heninger, G.R. Use of a statistical significance criterion in drawing inferences about hemispheric dominance for language function from dichotic listening data. *Brain and Language*, 1981, *13*, 13–18.

White, K., & Ashton, R. Handedness assessment inventory. *Neuropsychologia*, 1976, *14*, 261–264.

White, R.W. Motivation reconsidered: The concept of competence. *Psychological Review*, 1959, *66*(5), 297–333.

Willerman, L. Activity level and hyperactivity in twins. *Child Development*, 1973, *44*, 288–293.

Wilson, L.F. Assessment of congenital aphasia. *In* Rappaport, S.R. (Ed.), *Childhood aphasia and brain damage*: Vol. II. Narberth, PA: Livingston Publishing Co., 1965, 7–52.

Winik, M., Brasel, J., & Rosso, P. Nutrition and cell growth. *In* Winik, M. (Ed.), *Nutrition and development*. New York: Wiley, 1972.

Winzer, M. *Children with exceptionalities. A Canadian perspective*. Scarborough, Ontario: Prentice-Hall, 1990.

Witelson, S.F. Early hemisphere specialization and interhemisphere plasticity: An empirical and theoretical review. *In* Segalowitz, S.J., & Gruber, F.A. (Eds.), *Language development and neurological theory*. New York: Academic Press, 1977, 213–287.

Witelson, S.F. Bumps on the brain: Right-left anatomic asymmetry as a key to functional lateralization. *In* Segalowitz, S.J. (Ed.), *Language functions and brain organization*. New York: Academic Press, 1983, 117–144.

Witelson, S.F., & Pallie, W. Left hemisphere specialization for language in the newborn. *Brain*, 1973, *96*, 641–646.

Witkin, H. Sex differences in perception. *Transactions of the New York Academy of Science*, 1949, *12*, 22–26.

Wittrock, M.C. (Ed.). *The brain and psychology*. New York: Academic Press, 1980a.

Wittrock, M.C. Learning and the brain. *In* Wittrock, M.C. (Ed.), *The brain and psychology*. New York: Academic Press, 1980b, 371–403.

Wolf, S., & Wolff, H.G. Evidence on the genesis of peptic ulcer in man. *Journal of the American Medical Association*, 1942, *120*, 670–675.

Wong, B.Y.L. Strategic behaviors in selecting retrieval cues in gifted, normal achieving and learning disabled children. *Journal of Learning Disabilities*, 1982, *15*, 33–37.

Woods, B.T., & Carey, S. Language deficits after apparent clinical recovery from childhood aphasia. *Annals of Neurology*, 1979, *6*, 405–409.

Woods, B.T., & Teuber, H.-L. Changing patterns of child-hood aphasia. *Annals of Neurology*, 1978, *3*, 273–280.

Wooldridge, D.E. *The machinery of the brain*. New York: McGraw-Hill, 1963.

Wright, K.L. The relative values of three reading programs in facilitation of reading acquisition amongst Grade Two students. Undergraduate Honors Thesis, Departmental Monograph, Department of Psychology, University of Victoria, Victoria, B.C., Canada, 1978.

Yerkes, R.M., & Dodson, J.D. The relation of strength of stimulus to rapidity of habit formation. *Journal of Comparative Neurology & Psychology*, 1908, *18*, 459–482.

Ysseldyke, J.E., & Algozzine, B. On making psychoeducational decisions. *Journal of Psychoeducational Assessment*, 1983, *1*(2), 187–195.

Yule, W., Lansdown, R., Millar, I.B., & Urbanowicz, M.A. The relationship between blood lead concentrations, intelligence and attainment in a school population. A pilot study. *Developmental Medicine and Child Neurology*, 1981, *23*, 567–576.

Yule, W., & Rutter, M. Epidemiology and social implications of specific reading retardation. *In* Knights, R.M., & Bakker, D.J. (Eds.), *The neuropsychology of learning disorders*. Baltimore: University Park Press, 1976, 25–39.

Zaidel, D., & Sperry, R.W. Lateralized tests for temporal sequential order in the left and right hemispheres of man. *Biology Annual Report* (California Institute of Technology), 1973, p. 54.

Zaidel, E. Linguistic competence and related functions in the right cerebral hemisphere of man following commissurotomy and hemispherectomy. Unpublished Ph.D. Dissertation, California Institute of Technology, 1973.

Zaidel, E. The split and half brains as models of congenital language disability. *In The neurological bases of language disorders in children: Methods and directions for research*. NINCDS Monograph No. 22. Bethesda, MD: U.S. Department of Health, Education, and Welfare, August 1979, 55–89.

Zamenhof, S., & van Marthens, E. Nutritional influences on prenatal brain development. *In* Gottlieb G. (Ed.), *Early influences, Vol. IV*. New York: Academic Press, 1978.

Zametkin, A.J., Nordahl, T.E., Gross, M., King, A.C., Semple, W.E., Rumsey, J., Hamburger, S., & Cohen, R. Cerebral glucose metabolism in adults with hyperactivity of childhood onset. *The New England Journal of Medicine*, 1990, *323*, 1361–1415.

Zametkin, A.J., & Rappaport, J.L. Neurobiology of attention deficit disorder with hyperactivity: Where have we come in 50 years? *Journal of the American Academy of Child & Adolescent Psychiatry*, 1987, *26*, 676–686.

Zangwill, O.L. *Cerebral dominance and its relation to psychological functions*. London: Oliver & Boyd, 1960.

Zangwill, O.L. Thought and the brain. *British Journal of Psychology*, 1976, *67*, 301–314.

Zentall, S.S., & Zentall, T.R. Optimal stimulation: A model of disordered activity and performance in normal and deviant children. *Psychological Bulletin*, 1983, *94*, 446–471.

Zurif, E.B., & Bryden M.P. Familial handedness and left-right differences in auditory and visual perception. *Neuropsychologia*, 1969, *7*, 179–188.

Index of Names

Subject Index